UNDERSTANDING AND MODULATING AGING

ANNALS OF THE NEW YORK ACADEMY OF SCIENCES
Volume 1067

UNDERSTANDING AND MODULATING AGING

Edited by
Suresh I. S. Rattan, Peter Kristensen, and Brian F. C. Clark

Published by Blackwell Publishing on behalf of the New York Academy of Sciences
Boston, Massachusetts
2006

Library of Congress Cataloging-in-Publication Data

International Association of Biomedical Gerontology. International
Congress (11th : 2005 : University of Aarhus)
     Understanding and modulating aging / edited by Suresh Rattan,
Peter Kristensen, and Brian F.C. Clark.
         p. cm. — (Annals of the New York Academy of Sciences,
ISSN 0077-8923; v. 1067)
     Includes bibliographical references and index.
     ISBN-13: 978-1-57331-599-9 (alk. paper)
     ISBN-10: 1-57331-599-0 (alk. paper)
     1. Aging—Congresses.   I. Rattan, Suresh I.S. II. Kristensen, Peter.
III. Clark, Brian F.C. (Brian Frederic Carl) IV. New York Academy of
Sciences. V. Series.
     [DNLM: 1. Aging—Congresses. 2. Life Expectancy—Congresses.
W1 AN626YL v.1067 2006 / WT 104 I587u 2006]
     Q11.N5 vol. 1067
     [QP86]
     500 s–dc22
     [612.6'7]
                                                              2006011951

The *Annals of the New York Academy of Sciences* (ISSN: 0077-8923 [print]; ISSN: 1749-6632 [online]) is published 28 times a year on behalf of the New York Academy of Sciences by Blackwell Publishing, with offices located at 350 Main Street, Malden, Massachusetts 02148 USA, PO Box 1354, Garsington Road, Oxford OX4 2DQ UK, and PO Box 378 Carlton South, 3053 Victoria Australia.

Information for subscribers: Subscription prices for 2006 are: Premium Institutional: $3850.00 (US) and £2139.00 (Europe and Rest of World).
Customers in the UK should add VAT at 5%. Customers in the EU should also add VAT at 5% or provide a VAT registration number or evidence of entitlement to exemption. Customers in Canada should add 7% GST or provide evidence of entitlement to exemption. The Premium Institutional price also includes online access to full-text articles from 1997 to present, where available. For other pricing options or more information about online access to Blackwell Publishing journals, including access information and terms and conditions, please visit www.blackwellpublishing.com/nyas.

Membership information: Members may order copies of the *Annals* volumes directly from the Academy by visiting www.nyas.org/annals, emailing membership@nyas.org, faxing 212-888-2894, or calling 800-843-6927 (US only), or +1 212 838 0230, ext. 345 (International). For more information on becoming a member of the New York Academy of Sciences, please visit www.nyas.org/membership.

Journal Customer Services: For ordering information, claims, and any inquiry concerning your institutional subscription, please contact your nearest office:
UK: Email: customerservices@blackwellpublishing.com; Tel: +44 (0) 1865 778315; Fax +44 (0) 1865 471775
US: Email: customerservices@blackwellpublishing.com; Tel: +1 781 388 8599 or 1 800 835 6770 (Toll free in the USA); Fax: +1 781 388 8232
Asia: Email: customerservices@blackwellpublishing.com; Tel: +65 6511 8000; Fax: +61 3 8359 1120
Members: Claims and inquiries on member orders should be directed to the Academy at email: membership@nyas.org or Tel: +1 212 838 0230 (International) or 800-843-6927 (US only).

Printed in the USA.
Printed on acid-free paper.

ANNALS OF THE NEW YORK ACADEMY OF SCIENCES

Volume 1067
May 2006

UNDERSTANDING AND MODULATING AGING

Editors
SURESH I. S. RATTAN, PETER KRISTENSEN, AND BRIAN F. C. CLARK

This volume is the result of a conference entitled **11th Congress of the International Association of Biomedical Gerontology (IABG): Understanding and Modulating Aging**, sponsored by the Danish Centre for Molecular Gerontology (DCMG), University of Aarhus, Denmark, and the International Association of Biomedical Gerontology, and held on August 13–16, 2005, in Aarhus, Denmark.

CONTENTS

Understanding and Modulating Aging meeting sponsors:

Major sponsors

- Danish Centre for Molecular Gerontology
- Aarhus University
- International Union of Biochemistry and Molecular Biology (IUBMB)

Additional funding

- AH Diagnostics
- *Biogerontology*
- Compounding Pharmacy Mierlo-Hout
- NOW: Nutrition for Optimal Wellness (Bloomington, IL)
- SENETEK plc.

Preface

Understanding and Modulating Aging

Biogerontology—the study of the biological basis of aging—has progressed tremendously, and it has now become an independent and respectable field of study and research. Numerous universities, medical institutes, and research centers throughout the world now offer full-fledged courses on the biology of aging. The pharmaceutical, cosmeceutical, and nutriceutical industry's ever-increasing interest in aging research and therapy is also highly apparent. Moreover, increased financial support by national and international financial agencies to biogerontological research has given much impetus to its further development.

Since 1985, the International Association of Biomedical Gerontology (IABG), founded by Professor Denham Harman, originator of the free radical theory of aging, has been holding the International Congress of the IABG every two years in different parts of the world, including Australia, Canada, Germany, Hungary, Japan, the UK, and the United States. The 11th IABG Congress, held at the University of Aarhus, Denmark (August 13 to 16, 2005), was a tremendous success in bringing together biogerontologists, bioethicists, researchers, students, clinicians, dieticians, and social gerontologists. With more than 110 participants from 15 countries in Europe, Asia, and America, the main areas of discussion and presentation of new research results included:

- biological and nonbiological factors affecting lifespan and the quality of life;
- ethical and social issues related to lifespan and health-span extension;
- novel areas of understanding aging—physiological, cellular, and molecular aspects;
- new technologies to understand and modulate aging;
- the latest successful approaches in the prevention and treatment of age-related diseases; and
- aging intervention, prevention, and modulation by genes, natural and synthetic molecules, and nutritional and lifestyle modifications.

Address for correspondence: Suresh I. S. Rattan, Danish Centre for Molecular Gerontology, Department of Molecular Biology, University of Aarhus, Gustav Wieds Vej 10C, DK8000 Aarhus-C, Denmark. Voice: +45 89 42 50 34 or +45 2899 2496 (mobile); fax: +45 86 12 31 78.
  e-mail: Rattan@mb.au.dk [*or*] sureshrattan@gmail.com
  www.sureshrattan.com

Ann. N.Y. Acad. Sci. 1067: xv–xvi (2006). © 2006 New York Academy of Sciences.
doi: 10.1196/annals.1354.001

The present volume of the *Annals of the New York Academy of Sciences* is in line with the past IABG congresses, for which invited lectures and original papers and posters presented at the congress were compiled and published. Previously published *ANYAS* volumes from the IABG congresses are:

- 4th Congress: Physiological Processes of Aging: Towards a Multi-causal Interpretation. *Annals of the New York Academy of Sciences*; vol. 673, 1992. Editors: N. Fabris, D. Harman, D.L. Knook, E. Steinhagen-Thiessen, and I. Zs.-Nagy.
- 5th Congress: Pharmacology of Aging Processes: Methods of Assessment and Potential Interventions. *Annals of the New York Academy of Sciences*; vol. 717, 1994. Editors: I. Zs.-Nagy, D. Harman, and K. Kitani.
- 6th Congress: Pharmacological Intervention in Aging and Age-Associated Disorders. *Annals of the New York Academy of Sciences*; vol. 786; 1996. Editors: K. Kitani, A. Aoba, and S. Goto.
- 7th Congress: Towards Prolongation of the Healthy Life Span: Practical Approaches to Intervention. *Annals of the New York Academy of Sciences*; vol. 854; 1998. Editors: D. Harman, R. Holliday, and M. Meydani.
- 8th Congress: Healthy Aging for Functional Longevity: Molecular and Cellular Interactions in Senescence. *Annals of the New York Academy of Sciences*; vol. 928; 2001. Editors: S.C. Park, E.S. Hwang, H.S. Kim, and W.Y. Park.
- 9th Congress: Increasing Healthy Life Span: Conventional Measures and Slowing the Innate Aging Process. *Annals of the New York Academy of Sciences*; vol. 959; 2002. Editor: D. Harman.
- 10th Congress: Strategies for Engineered Negligible Senescence. *Annals of the New York Academy of Sciences*; vol. 1019; 2004. Editor: A.D.N.J de Grey.

The organizational success of the 11th IABG was assured by generous financial support from the following:

- The faculties of science and medicine, University of Aarhus, Denmark;
- Danish Centre for Molecular Gerontology, University of Aarhus, Denmark;
- International Union of Biochemistry and Molecular Biology (IUBMB);
- The journal *Biogerontology*, Springer Verlag, the Netherlands;
- Senetek PLC, USA and Denmark;
- NOW, manufacturer of vitamins, minerals, and herbs, USA;
- Compounding Pharmacy Mierlo-Hout, the Netherlands; and
- AH Diagnostics, Denmark.

—SURESH I. S. RATTAN
—PETER KRISTENSEN
—BRIAN F. C. CLARK

Aging is No Longer an Unsolved Problem in Biology

ROBIN HOLLIDAY

Australian Academy of Science, Canberra, Australia

ABSTRACT: For much of the 20th century, the accumulation of a considerable amount of information about the processes of aging did not reveal the underlying mechanisms. Toward the end of that century, the biological basis for aging became very much clearer. It became apparent that the best strategy for animals' survival was to develop to an adult, but not to invest resources in maintaining the body, or soma, indefinitely. In their natural environment, animals do not survive environmental hazards (predators, disease, starvation, and drought) to reach a long life span. There is thus a trade-off between the investment of resources in reproduction, and the survival time of the soma. At a stroke, this solves the problem of different rates of aging in different species, because those that develop and reproduce fast also have short life spans, and those that develop and reproduce slowly have long life spans. This difference is due to actual resources invested in the maintenance of the adult soma. There is now much evidence that long-lived mammals have much more efficient maintenance mechanisms than short-lived mammals. Thus, aging can be defined as the eventual failure of maintenance. It also became apparent that many different maintenance mechanisms exist, and that these depend on very many genes and a considerable investment in metabolic resources. Most individual theories of aging revolve around the failure of a given maintenance system, but as there are many of these, it is likely that most of the important theories have some degree of truth. A broad interpretation of the different degenerative changes during senescence should therefore be adopted, with the major conclusion that aging is multicausal. It is also evident that the evolved design of many components of complex animals is incompatible with indefinite survival. We can therefore conclude that this evolved design is intrinsically related to the fact of aging. This in turn means that aging cannot be reversed, although it may be modulated, as, for example, by calorie restriction.

KEYWORDS: evolution; maintenance; repair; damage; longevity

Address for correspondence: Robin Holliday, 12 Roma Court, West Pennant Hills, NSW 2125, Australia. Voice: +61-2-9873-3476; fax: +61-2-9871-2159.
e-mail: RandL.Holliday@bigpond.com

Ann. N.Y. Acad. Sci. 1067: 1–9 (2006). © 2006 New York Academy of Sciences.
doi: 10.1196/annals.1354.002

INTRODUCTION

In 1951, Peter Medawar delivered an inaugural professorial lecture at University College, London, entitled "An unsolved problem in biology." The unsolved problem was aging. The content was wide ranging and the published lecture became very influential.[1] Medawar appointed Alex Comfort to carry out research on aging, and as an aid to research he wrote a book, *The Biology of Senescence*, published in 1956.[2] Later, revised editions[3,4] were published in 1964 and 1979, and this third edition cited approximately 1,750 references. Many other reviews on aging have been published but most notable among these was that by Caleb Finch, *Longevity, Senescence and the Genome*, published in 1990, with nearly 700 pages of text and approximately 4,000 references.[5] Neither Comfort's nor Finch's books came to any strong conclusions about the biological reasons for aging. Indeed, during most of the second half of the 20th century, the field could be said to be in an unsatisfactory state. One reason for this was that there were many different theories of aging that seemed to be competing with each other. Moreover, a single theory of aging implied that there was a single cause, and as time went on this became less and less plausible. There was a huge amount of information from a large variety of experimental systems, but much of this was hard to interpret. One puzzling feature of mammalian aging was the fact that the senescent phenotype of different species was quite similar, even though the longevity of these species varied by about 30-fold. Thus, similar chemical or biochemical changes, such as the cross-linking of collagen, were occurring at very different rates.

Then, at the end of the 20th century, all this information began to fall into place, and the biological reasons for aging became very well understood. It was no coincidence that three books on aging were published in the mid-1990s, which all had positive titles. These were Hayflick's *How and Why We Age*,[6] Holliday's *Understanding Aging*,[7] and Austad's *Why We Age*.[8] There was also a more popular book: Kirkwood's *Time of Our Lives*.[9] These books are by no means similar, but they all reach the same conclusion, namely, that biologists now well understand the biological reasons for aging in animals. It is therefore no longer an unsolved problem of biology.

Some scientific discoveries are accepted almost immediately, and good examples are the discovery of the structure of DNA by Watson and Crick, and the polymerase chain reaction (PCR). Other discoveries lie latent for many years before they are recognized. This was the case for Wegener's proposals about continental drift, and even more well known, Mendel's discovery of the laws of inheritance. Unfortunately, the solving of the problem of aging will come into this second category. It is unlikely that it will be widely recognized either by scientists or the public at large, and people will go on speculating about the mysteries of aging for a long time to come. A lot that is written about aging now is biological nonsense, and that will undoubedly be true in the future as well.

AGING AND THE NATURAL ENVIRONMENT

In his lecture Medawar[1] was the first to point out that animals rarely become senescent in a natural environment, because they normally die from predation, disease, starvation, or drought. The life span of small ground-living mammals is particularly short. Even in gray squirrels, which can escape predators by climbing trees, survival after 1 year is only about 30%, and after 4 years is about 6–7%.[7,10] In the protected environment of a zoo, these animals can live for up to 20 years. Darwin well understood that mortality is very high in natural environments, and that only a proportion of animals survive long enough to breed. His theory of natural selection is based on the principle of the survival of the fittest. As we will see, the mortality of mammals in their natural environments varies considerably between species, and this determines evolutionary trends.

THE MULTIPLE CAUSES OF AGING

In protected environments, animals can reach their maximum life spans, and it is now very clear that their senescence, aging, and death have multiple causes. These include the accumulation of genetic damage or mutations in genes, chromsomes, and mitochondria; the deposition of lipofuscin and advanced glycation endproducts (AGEs) in many cell and tissue locations; the cross-linking of collagen and elastin, other abnormal modifications of proteins, and the accumulation of insoluble aggregates; damage by reactive oxygen species (ROS) in many contexts; loss of immune functions and autoimmunity; a decline in muscle strength; osteoporosis and osteoarthritis; inflammatory damage to tissues; hormone imbalance and a decline in homeostasis; epigenetic abnormalities, including the loss or gain of DNA methylation, and finally, a greatly increased incidence of tumors. All these can bring about a failure of major organ systems, such as the heart and major blood vessels, the brain and sensory organs, and so on. It is striking that the major theories of aging relate to particular causes of aging, such as the free radical theory, the somatic mutation theory, the mitochondrial theory, theories that relate to the accumulation of abnormal proteins, the immunologic theory, and several others.[4–7] If we accept the fact that there are multiple causes of aging, then it follows that many of the important theories of aging have some truth, and it is important to have a global view of both theories and causes of aging.

Aging is also directly related to the evolved design of the organism. It is clear that mammals and birds, as well as many of their precursors during evolution, have tissue and organ systems that can "last a lifetime," but certainly cannot last indefinitely. For example, the heart is a very efficient pump, but both it and the major blood vessels have very limited capacity for repair. The brain consists of innumerable neurons, most of which cannot be replaced. Eventually, brain cells are lost, and there is accumulation of abnormal peptides in plaques, as well as neurofibrillary tangles. The lens of the eye consists of crystallins that cannot be replaced, and eventually lose transparency. The retina continually turns over photoreceptors, and the ability to remove all this material eventually becomes impaired, with loss of retinal function. Joints cannot maintain a steady state, and often become damaged through continuous use. Finally, the wearing out of teeth provides an instructive example. Many herbivores, such as horses, have teeth that wear out through a lifetime of grazing. They are genetically programmed to last a lifetime, but suffer from wear and tear. This illustrates the fact that there is no real distinction between so-called programmed aging and the aging that is due to wear and tear. In humans, of course, the wearing out of teeth is circumvented by dental care, and some herbivores have incisor teeth that grow continuously throughout life.

It has been suggested that some vertebrates that continually increase in size, such as some large fish and reptiles, avoid the features of aging found in mammals and birds. This is open to serious question because age-related changes in these long-lived animals are poorly documented, and it cannot be disputed that their actual life spans are a tiny fraction of evolutionary time. A crucial feature of the evolved design of mammals and birds, as well as invertebrates, such as many insects and nematodes, is that post-mitotic cells cannot be expected to survive indefinitely. There are many events that can end the life of a cell, and it is therefore unreasonable to expect any to remain alive for ever.

MAINTENANCE OF THE ORGANISM

Why do mammalian and bird species live as long as they do? The answer depends on the efficiency of cell, tissue, and organ maintenance in each species.[7] Maintenance mechanisms are very extensive, and consume considerable resources. Moreover, as time goes on we learn more about the overall details of each mechanism and its relative importance in preserving the body or soma, and its role in maintaining a potentially immortal germ line. Thirteen separate mechanisms can now be identified:

1. the multiple pathways of DNA repair, which are vital for the removal of spontaneous lesions in DNA;
2. the defenses against oxygen-free radicals, which include antioxidants and enzymes;
3. the removal of defective proteins by proteases;
4. protein repair, such as the renaturation of proteins by chaperones, and the enzymic reversal of oxidization of amino acids;
5. the accuracy of synthesis of macromolecules, which depends on proof-reading mechanisms;
6. the immune response against pathogens and parasites;

7. the detoxification of harmful chemicals in the diet by the monooxyge-nase enzymes coded for by the P450 gene superfamily;
8. wound healing, blood clotting, and the healing of broken bones and torn ligaments;
9. physiological homeostasis, including temperature control;
10. the epigenetic stability of differentiated cells, and the defenses against neoplastic transformation;
11. apoptosis, which is the means of removing unwanted or damaged cells;
12. the storage of fat, to allow animals to survive in the absence of food; and
13. grooming of fur or feathers, which removes external parasites, dirt, and debris.

All these mechanisms depend on a large number of genes. For example, at least 1,000 genes are required for the immune system (P. Hodgkin, personal communication), and 150 genes for DNA repair (T. Lindahl, personal communication). Also, most of the maintenance mechanisms are the matter of scientific disciplines in their own right, so their understanding all depends on considerable biological and biochemical knowledge.

THE ALLOCATION OF RESOURCES

The energy and metabolic resources available to any animal must be divided between three fundamental features of life. The first comprises basic metabolism, which includes biochemical synthesis; respiration; cell turnover; movement; feeding, digestion, and excretion. The second is reproduction, which depends in mammals on the gonads, gametes, and sex; gestation and development; suckling; care of offspring, and growth to the adult. The third is maintenance, namely all the 13 functions listed in the previous section.

Whereas basic metabolism is essential for all animals, the extent of investment in reproduction and maintenance can vary between species. This is the trade-off known as the disposable soma theory of aging.[11-14] It states that increased investment in reproduction results in less investment in maintenance, and this reduces life span. More investment in maintenance and less in reproduction results in an increase in life span. The evolved balance between the two depends on the life history strategy and ecological niche of the species. It is predicted that there is an inverse relationship between the maximum potential number of offspring a female can produce during her lifetime and the maximum life span in a protected environment. This was confirmed for 47 mammalian species in which adequate data are available.[7,15] Of course, in natural environments females almost never achieve their full reproductive potential, nor do they reach their maximum life span. It should be noted that although this trade-off applies to females, males have the same genotypes (apart from the Y chromosome), so the same evolutionary forces will apply to them.

There have been many comparative studies that demonstrate that long-lived species have more efficient maintenance mechanisms than short-lived species. These have been comprehensively reviewed elswhere,[7] and since that time more evidence has been published.[16] Only a few examples are mentioned here: the same chemical cross-links in collagen occur much more quickly in bovine than human skin.[17] In rats, carcinomas arise far more frequently than they do in humans, with an approximately 30-fold difference in the rate of onset.[18] Also, somatic mutations in lymphocytes increase about 10-fold during the life span of mice and humans. However, this increase occurs over about 3 years in the mouse, and 80 years in humans.[19] It has been shown that the defenses against ROS in a long-lived bird, the pigeon, are much more efficient than those in the short-lived rat, a mammal of similar size and metabolic rate.[20] A similar difference is seen between small long-lived birds (canary and parakeet) and the mouse.[21] Many studies on DNA repair and DNA metabolism confirm a relationship between longevity and efficiency of maintenance.[7]

THE MODULATION OF AGING

It is very well known that calorie restriction in rodents substantially increases their life span, and it also greatly reduces their fecundity. This is probably an evolutionary adaptation, particularly in ground-living mammals which have a variable supply of food.[22–23] When food is absent or limited , it would be disadvantageous for females to breed, and better to invest available resources in maintenance and survival. When food becomes available, reproduction can then occur. The overall effect with a variable or limited food supply is to increase the life span.

Mutations in genes that increase longevity (in so-called gerontogenes) are likely to have deleterious effects on the phenotype, such as loss of fertility. Such animals would not compete with wild-type animals in a natural environment. It is therefore likely that any treatment that increases longevity comes at a cost. For example, there may be ways and means of reducing metabolic rate, or reducing temperature, or increasing sleep, all of which could conceivably increase longevity.

THE MODULATION OF AGING BY NATURAL SELECTION

With regard to life span, there have been two very different trends in mammalian evolution.[24] If the mortality increases, perhaps on account of a change in environment or the appearance of a new predator, then the population will decline. There will then be selection for earlier development and reproduction, with an increase in the number of offspring. Usually such animals become smaller. An excellent example of this trend is seen in the carnivores, with the evolution of small stoats and weasels. These develop rapidly, have large and frequent litters, and in captivity have a short life span. In their natural environment, their high mortality is largely due to shortage of prey. The opposite trend is illustrated by the very well-documented evolution of the horse. Primitive horses were about the size of a hare, but during the course of evolution their size gradually increased. This increase could also be associated with slower development, fewer offspring, and a longer life span. In this case, a reduction in mortality would result in the selection of the longest-living females that have, on average, the most offspring. This trend occurred in pachyderms, large whales, and the higher primates. Thus, the evolution of longevity ultimately depends on environmental mortality, and the ecological niche the species inhabits. It should also be realized that over long periods of time, the different causes of aging will become synchronized by natural selection.[25]

ANIMAL IMMORTALITY

An immortal animal must have the means to regenerate or replace cells and tissues that become damaged, or show signs of aging. Such regenerative powers are seen in a few simple animals, such as Hydra, some coelenterates, and flatworms. Aging is of ancient origin, since most differentiated invertebrates have finite life span. Many insects, and also nematodes, consist of post-mitotic cells, apart from germ cells. Since their cells cannot be replaced, they have clearly defined life spans. What would be the properties of more complex animals that could live indefinitely? Again, they would have to be capable of regenerating essential parts of the body; for example, with regard to the circulatory system, they would need two hearts and sets of major blood vessels. Then, as one declined in function, the second would start up, while the first would be repaired, then the second would be repaired, and so on. This would provide, in effect, a steady-state system with infinite survival time. It is much harder to see how such repair or regeneration could apply to the brain, in which long-lived neurons encapsulate experience and memory. The fact is that higher animals have simply not evolved that way because many of their phenotypic features demonstrate that many parts of the body have a finite life span. The evolved design of the body means that it has also a limited lifetime, and the reason for this is that it is counterproductive for animals to preserve their body, or soma, in environments where very few of them will survive for a long period. To put it another way, any animal that could preserve its soma indefinitely would have to invest so many resources that its Darwinian fitness would be lesser than that of an animal that has finite survival time.

CONCLUSIONS

The main conclusion is that after many decades of uncertainty, the biological reasons for aging became clear at the end of the 20th century. There are multiple causes of aging synchronized by natural selection, and the rate of aging and longevity in any given species depends on the failure of cell, tissue, and organ maintenance. There is now much evidence from comparative studies that efficiency of maintenance is correlated with maximum life span. Also, in mammals there is a clear inverse relationship between fecundity and longevity.

Although it may be possible to modulate life span, it is unreasonable to suppose that all the different causes of aging could be reversed. There is much discussion at present about anti-aging medicine. Ronald Klatz, in *Advances in Anti-Aging Medicine*, writes: "Within the next 50 years or so, assuming an individual can avoid becoming the victim of major trauma or homicide, it is entirely possible that he or she will be able to live virtually for ever."[26] This is biological nonsense, and reveals a complete ignorance of the field of gerontology, and why animals age. Unfortunately, despite our new understanding of aging, people will continue to misunderstand it for a long while to come.

ACKNOWLEDGMENTS

I thank Leonard Hayflick for much discussion, exchange of information, and for his agreement that aging is no longer an unsolved problem in biology.

REFERENCES

1. MEDAWAR, P.B. 1952. An Unsolved Problem in Biology. Lewis, London. Reprinted in Medawar, P.G., 1981.The Uniqueness of the Individual. Dover, New York.
2. COMFORT, A. 1956. The Biology of Senescence. Routledge and Kegan Paul. London.
3. COMFORT, A. 1964. Aging: the Biology of Senescence. Routledge and Kegan Paul. London.
4. COMFORT, A. 1979. The Biology of Senescence. Churchill Livingstone. Edinburgh and London.
5. FINCH, C. 1990. Senescence, Longevity and the Genome. The University of Chicago Press. Chicago.
6. HAYFLICK, L. 1994, 1996. How and Why We Age. Ballantine Books. New York.
7. HOLLIDAY, R. 1995. Understanding Aging. Cambridge University Press. Cambridge.
8. AUSTAD, S.N. 1997. Why We Age. John Wiley. New York.
9. KIRKWOOD, T. 1999. Time of Our Lives. Oxford University Press.
10. GURNELL, J. 1987. The Natural History of Squirrels. Christopher Helm. London.
11. KIRKWOOD, T.B.L. 1977. Evolution of aging. Nature **270:** 301–304.
12. KIRKWOOD, T.B.L. 2002. Evolution of aging. Mech. Age Dev. **123:** 737–745.
13. KIRKWOOD, T.B.L. & R. HOLLIDAY. 1979. The evolution of longevity. Proc. Roy. Soc. B. **205:** 532–546.
14. KIRKWOOD, T.B.L. & R. HOLLIDAY. 1986. Aging as a consequence of natural selection. *In* Biology of Human Aging. K.J. Collins & A.H. Bittles, Eds.: 1–16. Cambridge University Press. Cambridge.

15. HOLLIDAY, R. 1994. Longevity and fecundity in eutherian mammals. *In* Genetics and the Evolution of Aging. M.R. Rose & C.E. Finch, Eds.: 217–225. Kluwer Academic. Dordrecht.
16. HOLLIDAY, R. 2004. The multiple and irreversible causes of aging. J. Geront. Biol. Sci. **59A:** 568–572.
17. YAMAUCHI, M., D.T. WOODLEY & G.L. MECHANIC. 1988. Aging and cross-linking of skin collagen. Biochem. Biophys. Res. Comm. **152:** 898–903.
18. AMES, B.N., R.L. SAUL, E. SCHWIERS, *et al.* 1985. Oxidative damage as related to cancer and aging: the assay of thymine glycol, thymidine glycol and hydroxymethyl uracil in human and rat urine. *In* Molecular Biology of Aging. R.S. Sohal, L.S. Birnbaum & R.G. Cutler, Eds.: 137–144. Raven Press. New York.
19. MORLEY, A.A. 1998. Somatic mutations and aging. Ann. N. Y. Acad. Sci. **854:** 20–22.
20. PAMPLONA, R., M. PORTERO-OTIN, J.R. REQUENA, *et al.* 1999. A low degree of fatty acid unsaturation leads to lower lipid peroxidation and lipoxidation-derived protein modification in heart mitochondria of the longevous pigeon than the short lived rat. Mech. Age Dev. **106:** 283–296.
21. PAMPLONA, R., M. PORTERO-ORTIN, D. RIBA, *et al.* 1999. Heart fatty acid unsaturation and lipid peroxidation, and aging rate are lower in the canary and parakeet than in the mouse. Aging Clin. Exp. Res. **11:** 44–49.
22. HOLLIDAY, R. 1989. Food, reproduction and longevity: is the extended lifespan of calorie restricted animals as evolutionary adaptation? BioEssays **10:** 125–127.
23. TURTURRO, A. & R.W. HART. 1991. Longevity assurance mechanisms and calorie restriction. Ann. N. Y. Acad. Sci. **621:** 363–372.
24. HOLLIDAY, R. 2003. The modulation of lifespan by natural selection. *In* Modulating Aging and Longevity. S.I.S. Rattan Ed.: 17–26. Kluwer Academic. Dordrecht.
25. MAYNARD SMITH, J. 1962. The causes of aging. Proc. Roy. Soc. B **157:** 115–127.
26. KLATZ, R.M. 1996 ed. Advances in Anti-Aging Medicine. Mary Ann Liebert. New York.

Free Radical Theory of Aging: An Update

Increasing the Functional Life Span

DENHAM HARMAN

Department of Medicine, University of Nebraska College of Medicine, 984635 Nebraska Medical Center, Omaha, Nebraska, 68198-4635, USA

ABSTRACT: Aging is the progressive accumulation of diverse, deleterious changes with time that increase the chance of disease and death. The basic chemical process underlying aging was first advanced by the free radical theory of aging (FRTA) in 1954: the reaction of active free radicals, normally produced in the organisms, with cellular constituents initiates the changes associated with aging. The involvement of free radicals in aging is related to their key role in the origin and evolution of life. Aging changes are commonly attributed to development, genetic defects, the environment, disease, and an inborn aging process (IAP). The latter produces aging changes at an exponentially increasing rate with age, becoming the major risk factor for disease and death for humans after the age of 28 years in the developed countries. In them the IAP limits human average life expectancy at birth (ALE-B)—a rough measure of the healthy life span—to about 85 years; few reach 100 years and only one is known to have lived to 122 years. In these countries, improvements in living conditions (ILC) have gradually raised ALE-Bs to 76–79 years, 6–9 years less than the limit imposed by aging, with no change in the maximum life span (MLS). The extensive studies based on the FRTA hold promise that ALE-B and the MLS can be extended, the ALE-B possibly by a few years, and the MLS somewhat less.

KEYWORDS: aging; mitochondria; mutations; free radicals; longevity; origin of life; evolution

INTRODUCTION

Aging is the progressive, more-or-less random, accumulation of diverse, deleterious changes[1,2,3]—first in the male and female gametes, then in the

Address for correspondence: Denham Harman, M.D., Ph.D., Department of Medicine, University of Nebraska College of Medicine, 984635 Nebraska Medical Center, Omaha, Nebraska, 68198-4635, USA. Voice: 402-559-4416; fax: 402-559-7330.
e-mail: vcerino@unmc.edu

Ann. N.Y. Acad. Sci. 1067: 10–21 (2006). © 2006 New York Academy of Sciences.
doi: 10.1196/annals.1354.003

developing zygote formed from them, and finally throughout the cells and tissues of the resulting individual—that increase the chance of disease and death with advancing age. Aging changes are commonly attributed to development, genetic defects, environment, disease, and an inborn aging process (IAP). These changes limit the human life expectancy at birth (ALE-B)—a rough measure of the healthy life span—to a maximum of about 85 years.

The human ALE-B is increased by improvements in general living conditions (ILC), e.g., better nutrition, housing, medical care. These efforts are becoming increasingly less effective;[4,5] this is illustrated in FIGURE 1 by the curves of the logarithm of the chance of death versus age for Swedish females for various periods from 1751 to 1992, and in FIGURE 2 by the increases in the ALE-B of the population of the United States from 1900 to 1996.[3] The chances for death in the developed countries are now near limiting values.

Thus, as living conditions in a population approach the optimum, the curve of the chance of death versus age shifts toward a limit determined by the sum of the irreducible contributions to the chance of death by aging changes that can be prevented to varying degrees by ILC (e.g., those due to nutrition or disease) and contributions that can be influenced little, if at all, by ILC (e.g., due to the IAP).

The Inborn Aging Process

Aging changes produced by the IAP are few early on in life but increase rapidly with age, as illustrated in FIGURE 3 by a plot of the chances for death in 1985 for the U. S. population as a function of age.[6] IAP changes are largely responsible for the now almost exponential rise in the limiting chances for death after about the age of 28 years in the developed countries. Only 1–2% of a cohort die before this age.[3] The IAP limits ALE-B to about 85 years, permits a growing few to live to 100 years, and maintains the maximum life span (MLS) at around 122 years.

Free Radical Theory of Aging

The basic chemical process underlying aging was advanced in 1954 by the free radical theory of aging (FRTA):[7,8] the reaction of active free radicals, normally produced in the organism, with cellular constituents. The FRTA, and the simultaneous discovery of the important, ubiquitous involvement of free radicals in endogenous metabolic reactions, arose[9] from a consideration of aging phenomena (in the light of chemical knowledge, including free radical chemistry), from the premise that a single common process, modifiable by genetic and environmental factors, was responsible for the aging and death of all living things.

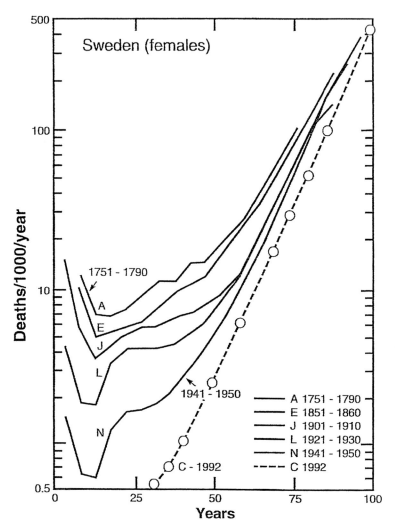

FIGURE 1. Age-specific death rates of Swedish females in various periods from 1751 to 1992. (Adapted from Jones' and the Sveriges Officiella Statistik.[5])

FRTA—An Update

1. 1972. The FRTA was first extended in 1972[10] with the suggestion that (1) most FRRs stemmed from superoxide radicals (SO) formed by the mitochondria in the course of normal metabolism and (2) the life span is determined primarily by the rate of free radical damage to mitochondria, apparently largely to mitochondrial DNA.
2. 1983. Consequences of mitochondrial aging[11] were discussed in 1983.

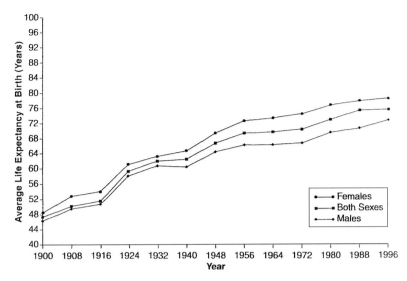

FIGURE 2. Average life expectancy at birth: United States, 1900–1996.

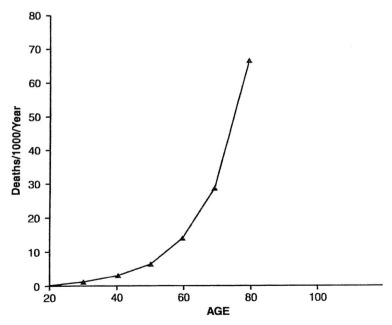

FIGURE 3. The chance of dying in 1985 as a function of age for the total population of the United States.

3. 1998. Later it became clear[12,13] that ILC increased ALE-B by decreasing the free radical reactions (FRRs) associated with suboptimal living conditions. The latter includes exposure of tissue to air.

   During surgery or trauma in the absence of measures to maintain normal tissue O_2 levels, antioxidant levels, such as that of serum ascorbic acid,[14] are depressed by tissue-derived FRRs. Thus limiting tissue exposure to air may have beneficial effects (e.g., on rate of recovery and the incidence of sepsis),[15] minimizing the expected shortening of the life spans. In accord with the foregoing are the beneficial effects of minimal access procedures in surgery[16] and those expected from antioxidant therapy.[17] In addition, the long-term postoperative cognitive dysfunction in older individuals[18] may reflect, in part, the exposure of the brain to lower-than-normal levels of antioxidants, such as ascorbic acid, during surgery.

4. 2002. Finally, it also became clear[19] that "aging" is the sum of the free radical damage associated with suboptimal living conditions plus that produced by the IAP.

Further support for the FRTA includes: (*a*) Genetically engineered mice that develop a 3–5-fold increase in the level of point mutations in mitochondrial DNA and increased amounts of deleted mtDNA have reduced life spans and premature onset of aging-related phenotypes.[20] (*b*) Transgenic mice that overexpress human catalase lived longer than controls.[21] (*c*) Comparing birds with mammals with similar metabolic rates, the much longer life spans of birds are related to a smaller diversion of O_2 to SO by the bird mitochondria.[22,23] Similarly, there is the difference in life spans between two closely related rodents.[24] (*d*) Life spans of different mammalian species are related to the rate of mitochondrial SO formation.[25] (*e*) The frequency of mitochondrial genotype, Mt5178A, in Japan is higher in centenarians than in healthy blood donors.[26] Since mitochondria are of maternal origin, siblings of centenarians live longer than normal.[27] (*f*) Mice genetically manipulated to accumulate high levels of mtDNA mutations had a significantly reduced life span and signs of premature aging.[28]

The FRTA suggests that measures to decrease (*a*) the rate of initiation of FRRs (e.g., by minimizing the presence of copper, iron, and other oxidant catalysts), and/or (*b*) the chain lengths of FRRs (e.g., with antioxidants such as vitamin E) can lower the rate of formation of aging changes, even under optimal living conditions, and in turn decrease the rate of aging and pathogenesis. Many studies now support this possibility.[2,29,30]

However, because the IAP increases exponentially with age it will progressively lower the rate of these decreases toward zero as the ALE-Bs approach the potential maximum of about 85 years.[2,3]

Nutrition has played a significant role in increasing ALE-B while having little or no effect on the MLS.[31] Future nutritional attempts to raise ALE-B further should be more effective using diets carefully selected to minimize free radical damage.[32]

Origin and Evolution of Life

The FRTA helped to focus interest on why free radical reactions are ubiquitous in living things. A reasonable explanation, as well as insight into the nature of the IAP, is provided by studies on the origin and evolution of life:[33] an overview is summarized in TABLE 1.

Life apparently arose spontaneously 3.5–4.0 billion years ago from amino acids, nucleotides, and other basic chemicals of living things. These building blocks were produced from simple reduced components (methane, hydrogen, ammonia, and water) of the primitive oxygen-free atmosphere by free radical reactions,[34–36] initiated mainly by ionizing radiation from the sun. The steady-state products, including the first protocells with simple self-replicating progenitors of DNA, reflected the innate chemical properties of the atoms and molecules from which they had been formed, as well as the environment in which they had been produced. The environment became warmer, and O_2 appeared in the atmosphere after the advent of blue-green algae, decreasing the intensity of ionizing radiation on Earth—eventually forming the "ozone shield." Precursors of life were the steady-state products of protocells that had been subjected to a long constant reiterative process. As the precursors

TABLE 1. Overview of the origin and evolution of life

Years ago	Main Events
3.5 billion	Basic chemicals of life formed by free radical reactions, largely initiated by ionizing radiation from the sun
	Life begins
	Excision repair and
	Recombinational repair
	Ferredoxin
	RH or $H_2S + CO_2–(h\upsilon) \rightarrow CH$
2.6 billion	Blue-green algae
	$H_2O–(h\upsilon) \rightarrow 2H + O_2$
1.3 billion	Atmospheric O_2 reaches 1% of present value
	Anaerobic prokaryotes disappear
	Eukaryotes become dominant cells
	Eukaryotes + blue-green algae $\rightarrow$ the green leaf plants
	Eukaryotes + a prokaryote able to reduce O_2 to $H_2O \rightarrow$ animal kingdom
	Emergence of multicellular organisms and plants
	Meiosis
500 million	Atmospheric O_2 reaches 10% of present value
	Ozone screen allows emergence of life from sea
56 million	Primates appear
5 million	Man

evolved and became more complex, one or more of them somehow acquired the characteristics of life, including the ability to internalize the initiation of free radical reactions.

Approximately 1.3 billion years ago the progenitor of the green plants acquired blue-green algae to assist with its energy needs, whereas that of the animal kingdom took in a prokaryote able to reduce O_2 to water. Subsequently, colonies of cells appeared that evolved into multicellular organisms and plants.

About 500 million years ago absorption of UV radiation by atmospheric oxygen reduced radiation reaching the surface to a level compatible with existence on land. Evolution then accelerated. Primates appeared about 65 million years ago, and man some 4–5 million years ago.

The Inborn Aging Process—Continued

The prokaryote acquired by the progenitor of the animal kingdom evolved into the mitochondrion.[37] Collectively, they are the IAP,[38,39] the major source of: (1) energy for metabolic needs and the activities of life, by using the conversion of ADP to ATP to capture energy released by the 4-electron reduction of O_2 to water during oxidative phosphorylation, and (2) superoxide radicals—largely responsible for the free radical reactions involved in mutations, disease, and death—by the one-electron reduction of O_2, using about 1–3% of the amount of O_2 consumed by oxidative phosphorylation. In addition, the mitochondria play a major role in apoptotic cell death.[40]

Further, all, or almost all, mitochondria are maternally inherited.[38] An individual's mitochondria in post-mitotic cells undergo free radical–induced changes with age;[11] only minor changes occur with age in the mitochondria of dividing cells.

Formation of SO in the course of normal metabolism apparently does not increase significantly with age,[39] while that of ATP declines on account of free radical damage. The latter may be largely responsible for the exponential nature of the mortality curve in a manner analogous to the autoxidation of a lipid containing an antioxidant:[41,42] the rate of oxidative change in the lipid is slow at first, becoming progressively faster as the antioxidant is consumed through the inhibition of free radical reactions. In living organisms the "antioxidant" level seemingly also decreases with age, as production of ATP for reductive synthesis (e.g., of glutathione and NADPH) declines as mitochondria age.

The relatively low free radical activity in early life permits growth and development of new offspring. These processes are slowed with age by the widespread continuous accumulation of IAP-associated free radical damage, including mutations, plus similar damage from ionizing radiation[43,45,46] and oxygen exposure,[44] as well as that produced by suboptimal living conditions.[19] This damage, incompletely repaired by processes dependent on ATP, is attributed to "Aging," and causes the transition into childhood, adolescence, adulthood, old age, and death. The transition rates determine longevity; evolution limits ALE-B of humans to about 85 years and the MLS to around 122 years. Efforts to decrease these rates will eventually be thwarted by the exponential nature of the IAP.

Thus, the IAP, a magnificent product of evolution, provides *with the aid of the growing accumulation of free radical damage with age*, for the development and birth of new individuals, mutations, activities during life and their eventual death. *Aging* is a growing expression with time of free radical damage from both endogenous and exogenous sources, incompletely repaired by processes dependant on ATP.

Slowing the IAP

Measures that can, or may, slow the rate of formation of aging changes with age, without significantly lowering normal ATP levels, include:

1. *Caloric restriction.* Increases in human longevity will be small with a tolerable level of restriction.[12] A recent study with *Drosophila melanogaster* concluded[47]: "Caloric restriction extends life span by slowing down the rate of normal aging."

2. *Compounds that compete with O_2 for access to "electron-rich areas" of the mitochondria.* Nitroxides compete with O_2 for electrons from the mitochondrial respiratory chain to form hydroxylamines[48] instead of superoxide radicals.

3. *Compounds that may decrease loss of mtDNA function with age.* (a) Levels of coenzyme Q_{10} decrease with age; dietary supplementation significantly increases them.[49] (b) Increased oxidative damage to mtDNA also decreases mitochondrial glutathione (GSH) content; reversed by oral antioxidants,[50] such as thiazolidine carboxylate, a *Ginkgo biloba* extract, and targeted antioxidants.[51] (c) Other measures directed at increasing mitochondrial GSH include supplementing the diet with GSH esters.[52] (d) The life span of *Drosophila melanogaster* was increased about 18% when maintained on a diet supplemented with either sodium or magnesium thiazolidine carboxylate.[53] (e) Increases in mitochondrial damage with age are decreased by supplementing the diet with a combination of acetyl-L-carnitine plus lipoic acid.[54,55]

4. *Genetic change.* (a) Efforts to determine the cause(s) for differences in O_2 diversion to SO (see above) may suggest measures to do so in humans. (b) In mice a homozygous mutation of p66[shc] increased life span by about 30%—around the same increase achievable by caloric restriction in the absence of any obvious defective phenotype.[56] (c) Similarly, increases in longevity demonstrated in the numerous and steadily increasing studies of mice and other model aging systems, e.g., yeast, *C. elegans*,

and *Drosophila* are compatible in most cases, if not all, with the possibility[57] that they are caused by lower levels of free radical reactions. (d) Genetic studies of premature aging syndromes are now also under way in an effort to increase longevity.[58–60] (e) Genetic changes that take place in early life may predispose to premature death. Some of these changes can be prevented, thus extending the "normal" life span.[12]

"Engineered negligible senescence"—This term has been suggested[61] for measures that may serve to remove or prevent the normal accumulation of aging changes.

COMMENT

Studies based on the FRTA have helped to increase the ALE-B; the exponential nature of the IAP blocks increases in MLS. However, growing knowledge of the IAP suggested potentially practical measures to increase the MLS discussed above; those directed at minimizing changes in early life and decreasing diversion of O_2 to SO might be the most productive. These efforts should also serve to focus further attention on the problems of old age[62,63] and how best to ameliorate them. The desire "to live long but not be old" is gradually being fulfilled.

Finally, the creation of life and its evolution on earth during the past 3.5 billion years is a truly remarkable example of what can be accomplished by chance through the continued interplay over time of energy, suitable molecules, simple chemical reactions, and environmental modulations. Energy sources on the earth initiated free radical reactions to create life from inert chemicals, starting with molecules of the primitive atmosphere. Then, by means of the same chemical reactions life evolved into chemically diverse complex forms.

The growing knowledge of evolution and aging permits modulation to some extent of the duration of life and its quality, as well as acceptance with equanimity, of the inevitable death mandated by evolution.

REFERENCES

1. KOHN, R.R. 1985. Aging and age-related diseases: normal processes. *In* Relation between Normal Aging and Disease. H.A. Johnson, Ed.: 1–44. Raven Press. New York.
2. HARMAN, D. 1994. Aging prospects for further increases in the functional life span. Age **17:** 119–146.
3. HARMAN, D. 2000. Antioxidant supplements: effect on disease and aging in the United States population. J. Am. Aging Assoc. **23:** 25–31.
4. JONES, H.R. 1955. The relation of human health to age, place and time. *In* Handbook of Aging and the Individual. J.E. Birren, Ed.: 333–363. University of Chicago Press. Chicago, IL.

5. SVERIGES OFFICIELLA STATISTIK. 1992. Befolknings-forandringar. 1987. Statistiska centralbyran, 114–115. Stockholm, Sweden.

6. NATIONAL CENTER FOR HEALTH STATISTICS. 1988. Vital Statistics of the United States. 1985. Life Tables, Vol. 2 (6). Hyattsville, MD (U.S. Dept. of Health & Human Services), PHS Pulb. No. 88-1104:9.

7. HARMAN, D. 1956. Aging: a theory based on free radical and radiation chemistry. J. Gerontol. Soc. **11:** 298–300.

8. HARMAN, D. 1992. Free radical theory of aging: history. *In* Free Radicals and Aging. I. Emerit & B. Chance Eds.: 1–10. Birkhauser. Basel.

9. KITANI, K. & G.O. IVY. 2003. "I thought, thought, thought for months in vain and suddenly the idea came"—an interview with Denham and Helen Harman. Biogerontolgy **4:** 401–412.

10. HARMAN, D. 1972. The biologic clock: the mitochondria? J. Am. Geriatr. Soc. **20:** 145–147.

11. HARMAN, D. 1983. Free radical theory of aging: consequences of mitochondrial aging. Age **6:** 86–94.

12. HARMAN, D. 1998. Free radical theory of aging: increasing the average life expectancy at birth and the maximum life span. J. Anti-Aging Med. **2:** 199–208.

13. HARMAN, D. 2000. Alzheimer's disease: a hypothesis on pathogenesis. J. Am. Aging Assoc. **23:** 147–161.

14. SCHORAH, C.J., C. DOWNING, A. PIRIPITSI, *et al.* 1996. Total vitamin C, ascorbic acid, and dehydroascorbic acid concentrations in plasma of critically ill patients. Am. J. Clin. Nutr. **63:** 760–765.

15. HOTCHKISS, R.S. & I.E. KARL. 2003. The pathophysiology and treatment of sepsis. New Engl. J. Med. **348:** 138–150.

16. REDMOND, H.P., R.W.G. WATSON, T. HOUGHTON, *et al.* 1994. Immune function in patients undergoing open vs laparoscopic cholecystectomy. Arch. Surg. **129:** 1240–1246.

17. CUZZOCREA, S., M.C. MCDONALD, H.M. FILIPE, *et al.* 2001. Effects of tempol, a membrane-permeable radical scavenger, in a rodent model of carrageenan-induced pleurisy. Eur. J. Pharmacol. **390:** 209–222.

18. MOLLER, J.T., P. CLUITMANS, L.S. RASMUSSEN, P. *et al.* 1998. Long-term postoperativae cognitive dysfunction in the elderly: ISPOCD1. Lancet **351:** 857–861.

19. HARMAN, D. 2002. Alzheimer's disease: role of aging in pathogenesis. Ann. N.Y. Acad. Sci. **959:** 384–395.

20. TRIFUNOVIC, A., A. WIREDENBERG, M. FALKENBERG, *et al.* 2004. Premature ageing in mice expressing defective mitochondrial DNA polymerase. Nature **429:** 417–423.

21. SCHRINER, S.E., N.J. LINFORD & G.M. MARTIN. 2005. Extension of murine life span by overexpression of catalase targeted to mitochondria. Science **308:** 1909–1911.

22. KU, H-H. & R.S. SOHAL. 1993. Comparison of mitochondrial proxidant generation and anti-oxidant defenses between rat and pigeon: possible basis of variation in longevity and metabolic potential. Mech. Ageing Dev. **72:** 7–76.

23. BARJA, G., S. CADENAS, C. ROJAS, *et al.* 1994. Low mitochondrial free radical production per unit O_2 consumption can explain the simultaneous presence of high longevity and high aerobic metabolic rate in birds. Free Radic. Res. **21:** 317–328.

24. SOHAL, R.S., H-H. KU & S. AGARWAL. 1993. Biochemical correlates of longevity in two closely related species. Biochem. Biophys. Res. Commun. **196:** 7–11.

25. KU, H-H., U.T. BRUNK & R.S. SOHAL. 1993. Relationship between mitochon-
    drial superoxide and hydrogen peroxide production and longevity of mammalian
    species. Free Radic. Biol. Med. **15:** 621–627.
26. TANAKA, M., J-S GONG, J. ZHANG, *et al.* 1998. Mitochondrial genotype associated
    with longevity. Lancet **351:** 185–186.
27. PERLS, T.T., E. BUBRICK, C.C. WAGER, *et al.* 1998. Siblings of centenarians live
    longer. Lancet **351:** 1560.
28. KUJOTH, G.C., A. HIONA, T.D. PUGH, *et al.* 2005. Mitochondrial DNA mutations,
    oxidative stress, and apoptosis in mammalian aging. Science **309:** 481–484.
29. HARMAN, D. 1993. Free radical involvement in aging: pathophysiology and thera-
    peutic implications. Drugs & Aging **3:** 60–80.
30. SOHAL, R.J., H-H KU, S. AGARWAL, *et al.* 1994. Oxidative damage, mitochondrial
    oxidant generation and antioxidant defenses during aging and in response to food
    restriction in the mouse. Mech. Ageing Dev. **74:** 121–133.
31. HARMAN, D. 1995. Role of antioxidant nutrients in aging: overview. Age **18:** 51–62.
32. AMES, B.N. 1999. Cancer prevention and the diet: help from single nucleotide
    polymorphisms. Proc. Natl. Acad. Sci. USA **96:** 12216–12218.
33. HARMAN, D. 1981. The aging process. Proc. Natl. Acad. Sci. USA **78:** 7124–
    7128.
34. OPARIN, A.I. 1953. Origin of Life. Translated by S. Morgulis, 3rd. ed., with addition
    of a new introduction by the translator. Dover Publications. New York.
35. MILLER, S.L. 1959. Formation of organic compounds on the primitive earth. *In*
    The Origin of Life. A.L. Oparin, Ed.: 123–135. Pergamon Press. London.
36. DAY, W. 1979. Genesis on Planet Earth. House of Talos. East Lansing, MI.
37. GRAY, M.W., G. BURGER & B.F. LANG 1999. Mitochondrial evolution: review.
    Science **283:** 1476–1481.
38. WALLACE, D.C. 1999. Mitochondrial disease in man and mouse: a review. Science
    283: 1482–1488.
39. BARJA, G. 1999. Mitochondrial oxygen radical generation and leak sites of pro-
    duction in states 4 and 3, organ specificity, and relation to aging and longevity.
    J. Bioenerg. Biomembr. **31:** 347–366.
40. ORRENIUS, S. 2004. Mitochondrial regulation of apoptotic cell death. Toxicol. Lett.
    149: 19–23.
41. LUNDBERG, W.O. 1962. Mechanisms (1962) *In* Lipids and Their Oxidation. H.W.
    Schultz, E.A. Day & R.O. Sinnhuber, Eds.: 31–50. The Avi Publishing Co.
    Westport.
42. AUGUSTIN, M.A. & S.K. BERRY. 1983. Effectiveness of antioxidants in refined,
    bleached and deodorized palm olein. J. Am. Oil Chem. Soc. **60:** 105–108.
43. UPTON, A.C. 1957. Ionizing radiation and the aging process: a review. J. Gerontol.
    12: 306–315.
44. GERSCHMAN, R. 1959. Oxygen effects in biological systems. *In* Proceedings of the
    21st International Congress of Physiological Sciences (August 9–15, Buenos
    Aires), pp. 222–226.
45. STREHLER, B.L. 1959. Origin and comparison of the effects of time and high-energy
    radiation on living systems. Quart. Rev. Biol. **34:** 117–142.
46. HARMAN, D. 1962. Role of free radicals in mutation, cancer, aging and the main-
    tenance of life. Radiat. Res. **16:** 753–763.
47. PLETCHER, S.D., S.J. MACDONALD, R. MARGUERIE, *et al.* 2002. Genome-wide tran-
    script profiles in aging and calorically restricted *Drosophila melanogaster.* Curr.
    Biol. **12:** 712–723.

48. QUINTANILHA, A.T. & L. PACKER. 1977. Surface localization of sites of reduction of spin-labeled molecules in mitochondria. Proc. Natl. Acad. Sci. USA **74:** 570–574.
49. MATTHEWS, R.T., L. YANG, S. BROWNE, *et al*. 1998. Coenzyme Q$_{10}$ administration increases brain mitochondrial concentrations and exerts neuroprotective effects. Proc. Natl. Acad. Sci. USA **95:** 8892–8897.
50. GARCIA DE LA ASUNCION, J., A. MILLAN, R. PLA, *et al*. 1996. Mitochondrial glutathione oxidation correlates with age-associated oxidative damage to mitochondrial DNA. FASEB J. **10:** 333–338.
51. KELSO, G.F., C.M. PORTEOUS, G. HUGHES, *et al*. 2002. Prevention of mitochondrial oxidative damage using targeted antioxidants. Ann. N. Y. Acad. Sci. **959:** 263–274.
52. MEISTER, A. 1994. Glutathione-ascorbic acid antioxidant system in animals. J. Biol. Chem. **269:** 9397–9400.
53. MIQUEL, J. & A.C. ECONOMOS. 1979. Favorable effects of the antioxidants sodium and magnesium thiazolidine carboxylate on the vitality and life span of *Drosophila* and mice. Exp. Gerontol. **14:** 279–285.
54. HAGEN, T., J. LIU, J. LYKKESFELDT, *et al*. 2002. Feeding acetyl-L-carnitine and lipoic acid to old rats significantly improves metabolic function while decreasing oxidative stress. Proc. Natl. Acad. Sci. USA **99:** 1870–1875.
55. AMES, B.N. 2004. Delaying the mitochondrial decay of aging. Ann. N.Y. Acad. Sci. **1019:** 406–411.
56. TRINEI, M., M. GIORGIO, A. CICALESE, *et al*. 2002. A p53-p66^{shc} signalling pathway controls intracellular redox status, levels of oxidation-damaged DNA and oxidative-stress induced apoptosis. Oncogene **21:** 3872–3878.
57. HARMAN, D. 2003. The free radical theory of aging. Antioxid. Redox. Signal. **5:** 557–561.
58. ERIKSSON, M., W.T. BROWN, L.B. GORDON, *et al*. 2003. Recurrent *de novo* point mutations in lamin A cause Hutchinson-Gilford progeria syndrome. Nature **423:** 293–298.
59. VASTAG, B. 2003. Cause of progeria's premature aging found: expected to provide insight into normal aging process. JAMA **289:** 2481–2482.
60. FOSSEL, M. 2003. The progerias: review. J. Anti-Aging Med. **6:** 123–138.
61. RIGA, D. 2003. SENS acquires SENSe: present and future anti-aging strategies. J. Anti-Aging Med. **6:** 231–236.
62. HARMAN, D. 2001. Aging: Overview. Ann. N.Y. Acad. Sci. **928:** 1–21.
63. PETERSON, P. 1999. Gray Dawn. 160–178. Times Books [a Division of Random House]. New York.

The Free Radical Fantasy

A Panoply of Paradoxes

RANDOLPH M. HOWES

The Johns Hopkins Hospital, Baltimore, Maryland, USA and University of Santo Tomas, Manila, Philippines

ABSTRACT: Overly exuberant and exaggerated past expectations and claims of the free radical theory have been quieted by extensive randomized, double-blind, controlled human studies. A half century of data demonstrates its lack of predictability and it has not been validated by the scientific method. Widespread use of antioxidants has failed to quell the current pandemic of cancer, diabetes, and cardiovascular disease or to stop or reverse the aging process. Electronically modified oxygen derivatives contribute to the modulation of cellular redox status, which is of primary importance in disease prevention and homeostasis.

KEYWORDS: oxidants; antioxidants; redox; free radical theory; aging; anti-aging, vitamins

INTRODUCTION

The basis for the free radical theory of Harman[1] is the belief that oxygen free radicals produce harmful oxidation products, which randomly accumulate with aging, and that they are responsible for more than 100 diseases and aging. This theory was further extended to especially apply to redox damage of the mitochondrion.[2]

Inherent in the free radical theory was the concept that the harmful effects of oxidized products could be diminished or alleviated by the judicious use of antioxidants. Although there was initially widespread enthusiasm for the antioxidant studies, it has become apparent, after 50 years of investigation, that the overall analysis of the data has failed to conclusively validate or confirm the free radical theory. The dream of stopping the aging process or of wiping out hordes of diseases with the use of antioxidants has turned into a meta-analytic nightmare for the sycophants of the free radical theory.

Address for correspondence: Randolph M. Howes, Adjunct Assistant Professor of Plastic Surgery, The Johns Hopkins Hospital, Baltimore, Maryland, USA and University of Santo Tomas, Manila, Philippines, 27439 Highway 441, Kentwood, LA 70444–8152. Voice: 985-229-3760; fax: 985-229-6955.

e-mail: rhowesmd@direcway.com
www.thepundit.com

Ann. N.Y. Acad. Sci. 1067: 22–26 (2006). © 2006 New York Academy of Sciences.
doi: 10.1196/annals.1354.004

Paradoxes are everywhere. Not only have antioxidants failed to stop disease and aging but also they may cause harm and mortality, which precipitated the stoppage of several large studies. A 2005 nutrition and supplement review in *JAMA* bolsters my position.[3] In my opinion, this scenario exemplifies the rise and fall of the free radical theory.

The following antioxidant studies have been conducted on more than 550,000 humans and have failed to lend credence to the free radical theory.

Alpha-Tocopherol/Beta-Carotene Cancer Prevention Study (ATBC) (1994)[4]: a study of pooled Finish male smokers (29,133 in all) found an 18% excess of lung cancer in participants receiving beta-carotene after 6 years and increased the incidence of cardiac death, hemorrhagic stroke, and the risk for major coronary events. This trial was stopped early.

Polyp Prevention Study Group (1994)[5]: Seven hundred and fifty-one patients completed this 4-year clinical trial. Neither β–carotene or vitamins C and E reduced the incidence of adenomas nor prevented any subtype of polyp.

The Beta-Carotene and Retinol Efficacy Trial (CARET) (1996)[6]: Smokers, former smokers, and workers exposed to asbestos (18,314) were given β–carotene and vitamin A for 4.0 years, and they had a 28% increase in lung cancer incidence. The trial was stopped 21 months early.

Physicians' Health Study I (PHS I) (1996)[7]: β–carotene, given to 22,071 U.S. male physicians, showed no differences in the incidence of malignant neoplasms, stroke, or cardiovascular disease or in overall mortality after 12 years of supplementation.

ATBC Substudy (1997)[8]: Men with prior myocardial infarction (1,862) took alpha-tocopherol and β-carotene for 5.3 years. There were no significant differences in major coronary events, but significantly more deaths from fatal coronary heart disease.

Antioxidant Vitamin Effect on Traditional CVD Risk Factors (1997)[9]: In 297 retired teachers, after 2–4 months of combined antioxidant supplements, showed no significant effect on systolic and diastolic blood pressures, fasting serum lipids (total cholesterol, high-density lipoprotein cholesterol, and low-density lipoprotein cholesterol) and fasting glucose.

The Nurses' Health Study (1998) and Folic Acid and Colon Cancer (1998)[10]: Women (88,756) taking vitamin C and β-carotene for 8 years did not have any reduction in heart disease risk. Multivitamins containing folic acid had no benefit with respect to colon cancer after 4 years of use and had no significant risk reductions after 5 to 9 or 10 to 14 years of use. Long-term use of multivitamins (for more than 15 years) may substantially reduce risk for colon cancer, perhaps on account of folic acid.

The Women's Health Study (1999)[11]: In 39,876 healthy women aged 45 years or older, there was no benefit from β–carotene, after 4.1 years, on the incidence of cancer, cardiovascular disease, or mortality.

The GISSI Trial (1999)[12]: Patients (11,324) with recent heart attacks showed no benefit from vitamin E supplements for up to 2 years. Results indicated that n-3 PUFA supplements, but not synthetic vitamin E, reduced long-term complications of myocardial infarction. The fish oil group had 15% decreased risk of death, nonfatal MI, and stroke.

The Health Professionals Follow-Up Study (1999)[13]: In this study 43,738 men were followed for 8 years. Vitamin E and C supplements and specific carotenoids did not reduce risk for stroke.

Meta-Analysis of Vitamin E in CVD, Ischemic Heart Disease (IHD), and Mortality (2000)[14]: Four randomized trails on 51,000 participants taking vitamin E or placebo for 1.4 to 6 years did not demonstrate a reduction in cardiovascular and IHD mortality or nonfatal myocardial infarction.

The Heart Outcomes Prevention Evaluation Study (HOPE) (2000)[15]: In this study 9,541 patients, at high risk for cardiovascular events or diabetes, were treated with vitamin E for 4.5 years, which had no effect on cardiovascular outcomes or stroke.

Age-Related Eye Disease Study Research Group (AREDS) (2001)[16]: All the 4,757 participants taking β–carotene and vitamins C and E had no effect on the 7-year risk of development or progression of age-related lens opacities or visual acuity loss.

Antioxidant Vitamins and U.S. Physician CVD Mortality (2002)[17]: Male U.S physicians (83,639) taking vitamin E, vitamin C, or multivitamins did not show a significant decrease in total CVD or CHD mortality.

The Women's Angiographic Vitamin and Estrogen (WAVE) Trial (2002)[18]: Four hundred and twenty-three postmenopausal women, with at least one 15% to 75% stenosis in the coronary artery, showed that neither HRT nor antioxidant vitamin supplements (vitamins C and E) provided any cardiovascular benefit. Instead, a potential for harm was suggested. Vitamin E supplements provided no benefit for cardiovascular mortality as reported in a 2003 review by Vivekananthan *et al.*[19], which included seven trials with 82,000 patients. A meta-analysis conducted in 2005, including more than 135,000 subjects, concluded that high doses of vitamin E increased mortality.[20]

The British Heart Protection Study, following 20,000 subjects for 5 years, found no benefit from a combination of vitamins E and C, and β–carotene, for heart disease, cancer, and several other conditions.[21] A study of more than 20,000 subjects found that vitamin E, vitamin C, and β-carotene supplementation resulted in small but significant increases in serum total cholesterol, low-density lipoprotein cholesterol, and triglyceride concentrations.[22]

Hopefully, for open-minded investigators, my point is made.

CONCLUSION

Randomized, double-blind, controlled trials in humans, which are the clinical "gold standard," have repeatedly shown that the free radical theory lacks predictability and fails to be confirmed by the scientific method.

Admittedly, there were likely many confounding variables in the antioxidant studies involving the use of other drugs, use of other dietary supplements, varying diets, varying environmental factors, presence or lack of exercise, degrees of obesity, varying dosage levels, varying antioxidant combinations, synthetic or natural vitamin sources, improperly combined study groups, use of improper exclusion criteria, flawed statistical methods, overgeneralization of findings, etc. Even though one can find positive antioxidant studies, the overall lack of predictability is undeniable.

I have formulated a new pro-oxidant protective paradigm to explain disease allowance and to stimulate new thinking regarding treatment.[23,24] Electronically modified oxygen derivatives (EMODs) support modulation of redox cycling and redox status, which are of utmost importance for disease prevention and maintaining cellular homeostasis.

In conclusion, extensive antioxidant studies have failed to confirm the free radical theory and antioxidant use may cause harm or accelerate one's demise. The free radical theory has fallen.

REFERENCES

1. HARMAN, D. 2000. Aging: overview. Ann. N.Y. Acad. Sci. **928:** 1–21.
2. HARMAN, D. 1972. "The biological clock: the mitochondria?" J. Am. Geriatr. Soc. **20:** 145–147.
3. LICHTENSTEIN, A.H. & R.M. RUSSELL. 2005. Essential nutrients: food or supplements? JAMA **294:** 351–358.
4. HEINONEN, O.P., J.K. HUTTUNEN, D. ALBANES & ATBC CANCER PREVENTION STUDY GROUP. 1994. The effect of vitamin E and beta carotene on the incidence of lung cancer and other cancers in male smokers. N. Engl. J. Med. **330:** 1029–1035.
5. GREENBERG, E.R., J.A. BARON & T.D. TOSTESON. 1994. A clinical trial of antioxidant vitamins to prevent colorectal adenoma. N. Engl. J. Med. **331:** 141–147.
6. OMENN, G.S., G.E. GOODMAN, M.D. THORNQUIST, *et al*. 1996. Effects of a combination of beta carotene and vitamin A on lung cancer and cardiovascular disease. N. Engl. J. Med. **334:** 1150–1155.
7. HENNEKENS, C.H., J.E. BURING, J.E. MANSON, *et al*. 1996. Lack of effect of long-term supplementation with beta carotene on the incidence of malignant neoplasms and cardiovascular disease. N. Engl. J. Med. **334:** 1145–1149.
8. RAPOLA, J.M., J. VIRTAMO, S. RIPATTI, *et al*. 1997. Randomized trial of alpha-tocopherol and beta-carotene supplements on incidence of major coronary events in men with previous myocardial infarction. Lancet **349:** 1715–1720.
9. MILLER, E.R. 3rd, L.J. APPEL, O.A. LEVANDER, *et al*. 1997. The effect of antioxidant vitamin supplementation on traditional cardiovascular risk factors. J. Cardiovasc. Risk **4:** 19–24.

10. GIOVANNUCCI, E., M.J. STAMPFER, G.A. COLDITZ, *et al.* 1998. Multivitamin use, folate, and colon cancer in women in the Nurses' Health Study. Ann. Intern. Med. **129:** 517–524.
11. LEE, I.M., N.R. COOK & J.E. MANSON. 1999. Beta-carotene supplementation and incidence of cancer and cardiovascular disease: Women's Health Study. J. Natl. Cancer Inst. **91:** 2102–2106.
12. GRUPPO ITALIANO PER LO STUDIO SOPRAVVIVENZA NELL'INFARTO MIOCARDICO. 1999. Dietary supplement with n-3 polyunsaturated acids and vitamin E after myocardial infarction: results of the GISSI-Prevention trial. Lancet **354:** 447–455.
13. ASCHERIO, A., E.B. RIMM, M.A. HERNAN, *et al.* 1999. Relation of consumption of vitamin E, vitamin C, and carotenoids to risk for stroke among men in the United States. Ann. Intern. Med. **130:** 963–970.
14. DAGENAIS, G.R., R. MARCHIOLI, S. YUSUF, *et al.* 2000. Beta-carotene, vitamin C, and vitamin E and cardiovascular diseases. Curr. Cardiol. Rep. **2:** 293–299.
15. YUSUF, S., G. DAGENAIS, J. POGUE, *et al.* 2000. Vitamin E supplementation and cardiovascular events in high risk patients: The Heart Outcomes Prevention Evaluation Study Investigators. N. Engl. J. Med. **342:** 154–160.
16. AREDS. 2001. A Randomized, Placebo-Controlled, Clinical Trial of High-Dose Supplementation with Vitamins C and E and Beta Carotene for Age-Related Cataract and Vision Loss: AREDS Report no. 9. 2001. Arch. Ophthalmol. **119:** 1439–1452.
17. MUNTWYLER, J., C.H. HENNEKENS, J.E. MANSON, *et al.* 2002. Vitamin supplement use in a low-risk population of US male physicians and subsequent cardiovascular mortality. Arch. Intern. Med. **62:** 1472–1476.
18. WATERS, D.D., E.L. ALDERMAN, J. HSIA, *et al.* 2002. Effects of hormone replacement therapy and antioxidant vitamin supplements on coronary atherosclerosis in postmenopausal women: a randomized controlled trial. JAMA **88:** 2432–2440.
19. VIVEKANANTHAN, D.P. *et al.* 2003. Use of antioxidant vitamins for the prevention of cardiovascular disease: meta-analysis of randomized trials. Lancet **361:** 2017–2023.
20. MILLER, E.R., R. PASTOR-BARRIUSO, D. DALAL, *et al.* 2005. Meta-analysis: high-dosage vitamin E supplementation may increase all-cause mortality. Ann. Intern. Med. **142:** 37–46.
21. COLLINS, R., J. ARMITAGE, S. PARISH, *et al.* 2002. MRC/BHF Heart Protection Study of cholesterol lowering with simvastatin in 20,536 high-risk individuals: a randomized placebo controlled trial. Lancet **360:** 7–22.
22. COLLINS, R., J. ARMITAGE, S. PARISH, *et al.* 2002. MRC/BHF Heart Protection Study of antioxidant vitamin supplementation in 20,536 high-risk individuals: a randomized placebo-controlled trial. Lancet **360:** 23–33.
23. HOWES, R.M. 2004. U.T.O.P.I.A.–Unified Theory of Oxygen Participation in Aerobiosis. Free Radical Publishing Co. Kentwood, LA.
24. HOWES, R.M. 2005. The Medical and Scientific Significance of Oxygen Free Radical Metabolism. Free Radical Publishing Co. Kentwood, LA.

Catabolic Insufficiency and Aging

ALEXEI TERMAN

Division of Experimental Pathology, Faculty of Health Sciences,
Linköping University, Linköping, Sweden

ABSTRACT: Cellular degradative processes, which include lysosomal (autophagic) and proteasomal degradation, as well as the activity of cytosolic and mitochondrial proteases, provide for a continuous turnover of damaged and obsolete biomolecules and organelles. Inherent insufficiency of these degradative processes results in progressive accumulation within long-lived postmitotic cells of biological "garbage" ("waste" material), such as indigestible protein aggregates, defective mitochondria, and lipofuscin (age pigment), an intralysosomal, polymeric, undegradable material. Intracellular "garbage" is neither completely catabolized, nor exocytosed to any considerable extent. Heavy lipofuscin loading of lysosomes, typical of old age, seems to pronouncedly decrease autophagic potential. As postulated in the mitochondrial–lysosomal axis theory of aging, this occurs on account of the transport of newly synthesized lysosomal enzymes to lipofuscin-loaded lysosomes rather than to active lysosomes/late endosomes, making the enzyme content of autophagolysosomes insufficient for proper degradation. Consequently, the turnover of mitochondria progressively declines, resulting in decreased ATP synthesis and enhanced formation of reactive oxygen species, inducing further mitochondrial damage and additional lipofuscin formation. With advancing age, lipofuscin-loaded lysosomes and defective mitochondria occupy increasingly larger parts of long-lived postmitotic cells, leaving less and less capability for normal turnover and ATP production, finally resulting in cell death.

KEYWORDS: aging; autophagy; lysosomes; mitochondria; mutations; oxidative stress

INTRODUCTION

Aging (senescence) is characterized by progressive accumulation of deleterious changes, resulting in gradual functional decline, decreased adaptability, and increased probability of disease and death. Increasing evidence links aging with continuous damage to biomolecules such as nucleic acids, proteins, and lipids. Such damage inevitably occurs even under favorable environmental

Address for correspondence: Alexei Terman, Division of Experimental Pathology, University Hospital, SE-58185 Linköping, Sweden. Voice: +46-13-221525; fax: +46-13-221529.
 e-mail: alete@inr.liu.se

Ann. N.Y. Acad. Sci. 1067: 27–36 (2006). © 2006 New York Academy of Sciences.
doi: 10.1196/annals.1354.005

conditions, first of all due to toxic effects of reactive oxygen species (ROS) that constantly form as side-products or normal mitochondrial respiration (extensively reviewed in references[1–3]). Glucose and other reducing sugars can contribute to molecular damage by reacting with amino groups of proteins and forming advanced glycation end products (AGEs), known to cause protein–protein cross-linking and mutations.[4,5] In addition, due to inherent instability, macromolecules can undergo spontaneous modifications such as DNA strand breaks or isomerization of protein amino acid residues.[6]

Aging occurs despite the fact that all components of organisms are continuously renewed. This means that even young individuals cannot renew themselves with perfect accuracy and, consequently, senescent changes gradually develop. The renewing mechanisms are thus inherently imperfect, although they may deteriorate further with years, resulting in the acceleration of the aging process.

Here I discuss the principal mechanisms that are responsible for imperfect renewal of biological systems and their progressive damage with age.

BIOLOGICAL RENEWAL MECHANISMS

Most damaged biological structures are effectively removed and replaced by newly synthesized ones. A number of complementary mechanisms are involved in the elimination of damaged intracellular structures. Cytosolic proteins, mainly short-lived, are decomposed by calpains[7] and proteasomes,[8] while mitochondrial proteins are degraded by matrix Lon[9] and membrane-embedded AAA[10] proteases. Lysosomes, acidic vacuolar organelles possessing several dozens of hydrolytic enzymes, can degrade not only various types of macromolecules, but also other organelles such as mitochondria.[11,12] Intralysosomal degradation of cells' own constituents is called autophagocytosis, or autophagy.[11,12]

Depending on how intracellular structures are delivered to lysosomes for degradation, three types of autophagy are recognized in mammalian cells. Macroautophagy is the most universal degradation pathway in which even relatively large organelles such as mitochondria can be turned over. Macroautophagy is associated with the sequestration of a portion of cytoplasm within a double membrane structure called autophagosome. The origin of the sequestration membrane in mammalian cells is not clearly defined. Both the *de novo* formation of the autophagosome membrane (as it occurs in yeast) and its development from other organelles such as endoplasmic reticulum or Golgi complex are considered possible.[11–13] Autophagosomes then fuse with lysosomes or late endosomes. In microautophagy, macromolecules or small organelles are delivered to lysosomes through invaginations of their membranes, while chaperone-mediated autophagy (CMA) is a selective degradation pathway for particular proteins.[11–13]

Renewal at tissue level involves division and differentiation of stem cells providing for replacement of worn-out or damaged cells. The rate of cell replacement varies dramatically between tissues. Neurons, cardiac myocytes, skeletal muscle fibers, and retinal pigment epithelial cells are very rarely replaced and therefore are called long-lived postmitotic (terminally differentiated) cells.[14] In contrast, mature enterocytes, epidermal keratinocytes, and peripheral blood cells are characterized by a high replacement rate and thus represent short-lived postmitotic cells.[14] Cell division is associated with intensive synthesis of new biological structures, resulting in the dilution of damaged cellular constituents.[15] This makes mitotic activity, especially repetitive (which is involved, in particular, in the differentiation and replacement of short-lived postmitotic cells), an efficient rejuvenation mechanism, being able to diminish the content of damaged material that had not been removed by autophagy and other intracellular renewal mechanisms. The antiaging role of cell division is supported by observations using various cell systems *in vivo*[16,17] and *in vitro.*[18,19]

IMPERFECT RENEWAL AND ACCUMULATION OF DAMAGED BIOLOGICAL STRUCTURES

Only those changes that accumulate are important for the progress of aging. Some early concepts of aging emphasized the role of biosynthetic errors in triggering senescence. The error catastrophe theory of aging represents an attempt to explain aging as a consequence of translational errors.[20] This theory has not been supported by further experiments, showing lack of propagation of such errors with age.[21,22] It should be pointed out that wrongly synthesized proteins would not accumulate if they were perfectly turned over. The somatic mutation theory of aging is another important concept implying a possible role of biosynthetic errors.[23,24] Although this theory failed to explain many manifestations of aging,[25] it is clear that certain senescent changes are mutation-related. Lethal mutations may contribute to the loss of cells, particularly in tissues with low proliferation rate. Nonlethal nuclear and mitochondrial mutations can accumulate with age. Some nuclear mutations result in the development of neoplasms, most commonly affecting tissues with high proliferation potential.[26] Mutated mitochondria can replicate in different cell types, affecting both short-lived and long-lived postmitotic cells (see next section).

Biological "garbage" ("waste" material) represents functionally worthless and often toxic structures that originate from damaged macromolecules and organelles and cannot be catabolized. The accumulation of biological "garbage" with age preferentially occurs within long-lived postmitotic cells, which are rarely replaced by newly differentiated cells. In contrast, short-lived cells do not accumulate substantial amounts of "garbage" and may only suffer the effect of certain mutations that propagate during cell division (see above). The role of postmitotic cells such as neurons and cardiac myocytes in vital brain and heart functions underlies the significance of "waste" accumulation in the overall aging process.

Intracellular "garbage" accumulates extra- and intralysosomally, reflecting imperfect autophagic sequestration and degradation, respectively. Intralysosomal "waste" material is called lipofuscin, or age pigment. Lipofuscin is neither degraded by lysosomal enzymes, nor exocytosed from cells to any substantial extent.[27,28] Even starving cells that intensely degrade their constituents for energy production and biosynthesis cannot catabolize lipofuscin.[29] Lipofuscin is largely composed of aldehyde-cross-linked protein and lipid residues and also contains some carbohydrates and traces of metals.[30] It is characterized by natural brown-yellow color, wide-spectrum autofluorescence, and high electron density when visualized by transmission electron microscopy.[30] Lipofuscin accumulation has been shown to inhibit cellular autophagic capacity[29] and to sensitize cells to oxidant-induced damage.[31]

Defective mitochondria and indigestible protein aggregates are the most typical and well-characterized forms of extralysosomal "garbage." Mitochondria in aged postmitotic cells are usually enlarged and structurally deteriorated, showing swelling and/or destruction of inner membranes, often resulting in the formation of amorphous material.[32,33] Extremely enlarged mitochondria are often called "giant."[32] Senescent mitochondria not only are defective in ATP production, but also produce increased amounts of ROS, thus enhancing biomolecular damage.[34] Fission and fusion events are also disturbed in aged mitochondria.[35]

Indigestible protein aggregates (aggresomes) most commonly occur in aged neurons. For instance, alpha-synuclein aggregates accumulate within aged dopaminergic neurons of substantia nigra, forming Lewy bodies,[36] while aggregates of hyperphosphorylated protein tau compose neurofibrillary tangles and argyrophilic grains in neuronal perikarya and processes, respectively.[37] Certain types of aggresomes increase dramatically in a number of age-related pathologic conditions, such as Lewy bodies in Parkinson's disease and neurofibrillary tangles in Alzheimer's disease.[38]

FIGURE 1 shows principal processes involved in the renewal of damaged biological structures as well as their malfunction leading to the aging process.

MECHANISMS OF BIOLOGICAL "GARBAGE" ACCUMULATION

Understanding of lipofuscinogenesis was favored by experimental manipulations *in vivo* and *in vitro* that accelerated or inhibited intralysosomal accretion of undegradable material. Oxidative stress, such as exposure of cells to high ambient oxygen concentrations or iron (which enhances ROS generation by activating Fenton reaction), increased lipofuscin formation, whereas administration of antioxidants or iron chelators inhibited it.[30] Furthermore, it has

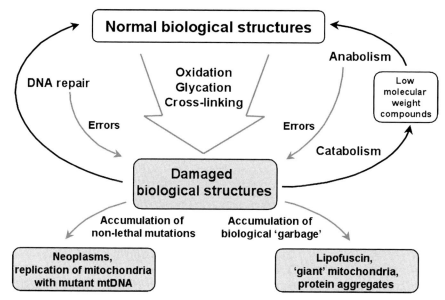

FIGURE 1. Scheme showing the role of imperfect turnover of biological structures in aging of long-lived postmitotic cells. Names of biological structures are framed; *arrows* represent biological processes. Names of normal and damaged structures are shown on white and gray backgrounds, respectively. *Black arrows* symbolize normal (adaptive) processes, while *gray arrows* indicate damage. Detailed explanations are given in the text.

been found that the prolonged inhibition of lysosomal enzymes dramatically enhances the formation of indigestible intralysosomal material,[39] especially when such inhibition is combined with oxidative stress.[28] These observations led to the conclusion that lipofuscin largely forms within lysosomes, as a result of iron-catalyzed oxidative modification of macromolecules undergoing autophagic degradation.[30,40] Autophagocytosed mitochondria, rich in oxidized matrix and membrane components, as well as in iron-containing proteins, are important sources of lipofuscin. In addition, mitochondria are the main cellular producers of ROS, including hydrogen peroxide that easily diffuses into lysosomes and participates in lipofuscinogenesis. In cells with active heterophagy, such as macrophages or retinal pigment epithelial cells, lipofuscin mainly originates from extracellular material.[30] It has been suggested that protein–protein cross-linking (in particular, by aldehyde bridges) plays an important role in lipofuscinogenesis, being responsible for its undegradability.[41]

Age-related accumulation of damaged mitochondria is most likely dependent on several different mechanisms. Initial mitochondrial damage apparently occurs secondary to ROS attack combined with insufficient functions of Lon and AAA proteases, as well as mitochondrial DNA (mtDNA) repair. The fact that defective mitochondria accumulate with age suggests that they either replicate faster than normal mitochondria, or somehow escape autophagy. The possibility of enhanced replication (clonal expansion) of damaged mitochondria is suggested by the fact that in some senescent cells mitochondria with single-type mtDNA mutations (homoplasmic mutations) completely replace normal organelles.[42,43] The clonal expansion hypothesis is additionally supported by findings of homoplasmic mtDNA mutations in intestinal epithelium[44] and malignant neoplasms,[45] in which active mitotic activity theoretically should result in the dilution of damaged structures. These findings, however, do not exclude the possibility of decreased autophagy of defective mitochondria. According to de Grey's SOS (for survival of the slowest) hypothesis, mutated mitochondria with deficient respiration might experience decreased oxidative damage to their membranes and, consequently, be less targeted for macroautophagy than would be normal organelles.[46] Although senescent mitochondria are generally known to produce increased amounts of ROS,[34] even the appearance of only one or a few mutated mitochondria with low ROS generation would be enough to initiate their selective accumulation. In support of the SOS hypothesis, some observations show selective mitochondrial autophagy. For example, ubiquitinated sperm mitochondria are selectively degraded in fertilized oocytes,[47] while the outer membrane protein Uth1p tags yeast mitochondria for autophagy.[48]

Only some senescent postmitotic cells, however, harbor mtDNA mutations (for instance, one out of seven cells in aged human heart),[43] suggesting that age-related mitochondrial changes may not necessarily depend on mtDNA damage.[49] It has been found that small cardiac myocyte mitochondria are autophagocytosed more actively than are large mitochondria, apparently because enlargement of organelles makes their autophagy more energy consuming.[33] This suggests that enlargement of some mitochondria may become an obstacle for their autophagic turnover, further promoting their damage and accumulation with age. Mitochondrial enlargement may initially occur as a consequence of oxidative damage to proteins or corresponding genes involved in mitochondrial fission. In support of this, mtDNA synthesis has been found to be suppressed in large mitochondria.[33] In aged postmitotic cells, mitochondrial turnover can also decrease secondary to lipofuscin overload (see next section).

Aggresomes form secondary to protein unfolding and misfolding associated with oxidative protein damage or mutations.[50] Apparently, certain types of damage make proteins more resistant to degradation and cause them to aggregate. It has been shown that while normal alpha-synuclein is degraded, at least partially, by CMA, its mutant form (typical of familial Parkinson's disease) is resistant to digestion and prone to aggregate.[51] Early alpha-synuclein aggregates may be still degradable by macroautophagy, which is, however, not efficient enough to prevent aggresome accumulation with years.[51] Conceivably, initial dysfunction of protein turnover systems including calpains, proteasomes, and autophagy may also be involved in aggresome formation.

BIOLOGICAL "GARBAGE" ACCUMULATION
AND CELL DEATH

There is increasing evidence that progressive accumulation of biological "waste" inevitably interferes with cellular functions, resulting in decreased adaptability and death of postmitotic cells.[14,52] Although loaded with "waste" material, aged postmitotic cells can still produce normal biomolecules and organelles, allowing them to temporarily maintain basic functions. Such compensatory production of new biological structures results in the increase of cell size, which, however, is limited because transport of nutrients and metabolites is complicated in large cells. Finally, compensatory mechanisms fail, and cells die.

The consequences of cellular waste accumulation have been recently studied using cultured human fibroblasts.[19] It has been found that prolonged administration of 3-methyladenine or leupeptin (which inhibits autophagic sequestration and degradation, respectively) gradually decreased viability of growth-arrested (confluent) fibroblasts, resulting in apoptotic or necrotic death. Dying cells appeared overloaded with biological "waste," mainly in the form of lipofuscin-like material and damaged mitochondria. Remarkably, inhibition of autophagy did not substantially affect viability of dividing (sub-confluent) cells, thus confirming the rejuvenative role of cell division. This work supports the idea that biological "garbage" accumulation is an important contributor to aging and death of postmitotic cells.

There are good reasons to believe that age-related accumulation of lipofuscin and defective mitochondria are interrelated and can enhance each other. It has been shown that autophagic capacity is diminished in lipofuscin-loaded cells,[29] most probably because a large fraction of lysosomal enzymes is allocated to lipofuscin-loaded lysosomes for futile trials to degrade the indigestible pigment. This complicates the turnover of defective mitochondria, and their accumulation increases. On the other hand, elevated ROS production by defective mitochondria would accelerate lipofuscinogenesis, further hampering mitochondrial turnover. In addition, lipofuscin accumulation would also promote generation of ROS due to deposition of iron within lipofuscin granules. This scenario, finally resulting in the death of aged postmitotic cells, is described in detail in the mitochondrial–lysosomal axis theory of aging.[52] In support of this theory, lipofuscin content, mitochondrial damage, and ROS production strongly correlated in cultured aged cardiac myocytes.[53]

Considering the role of biological "garbage" accumulation in the aging process, stimulating cellular degradative pathways, first of all through autophagy, may become a prospective anti-aging strategy, which can be used in combination with antioxidants and iron chelators.[54] In support of this view, autophagy has been found enhanced in calorie-restricted animals,[55] as well as in long-lived *C. elegans* mutants.[56] A more challenging anti-aging approach might involve transfection of cells with genes coding for xenohydrolases, that is, bacterial and fungal enzymes that can degrade substances resistant to lysosomal hydrolases.[57]

REFERENCES

1. HARMAN, D. 1992. Free radical theory of aging. Mutat. Res. **275:** 257–266.
2. SOHAL, R.S. & R. WEINDRUCH. 1996. Oxidative stress, caloric restriction, and aging. Science **273:** 59–63.
3. CADENAS, E. & K.J. DAVIES. 2000. Mitochondrial free radical generation, oxidative stress, and aging. Free Radic. Biol. Med. **29:** 222–230.
4. LEE, A.T. & A. CERAMI. 1992. Role of glycation in aging. Ann. N.Y. Acad. Sci. **663:** 63–70.
5. BROWNLEE, M. 1995. Advanced protein glycosylation in diabetes and aging. Annu. Rev. Med. **46:** 223–234.
6. HIPKISS, A.R. 2003. Non-oxidative modification of DNA and proteins. *In* Aging at the Molecular Level. T. von Zglinicki, Ed.: 145–177. Kluwer. Dordrecht.
7. SORIMACHI, H., S. ISHIURA & K. SUZUKI. 1997. Structure and physiological function of calpains. Biochem. J. **328:** 721–732.
8. WOJCIK, C. & G.N. DEMARTINO. 2003. Intracellular localization of proteasomes. Int. J. Biochem. Cell Biol. **35:** 579–589.
9. BAKALA, H., E. DELAVAL, M. HAMELIN, *et al.* 2003. Changes in rat liver mitochondria with aging. Lon protease-like reactivity and N(epsilon)-carboxymethyllysine accumulation in the matrix. Eur. J. Biochem. **270:** 2295–2302.
10. ARNOLD, I. & T. LANGER. 2002. Membrane protein degradation by AAA proteases in mitochondria. Biochim. Biophys. Acta **1592:** 89–96.
11. CUERVO, A.M. 2004. Autophagy: many paths to the same end. Mol. Cell. Biochem. **263:** 55–72.
12. LEVINE, B. & D.J. KLIONSKY. 2004. Development by self-digestion: molecular mechanisms and biological functions of autophagy. Dev. Cell **6:** 463–477.
13. FENGSRUD, M., M.L. SNEVE, A. OVERBYE, *et al.* 2004. Structural aspects of mammalian autophagy. *In* Autophagy. D.J. Klionsky, Ed.: 11–25. Landes Bioscience. Georgetown, TX.
14. TERMAN, A. & U.T. BRUNK. 2004. Aging as a catabolic malfunction. Int. J. Biochem. Cell Biol. **36:** 2365–2375.
15. SHELDRAKE, A.R. 1974. The ageing, growth and death of cells. Nature **250:** 381–385.
16. MARTINEZ, D.E. 1996. Rejuvenation of the disposable soma: repeated injury extends lifespan in an asexual annelid. Exp. Gerontol. **31:** 699–704.
17. MARTINEZ, D.E. 1998. Mortality patterns suggest lack of senescence in hydra. Exp. Gerontol. **33:** 217–225.
18. CAMPISI, J., G.P. DIMRI, J.O. NEHLIN, *et al.* 1996. Coming of age in culture. Exp. Gerontol. **31:** 7–12.
19. STROIKIN, Y., H. DALEN, U.T. BRUNK, *et al.* 2005. Testing the "garbage" accumulation theory of ageing: mitotic activity protects cells from death induced by inhibition of autophagy. Biogerontology **6:** 39–47.
20. ORGEL, L.E. 1973. Ageing of clones of mammalian cells. Nature **243:** 441–445.
21. GALLANT, J. & L. PALMER. 1979. Error propagation in viable cells. Mech. Ageing Dev. **10:** 27–38.

22. HARLEY, C.B., J.W. POLLARD, J.W. CHAMBERLAIN, *et al.* 1980. Protein synthetic errors do not increase during aging of cultured human fibroblasts. Proc. Nat. Acad. Sci. USA **77:** 1885–1889.

23. CURTIS, H.J., J. TILLEY, C. CROWLEY, *et al.* 1966. The role of genetic factors in the aging process. J. Gerontol. **21:** 365–368.

24. BURNET, F.M. 1973. A genetic interpretation of ageing. Lancet **2:** 480–483.

25. KIRKWOOD, T.B. 1989. DNA, mutations and aging. Mutat. Res. **219:** 1–7.

26. CAMPISI, J. 2003. Cancer and ageing: rival demons? Nat. Rev. Cancer **3:** 339–349.

27. TERMAN, A. & U.T. BRUNK. 1998. On the degradability and exocytosis of ceroid/lipofuscin in cultured rat cardiac myocytes. Mech. Ageing Dev. **100:** 145–156.

28. TERMAN, A. & U.T. BRUNK. 1998. Ceroid/lipofuscin formation in cultured human fibroblasts: the role of oxidative stress and lysosomal proteolysis. Mech. Ageing Dev. **104:** 277–291.

29. TERMAN, A., H. DALEN & U.T. BRUNK. 1999. Ceroid/lipofuscin-loaded human fibroblasts show decreased survival time and diminished autophagocytosis during amino acid starvation. Exp. Gerontol. **34:** 943–957.

30. TERMAN, A. & U.T. BRUNK. 2004. Lipofuscin. Int. J. Biochem. Cell Biol. **36:** 1400–1404.

31. TERMAN, A., N. ABRAHAMSSON & U.T. BRUNK. 1999. Ceroid/lipofuscin-loaded human fibroblasts show increased susceptibility to oxidative stress. Exp. Gerontol. **34:** 755–770.

32. BEREGI, E., O. REGIUS, T. HUTTL, *et al.* 1988. Age-related changes in the skeletal muscle cells. Z. Gerontol. **21:** 83–86.

33. TERMAN, A., H. DALEN, J.W. EATON, *et al.* 2003. Mitochondrial recycling and aging of cardiac myocytes: the role of autophagocytosis. Exp. Gerontol. **38:** 863–876.

34. SOHAL, R.S. & B.H. SOHAL. 1991. Hydrogen peroxide release by mitochondria increases during aging. Mech. Ageing Dev. **57:** 187–202.

35. JENDRACH, M., S. POHL, M. VOTH, *et al.* 2005. Morpho-dynamic changes of mitochondria during ageing of human endothelial cells. Mech. Ageing Dev. **126:** 813–821.

36. BENNETT, M.C. 2005. The role of alpha-synuclein in neurodegenerative diseases. Pharmacol. Ther. **105:** 311–331.

37. HARDY, J. & D.J. SELKOE. 2002. The amyloid hypothesis of Alzheimer's disease: progress and problems on the road to therapeutics. Science **297:** 353–356.

38. THAL, D.R., K. DEL TREDICI & H. BRAAK. 2004. Neurodegeneration in normal brain aging and disease. Sci. Aging Knowledge Environ. 2004: pe26.

39. IVY, G.O., F. SCHOTTLER, J. WENZEL, *et al.* 1984. Inhibitors of lysosomal enzymes: accumulation of lipofuscin-like dense bodies in the brain. Science **226:** 985–987.

40. BRUNK, U.T., C.B. JONES & R.S. SOHAL. 1992. A novel hypothesis of lipofuscinogenesis and cellular aging based on interactions between oxidative stress and autophagocytosis. Mutat. Res. **275:** 395–403.

41. KIKUGAWA, K., T. KATO, M. BEPPU, *et al.* 1989. Fluorescent and cross-linked proteins formed by free radical and aldehyde species generated during lipid oxidation. Adv. Exp. Med. Biol. **266:** 345–357.

42. OZAWA, T. 1997. Genetic and functional changes in mitochondria associated with aging. Physiol. Rev. **77:** 425–464.

43. KHRAPKO, K., N. BODYAK, W.G. THILLY, *et al.* 1999. Cell-by-cell scanning of whole mitochondrial genomes in aged human heart reveals a significant fraction of myocytes with clonally expanded deletions. Nucleic Acids Res. **27:** 2434–2441.
44. TAYLOR, R.W., M.J. BARRON, G.M. BORTHWICK, *et al.* 2003. Mitochondrial DNA mutations in human colonic crypt stem cells. J. Clin. Invest. **112:** 1351–1360.
45. HOCHHAUSER, D. 2000. Relevance of mitochondrial DNA in cancer. Lancet **356:** 181–182.
46. DE GREY, A.D. 1997. A proposed refinement of the mitochondrial free radical theory of aging. BioEssays **19:** 161–166.
47. SUTOVSKY, P., R.D. MORENO, J. RAMALHO-SANTOS, *et al.* 1999. Ubiquitin tag for sperm mitochondria. Nature **402:** 371–372.
48. KISSOVA, I., M. DEFFIEU, S. MANON, *et al.* 2004. Uth1p is involved in the autophagic degradation of mitochondria. J. Biol. Chem. **279:** 39068–39074.
49. DE GREY, A.D. 2004. Mitochondrial mutations in mammalian aging: an over-hasty about-turn? Rejuvenation Res. **7:** 171–174.
50. GRUNE, T., T. JUNG, K. MERKER, *et al.* 2004. Decreased proteolysis caused by protein aggregates, inclusion bodies, plaques, lipofuscin, ceroid, and "aggresomes" during oxidative stress, aging, and disease. Int. J. Biochem. Cell Biol. **36:** 2519–2530.
51. CUERVO, A.M., L. STEFANIS, R. FREDENBURG, *et al.* 2004. Impaired degradation of mutant alpha-synuclein by chaperone-mediated autophagy. Science **305:** 1292–1295.
52. BRUNK, U.T. & A. TERMAN. 2002. The mitochondrial-lysosomal axis theory of aging: accumulation of damaged mitochondria as a result of imperfect autophagocytosis. Eur. J. Biochem. **269:** 1996–2002.
53. TERMAN, A., H. DALEN, J.W. EATON, *et al.* 2004. Aging of cardiac myocytes in culture: oxidative stress, lipofuscin accumulation, and mitochondrial turnover. Ann. N.Y. Acad. Sci. **1019:** 70–77.
54. PERSSON, H.L., Z. YU, O. TIROSH, *et al.* 2003. Prevention of oxidant-induced cell death by lysosomotropic iron chelators. Free Radic. Biol. Med. **34:** 1295–1305.
55. BERGAMINI, E., G. CAVALLINI, A. DONATI, *et al.* 2003. The anti-ageing effects of caloric restriction may involve stimulation of macroautophagy and lysosomal degradation, and can be intensified pharmacologically. Biomed. Pharmacother. **57:** 203–208.
56. MELENDEZ, A., Z. TALLOCZY, M. SEAMAN, *et al.* 2003. Autophagy genes are essential for dauer development and life-span extension in *C. elegans*. Science **301:** 1387–1391.
57. DE GREY, A.D. 2002. Bioremediation meets biomedicine: therapeutic translation of microbial catabolism to the lysosome. Trends Biotechnol. **20:** 452–455.

Methionine Sulfoxide Reductases

Relevance to Aging and Protection against Oxidative Stress

FILIPE CABREIRO,[a] CÉDRIC R. PICOT,[a,b] BERTRAND FRIGUET,[a] AND ISABELLE PETROPOULOS[a]

[a]*Laboratoire de Biologie et Biochimie Cellulaire du Vieillissement, Université Paris7-Denis Diderot, 2 place Jussieu, Tour 33–23, 1er étage, CC 7128, 75251 Paris Cedex 05, France*

[b]*LVMH-Recherches, Laboratoires R & D, Branche Parfums-Cosmétiques, 45804 Saint-Jean-de-Braye Cedex, France*

ABSTRACT: Proteins are subject to modification by reactive oxygen species (ROS), and oxidation of specific amino acid residues can impair their biological function, leading to an alteration in cellular homeostasis. Methionine is among the amino acids the most susceptible to oxidation by almost all forms of ROS, resulting in both S and R diasteroisomeric forms of methionine sulfoxide. These modifications can be repaired specifically by the peptide methionine sulfoxide reductase A and B enzymes (MsrA and MsrB), respectively. MsrA has been detected in several organisms going from prokaryotes to eukaryotes. MsrA is tightly implicated in protection against oxidative stress and in protein maintenance, which is critical in the aging process. Several studies have shown that overexpression of MsrA led to an increased resistance against oxidative stress, while MsrA null mutants are more sensitive toward oxidative stress. Since oxidative damage is a key factor in aging, overexpression of MsrA in some organisms led to an increased life span whereas deletion of the gene led to the opposite. MsrA could also be involved, by regulating the function and/or expression of target proteins, in ROS-mediated signal transduction. In fact, changes in gene expression, including certain oxidative stress–response genes, have been observed when MsrA is overexpressed. This review elaborates on the current knowledge in the implication of the Msr system in protection against oxidative stress and aging.

KEYWORDS: oxidative stress; aging; oxidized protein; methionine oxidation; repair enzymes; MsrA

Address for correspondence: Bertrand Friguet, Laboratoire de Biologie et Biochimie Cellulaire du Vieillissement, Université Paris 7-Denis Diderot, 2 place Jussieu, Tour 33-23, 1er étage, CC 7128, 75251 Paris Cedex 05. Voice/fax: 33-1-44 27 82 34.
  e-mail: bfriguet@paris7.jussieu.fr

Ann. N.Y. Acad. Sci. 1067: 37–44 (2006). © 2006 New York Academy of Sciences.
 doi: 10.1196/annals.1354.006

INTRODUCTION

According to the free radical theory of aging, aerobic respiration leads to the production of reactive oxygen species (ROS), which induces oxidative damage to molecular macromolecules such as proteins, lipids, and DNA, hence contributing to the aging process.[1] Protein oxidative modifications that can be repaired *in vivo* are those resulting from the oxidation of the sulfur-containing amino acids, such as cysteine and methionine. Methionine residues are particularly susceptible to oxidation by almost all forms of ROS,[2] resulting in both S and R diasteroisomeric forms of methionine sulfoxide (MetO). These modifications can be reversed specifically by the peptide methionine sulfoxide reductase A and B enzymes, respectively.[3–7] In this review, the role of MsrA in protection against different types of induced oxidative stress is first discussed. The effects of overexpressing and deleting MsrA in oxidative stress protection and lifespan and its possible role in modulating the expression of other proteins are also discussed.

METHIONINE SULFOXIDE REDUCTASES AND PROTECTION AGAINST OXIDATIVE STRESS

After oxidative stress, the combined action of MsrA and MsrB is essential for reducing the complete content of free as well as protein-bound MetO, given the presence of two diasteroisomeric forms of MetO.[8] The resulting oxidized MsrA and/or MsrB are then reduced back to the native form by the action of the thioredoxin/thioredoxin reductase system *in vivo*.

In mammals, MsrA is encoded by a single gene and was found present in the cytosol,[9] in the mitochondria,[9,10] and in the nucleus.[11] Its expression was found in almost all human tissues with the exception of leukemia and lymphoma cell lines.[5] MsrB enzymes are encoded by three different genes and their products are designated MsrB1 (SelX), a selenoprotein present in the nucleus and the cytosol; MsrB2 (CBS-1), localized in the mitochondria; and MsrB3A/B, generated by alternative splicing. These gene products are targeted to the endoplasmic reticulum and to the mitochondria, respectively.[12] MsrA and MsrB are low molecular weight proteins showing molecular masses of approximately 25 kDa for MsrA, and 12 kDa for MsrB1, 20 kDa for MsrB2 and 20 kDa for MsrB3A/B. Interestingly, all MsrB enzymes are dependent on zinc.[13,14] MsrA is a well-conserved enzyme found in eukaryotes, bacteria, and to a lesser extent in Archeabacteria. MsrB are less highly conserved proteins that are not present in a number of bacteria and archaebacteria. Kryukov *et al.* have analyzed the completely sequenced genome of several bacteria, archaebacteria, and eukaryotes to determine the identities of the genes flanking the MsrA and MsrB genes.[13] The fact that numerous cases of clustering were observed between the two genes suggests that their patterns of expression are correlated. In some cases, the two genes are fused, encoding a single protein with two independent domains, each showing methionine sulfoxide reductase (MsrA or MsrB) activity.

Several studies were realized in different bacteria to study the role of MsrA in protection against oxidative stress. Absence of MsrA expression turns *Escherichia coli* more sensitive to growth inhibition caused by H_2O_2, suggesting that methionine in proteins can be a primary target for H_2O_2 oxidation.[15] This inhibition was reversed by the transformation of the mutant strain with a plasmid containing the MsrA wild-type gene from *E. coli* as well as the MsrA gene from *Mycobacterium tuberculosis*.[15,16] It was also shown that *E. coli* mutant strains are sensible to oxidative damage from reactive nitrogen intermediates (RNI).[16] Studies done by Singh *et al.*[17] demonstrated an increased susceptibility of *S. aureus* to oxidative stress. An insertional mutation in one of the MsrA genes led to increased susceptibility of the mutant to H_2O_2 compared to the parental strain, suggesting an important physiological role of the Msr system. Macrophages and other cells of the immune system are capable of producing high levels of ROS and RNI as a host defense against microorganisms. In such a harsh environment, the MsrA mutant strain of *Mycobacterium smegmatis* was much more sensitive to H_2O_2 than the parental strain, suggesting that MsrA plays an important role in the intracellular survival of *M. smegmatis* within macrophages.[18] From this point of view, MsrA can be seen as a virulence determinant that is important for the survival of the microorganism inside macrophages. MsrA has been also implicated in the protection of *Ochrobactrum anthropi* from ROS produced during the oxidative metabolism of aromatic substrates as phenol and 4-chlorophenol.[19] As we can see from these studies, bacteria are highly dependent on MsrA to counteract the damaging effects of oxidative stress, to increase their virulence, and consequently for their survival in diverse natural niches.

In yeast, MsrA null mutants are not capable of reducing protein-bound MetO and retain only 33% of their activity toward free MetO when compared to their parental strains. In normal conditions, both strains do not show significant differences in growth while, when submitted to the presence of H_2O_2, MsrA null mutants show increased growth delay, compared to the parental strain.[20] These results are in agreement with those obtained for *E. coli*.[15] In addition, overexpression of MsrA in yeast led to levels of free and protein-bound MetO that were 16.7% and 66% lower than those measured in the parental strain, respectively. It also led to increased resistance to toxic concentrations of H_2O_2.[21] Aging in *S. cerevisiae* can be modulated by the Msr system, pointing to an important role in the balance between ROS and antioxidant systems in the regulation of aging under aerobic conditions, but not in anaerobic conditions.[22]

During the dark period of *A. thaliana*, there is an increased accumulation of ROS, indicating that these plants are exposed to high levels of oxidative stress during the night. Bechtold *et al.* have shown that the Msr system is important in the repair of oxidized proteins to prevent cellular oxidative damage accumulation, minimizing protein turnover under conditions of limited energy provision.[23]

Resistance to oxidative stress and decrease of oxidative damages are believed to be key elements in determining the life span of organisms. Overexpression of MsrA in the nervous system of invertebrates such as *D. melanogaster* led to transgenic animals being more resistant to paraquat-induced oxidative stress with a markedly extended life span. In this work, it was suggested that life-span extension is caused by the antioxidant action of MsrA.[24]

METHIONINE SULFOXIDE REDUCTASES, PROTEIN OXIDATIVE DAMAGE, AND AGING

In proteins, amino acid residues under the action of severe oxidative stress can suffer a conversion into irreversible oxidation products such as protein carbonyls. Protein carbonyls are usually assumed as a marker of oxidative stress and aging.[25] Moskovitz *et al.* have shown that MsrA null mutant mice present a higher level of protein carbonyls than the wild-type when exposed to hyperoxia, which indicates increased sensitivity toward oxidative stress. These mutant strains also exhibit a shortened lifespan when compared to the wild-type under conditions of hyperoxia and normoxia.[26] The effects of oxidative stress caused by alterations in the oxygen concentration were also verified in neuronal PC12 cells. Under brief hypoxia/reoxygenation, MsrA overexpression protects against injury by preventing the increase of ROS level in the cell after hypoxia and reoxygenation.[27] The opacity of the human lens cell is related to oxidative stress, with methionine sulfoxide being one of the major oxidative stress products. In fact, overexpression of MsrA in HLE lens cells confers increased resistance to H_2O_2-induced stress whereas siRNA MsrA gene silencing led to increased sensitivity toward added oxidative stress. Silencing of the gene also pointed out an important role of MsrA for lens cell viability even in the absence of exogenously added stress, suggesting that MsrA is important for normal lens cell function.[28] The protecting role of MsrB against oxidative stress was also stressed out in human lens cells. Silencing of all or individual MsrB genes led to increased oxidative stress-induced cell death, indicating that MsrB together with MsrA is also implicated in human lens cell viability.[29]

We have shown that when WI-38 human fibroblasts were exposed to low concentrations of H_2O_2, a mild stress treatment, both MsrA and CBS-1 genes were upregulated, suggesting that these genes are necessary for cellular stress defense. On the other hand, decreased expression of MsrA and CBS-1 was also observed associated with replicative senescence. These results suggest that downregulation of MsrA and CBS-1 can alter the redox homeostasis of the cell, hence contributing to the accumulation of oxidative damage associated with senescence.[30] Recently, we have shown that overexpression of MsrA in WI38-SV40 human fibroblasts protects them against H_2O_2-mediated stress.

MsrA-overexpressing cells presented increased survival after an H_2O_2 oxidative stress. This was accompanied by lower levels of intracellular ROS and carbonyl content, pointing to a prevention against accumulation of protein oxidative damage.[31]

MsrA could also be involved in the activity regulation of target proteins such as calmodulin,[32-34] *D. melanogaster* shaker K^+ channel,[35] and the α isoform of the inhibitory protein κB.[36] Some of these proteins, whose activity and function are regulated by MsrA, are involved in ROS-mediated signal transduction. In fact, the cellular H_2O_2 response (i.e., changes in gene expression including oxidative stress response genes) is modified when MsrA is deleted or overexpressed in yeast. In the first situation, peroxisomal and cytosolic catalase and mitochondrial thioredoxin genes were found to be downregulated, whereas the genes for glutathione peroxidase, manganese and copper–zinc superoxide dismutase, flavohemoglobin, and thiol-specific antioxidant genes were upregulated. In the case of MsrA overexpression, peroxisomal catalase, manganese superoxide dismutase, flavohemoglobin, cytochrome c peroxidase, and the yap-1 transcription factor genes were downregulated. In contrast, mitochondrial thioredoxin, gluthatione peroxidase, and the copper chaperone genes were upregulated.[22] In mammals, $MsrA^{-/-}$ null double mutant mice are less able to upregulate expression of thioredoxin reductase under hyperoxia.[26] It was also shown that in $MsrA^{-/-}$ mice, there is a loss in MsrB activity, correlated with decrease in levels of MsrB expression, revealing interplay between MsrA and other proteins. In a recent work using proteomic analysis, we have studied the modulation of protein expression compared to control cells. We also analyzed the expression profile of control cells compared to MsrA-overexpressing cells submitted to H_2O_2 to better understand the relationship between protection against oxidative stress and MsrA overexpression. We have found that six proteins present a modification of their expression in MsrA-overexpressing cells and were identified by mass spectrometry as redox enzymes, structural and regulatory proteins. Interestingly, only one of the previously identified six proteins showed an altered expression when we submitted the same cells to an H_2O_2-induced oxidative stress.

CONCLUSION

Taken together, all the results reported in this review show that the survival of bacteria, yeast, and mammals is dependent on MsrA ability to reverse oxidized methionine. In fact, methionine oxidation modulates the biological activity of some proteins, pointing to an important role for MsrA in protein activity regulation. Moreover, the Msr system also seems to be highlighted in maintaining the reduced state of the N-terminal Met of newly synthesized proteins. The reversal of this oxidation seems essential for cell viability since oxidized methionine residues in the N-terminal of nascent chains could be a lethal event.[37] As proposed by Levine *et al*,[38] MsrA could reduce the intracellular level of ROS, scavenging them through a cyclic oxidation/reduction mechanism. Cyclic oxidation/reduction of exposed methionines could counteract the damaging effects of oxidative stress. In fact, we observed that the decrease in the protein carbonyl content in WI-38 SV40 fibroblasts overexpressing MsrA was accompanied by a decrease in the level of intracellular ROS.[31] In accordance with other studies that suggested an interplay between MsrA and other proteins, we have recently shown that overexpression of MsrA in fibroblast cells alters the expression of some proteins. Altogether, these findings point to a complex mechanism of MsrA in cellular protection against oxidative stress and reinforce its role in the aging process.

ACKNOWLEDGMENTS

The research at our laboratory is supported by funds from MENRT (Université Paris 7) and by a European 6th Framework Program Grant–Zincage–(FOOD-CT-2003–506850).

REFERENCES

1. HARMAN, D. 1956. Aging: a theory based on free radical and radiation chemistry. J. Gerontol. **11:** 298–300.
2. VOGT, W. 1995. Oxidation of methionyl residues in proteins: tools, targets, and reversal. Free Radic. Biol. Med. **18:** 93–105.
3. GRIMAUD, R. *et al.* 2001. Repair of oxidized proteins. Identification of a new methionine sulfoxide reductase. J. Biol. Chem. **276:** 48915–48920.
4. JUNG, S. *et al.* 2002. Activity, tissue distribution and site-directed mutagenesis of a human peptide methionine sulfoxide reductase of type B: hCBS1. FEBS Lett. **527:** 91–94.
5. KUSCHEL, L. *et al.* 1999. Molecular cloning and functional expression of a human peptide methionine sulfoxide reductase (hMsrA). FEBS Lett. **456:** 17–21.
6. LESCURE, A. *et al.* 1999. Novel selenoproteins identified *in silico* and *in vivo* by using a conserved RNA structural motif. J. Biol. Chem. **274:** 38147–38154.
7. WEISSBACH, H. *et al.* 2002. Peptide methionine sulfoxide reductase: structure, mechanism of action, and biological function. Arch. Biochem. Biophys. **397:** 172–178.
8. BAR-NOY, S. & J. MOSKOVITZ. 2002. Mouse methionine sulfoxide reductase B: effect of selenocysteine incorporation on its activity and expression of the seleno-containing enzyme in bacterial and mammalian cells. Biochem. Biophys. Res. Commun. **297:** 956–961.
9. VOUGIER, S., J. MARY & B. FRIGUET. 2003. Subcellular localization of methionine sulphoxide reductase A (MsrA): evidence for mitochondrial and cytosolic isoforms in rat liver cells. Biochem. J. **373:** 531–537.
10. HANSEL, A. *et al.* 2002. Mitochondrial targeting of the human peptide methionine sulfoxide reductase (MSRA), an enzyme involved in the repair of oxidized proteins. FASEB J. **16:** 911–913.

11. KIM, H.Y. & V.N. GLADYSHEV. 2005. Role of structural and functional elements of mouse methionine-S-sulfoxide reductase in its subcellular distribution. Biochemistry **44:** 8059–8067.

12. KIM, H.Y. & V.N. GLADYSHEV. 2004. Methionine sulfoxide reduction in mammals: characterization of methionine-R-sulfoxide reductases. Mol. Biol. Cell. **15:** 1055–1064.

13. KRYUKOV, G.V. *et al.* 2002. Selenoprotein R is a zinc-containing stereo-specific methionine sulfoxide reductase. Proc. Natl. Acad. Sci. USA **99:** 4245–4250.

14. KUMAR, R.A. *et al.* 2002. Reaction mechanism, evolutionary analysis, and role of zinc in *Drosophila* methionine-R-sulfoxide reductase. J. Biol. Chem. **277:** 37527–37535.

15. MOSKOVITZ, J. *et al.* 1995. *Escherichia coli* peptide methionine sulfoxide reductase gene: regulation of expression and role in protecting against oxidative damage. J. Bacteriol. **177:** 502–507.

16. ST JOHN, G. *et al.* 2001. Peptide methionine sulfoxide reductase from *Escherichia coli* and *Mycobacterium tuberculosis* protects bacteria against oxidative damage from reactive nitrogen intermediates. Proc. Natl. Acad. Sci. USA **98:** 9901–9906.

17. SINGH, V.K. *et al.* 2001. Molecular characterization of a chromosomal locus in *Staphylococcus aureus* that contributes to oxidative defence and is highly induced by the cell-wall-active antibiotic oxacillin. Microbiology. **147:** 3037–3045.

18. DOUGLAS, T. *et al.* 2004. Methionine sulfoxide reductase A (MsrA) deficiency affects the survival of *Mycobacterium smegmatis* within macrophages. J. Bacteriol. **186:** 3590–3598.

19. TAMBURRO, A. *et al.* 2004. Expression of glutathione S-transferase and peptide methionine sulphoxide reductase in *Ochrobactrum anthropi* is correlated to the production of reactive oxygen species caused by aromatic substrates. FEMS Microbiol. Lett. **241:** 151–156.

20. MOSKOVITZ, J. *et al.* 1997. The yeast peptide-methionine sulfoxide reductase functions as an antioxidant *in vivo*. Proc. Natl. Acad. Sci. USA **94:** 9585–9589.

21. MOSKOVITZ, J. *et al.* 1998. Overexpression of peptide-methionine sulfoxide reductase in *Saccharomyces cerevisiae* and human T cells provides them with high resistance to oxidative stress. Proc. Natl. Acad. Sci. USA **95:** 14071–14075.

22. KOC, A. *et al.* 2004. Methionine sulfoxide reductase regulation of yeast lifespan reveals reactive oxygen species-dependent and -independent components of aging. Proc. Natl. Acad. Sci. USA **101:** 7999–8004.

23. BECHTOLD, U., D.J. MURPHY & P.M. MULLINEAUX. 2004. Arabidopsis peptide methionine sulfoxide reductase2 prevents cellular oxidative damage in long nights. Plant Cell. **16:** 908–919.

24. RUAN, H. *et al.* 2002. High-quality life extension by the enzyme peptide methionine sulfoxide reductase. Proc. Natl. Acad. Sci. USA **99:** 2748–2753.

25. BERLETT, B.S. & E.R. STADTMAN. 1997. Protein oxidation in aging, disease, and oxidative stress. J. Biol. Chem. **272:** 20313–20316.

26. MOSKOVITZ, J. *et al.* 2001. Methionine sulfoxide reductase (MsrA) is a regulator of antioxidant defense and lifespan in mammals. Proc. Natl. Acad. Sci. USA **98:** 12920–12925.

27. YERMOLAIEVA, O. *et al.* 2004. Methionine sulfoxide reductase A protects neuronal cells against brief hypoxia/reoxygenation. Proc. Natl. Acad. Sci. USA **101:** 1159–1164.

28. KANTOROW, M. *et al*. 2004. Methionine sulfoxide reductase A is important for lens cell viability and resistance to oxidative stress. Proc. Natl. Acad. Sci. USA **101:** 9654–9659.
29. MARCHETTI, M.A. *et al*. 2005. Methionine sulfoxide reductases B1, B2, and B3 are present in the human lens and confer oxidative stress resistance to lens cells. Invest. Ophthalmol. Vis. Sci. **46:** 2107–2112.
30. PICOT, C.R. *et al*. 2004. The peptide methionine sulfoxide reductases, MsrA and MsrB (hCBS-1), are downregulated during replicative senescence of human WI-38 fibroblasts. FEBS Lett. **558:** 74–78.
31. PICOT, C. *et al*. 2005. Overexpression of MsrA protects WI-38 SV40 human fibroblasts against H_2O_2-mediated oxidative stress. Free Radic. Biol. Med. **39:** 1332–1341.
32. BARTLETT, R.K. *et al*. 2003. Oxidation of Met144 and Met145 in calmodulin blocks calmodulin dependent activation of the plasma membrane Ca-ATPase. Biochemistry **42:** 3231–3238.
33. SUN, H. *et al*. 1999. Repair of oxidized calmodulin by methionine sulfoxide reductase restores ability to activate the plasma membrane Ca-ATPase. Biochemistry **38:** 105–112.
34. VOUGIER, S. *et al*. 2004. Essential role of methionine residues in calmodulin binding to *Bordetella pertussis* adenylate cyclase, as probed by selective oxidation and repair by the peptide methionine sulfoxide reductases. J. Biol. Chem. **279:** 30210–30218.
35. CIORBA, M.A. *et al*. 1997. Modulation of potassium channel function by methionine oxidation and reduction. Proc. Natl. Acad. Sci. USA **94:** 9932–9937.
36. KANAYAMA, A. *et al*. 2002. Oxidation of IκBα at methionine 45 is one cause of taurine chloramine-induced inhibition of NF-kappa B activation. J. Biol. Chem. **277:** 24049–24056.
37. CHANG, S.Y., E.C. McGARY & S. CHANG. 1989. Methionine aminopeptidase gene of *Escherichia coli* is essential for cell growth. J. Bacteriol. **171:** 4071–4072.
38. LEVINE, R.L. *et al*. 1996. Methionine residues as endogenous antioxidants in proteins. Proc. Natl. Acad. Sci. USA **93:** 15036–15040.

Inadequate Intensity of Various Components of Total Environmental Signals Can Lead to Natural Aging

ALEXANDER V. KHALYAVKIN[a] AND ANATOLI I. YASHIN[b]

[a]Institute of Biochemical Physics of RAS, Moscow, Russia
[b]Center for Demographic Studies, Duke University, Durham, NC, USA

ABSTRACT: We suppose that natural aging derives from an inevitable shift in certain parameters of physiological control systems under the influence of inadequate environmental conditions, which are not able to fully induce an organism's "optimal" existence in the self-maintenance mode. In this case the rate of aging is proportional to the multidimensional difference between the cues from evolutionarily designed adequate habitat and signals from the real environment. The negative correlation between parameters of Gompertzian mortality (and some other published findings) is compatible with this view. Here we discuss examples from intracellular to organism level in order to show that adequate patterns of outer signals can reverse some aging manifestations.

KEYWORDS: primary cause of aging; aging plasticity; rate of aging; deceleration of senescence; reversibility of aging; signaling; environmental influences; intracellular microenvironment

The role of signaling in the control of aging is very important.[1] Here we propose that an organism's senescence is not only controlled by cues received from the environment, but also originates from the cues' inadequate intensity and composition. We suppose that natural aging stems from an inevitable shift in certain parameters of physiological control systems under the influence of inadequate environmental conditions, which are not able to fully induce the organism's "optimal" existence in the self-maintenance mode. In this case the rate of aging is proportional to the multidimensional difference between cues from evolutionarily designed adequate habitat and signals from the real environment. The negative correlation between parameters of Gompertzian mortality[2–4] (and some other findings) is compatible with this view. For example, the external milieu for mitochondria is intracellular microenvironment. The mtDNA transplantation from elderly humans to young ones have shown that

Address for correspondence: Alexander V. Khalyavkin, Ph.D., Institute of Biochemical Physics of RAS, 4 Kosygin St, Moscow 119991, Russia. Voice: +7 095 422-7164; fax: +7 095 137-4101.
e-mail: ab3711@mail.sitek.net

Ann. N.Y. Acad. Sci. 1067: 45–46 (2006). © 2006 New York Academy of Sciences.
doi: 10.1196/annals.1354.007

the old molecules of mtDNA remain functionally preserved.[5] Transplantation of HeLa nuclei to cells of elderly men also restores activity of old mitochondria.[5] This means that age-related reduction of activity in mitochondria does not occur from the mutation-accumulation in mtDNA, but is induced by extramitochondrial signals. A similar remarkable result was recorded at the cellular level.[6] The same phenomenon of functional reversibility is known from experiments with the transplantation of old ovaries to a young recipient,[7] as well as with the transfer of fetal hypothalamus to an old recipient,[8] or via artificial irritation of old hypothalamus.[9] Such stimulation fills the deficiency of aforementioned adequate environmental signals. Therefore, different sets of outer cues can either evoke senescence or even reverse some aging manifestations. The last case is a special variant of the so-called negative senescence,[10] when a potentially ageless organism, which was senescent in a nonsupportive environment[4] starts to restore lost *status quo* via positive external influences.

REFERENCES

1. KENYON, C. 2005. The plasticity of aging: insights from long-lived mutants. Cell **120:** 449–460.
2. STREHLER, B.L. & A.S. MILDVAN. 1960. General theory of mortality and aging. Science **132:** 14–21.
3. YASHIN, A.I., I.A. IACHINE & A.S. BEGUN. 2000. Mortality modeling: a review. Math. Popul. Stud. **8:** 305–332.
4. KHALYAVKIN, A.V. 2001. Influence of environment on the mortality pattern of potentially non-senescent organisms: general approach and comparison with real populations. Adv. Gerontol. **7:** 46–49.
5. HAYASHI, J.-I., O. OHTA, Y. KAGAWA, *et al.* 1994. Nuclear but not mitochondrial genome involvement in human age-related mitochondrial dysfunction: functional integrity of mitochondrial DNA from aged subjects. J. Biol. Chem. **269:** 6878–6883.
6. CONBOY, I.M., M.J. CONBOY, A.J. WAGERS, *et al.* 2005. Rejuvenation of aged progenitor cells by exposure to a young systemic environment. Nature **433:** 760–764.
7. KUSHIMA, R.K., K. KAMIO & Y. OKUDA. 1961. Climacterium, climacteric disturbance and rejuvenation of sex centers. Tohoku J. Exp. Med. **74:** 113–129.
8. HUANG, H.H., J.Q. KISSANE & E.J. HAWRYLEWICZ. 1987. Restoration of sexual function and fertility by fetal hypothalamus transplant in impotent aged male rats. Neurobiol. Aging **8:** 465–472.
9. CLEMENS, J.A., Y. AMENOMORI, T. JENKINS, *et al.* 1969. Effects of hypothalamic stimulation, hormones, and drugs on ovarian function of old female rats. Proc. Soc. Biol. Exp. Med. **132:** 561–563.
10. VAUPEL, J.W., A. BAUDISCH, M. DOLLING, *et al.* 2004. The case for negative senescence. Theor. Popul. Biol. **65:** 339–351.

Cellular Redox Regulation and Prooxidant Signaling Systems

A New Perspective on the Free Radical Theory of Aging

ANTHONY W. LINNANE AND HAYDEN EASTWOOD

Centre for Molecular Biology and Medicine, Epworth Medical Centre, Richmond, (Melbourne) Victoria 3121, Australia

ABSTRACT: The overarching role of coenzyme Q_{10} in gene regulation, bioenergy formation, cellular redox poise regulation, and hydrogen peroxide formation is presented. Coenzyme Q_{10} has a central role acting as a prooxidant in the generation of H_2O_2. Contrary to the dogma that superoxide and H_2O_2 formation are highly deleterious to cell survival this premise is rejected. Data are discussed that continuous superoxide and hydrogen peroxide formation are essential for normal cell function and that they play a major role in subcellular redox state modulation. It is the prooxidant activity of the so-called antioxidants that may be responsible for previously claimed benefits for high doses of oxido-reduction nutritional supplements such as alpha lipoic acid and coenzyme Q_{10}. Oxygen-free radical formation is essential for the biological function and is not a direct causation of the mammalian aging process; aging is a multisystem stochastic process.

KEYWORDS: coenzyme Q_{10}; redox poise; gene regulation; metabolic regulation; hydrogen peroxide; prooxidants; antioxidants; aging

INTRODUCTION

This article summarizes some of our earlier work[1–4] and further elaborates our concepts relating to the free radical theory of aging. Interest in superoxide formation and its putative toxic effects on cells and whole organisms, ranging from yeasts to man, has been the subject of intense study for many decades. In 1956 Denham Harman was the first to propose the visionary free radical theory of aging. This concept received strong support in the 1970s from voluminous studies, but particularly from the mitochondrial studies of Chance

Address for correspondence: Anthony W. Linnane, Centre for Molecular Biology and Medicine, Epworth Medical Centre, 185–187 Hoddle Street, Richmond, Victoria 3121, Australia. Voice: +61-3-9426-4200; fax: +61-3-9426-4201.

e-mail: tlinnane@cmbm.com.au

Ann. N.Y. Acad. Sci. 1067: 47–55 (2006). © 2006 New York Academy of Sciences.

doi: 10.1196/annals.1354.008

and colleagues, who demonstrated the formation of high concentrations of superoxide and H_2O_2 by respiratory chain-inhibited organelles as well as by microsomes and by peroxisomes.[5,6] On the basis of those studies, they estimated 1–3% of inspired oxygen was metabolized to superoxide and hydrogen peroxide, thereby generating a continual supply of high concentrations of potentially toxic products. Coenzyme Q_{10} semiquinone was shown to be the major source of the superoxide. There is indisputable evidence of the formation of a range of macromolecular oxidation products encompassing lipids, nucleic acids, and proteins, presumably arising from oxygen free radical activity. However, counterbalancing oxygen radical damage, there exists a wide range of enzyme repair and small molecule scavenging systems for the prevention of the potential ravages of oxygen metabolic toxicity. Also, over time a progressive accumulation of oxidatively damaged molecules is not observed. Studies by a number of laboratories indicate that earlier work has overestimated the quantum of formation of superoxide and hydrogen peroxide by respiring mitochondria by more than two orders of magnitude. Indeed, the formation of superoxide and hydrogen peroxide is barely detectable in normally respiring (uninhibited) mitochondria.[7,8]

Accepted dogma has been that superoxide and H_2O_2 formation are highly deleterious to cell survival and that they play a major causative role in the aging process. According to this view an intervention to prevent their formation by the administration of antioxidants constitutes a major therapy for the amelioration of the aging process and age-associated diseases. We question this premise; indeed, the so-called antioxidants may be physiologically acting as prooxidants and therein, as high-dose nutritional supplements, may lie their proposed beneficial effects—effects that in any event have yet to be unequivocally established some 50 years since the original proposal. Our proposal finds support in the recent report that alpha lipoic acid, when administered to rats, acts as a prooxidant and not an antioxidant.[9] The possibility must be considered that any physiological beneficial effects attributed to antioxidants are actually the reverse.

Here we elaborate upon the role that superoxide and H_2O_2 formation have in normal cellular function and their beneficial requisite for subcellular redox modulation and that their actions are central to normal cellular energy and metabolic regulation. We further propose that the conventional support and use of antioxidant therapy is flawed; indeed, if such treatment were effective in interfering with the primary formation of superoxide and H_2O_2, the outcome would be potentially catastrophic. There is a need for a more balanced and rigorous approach to the role of oxygen free radicals and H_2O_2 in the physiological process of aging rather than a seemingly endless effort to prove a preconceived 50-year old concept. There has been an overemphasis on the potential extent of oxidative damage and a lack of appropriate appreciation that the fluctuating subcellular redox state of cells and superoxide and H_2O_2 formation constitute a major regulatory signaling system important for normal cell function and metabolism. Although excessive superoxide production, if it occurs, may lead to undesirable long-term effects, to date such an unequivocal demonstration is lacking in mammalian subjects.

Our proposals can be best illustrated by a consideration of coenzyme Q_{10} and its overarching role in metabolic function and particularly its role in redox regulation and superoxide formation.

THE OVERARCHING CELLULAR REGULATION ROLE OF COENZYME Q_{10}

We have earlier summarized, as outlined in FIGURE 1, the global functions of coenzyme Q_{10} in relation to subcellular bioenergy systems, redox poise, metabolic flux modulation, gene regulation, and oxygen radical formation.[4] Specifically, coenzyme Q_{10} is known to occur in all subcellular membranes and has a functional role in many known membrane oxido-reductase systems therein: mitochondria, lysosomes, plasmalemma, and the Golgi apparatus. In essence, it is coenzyme Q_{10}'s particular subcellular redox poise (ratio of reduced to oxidized form) changes that determine its key metabolic control function. The redox poise of coenzyme Q_{10} in the various membranes will fluctuate continuously as an expression of the metabolic processes being carried out at any given time, within the various subcellular compartments, to produce a particular localized redox poise, resulting in a signaling process. This process together with coenzyme Q_{10}'s acting as a prooxidant will produce superoxide

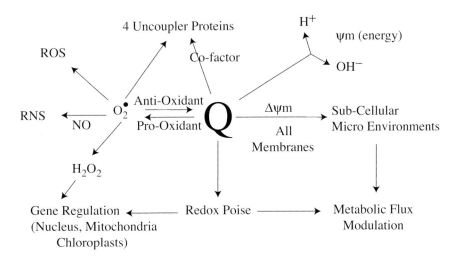

FIGURE 1. Coenzyme Q_{10}: its overarching role in energy generation, metabolic flux modulation, gene regulation. (From Linnane and Eastwood. Reprinted with permission from Elsevier.)

anion and the known mitogen H_2O_2, which then functions as a second messenger to inform the nucleus and mitochondria (chloroplasts) of the need for appropriate gene expression/regulation.

In addition to playing a major role in the mitochondrial electron transport system for the generation of biological energy, coenzyme Q_{10} also plays a role in other membrane oxido-reductase systems, contributing to their specific membrane potentials. Conversely, it is a major component of energy dissipation systems via the uncoupler proteins acting both as a cofactor proton carrier and by the generation of superoxide, which also activates the system. The biological role of coenzyme Q_{10} is thus complex, but its functions serve to highlight the role of cellular redox regulation as a major key to cellular well-being (cf.[4] for discussion and further details as outlined in FIG. 1).

CELLULAR FUNCTIONS OF COENZYME Q_{10} AND HYDROGEN PEROXIDE

On account of space limitations we summarize in TABLE 1 the cellular functions of coenzyme Q_{10} and the second messenger role of the mitogen H_2O_2. The attributions may be consulted for details and only three items are further considered here for elaboration:

1. *Vectorial formation of hydrogen peroxide by mitochondria*. FIGURE 2 summarizes some observations of St Pierre and colleagues[8] demonstrating that only very low levels of H_2O_2 are produced by normal respiring rat

TABLE 1. Cellular functions of coenzyme Q_{10} and the role of hydrogen peroxide as a second messenger

- Coenzyme Q_{10} electron transport/energy systems mitochondria/plasma membrane/Golgi/lysosomes/chloroplasts (plastoquinone).[10-14]
- Coenzyme Q_{10} occurs in all cellular membranes; its redox poise[a] influences membrane potential Ψ_m values.
- H_2O_2 formed by respiring mitochondria has been overestimated by about two orders of magnitude.[7,8]
- H_2O is a redox poise second messenger mitogen.[15,16]
- Coenzyme Q_{10} is an antioxidant and also acts as a prooxidant to generate superoxide and H_2O_2. There is an essential cellular requirement for small regulated amounts of H_2O_2.[4]
- Coenzyme Q_{10} acts as a gene regulator (with H_2O_2 acting as its second messenger).[4]
- Uncoupler proteins 1,2,3 (Ref. 4) are proton translocators lowering Ψ_m and require fatty acid substrate and coenzyme Q_{10} as a cofactor. Superoxide is an activator of the uncoupler protein family.[17,18]
- Coenzyme Q_{10} is a cofactor required for protein SH $\leftrightarrow$ S-S interconversions. Cell compartments: cytosol — SH; other –S-S–.[19]
- Plastoquinone (coenzyme Q_{10} analogue) redox poise regulates chloroplast and nuclear gene transcription.[13,20,21]

[a]Redox poise: ratio of oxidized to reduced form at any instant in time.

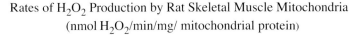

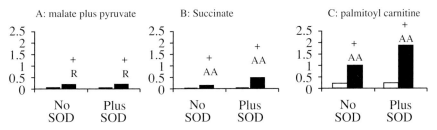

Mitochondrial Vectorial H₂O₂ Formation
Complex I: release superoxide into matrix
Complex III: (muscle) and Fatty Acid Oxidation: release superoxide into cytoplasm.

FIGURE 2. Superoxide and vectorial hydrogen peroxide formation by mitochondria. Rotenone (R), antimycin A (AA), superoxide dismutase (SOD). (Modified from St. Pierre et al.[8])

skeletal muscle mitochondria. The levels of H_2O_2 formed are increased when the mitochondria are inhibited by rotenone and antimycin A, consistent with earlier reports. Complex I, H_2O_2 production is insensitive to added superoxide dismutase, which indicates that the H_2O_2 formed is vectorially released into the matrix. By contrast, H_2O_2 formed with succinate or palmitoyl carnitine as substrates is enhanced by the addition of SOD, indicating that H_2O_2 arising from their oxidation is targeted to the cytoplasm. These authors also reported that rat heart mitochondria oxidizing fatty acid release H_2O_2 into the matrix, unlike the skeletal muscle results. We interpret these observations to suggest that second messenger H_2O_2 vectorial release is tissue specific, in keeping with the different metabolic needs of individual tissues for the regulation of their specific metabolisms.

2. *Redox poise modulation of chloroplast respiration determines chloroplast DNA expression.* FIGURE 3 is an overview summary of a report by Pfannschmidt and colleagues[13] showing that, by the use of the inhibitors DCMU and DBMIB, the redox poise of plastoquinone was modulated during specific light activation of photosystems I or II. Study of photosystem proteins synthesized revealed that the oxidized form of plastoquinone favored the synthesis of proteins of chloroplast photosystem II; by contrast, the reduced form favored the synthesis of proteins of photosystem I. Plastoquinone is a coenzyme Q analogue: it acts in a similar mode to coenzyme Q_{10} as a mobile electron carrier between the chloroplast electron carrier systems comprising the two photosystems. Clearly, the redox poise of the overall system signals specific gene regulation/expression.

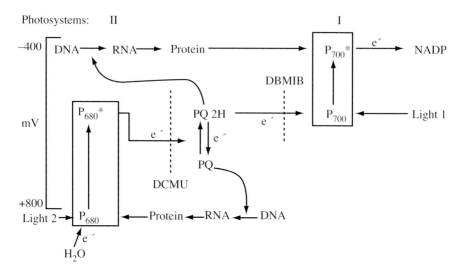

FIGURE 3. Redox regulation of transcription control of chloroplast gene expression. DCMU (3-[3′,4′-dichlorophenyl]-1,1′-dimethyl urea) inhibits electron flow from photosystem II into the plastoquinone pool. DBMIB (2,5-dibromo-3-methyl-6-isopropyl-benzoquinone) inhibits the oxidation of plastoquinol by photosystem I. (Summarized from Pfannschmidt et al.[13])

We would suggest that H_2O_2 arises from the semiquinone form of plastoquinone and acts as the second messenger for the activation of appropriate genes encoded in chloroplast DNA. It is particularly noteworthy that two earlier publications[20,21] reporting on algal activity have reported that cellular redox poise plays a key role in regulating plant cell nuclear gene expression.

3. *Cellular redox poise determines cell differentiation pathways.* The major importance of redox regulation in cell differentiation is underscored by the work of Smith and colleagues[22] and the observations arising from that study are summarized in TABLE 2.

Rat glial oligodendrocyte/astrocyte progenitor cells were grown under conditions to establish a more oxidizing or reducing intracellular redox state. The more oxidizing cytoplasmic environment induced by growth factors such as thyroid hormone and bone morphogenic protein 4, and the chemical oxidant *tert*-butyl hydroperoxide favored cell differentiation to oligodendrocyte formation. By contrast, a more reducing cytoplasmic environment induced by growth in the presence of a basic fibroblast growth factor, platelet-derived growth factor, or their combination favored the maintenance of the progenitor cells. The article[22] details the use of various chemical and growth factor combinations interacting to produce a range of redox poise states to have a marked influence on the number and

TABLE 2. Redox state: central modulator of self-renewal and differentiation of glial precursor cell

| Culture additions | Intracellular redox environment | | Predominant cell type formed |
	Reducing	Oxidizing	
Tert-butyl hydroperoxide	—	+	Oligodendrocytes
N-acetyl cysteine	+	—	Progenitor 0–2A cells
Thyroid hormone	—	+	Oligodendrocytes
Bone morphogenic protein 4	—	+	Astrocytes
Basic fibroblast growth factor	+	—	Progenitor 0–2A cells
Platelet-derived growth factor	+	—	Progenitor 0–2A cells
Platelet-derived growth factor plus basic fibroblast growth factor	+	—	Only progenitor 0–2A cells

Rat glial oligodendrocytes—type-2 (0–2A) astrocyte progenitor cells were cultured in the presence of the additions indicated to modulate the intracellular redox poise. Cellular redox changes (states) were determined by rosamine fluorescence; relatively small redox changes have profound outcomes. Data are summarized from Smith *et al.*[22]

rate of formation of progenitor cells or their differentiation into astrocytes or oligodendrocytes. Even small changes in redox poise had a profound influence on outcomes.

Finally, it may be remarked that there is an extensive literature on the role of oxygen radicals and signaling reviewed by Finkel,[14] and Rhee[15] has reviewed redox signaling with hydrogen peroxide as an intracellular messenger.

CONCLUSION

Respirating mitochondria normally produce only trace amounts of H_2O_2 contrary to early reports of a large amount of H_2O_2 formation (<0.1 nmol H_2O_2/min/mg protein rat muscle mitochondria)[8] compared with levels in excess of two orders of magnitude higher.[5,6] H_2O_2 is an ideal second messenger as it can readily diffuse throughout the cell, it is nontoxic except at excessive concentrations, and it is an established mitogen. H_2O_2 is generated at many subcellular locations other than mitochondria, and therefore can serve as a fundamental messenger, signaling the redox poise at various subcellular locales at any given time.[4]

Subcellular redox poise is a major regulatory factor of cell growth, differentiation, and metabolic function.

Consideration of the overarching role of coenzyme Q_{10} in cellular metabolism and regulation via its prooxidant activity to produce H_2O_2 leads to a reassessment of the role of so-called antioxidants in metabolism and the aging process.

It is proposed that the concept of clinical use of antioxidants for the treatment of disease and aging as an overriding concept is incorrect. If antioxidants functioned to significantly scavenge cellular H_2O_2, the outcome would be a physiological catastrophe. Claimed benefits for antioxidant treatments are more likely to be due to their roles as prooxidants.

REFERENCES

1. LINNANE, A.W. *et al*. 1995. The universality of bioenergetic disease and amelioration with redox therapy. Biochim. Biophys. Acta **1271**: 191–194.
2. LINNANE, A.W. *et al*. 2002. Aging and global function of coenzyme Q_{10}. Ann. N.Y. Acad. Sci. **959**: 396–411.
3. LINNANE, A.W. *et al*. 2002. Cellular redox activity of coenzyme Q_{10}: effect of Co Q_{10} supplementation on human skeletal muscle. Free Radic. Res. **36**: 445–453.
4. LINNANE, A.W. & H. EASTWOOD. 2004. Cellular redox poise modulation; the role of coenzyme Q_{10}, gene and metabolic regulation. Mitochondrion **4**: 779–789.
5. BOVERIS, A. & B. CHANCE. 1973. The mitochondrial generation of hydrogen peroxide. Biochem. J. **134**: 707–716.
6. BOVERIS, A. *et al*. 1972. The cellular production of hydrogen peroxide. Biochem. J. **128**: 617–630.
7. STANIEK, K. & N. NOHL. 2000. Are mitochondria a permanent source of reactive oxygen species? Biochim. Biophys. Acta **1460**: 268–275.
8. ST-PIERRE, J. *et al*. 2002. Topology of superoxide production from different sites in the mitochondrial electron transport chain. J. Biol. Chem. **277**: 44784–44790.
9. CAKATAY, M. & R. KAYALI. 2005. Plasma protein oxidation in aging rats after alpha-lipoic acid administration. Biogerontology **6**: 87–93
10. CRANE, F.L. *et al*. 1957. Isolation of a quinone from beef heart mitochondria. Biochim. Biophys. Acta **25**: 220–221.
11. CRANE, F.L. *et al*. 1994. Coenzyme Q_{10} in Gogli apparatus membrane redox activity and proton uptake. *In* Biomedical and Clinical Aspects of Coenzyme Q_{10}. K. Folkers and Y. Yamamura, Eds.: Vol. **4**: 77–85. Elsevier. Amsterdam.
12. CRANE, F.L. *et al*. 1994. Coenzyme Q_{10}, plasma membrane oxidase and growth control. Mol. Aspects Med. **15**: 1–11.
13. PFANNSCHMIDT, T., A. NILSSON & J. ALLEN. 1999. Photosynthetic control of chloroplast gene expression. Nature **397**: 625–628.
14. GILLE, L. & H. NOHL. 2000. The existence of a lysosomal redox chain and the role of ubiquinone arch. Biochem. Biophys. Acta **375**: 347–354.
15. FINKEL, T. 1998. Oxygen radicals and signaling. Cell Biol. **10**: 248–253
16. RHEE, S. 1999. Redox signaling: hydrogen peroxide as intracellular messenger. Exp. Mol. Med. **31**: 53–59.
17. ECHTAY, K.S., E. WINKLER & M. KLINGENBERG. 2000. Coenzyme Q_{10} is a obligatory co-factor for uncoupling protein function. Nature **408**: 609–613.
18. ECHTAY, K.S. *et al*. 2002. Superoxide activates mitochondrial uncoupling proteins. Nature **415**: 96–99.
19. BADER, M. *et al*. 2000. Disulfide bonds are generated by quinone reduction. J. Biol. Chem. **275**: 26082–26088.
20. MAXWELL, D., D. LAUDENBACH & N. HUNTER. 1995. Redox regulation of light-harvesting complex II and cab mRNA abundance in *Dunaliella salina*. Plant Physiol. **109**: 787–795.

21. ESCOUBAS, J. *et al.* 1995. Light intensity regulation of cab gene transcription is signaled by the redox state of the plastoquinone pool. Proc. Natl. Acad. Sci. USA **92:** 10237–10241.

22. SMITH, J. *et al.* 2000. Redox state is a central modulator of the balance between self-renewal and differentiation in a dividing glial precursor cell. Proc. Natl. Acad. Sci. USA **97:** 10032–10037.

Human Immunosenescence

Does It Have an Infectious Component?

G. PAWELEC,[a] S. KOCH,[a] C. FRANCESCHI,[b] AND A. WIKBY[c]

[a]University of Tübingen Medical School, Center for Medical Research,
ZMF, Waldhörnlestr 22, D-72072 Tübingen, Germany

[b]University of Bologna, Department of Experimental Pathology,
via S. Giacomo 12, I-40126 Bologna, Italy

[c]Department of Natural Science and Biomedicine, School of Health Sciences,
Jönköping University, 551 11 Jönköping, Sweden

ABSTRACT: The rate of acceleration of the frequency of death due to cardiovascular disease or cancer increases with age from middle age up to around 75–80 years, plateauing thereafter. Mortality due to infectious disease, however, does not plateau, but continues to accelerate indefinitely. The elderly are particularly susceptible to novel infectious agents such as SARS, as well as to previously encountered pathogens. Why is this? The elderly commonly possess oligoclonal expansions of T cells, especially of CD8 cells, which, surprisingly, are associated with cytomegalovirus (CMV) seropositivity. This in turn is associated with many of the same phenotypic and functional alterations to T cell immunity that have been suggested as biomarkers of immune system aging. We suggest that, in fact, CMV, not age *per se*, is the prime driving force behind many or most of the oligoclonal expansions and altered phenotypes and functions of CD8 cells in the elderly. Thus, the manner in which CMV and the host immune system interact (over which period? on which genetic background? with which co-infections?) is critical in determining the "age" of adaptive immunity and hence human longevity. In this respect, immunosenescence is infectious.

KEYWORDS: immunosenescence; CD8 T lymphocyte; cytomegalovirus; longitudinal study

WHAT IS IMMUNOSENESCENCE?

Immunosenescence is the term used to designate dysfunctional immunity in the elderly, characterized especially by perturbations of the T lymphocyte

Address for correspondence: G. Pawelec, University of Tübingen Medical School, Center for Medical Research, ZMF, Waldhörnlestr. 22, D-72072 Tübingen, Germany. Voice: 0049-7071-2982805; fax: 0049-7071-294677.

e-mail: graham.pawelec@uni-tuebingen.de
www.medizin.uni-tuebingen.de/t-cia

Ann. N.Y. Acad. Sci. 1067: 56–65 (2006). © 2006 New York Academy of Sciences.
doi: 10.1196/annals.1354.009

system (reviewed in Ref. 1). These are manifest as increasing frequencies of cells previously exposed to antigen ("memory" cells) and decreasing frequencies of cells able to recognize and combat sources of new antigens ("naïve" cells). The accumulated memory cells may fill the "immunological space," resulting in a shrunken T cell repertoire for new antigens; we believe that this situation contributes to the increased susceptibility of the elderly to infectious disease and possibly cancer, owing to decreased efficiency of immunosurveillance. A striking example of this was recently provided by the finding that the novel pathogen responsible for SARS was rarely fatal in young people but had >50% mortality in the elderly. This phenomenon is not limited to newly arising pathogens and has been clearly shown for several other important pathogens, such as those causing influenza, currently responsible for one-quarter of deaths of people over 65 years in the United States[2]—and this without the presently feared H5N1 pandemic. The hallmark of T cell–mediated adaptive immunity is a lag phase while the antigen is captured, processed, and presented, most usually by dendritic cells, and then rapid extensive clonal expansion on first contact with these antigen-presenting cells, followed by clonal contraction on antigen clearance, and generation of long-term memory. Although higher frequencies of memory cells specific for a particular antigen do accumulate, they are qualitatively different from naïve cells and the characteristically rapid and extensive reinduction of functional immunity on antigen rechallenge can be accomplished without maintaining such large numbers of memory cells that they contribute markedly to filling the "immunological space." However, in cases where the antigen cannot be cleared, as in persistent infection and cancer, "clonal exhaustion" may occur, characterized by tolerance induction mediated either by clonal deletion of antigen-specific T cells or by the induction of anergy (i.e., the antigen-specific T cells remain present but fail to function fully). On the basis of data from longitudinal studies, we believe[3] that the latter process commonly occurs and does not merely compromise the response to that particular pathogen, but has much more far-reaching effects on the response to all others, according to the following hypothesis.

Hypothesis: The infectious agent Cytomegalovirus is materially involved in the development of immunosenescence.

Cytomegalovirus (CMV) is a persistent activating virus of the β-herpesvirus family, which resides in the myeloid cell compartment but may also infect other cell types. Infection may occur perinatally via mother's milk, or at any time thereafter via intimate contact of various kinds. In most Western populations, the majority of people are infected by middle age, and finding uninfected individuals >65 years of age can be a challenge. Infection generally seems to pass unnoticed in immunocompetent hosts, with T cell memory rapidly established and persisting for life. However, recent surveys suggest that active CMV infection even in immunocompetent hosts may not in fact be quite as asymptomatic as previously assumed—over half of infected patients may suffer malaise and fever, and have abnormal liver function tests.[4] Earlier reports had suggested that CMV reactivation did occur and was actually age-associated, although still well controlled,[5] analogous to the well-known age-associated reactivation of the related Varicella zoster virus causing shingles. The critical importance of maintaining immunosurveillance against CMV is underlined by the severe consequences of reactivation in immunosuppressed individuals, such as AIDS patients and hematopoietic stem cell recipients, who commonly suffer serious, even fatal, CMV disease.

Earlier studies on the composition of the different T cell subsets indicated that CMV infection markedly altered their ratios[6] and reported expansions of CD8[+]CD57[+] subsets in CMV-seropositive individuals. Increases of cells with this same phenotype were independently found to be associated with increasing age in other studies. It was eventually realized that the age-associated increase in the numbers of CMV-seropositive donors paralleled such changes and could actually be responsible for them, not aging *per se.*[7] Since then, a large number of studies have sought to define T cell subset changes in CMV infection and in aging, and generally speaking, the similarities between the two have been confirmed. This strongly implicates viral infection as the driving force behind some of the most marked changes that have been determined as "biomarkers of aging" in the human immune system.[3]

CMV-SPECIFIC CD8 CELLS

Many years ago, age-associated clonal expansions of CD8 cells were noted in middle-aged and elderly people.[8] In almost all cases where this has been examined, it transpired that such clonal expansions, or the degree to which they occurred, were associated with CMV-seropositivity.[9,10] By means of HLA/CMV peptide tetramers to identify CD8 cells carrying receptors for an immunodominant epitope of the HCMV pp65 protein (NLVPMVATV, binding HLA-A2), we have established the frequencies, surface marker phenotypes, and some of the functional characteristics of these cells.[11–13] It was found that they are a mixture of CD45RA-positive and CD45RA-negative populations in both young and old. However, the proportion of cells expressing the important costimulatory molecule CD28 is very low in the elderly ($<10\%$ on average) and relatively high ($>75\%$ on average) in the young.[3] Furthermore, a fairly high proportion of CMV-specific CD8 cells in the young are still included in the phenotypically naïve subpopulation (CCR7[+]CD45RA[+]), but in the elderly most have a more differentiated phenotype commonly associated with effector memory cells (CCR7-negative, CD45RA-low) or effector cells (CCR7-negative CD45RA[+]) cells.[3] Differences between young and old donors' CMV-specific cells may be due to more extended periods of persistent infection in the latter, although certain alterations appear to occur very rapidly on infection, within 8 weeks in one individual with primary CMV infection,[14] perhaps rendering this explanation unlikely. No details were given on this single patient, who may not have been healthy. However, it has also been reported that in congenital CMV infection, CD28 expression is already decreased in fetal CD8 T cells, indicating that this virus induces a rapid shift from naïve phenotype to effector memory and effector phenotype[15]—although here with the proviso that the fetal immune system is very different from that of the adult. If the differences between young and old are not caused only by duration of infection, we may need to look at differences in the immune ecology of the young and old to explain and understand these changes.

We and others have examined several different young and old populations regarding the frequencies of CMV-specific cells, as detected by tetramers.[11–17] In the extremely valuable and informative Swedish OCTO and NONA longitudinal studies, we were able to distinguish what we dubbed an "immune risk phenotype" (IRP)[18] predictive of 2- and 4-year mortality in these free-living very elderly,[9,10,19–21] which was, importantly, independent of current health status and also applicable to less than perfectly healthy individuals.[22] As summarized in TABLE 1, one important component of the IRP is CMV-seropositivity; this correlates with frequencies of A2/NLVPMVATV tetramer-positive cells, with IRP elderly having on average higher numbers of such cells.[11–13] However, the IRP group consists of individuals with a wide range of such CMV-specific cells, so that there is a great deal of intraindividual variation and, as one might expect, there must be other reasons for their belonging to this group in addition to CMV status. Our studies mentioned above were conducted only on HLA-A2+ donors, using tetramers detecting TCR specific for just one, albeit immunodominant, CMV epitope. It is therefore all the more impressive that

TABLE 1. Immune status in very elderly IRP and non-IRP donors

Alterations with age	
non-IRP	IRP
Marker and cells	
CD4:CD8 > 1	CD4:CD8 < 1
T cell proliferation	T cell proliferation ↓
CD28 ↑	CD28 ↓
CD57 ↓	CD57 ↑
CD45RA ↑	CD45RA ↓
CD45RO ↓	CD45RO
KLR-G1 ↓	KLR-G1 ↑
Cytokines and growth factors	
IL-2 ↑	IL-2 ↓
IL10 →	IL-10 →
IFN-γ ↑	IFN-γ ↓
CMV/EBV status	
CMV+/lower frequencies	CMV+/higher frequencies
Mostly KLR-G1+	Mostly KLR-G1+
EBV+/lower frequencies	EBV+/higher frequencies

such correlations could be seen at all. We have also begun to examine two different CMV epitopes presented in the context of HLA-B7, because it was reported that in donors carrying both A2 and B7, all T cell responses were directed to the latter[16] (we have confirmed that this is generally true, but for unknown reasons rare donors who are A2- and B7-positive do possess CD8 clonal expansions restricted by both [Koch *et al.*, unpublished results]). Therefore, elderly persons in the IRP group with small numbers of A2/NLVPMVATV tetramer-positive cells could be harboring clonal expansions restricted by B7 instead. Of course, the same considerations apply to other HLA alleles and other CMV epitopes; and such studies must be extended to CD4 cells as well, since the CD8 are responsive to "help" from such MHC class II–restricted cells.

FUNCTIONS OF CMV-SPECIFIC CD8 CELLS IN THE YOUNG AND OLD

The emerging analyses every 2 years from the OCTO/NONA studies mentioned above clearly showed that CMV-seropositivity and CMV-specific CD8 cell accumulation were associated with the IRP and contributed to increased mortality in the very old. If these differences are not solely due to the relatively trivial factor of duration of infection, other factors must be taken into account. There may very well be genetic influences determining the efficacy with which the immune system deals with CMV (e.g., the apparent immune response gene susceptibility function of HLA-DR7 in organ transplant recipients or AIDS patients, where otherwise occult genetic influences are revealed under immunosuppression[23,24]). The past history of the individual regarding exposure to other infectious agents may also be critical in determining the long-term outcome of CMV infection, especially in terms of setting an agenda of pro- or anti-inflammatory status as a result of gene/environment interactions.

The question remains as to why these clonal expansions of CMV-specific cells and, to a lesser extent, also Epstein–Barr virus (EBV)-specific cells[25] are associated with shorter survival. One major finding is that many of the CMV-specific cells in the elderly appear to be anergic and apoptosis-resistant. That is, they can be stimulated by mitogens, but not by cognate antigen, to secrete cytokines such as IFN-γ. As may often be the case with anergic cells, they appear also to be relatively resistant to apoptosis, either occurring spontaneously in culture, or being induced. The clonal expansions seen in the elderly, predominantly in the IRP elderly, contain a majority of such dysfunctional cells; nonetheless, they also contain sufficient functional CMV-specific cells to maintain immunosurveillance and control CMV disease. In fact, the elderly possess, on average, larger absolute numbers of functional CMV-specific cells than do the young. The problem as we see it is not the presence or absence of functional CMV-specific cells, but the accumulation of dysfunctional cells

TABLE 2. Summary of immunological parameters for T cells of young, old, and centenarian donors

Paramaters/age group	Young (<40 Years)	Old (>65 years)	Centenarian (100 years)
T cells in general			
CD4:CD8 ratio	>1	<1 or >1	nt
KLR-G1+ T cells	Low	High	Low
A2 and B7/CMV-specific T cells			
Number of functional CMV-specific CD8 cells	+	+	+
A2/CMV-NLV-specific T cells	+	+	+
B7/CMV-TPR-specific T cells	+	+	nt
B7/CMV-RPH specific T cells	+	+	nt
Clonal expansion of CMV-specific CD8 cells	−	+	−
Fraction of CMV-specific cells KLR-G1-positive	Low	High	Low
Functional status/IFN-γ secretion/apoptosis			
Antigen responsiveness (IFN-γ secretion)	+	−	nt
Mitogen responsiveness (IFN-γ secretion)	+	+	nt
Apoptosis resistance	Low	High	nt

that are absent both in the young and in the non-IRP elderly.[3] However, it is still unclear to what extent the accumulation of CMV-specific CD8 T cells may be a major factor significantly contributing to the global process of immunosenescence (see TABLE 1). It is conceivable that such apoptosis-resistant cells exert suppressive activity on bystander cells; they may also fill the "immunological space" and block release of naïve T cells to the periphery. Because the thymus produces fewer new T cells with increasing age, it has been assumed that peripheral T cell expansion is required to maintain cell numbers in the elderly. However, our scenario is that the persistence of large accumulations of CMV-specific clones reduces or prevents the generation of naïve cells by a process of negative feedback inhibition. Even if the thymus was still functioning in the elderly (and usually it is architecturally and functionally much compromised, but can still retain some function, as shown by enumerating recent thymic emigrants[26]), homeostatic mechanisms maintaining stable cell numbers in the periphery (i.e., in the "immunological space") might prevent their release (FIG. 1). From this, it would be predicted that CMV-seropositivity would be associated with poorer responses to other pathogens. There are several data consistent with this prediction: for example, changes in the EBV-specific response with age are much smaller than those to CMV in the majority of donors (who are, of course, CMV-positive),[25] whereas in CMV-seronegative donors the response to EBV increases significantly with age.[27] Other indications that CMV may hinder immune responses to other pathogens in clinically important situations are the poorer responses to influenza vaccination[28] and failure to control HIV in progression to AIDS[29] in CMV-seropositive donors.

Another way of asking whether the accumulation of CMV-specific clonal expansions is deleterious in the elderly is to consider whether they occur, or

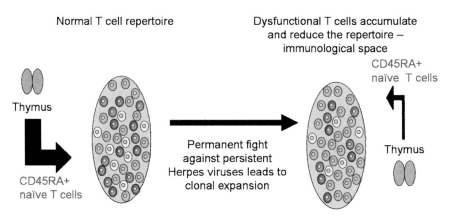

FIGURE 1. Consequences of persistent viral infections on the T cell repertoire of aged individuals. Young and healthy persons are able to produce more naïve cells and provide a large repertoire against different pathogens. Chronic antigenic stress caused by persistent viruses, especially HCMV or EBV, and thereby triggered clonal expansions, leads to an age-associated accumulation of mostly dysfunctional antigen-specific CD8+ T cells. To maintain peripheral T cell homeostasis, feedback inhibition reduces thymic output, which is already compromised in the elderly. The result is a shrunken repertoire of naïve cells specific for other pathogens.

occur to the same extent, in the "successfully" aged (TABLE 2). As has been noted for several of the age-associated changes observed in T cells, centenarian donors as an example of the successfully aged have a CMV repertoire more similar to that of the young than the old. We found a mean of only 1.54% A2/NLVPMVATV tetramer-positive CD8 cells in centenarians, which is very similar to that in the young.[30] Moreover, of these, only about half carried the killer-like lectin receptor-G1 (KLR-G1), which appears to represent end-stage differentiated cells without proliferative capacity.[31] KLR-G1 is expressed not only by peripheral NK, but also by T cells, and contains an inhibitory ITIM motive, suggesting that it is therefore an inhibitory NK receptor. In recent studies, it was shown that the poor proliferative capacity of KLR-G1+ T cells was limited to those coexpressing another "senescence" marker, CD57, which lacks CD28.[32] In the case of the CMV-specific cells, we could show that KLR-G1 expression increased with age and nearly all CMV-specific cells carry this receptor.[11] Because KLR-G1+ cells are more resistant than KLR-G1− cells to either spontaneous or induced apoptosis *in vitro* (Koch *et al.*, unpublished results), we hypothesize that apoptosis-resistant KLR-G1+ CD8 cells accumulate in the very old, aged 80–95 years, and acquire dysfunctional characteristics associated with the IRP. Compared with a sample of very old, the prevalence of IRP and associated increases of CMV-specific cells might decline in a sample of centenarians by selective mortality, because survival in those aged 80–95 years occurs preferentially in the non-IRP individuals.

CONCLUSION

We believe that it is now established beyond reasonable doubt that the "harmless" herpesvirus CMV exerts a greatly deleterious effect on T cell immunity in aging and that the way in which the immune system copes with persistent infection with this virus contributes critically to immune status in aging and thereby to healthful longevity. We suggest that the marked accumulation of dysfunctional apoptosis-resistant anergic CD8 T cells recognizing pp65-derived viral epitopes materially contributes to this state of affairs. These cells secrete interferon-γ after stimulation with strong nonspecific mitogenic agents but cannot proliferate and are apoptosis-resistant. In contrast, their ability to secrete interferon-γ after stimulation with specific CMV antigen is hugely reduced (a hallmark of anergic cells). Although the elderly as a group possess larger numbers of these cells than the young or middle-aged, there is a great deal of intraindividual variation and such clonal expansions are notably less extensive in the very elderly, who do not fall into what we call the "immune risk category." They are also less prevalent in centenarians ("successfully" aged). The percentage of CMV-specific cells expressing KLRG-1, which has been associated with senescence and resistance to apoptosis, is higher in the at-risk elderly donors than in centenarians or younger people. Strict homeostatic control of peripheral T cell numbers may prevent any residual functional thymic output of naïve T cells due to negative feedback from these accumulated dysfunctional cells, and a shrinking T cell repertoire results. This contributes to increased susceptibility to other infectious diseases, especially newly encountered pathogens, and hence increased morbidity and mortality. This may explain why the rate of fatalities due to SARS was 3% in persons under 40 years of age, but 55% in those over 60 years, an odds ratio of 20![33]

ACKNOWLEDGMENTS

This study was supported by EU contracts QLK6-CT2002–02283, "T Cells in Ageing, T-CIA" (see www.medizin.uni-tuebingen.de/t-cia/), FP6–506850 "ZINCAGE" (see www.zincage.org) and by the Deutsche Forschungsgemeinschaft (SFB 685).

REFERENCES

1. PAWELEC, G. *et al*. 2002. T cells and ageing: January 2002 update. Front. Biosci. **7:** d1056–d1183.
2. GROSS, P.A. *et al*. 1995. The efficacy of influenza vaccine in elderly persons: a meta-analysis and review of the literature. Ann. Intern. Med. **123:** 518–527.
3. PAWELEC, G. *et al*. 2005. Human immunosenescence: is it infectious? Immunol. Rev. **205:** 257–268.

4. WREGHITT, T.G. *et al.* 2003. Cytomegalovirus infection in immunocompetent patients. Clin. Infect. Dis. **37:** 1603–1606.

5. MCVOY, M.A. & S.P. ADLER. 1989. Immunologic evidence for frequent age-related cytomegalovirus reactivation in seropositive immunocompetent individuals. J. Infect. Dis. **160:** 1–10.

6. GRATAMA, J.W. *et al.* 1987. Effects of herpes virus carrier status on peripheral T lymphocyte subsets. Blood **70:** 516–523.

7. LOONEY, R.J. *et al.* 1999. Role of cytomegalovirus in the T cell changes seen in elderly individuals. Clin. Immunol. **90:** 213–219.

8. POSNETT, D.N. *et al.* 1994. Clonal populations of T cells in normal elderly humans: the T cell equivalent to 'benign monoclonal gammapathy.' J. Exp. Med. **179:** 609–618.

9. OLSSON, J. *et al.* 2000. Age-related change in peripheral blood T-lymphocyte subpopulations and cytomegalovirus infection in the very old: the Swedish longitudinal OCTO immune study. Mech. Ageing Dev. **121:** 187–201.

10. WIKBY, A. *et al.* 2002. Expansions of peripheral blood CD8 T-lymphocyte subpopulations and an association with cytomegalovirus seropositivity in the elderly: the Swedish NONA immune study. Exp. Gerontol. **37:** 445–453.

11. OUYANG, Q. *et al.* 2003. Age-associated accumulation of CMV-specific CD8+ T cells expressing the inhibitory killer cell lectin-like receptor G1 (KLRG1). Exp. Gerontol. **38:** 911–920.

12. OUYANG, Q. *et al.* 2003. Large numbers of dysfunctional CD8+ T lymphocytes bearing receptors for a single dominant CMV epitope in the very old. J. Clin. Immunol. **23:** 247–257.

13. OUYANG, Q. *et al.* 2004. Dysfunctional CMV-specific CD8(+) T cells accumulate in the elderly. Exp. Gerontol. **39:** 607–613.

14. WILLS, M.R. *et al.* 2002. Identification of naive or antigen-experienced human CD8(+) T cells by expression of costimulation and chemokine receptors: analysis of the human cytomegalovirus-specific CD8(+) T cell response. J. Immunol. **168:** 5455–5464.

15. KOMATSU, H. *et al.* 2003. Population analysis of antiviral T cell responses using MHC class I-peptide tetramers. Clin. Exp. Immunol. **134:** 9–12.

16. KHAN, N. *et al.* 2002. Cytomegalovirus seropositivity drives the CD8 T cell repertoire toward greater clonality in healthy elderly individuals. J. Immunol. **169:** 1984–1992.

17. ALMANZAR, G. *et al.* 2002. Long-term cytomegalovirus infection leads to significant changes in the composition of the CD8+ T-cell repertoire, which may be the basis for an imbalance in the cytokine production profile in elderly persons. J. Virol. **79:** 3675–3683.

18. PAWELEC, G., F.G. FERGUSON & A. WIKBY. 2001. The SENIEUR protocol after 16 years. Mech. Ageing Dev. **122:** 132–134.

19. WIKBY, A. *et al.* 1994. Age-related changes in immune parameters in a very old population of Swedish people: a longitudinal study. Exp. Gerontol. **29:** 531–541.

20. FERGUSON, F.G. *et al.* 1995. Immune parameters in a longitudinal study of a very old population of Swedish people: a comparison between survivors and nonsurvivors. J. Gerontol. Biol. Sci. B **50:** 378–382.

21. WIKBY, A. *et al.* 2005. An immune risk phenotype, cognitive impairment and survival in very late life: the impact of allostatic load in Swedish octo- and nonagenarian humans. J. Gerontol. B **60:** 556–565.

22. NILSSON, B.O. *et al.* 2003. Morbidity does not influence the T-cell immune risk phenotype in the elderly: findings in the Swedish NONA immune study using sample selection protocols. Mech. Ageing Dev. **124:** 469–476.

23. BLANCHO, G. *et al.* 1992. The influence of HLA A-B-DR matching on cytomegalovirus disease after renal transplantation. Evidence that HLA-DR7-matched recipients are more susceptible to cytomegalovirus disease. Transplantation **54:** 871–874.

24. SCHRIER, R.D. *et al.* 1995. Immune predispositions for cytomegalovirus retinitis in AIDS. The HNRC Group. J. Clin. Invest. **95:** 1741–1746.

25. OUYANG, Q. *et al.* 2003. An age-related increase in the number of CD8+ T cells carrying receptors for an immunodominant Epstein-Barr virus (EBV) epitope is counteracted by a decreased frequency of their antigen-specific responsiveness. Mech. Ageing Dev. **124:** 477–485.

26. DOUEK, D.C. & R.A. KOUP. 2000. Evidence for thymic function in the elderly. Vaccine **18:** 1638–1641.

27. KHAN, N. *et al.* 2004. Herpesvirus-specific CD8 T cell immunity in old age: cytomegalovirus impairs the response to a coresident EBV infection. J. Immunol. **173:** 7481–7489.

28. TRZONKOWSKI, P. *et al.* 2003. Association between cytomegalovirus infection, enhanced proinflammatory response and low level of anti-hemagglutinins during the anti-influenza vaccination: an impact of immunosenescence. Vaccine **21:** 3826–3836.

29. SINICCO, A. *et al.* 1997. The influence of cytomegalovirus on the natural history of HIV infection: evidence of rapid course of HIV infection in HIV-positive patients infected with cytomegalovirus. Scand. J. Infect. Dis. **29:** 543–549.

30. KOCH, S. *et al.* 2005. CMV and T cell immunosenescence. Mech. Ageing Dev. In press.

31. VOEHRINGER, D. M. KOSCHELLA & H. PIRCHER. 2002. Lack of proliferative capacity of human effector and memory T cells expressing killer cell lectinlike receptor G1 (KLRG1). Blood **100:** 3698–3702.

32. IBEGBU, C.C. *et al.* 2005. Expression of killer cell lectin-like receptor G1 on antigen-specific human CD8+ T lymphocytes during active, latent, and resolved infection and its relation with CD57. J. Immunol. **174:** 6088–6094.

33. LEUNG, G.M. *et al.* 2004. The epidemiology of severe acute respiratory syndrome in the 2003 Hong Kong epidemic: an analysis of all 1755 patients. Ann. Intern. Med. **141:** 662–673.

Aging in Mouse and Human Systems

A Comparative Study

LLOYD DEMETRIUS

*Department of Organismic and Evolutionary Biology, Harvard University,
Cambridge, Massachusetts 02138, USA*

Max Planck Institute for Molecular Genetics, 14195 Berlin, Germany

ABSTRACT: This article discusses the significance of mouse models as a basis for elucidating the aging process in humans. We identify certain parallels between mouse and human systems and review the theoretical and empirical support for the claim that the large divergence in the rate of aging between the two species resides in differences in the stability of their metabolic networks. We will show that these differences in metabolic stability have their origin in the different ecological constraints the species experience during their evolutionary history. We exploit these ideas to compare the effect of caloric restriction on murine and human systems. The studies predict that the large increases in mean life span and maximum life-span potential observed in laboratory rodents subject to caloric restriction will not obtain in human populations. We predict that, in view of the different metabolic stability of the two systems, caloric restriction will have no effect on the maximum life-span potential of humans, and a relatively minor effect on the mean life span of nonobese populations. This article thus points to certain intrinsic limitations in the use of mouse models in elucidating the aging process in humans. We furthermore contend the view that these limitations can be mitigated by considering the metabolic stability of the two species.

KEYWORDS: aging; metabolic stability; entropy; caloric restriction

INTRODUCTION

Maximal life-span potential is defined as the maximum observed life span of a species. This value is usually obtained with animals living under favorable conditions where the factors that induce extrinsic mortality are considerably reduced. There is about a 50-fold range of maximum life-span potential for the mammalian species. Mice and humans with a maximum life-span potential of

Address for correspondence: Lloyd Demetrius, Department of Organismic and Evolutionary Biology, Harvard University, Cambridge, Massachusetts, 02138 U.S.A.
e-mail: ldemetr@fas.harvard.edu

Ann. N.Y. Acad. Sci. 1067: 66–82 (2006). © 2006 New York Academy of Sciences.
doi: 10.1196/annals.1354.010

4 years and 120 years, respectively, are at two extremes of the longevity continuum. In spite of these large differences in life span, mouse models constitute one of the primary systems in studies of human longevity. The prevalence of mouse models in the analysis of age-related diseases and the rate of aging in humans has a biological rationale.

Mouse and human cells are endowed with a similar molecular apparatus that regulates differentiation and death. The cells are also similar in the molecular mechanisms by which they execute basic cellular processes. Mice and humans also share organs and systemic physiology and show a certain consistency in disease pathogenesis. Comparative studies of cancer pathogenesis, for example, show that mouse tumors have histological features similar to those of comparable human tumors and that the frequency of cancer is similar in spite of the large differences in life span. In addition, mice acquire mutations in an equivalent spectrum of protooncogenes and tumor suppressor genes.[1]

The problem this article addresses is: Are these similarities in cellular processes and disease pathogenesis sufficiently robust that experimental findings from mouse models can be extrapolated to study aging in human systems?

Aging, in its broadest sense, is the progressive and irreversible loss of function accompanied by increasing mortality with advancing age.[2] The rate of senescence can be defined as the rate at which the various physiological processes decline. In order to evaluate the significance of mouse models in the analysis of aging, the question that needs to be addressed is: Is the aging process in mouse and human systems defined by equivalent rates of senescence, and concomitantly, homologous molecular mechanisms?

This problem was initially discussed in Demetrius,[3] where we argued that mice and humans, in spite of certain similarities in system physiology and age-associated disease pathogenesis, will be defined by distinct differences in their rates of senescence. Consequently, the mechanisms underlying the aging process in the two systems will be similar.

This article will further develop this argument by delineating the physiological and demographic basis for the claim that mice and human systems will be defined by critical differences in their aging processes. We propose a molecular mechanism and provide an evolutionary rationale for these species-specific differences in the rates of aging: The models we propose point to certain intrinsic limitations in the use of mouse models to study human longevity.

This review is organized around two concepts: (i) metabolic stability, a molecular property which pertains to the regulatory network that defines the metabolic pathway in cells, and (ii) evolutionary entropy, a population property that describes the demographic network that defines a population of replicating organisms.

The concept of metabolic stability was originally introduced in an analytic theory of longevity to provide a molecular mechanism for the large variation in life span observed between species.[4]

Metabolic stability, roughly speaking, describes the capacity of the metabolic network to maintain steady-state values of redox couples in response to random perturbations in the rates of enzymatic processes. The significance of this concept in studies of aging resides in the metabolic stability-longevity principle. This asserts that metabolic stability is the prime determinant of the rate of aging and is positively correlated with the maximal life-span potential of a species. Accordingly, strongly stable networks will be defined by slow rates of aging, whereas weakly stable networks will be defined by rapid rates of aging.[3,4]

The concept of evolutionary entropy was introduced to provide an evolutionary rationale for the large differences in species life span.[4] Evolutionary entropy, a function of the age-specific fecundity and mortality of individuals in a population, predicts the outcome of competition between a rare mutant and the wild type.[5] This life-history parameter characterizes demographic stability, which is the ability of the population to maintain steady-state values of population size in the face of random perturbations in age-specific birth and death rates.[6] Evolutionary entropy is the cornerstone of a class of dynamical models—directionality theory—which studies changes in the genotypic and phenotypic composition of populations under mutation and selection.

This article is organized as follows. We first contrast mouse and human systems in terms of their physiology, disease pathogenesis, and life history. We exploit this contrast to show that mouse and human systems will be defined by decisive differences in their rates of aging. The molecular mechanisms underlying these differences and their evolutionary basis are then delineated. These developments are then exploited to analyze the effect of interventions such as caloric restriction on the mean and maximum life span in mammalian species. Finally, we contrast the new theory of aging described in this article with earlier studies of the senescent process: the metabolic rate–oxidative stress theory proposed by Harman[7] and the evolutionary theory of senescence advanced by Medawar,[8] Williams,[9] and Hamilton.[10]

COMPARATIVE BIOLOGY: MICE VERSUS HUMANS

Mice share genes, organ systems, and systemic physiology with humans. The species, however, differ significantly in terms of physiological properties, disease pathogenesis, and life-history attributes. We will briefly summarize the nature and extent of these differences and discuss their implications in understanding the divergences in the rate of aging in the two species.

1. *Physiological properties*: Mice and human systems are known to show significant differences in the production rate of reactive oxygen species (ROS)—a term used to describe molecular species, such as superoxide radical, hydrogen peroxide, and hydroxyl-free radical. ROS are involved

as specific signaling molecules under physiological conditions and also act as an essential host defense mechanism against infection.[11–13] Decreased levels of ROS may therefore interfere with the physiological role of oxidants in cellular signaling and host defense. Increased levels of ROS, however, can lead to random damage to proteins, lipids, and DNA. The existence of both positive and deleterious effects of ROS suggests that regulating overall levels of ROS will be a critical factor in aging, and that the capacity to maintain ROS within certain prescribed bounds will be an important element in determining longevity.[4] This capacity will to a large extent depend on factors such as (*a*) proton conductance (*b*) metabolic efficiency, and (*c*) the proton motive force, parameters that are involved in ROS production. These parameters depend, among other features, on the phospholipid composition of the biomembrane—a property that is known to differ between mice and human species.[14] We can therefore conclude that mice and humans, in spite of similarities in the basic molecular processes, will be described by differences in their capacity to maintain stable concentrations of ROS. Consequently, these organisms will be characterized by significant disparities in their rate of aging.

2. *Pathogenesis*: In addition to the differences in the physiological properties of the two species, there exist striking dissimilarities in disease pathogenesis, assessed, for example, in terms of cancer incidence and susceptibility.[15,16] Although the dynamics of tumor progression from benign to malignant state is similar in both rodent and human cancers, there exist significant differences in both the nature of the cancer and the susceptibility of individuals to the disease. In mice, mesenchymal and hematopoietic malignancies prevail and the incidence of invasive cancer increases exponentially with age. In humans, the nature of the cancer and its invasive dynamics are highly age-dependent. Sarcomas and lymphomas are the prevalent malignancies in children, and the incidence of cancer increases linearly with age. Among adults, epithelial carcinomas predominate. Invasive cancer increases exponentially with age from age 40 to 80 years. Beyond the age of 80 years, the incidence of cancer becomes independent of age.[17,18] These differences in the rate of pathogenesis of the two species indicate that the senescence process in mice and humans is driven by qualitatively different mechanisms.

3. *Life history*: The term *life history* refers to a population-level property. It describes the age-specific fecundity and mortality of the individuals in a population. Enormous variability in life history traits exist between species. The variability in life history can be described in terms of the following demographic variables: age of sexual maturity, size of progeny sets, and reproductive span. These parameters show a large range of variation between species. Within the mammalian lineage, the range of

TABLE 1. Life-history variation in mammals

Demographic property	Mammals' range of variation	Mice	Humans
Age of sexual maturity	9 days–13 years	35–50 months	13 years
Litter size	1–16	4–8	1
Reproductive span	1 year–35 years	2 years	35 years

variation and the corresponding values for mice and humans are shown in TABLE 1.[19]

Analysis of demographic models shows that this life-history variability can be characterized in terms of the parameter, evolutionary entropy, a function of age-specific fecundity and mortality distribution. Entropy characterizes the variability in the age at which individuals reproduce and die. The demographic parameter is an information-theoretic measure that describes the uncertainty in the age of the mother of a randomly chosen newborn. High-entropy systems distribute their reproductive activity throughout different stages of their life cycle. These populations are defined by late age of sexual maturity, small litter size, and broad reproductive span. Low-entropy systems concentrate their reproduction at a single stage in their life cycle. These populations are defined by early age of sexual maturity, small litter size, and narrow reproductive span.

The significance of evolutionary entropy in studies of aging resides in the fact that entropy is positively correlated with maximum life-span potential, the life span of an organism in a protected environment.[4]

Mice (a low-entropy species), and humans (a high-entropy species) occupy different poles of the entropy continuum. This property, together with the positive correlation between entropy and maximum life span, provides further support for the proposition that mice and humans, in spite of similarities at the genetic, molecular, and cellular levels, will be sharply divergent in their rates of aging.

METABOLIC STABILITY: A MOLECULAR MECHANISM OF AGING

The large divergences in physiological properties, disease pathogenesis, and life-history properties entail that mice and human systems, in spite of congruencies at the molecular and cellular level, will be defined by significant differences in their rate of aging.

The question of interest now becomes: What is the molecular mechanism that underlies these divergences in the rate of senescence? Can this variability be explained in terms of processes at the cellular level? These issues, as shown in Ref. 3, can be addressed in terms of the concept of metabolic stability, a measure of the robustness of the regulatory networks that are involved in cell metabolism.[4]

Metabolic Networks, Metabolic Stability, and Life Span

The term *metabolic stability* refers to the capacity of the metabolic network to control and maintain an adequate redox balance in the face of random perturbations in the reaction rates of the underlying enzymatic processes. This concept is the fundamental notion in the new theory of longevity proposed in Ref. 4. According to this theory, the senescence-related loss of function at the organismic level is due to the dysregulation of the steady-state values of redox couples. The model contends that deviations from redox balance are an intrinsic property of all metabolic processes. These deviations derive from the chance perturbations in enzymatic reaction rates that characterize all metabolic systems where the concentration of reacting species is extremely low. We postulate that the effect of these random perturbations will accumulate over time and lead ultimately to the impairment of cellular signaling, the dysregulation of ontogenetic events, and cell death. Accordingly, senescence is the result of spontaneous changes in the metabolic condition of the cell during normal development.

In the context of this model, cell death is the result of a complete dysregulation of the regulatory networks—a state of metabolic instability. The time that elapses before this condition is attained will depend on the ability of the system to maintain cellular homeostasis in the face of random perturbations in the enzymatic reaction rates. The ability to maintain the homeostatic condition and thus decelerate the aging process can be enhanced by factors such as DNA repair. However, maximal life-span potential will be positively correlated with metabolic stability. The spontaneous nature of the process, which induces cellular dysregulation, entails that metabolic stability is not simply correlated with life span, but is a critical determinant of longevity.

These observations can be qualitatively annotated in terms of what we call the metabolic stability–longevity principle: The metabolic stability of an organism, which is its capacity to maintain steady-state concentration of redox couples in the face of random perturbations in the enzymatic reaction rates, is the prime determinant of organismic longevity.[4]

Two important implications follow immediately from this principle:

I. The metabolic stability of an organism will be a decreasing function of age.
II. The metabolic stability of an organism will be positively correlated with maximum life-span potential.

Studies consistent with (I) are the empirical investigations using *C. elegans*, which show that ATP/AMP ratio, a metabolic marker of stability, decreases with age and that organisms with a larger ATP:AMP ratio live longer.[20] Analyses consistent with (II) are comparative studies of fibroblast cells from several mammalian species, showing the relation between species life span and cell stress resistance.[21] These investigations show that the ability of cells to tolerate

oxidative stress, a physiological marker of metabolic stability, is positively correlated with life span.

ENTROPY: THE EVOLUTIONARY RATIONALE

The metabolic stability–longevity principle provides a basis for predicting the metabolic stability of the cellular network of a species from its life
span. Long-lived species, such as humans, will be described by highly stable networks—metabolic systems that have a strong capacity for homeostatic
regulation. Short-lived species, such as mice, will be characterized by weakly
stable networks—systems with a weak capacity to maintain their homeostatic
condition.

The problem we now address is: Can these species-specific differences in
metabolic stability be explained in evolutionary terms? In other words, are the
highly and weakly stable networks of humans and mice, respectively, the result
of the process of mutation and natural selection? This problem can be resolved
by appealing to directionality theory, a class of evolutionary models based on
the concept of entropy as the measure of Darwinian fitness.[22]

Directionality Theory and the Evolution of Life History

Directionality theory distinguishes between species in terms of the nature
and intensity of fluctuations in population numbers. The term *equilibrium
species* describes species that spend the major part of their evolutionary history in the stationary growth phase or with a population size that fluctuates
around some constant value. These species are subject to ecological conditions
that provide limited but constant resources. Humans are a canonical example
of an equilibrium species. Humans have clearly increased in size as they moved
from the hunter-gathering state, to the agricultural phase, and then to industrial-
ized populations: However, population growth rate during the hunter-gathering
phase, a period that represent 99% of human history, ranged between 0.007
and 0.0015 per thousand per year. The large increases in growth rate (0.36 per
1,000) at the establishment of agriculture 10,000 years ago, and the explosion
in growth rate (0.56 per 1,000) since 1750, have occurred during periods that
represent 1% of human evolutionary history.[23]

The term *opportunistic species* refers to populations that are subject to large
and irregular fluctuations in population size. These species are typically subject
to conditions where the resources are ample but intermittently available. Wild
mice are a typical example of the opportunistic state. Population size in these
species reflects resource conditions that are highly variable, and hence large
irregular fluctuations in numbers will be common.

Directionality theory revolves around the proposition that Darwinian fitness,
the demographic property that determines the outcome of competition between

a mutant allele and the resident type, is characterized by the robustness or the demographic stability of the population. This notion of stability refers to the rate at which a population returns to its original size after a random perturbation in its age-specific birth and death rate. Strongly stable or *robust* systems are populations described by a rapid rate of return to their steady-state condition. These populations have a strong capacity for the homeostatic regulation of their numbers. Weakly stable or *flexible* systems are populations characterized by a slow rate of return to their steady state. Such systems have a correspondingly weak capacity to maintain their size in the face of chance perturbations in the individual birth and death rates. Directionality theory exploits certain analytic properties of the entropy function to predict that (*a*) among equilibrium species, mutations that increase demographic stability will have a selective advantage, as they increase the capacity of the population to efficiently exploit the limited but constant resources that define their environmental condition; but (*b*) in opportunistic species, mutations that decrease demographic stability will now have a selective advantage as they enhance the ability of the population to exploit the large variation in resource availability that defines their environmental state. The theory postulates that the dynamics of the evolutionary process of mutation and natural selection will induce changes in the life-history characteristics of the species over time, as mutant alleles replace ancestral types in response to the prevailing selective constraints. The major predictions of the theory are as follows:

A. Evolution in equilibrium species will be described by an increase in entropy. These species will be characterized by the following life-history properties: late age of sexual maturity, small progeny sets, broad reproductive span, and long life span.
B. Evolution in opportunistic species will be described by a decrease in entropy. These species will be defined by: early age of sexual maturity, large progeny sets, narrow reproductive span, and short life span.

Metabolic Stability and Directionality Theory

The evolutionary dynamics of metabolic stability can be predicted from directionality theory. The basis for the prediction resides in the tight coupling between processes at the cellular, individual, and population levels of biological organization. The dynamics of the metabolic network determine the life-history features of the population. Changes in the topology and kinetics of the network will result in changes in the individual birth and death rates. Variations that increase the robustness of the network will have a corresponding effect on the robustness or stability of the population. Consequently, changes in metabolic stability and evolutionary entropy will be positively correlated. This correlation implies that the directionality principles for evolutionary entropy

TABLE 2. Physiological and demographic properties for equilibrium and opportunistic species

Physiological and demographic properties	Equilibrium species	Opportunistic species
Metabolic stability	Strong	Weak
Demographic stability	Large	Small
Rate of senescence	Slow	Fast
Maximum life-span potential	Large	Short

can be invoked to predict evolutionary changes in metabolic stability. Accordingly, equilibrium species will be described by metabolic networks that are highly resilient with respect to random perturbations in the enzymatic reaction rates, whereas opportunistic species will be defined by metabolic networks that are highly sensitive to random fluctuations in the reaction rates.

The relationship between the physiological and demographic attributes of equilibrium species (humans) and opportunistic species (mice) are summarized in TABLE 2.

This analysis based on directionality theory provides an evolutionary rationale for the empirical observation that humans, a typical equilibrium species, consist of cells that are highly stress-resistant, whereas mice, a typical opportunistic species, are composed of cells whose metabolic dynamics are highly sensitive to random perturbations. The large differences in stability of the metabolic network in humans and mice have their origin in the different ecological constraints that these species have endured.

DIETARY RESTRICTION: EQUILIBRIUM
AND OPPORTUNISTIC SPECIES

Dietary restriction (DR), the extension of life span by reduced nutrient intake without malnutrition, is often invoked as the canonical method for interventions that modulate life span. The life-span extension effects of DR go back to the pioneering experiment on rats by McCay et al.[24] Since the time of these experiments, some form of food restriction has been shown to increase life span in a variety of organisms, including yeast, nematodes, fruit flies, and mice.[25] The mechanisms that are responsible for increased longevity, however, have not been fully elucidated. Dietary restriction, however, has been shown to increase the efficiency of a number of key enzymes in intermediary metabolism.[26] We have appealed to this empirical fact and invoked the metabolic longevity principle to suggest a mechanism for the action of DR on life span.[4] The models predict that DR extends life span by increasing the stability of the metabolic networks.

Support for this mode of action of DR derives from studies of a genome-wide microarray expression analysis of genes in the liver.[27] The liver is the central organ for the regulation of glucose homeostasis. Accordingly, it has a major effect on metabolic regulation during aging. A common effect of aging in liver is the induced expression of a number of stress-response genes—a condition that reduces the homeostatic capability of the organ. The experimental design reported in Cac *et al.*[27] showed that DR opposed the age-related induction of stress-response genes and inflammatory genes. This can be considered as an enhancement of homeostatic regulation, and hence an increase in the stability of the metabolic network.

The proposition that dietary restriction acts by increasing metabolic stability, and the observation that equilibrium and opportunistic species differ significantly in terms of this property, entails that the response to DR will be contingent on the equilibrium or opportunistic status of the species.

Equilibrium species have evolved to increase metabolic stability because this property enhances the capacity to adapt to the limited resource conditions these species have endured during their evolutionary history. These species will therefore be defined by a metabolic stability close to its maximal value. This implies that any further increase in metabolic stability that DR may induce will be relatively small.

Opportunistic species, by contrast, have evolved to decrease metabolic stability as this condition facilitates their capacity to adapt to the highly variable resource conditions that characterize the environmental constraints these species experience. Opportunistic species will be characterized by weak metabolic stability. Consequently, DR, when imposed on opportunistic species, will result in decisive increases in metabolic stability.

A central tenet in this new theory of longevity is that metabolic stability and longevity are positively correlated. In view of this correlation we can infer that in equilibrium species DR will have no significant effect on maximum life-span potential. DR will, however, have an effect on mean life span. The effect will be induced by the reduction in the incidence of age-related diseases, which include neoplasia, cardiovascular disease, and diabetes. These effects, however, will be relatively small since they will not involve any changes in the rate of aging.

We can furthermore infer that in the case of opportunistic species, the effect of DR on both the maximum life-span potential and the mean life span may be significant. This derives from the fact that opportunistic species are defined by weak metabolic stability. DR may induce appreciable increases in this property, thereby decelerating the rate of aging.

DR in Humans and Mice

Humans are the canonical equilibrium species. *Homo sapiens* has been subject to ecological constraints that ensure a stationary or very slow population growth throughout most of its evolutionary history. Humans will therefore evolve a life-history schedule defined by high entropy. This prediction is consistent with the following life-history characteristics of humans: late sexual maturity, small litter size, and a long maximum life-span potential (~120 years). The high-entropy condition implies that humans will be characterized by metabolic networks whose stability is close to the maximal condition.

DR increases longevity by increasing the metabolic stability of the regulatory networks. We can therefore infer that, in the case of humans, a species close to the condition of maximal metabolic stability, DR will have negligible effect on stability, and hence no effect on maximum life span. However, DR may have an effect on mean life span. Mean life span is simply a measure of our ability to minimize premature death. DR can influence mean life span by simply reducing the incidence of diseases such as diabetes, atherosclerosis, and hypertension. These changes, however, will result in an increase in life span of only about 3–5 years—a moderate effect. Since DR will have a negligible effect on metabolic stability, it will exert no effect on the rate of aging and hence induce no changes in the human senescence process.

Mice are classical examples of opportunistic species. These organisms have been subject to ecological constraints defined by large variations in resource abundance. These species will therefore evolve a life history defined by high entropy. This situation is consistent with the following life-history characteristics of mice: early sexual maturity, large litter size, and a short maximum life span potential of ~4 years. The low-entropy condition entails that mice will be characterized by metabolic networks whose stability is close to the minimal condition. Since DR increases longevity by increasing metabolic stability, we can infer that in the case of mice, DR, by causing significant increases in metabolic stability, will influence the rate of aging and thereby induce changes in both the maximum and the mean life span. The studies described on laboratory mice and reported by McKay *et al.*[24] are consistent with this prediction.

DR in Rhesus Monkeys

We should point out at this juncture the ongoing longitudinal studies of caloric restriction on life span in rhesus monkeys.[28] These studies indicate lower incidence of disease risk and less incidence of age-related diseases in DR monkeys compared to controls: Rhesus monkeys share 92% gene homology with humans. Many biological similarities in the profile of aging also exist between the two species. These similarities have suggested to many researchers that DR in humans may result in increases in mean and maximum life span comparable to the increases that may subsequently be observed in rhesus monkeys. We contend, however, that although rhesus monkeys and humans are equilibrium species and should therefore show comparable aging patterns, the effect of DR on mean and maximum life span in the two species will be quantitatively quite distinct. The reasons for this are as follows: Rhesus monkeys and humans, although both equilibrium species, are described by significant differences in life-history patterns. In rhesus monkeys, sexual maturity occurs at 3 to 5 years of age, mean life span is 25 years, and estimated maximum life span is 40 years. Hence rhesus monkeys will have an inferior evolutionary entropy, and consequently weaker metabolic stability than humans. Our analysis thus predicts that DR will induce changes in longevity in rhesus monkeys. These changes however, will be less pronounced than those recorded in mice—an opportunistic species—but significantly more pronounced than any changes that may occur in humans.

THE ORIGIN AND EVOLUTION OF LONGEVITY: A COMPARISON OF MODELS

Our comparative study of mice and human systems has been based on a new analytic theory of longevity that proposes a molecular mechanism for senescence, and postulates an evolutionary rationale for the species-specific differences in rates of aging.

The studies of the molecular mechanism are based on the metabolic stability concept. Our analysis has been organized around the stability–longevity principle, which asserts that metabolic stability is the prime determinant of life span.

The studies that were aimed at explaining species differences in the rate of senescence were based on directionality theory. The analysis in this case is now organized around an entropic principle. This contends that entropy predicts the outcome of competition between the mutant type and the ancestral population. Competitive success, however, is mediated by the demographic characteristics of the population. In equilibrium species, mutants with higher entropy will be selectively advantageous, whereas in opportunistic species, mutants with lower entropy will prevail.

Entropy characterizes the demographic stability or robustness of the population. Hence the entropic principle can be reformulated to assert that high demographic stability or strong robustness determines competitive success in equilibrium species, whereas weak demographic stability or flexibility confers a selective advantage in opportunistic species.

The theory we have outlined in comparing the aging process in mice and humans provides answers to two fundamental questions:

1. Why do organisms undergo progressive and irreversible physiological decline after the reproductive phase of life ceases?
2. Why do life span and the rate of aging vary between species?

Problems pertaining to how and why we age have attracted the attention of several generations of biologists. Hence, it is of some interest to view the theory described in this article with earlier efforts that have been proposed to understand the molecular mechanism and evolutionary rationale of the senescence process.

Rate of Living and Oxidative Stress

Early efforts to delineate how we age have their origin in the phenomenological models of Pearl,[29] expressed in terms of the rate-of-living theory, and the molecular mechanism proposed by Harman,[8] in terms of free radicals. The rate-of-living theory was inspired by the following empirical observation: Lifetime energy expenditure does not vary significantly between species.[30] Pearl invoked this empirical study, based on a small group of nonprimate mammals, to propose a general tenet: species life span should be inversely correlated with mass-specific metabolic rate.

Harman[8] provided a molecular basis for the rate-of-living theory. He postulated that free radicals, endogenously generated during normal oxygen consumption in mitochondria, will cause permanent damage to DNA and lipids. The accumulation of this damage is manifested as aging.

The rate-of-living tenet and the free radical model, however, are not necessarily equivalent, since metabolic rate and ROS production rate are not always positively correlated. Both theories, however, are similar in that they postulate that production rate of biomolecules is the prime determinant of the rate of aging.

Empirical observations do not conform to either of these two theories. As regards the rate-of-living theory, considerable variation in life span, exists that cannot be explained by variation in metabolic rate. For example, birds live much longer than mammals although they have similar metabolic rate.[31] As regards the free radical theory, certain inconsistencies have also been recognized: There exists a 7-fold difference between the life span of pigeons and rats; however, ROS production by rat mitochondria is only slightly greater than that of pigeon mitochondria.[14] Bird–mammal comparisons lead to similar anomalies. As noted in Herrero and Barja[32] there is a 7-fold difference in life span between parakeet and mouse; however, the ratio of H_2O_2 production to respiration in heart mitochondria was the same in the both species.

These inconsistencies thus question the validity of the oxidative stress theory as a model for the origin of aging. The difficulties raised by the notion that production rate of metabolic species is a determinant of aging becomes quite evident in the context of the free radical theory. This theory postulates that the production rate of ROS is the prime determinant of the rate of aging. However, ROS has two kinds of effects on metabolic activity.[12,13] First, these small diffusible molecular species can interact with DNA and RNA to impair function. The molecules are also known to act as second messengers in signal transduction. Hence *increased* production may impair metabolism, thus leading to cell death, and concomitantly, *decreased* production may compromise signal transduction and disrupt cell regulation.[12] These observations argue against the production rate of ROS as being the primary determinant of longevity, and suggest that the ability to maintain ROS within certain range of values may be more critical.

Darwinian Fitness and the Malthusian Parameter

The efforts to understand why we age have their source in the models of Medawar,[9] Hamilton,[11] and Williams.[10] The approaches of these authors differ significantly in methodology and analytical rigor. The models proposed, however, do share a common conceptual framework; namely the notion that the population growth rate or the Malthusian parameter characterizes Darwinian fitness.

The claim that fitness is determined by the rate of increase of population numbers goes back to Fisher[33] and has been the driving force in most studies of population genetics and ecology. Empirical and theoretical studies, however, do not support the Malthusian parameter as the measure of Darwinian fitness. Data from studies of invasion in a wide variety of organisms, both vertebrates and invertebrates, indicate that the population growth rate is not the main determinant of invasion success. These investigations show that the probability of the establishment of an invader is highly correlated with the amplitude of population fluctuations.[34] Analytical studies of invasion dynamics based on diffusion processes show that the rate at which a population returns to its original size after a random perturbation, a property measured by evolutionary entropy, predicts invasion success. These studies also show that the rate at which population numbers increase in size is a predictor of invasion success only in the case of populations of effectively infinite size.[35]

Production Rate and Dynamic Stability

The oxidative stress theory and the Malthusian theory of senescence may be called *production rate* theories. Both postulate that the rate at which certain metabolic and demographic processes operate is the driving mechanism that underlies the ability of these processes to adapt to the environmental conditions which modulate the dynamics of evolution. The metabolic stability theory of aging and the entropic model may be called *stability* theories. They contend that the rate at which certain metabolic and demographic processes return to their steady-state condition after a random perturbation is the central mechanism that determines the ability of these processes to respond to environmental and evolutionary constraints.

Empirical observations and analytical studies have pointed to the inconsistencies in production rate theories as a paradigm for the understanding of adaptation in the biological processes that underlie senescence. The explanatory and predictive power of models based on stability concepts underscores the range and scope of metabolic stability-entropic factors in understanding the mechanism and evolutionary rationale of senescence. This contrast between production rate and stability theories points to the significance of homeostatic regulation as the primary mechanism for explaining diversity and adaptation in biological systems.

CONCLUSIONS

Mouse models of senescence in human populations have become a central element in many types of biomedical research. The significance of this system derives from its experimental accessibility and the fact that mice share organ systems, systemic physiology, and genes with humans.

We have addressed the question: To what extent can one extrapolate from experimental observations on mouse models to predict the dynamics of the senescent process in humans? The argument developed in this article shows that any effort to exploit murine systems to elucidate human aging or the human disease process must take into account the vast differences in the metabolic stability of the cells that compose the two species. These differences in metabolic stability derive from the contrasting evolutionary history of the species and the environmental constraints they have experienced. An understanding of this history, and its signature at the cellular level, robustness of the metabolic network, are thus crucial in elucidating human aging and human disease pathogenesis from mouse models.

REFERENCES

1. BALMAIN, A. & C. HARRIS. 2000. Carcinogenesis in mouse and human cells: parallels and paradoxes. Carcinogenesis 21: 371–347.
2. SOHAL, R.S. & R. WEINDRUCH. 2001. Oxidative stress, caloric restriction and aging. Science 273: 59–63.
3. DEMETRIUS, L. 2005. Of mice and men. EMBO Reports 6: 539–544.
4. DEMETRIUS, L. 2004. Caloric restriction, metabolic rate and entropy. J. Gerontol. Biol. Sci. 59A: 902–915.
5. DEMETRIUS, L. 1991. Mortality plateaus and directionality theory. Proc. Royal. Soc. London B. 268: 2029–3037.
6. DEMETRIUS, L., M. GUNDLACH & G. OCHS. 2004. Complexity and stability in population models. Theor. Pop. Biol. 65: 211–225.
7. HARMAN, D. 1956. Aging: a theory based on free radical and radiation chemistry. J. Gerontol. 11: 298–300.
8. MEDAWAR, P.B. 1952. An Unsolved Problem of Biology. H. K. Lewis. London.
9. WILLIAMS, G.C. 1999. Pleiotropy, natural selection and the evolution of aging. Evolution 11: 398–411.

10. HAMILTON, W.D. 1966. The moulding of senescence by natural selection. J. Theor. Biol. **12:** 12–45.

11. FINKEL, T. 2003. Oxidant signals and oxidative stress. Curr. Opin. Cell Biol. **15:** 247–254.

12. FINKEL, T. & N.J. HOLBROOK. 2000. Oxidants, oxidative stress and the biology of aging. Nature **408:** 239–243.

13. LANDER, H.M. 1997. An essential role for free radicals and derived species in signal transduction. FASEB J. **11:** 118–124.

14. HULBERT, A.J. On the importance of fatty acid composition of membranes for aging. J. Theor. Biol. **234:** 277–288.

15. HOLLIDAY, R. 1996. Neoplastic transformation: the contrasting stability of human and mouse cells. Cancer Surv. **26:** 103–115.

16. RANGARAJAN, A. & R.A. WEINBERG. 2003. Comparative biology of mouse versus human cells: modelling human cancer in mice. Nat. Rev. **3:** 952–959.

17. DEPINHO, R.A. 2000. The age of cancer. Nature **408:** 248–253.

18. PIANTANELLI, L. 1988. Cancer and aging: from the kinetics of biological parameters to the kinetics of cancer incidence and mortality. Ann. N. Y. Acad. Sci. **521:** 99–109.

19. AUSTAD, S.N. 1998. Comparing aging and life histories in mammals. Exp. Gerontol. **32:** 22–38.

20. APFELD, J., G. O'CONNOR, T. MCDONAGH, et al. 2004. The AMP-activated protein kinase AAK-2 links energy levels and insulin-like signals to lifespan in C. elegans. Genes Dev. **18:** 3004–3009.

21. KAPATHI, P., M.E. BOUILTON & T.B. KIRKWOOD. 1999. Positive correlation between mammalian life span and cellular resistance to stress. Free Radic. Biol. Med. **26:** 495–500.

22. DEMETRIUS, L. 1997. Directionality principles in thermodynamics and evolution. Proc. Natl. Acad. Sci. USA **24:** 3491–3498.

23. COALE, A.J. 1974. The history of the human population. Sci. Am. **231:** 41–51.

24. MCKAY, C.M., M. F. CROWELL & L.A. MAYNARD. 1935. The effect of retarded growth upon the length of life span and upon ultimate body size. J. Nutr. **10:** 63–79.

25. WEINDRUCH, R. & R.L. WALFORD. 1988. The Retardation of Aging and Disease by Dietary Restriction. Charles C Thomas. Springfield, IL.

26. HOUTHOOFD, K., P. BRAECKMAN, et al. 2002. Axenic growth up regulates mass-specific metabolic rate, stress resistance and extends life span in C. elegans. Exp. Gerontol. **37:** 1369–1376.

27. CAO, S.X., J. M. DHABHI, P. L. MOTE, et al. 2001. Genomic profiling of short and long term caloric restriction effects in the liver of aging mice. Proc. Natl. Acad. Sci. USA **98:** 2029–2037.

28. ROTH, G.S. et al. 2004. Aging in rhesus monkeys: relevance to human health interventions. Science **305:** 1423–1426.

29. PEARL, R. 1928. The Rate of Living. University of London Press. London.

30. RUBNER, M. 1908. Das Problem der Lebensdauer. Berlin, Germany.

31. HOLMES, D.H. & S.N. AUSTAD. 1995. Birds as animal models for the comparative biology of aging: a prospectus. J. Gerontol. **50:** 59–66.

32. HERRERO, A. & G. BARJA. 1998. H_2O_2 production of heart mitochondria and aging rate are slower in canaries and parakeets than in mice: signs of free radical generation and mechanisms involved. Mech. Aging. Dev. **103:** 133–146.

33. FISHER, R.A. 1990. The Genetical Theory of Natural Selection. Clarendon Press, Oxford.
34. LAWTON, J. & T. BROWN. 1986. The population and community ecology of invading insects. Phil. Trans. R. Soc. B. **314:** 607–617.
35. DEMETRIUS, L. 2001. Mortality plateaus and directionality theory. Proc. R. Soc. **268:** 2029–2037.

Extrapolaholics Anonymous

Why Demographers' Rejections of a Huge Rise in Cohort Life Expectancy in This Century are Overconfident

AUBREY D.N.J. DE GREY

Department of Genetics, University of Cambridge, Cambridge, UK

ABSTRACT: Criticisms of demographers by other demographers have become frequent in scientific literature, generally consisting of accusations that trends observed in the recent past have been extrapolated unjustifiably into the future. Demographers, along with their colleagues in the actuarial profession, are in an invidious position in this regard, knowing full well that extrapolation is almost always only minimally justifiable, but knowing also that their readers, colleagues, and sources of funding tend to be much more interested in the future than in the past. It is unfortunate that, while actuaries typically resolve this dilemma by emphasizing the limitations of their methods and thereby lowering expectations that their predictions will be accurately fulfilled, demographers are more prone to respond combatively, attempting to reinforce the credibility of their extrapolations by recourse to data from areas in which their expertise is less tested, such as biology. This is valuable in that it raises the profile of the debate on the likely rate of scientific progress relevant to mortality rates, but it also runs the risk of lowering the technical quality of that debate, by telling policy makers and the public what they want to hear and thereby entrenching their expectations without recourse to the relevant biological facts. Extrapolations based on plausible sequences of scientific advances and the sociopolitical responses to them, summarized in this article, have led to the prediction of four-digit life expectancies of cohorts born in the 21st century and possibly even in the 20th. This prediction has attracted inevitable ridicule from prominent demographers, but being founded on science and sociology rather than on history it may be much more reliable than the extrapolations that those demographers presently prefer.

KEYWORDS: longevity; extrapolation; rejuvenation therapies; timeframes; life tables; longevity escape velocity

Address for correspondence: Aubrey D.N.J. de Grey, Department of Genetics, University of Cambridge, Downing Street, Cambridge CB2 3EH, UK. Voice: +44 1223 366197; fax: +44 1223 333992.

e-mail: ag24@gen.cam.ac.uk

http://www.sens.org

Ann. N.Y. Acad. Sci. 1067: 83–93 (2006). © 2006 New York Academy of Sciences.

doi: 10.1196/annals.1354.011

DEMOGRAPHERS' LOVE–HATE RELATIONSHIP WITH EXTRAPOLATION

The public's interest in the postponement of aging and death is perhaps greater now than ever. This is manifest not only in an insatiable appetite for documentaries and news articles on the work of biogerontologists, but also in an intense demand for prediction of how long those of a given age today are likely to live. The latter topic is the province of the demographer.

Unfortunately, such extrapolation depends on assumptions that can be very easily challenged. Demographers have nonetheless felt it necessary to make these predictions—which have varied widely[1,2]—given the aforementioned thirst for them. Especially dangerous, in my view, are extrapolations (or critiques of others' extrapolations) based on misuse of biology. The demographer most identified with such arguments at present, Jay Olshansky, has authored or coauthored a number of popular pieces,[3-5] one of which[3] suggested various ways—many of them clearly beyond the realm of foreseeable medical science, even setting aside their aesthetic shortcomings—in which the human body might hypothetically be "redesigned" to make it age more slowly and thus live longer. The rhetorical nature of such speculation is obvious to any biologist and was not disguised, but yet was overlooked by some commentators, who treated these publications as presenting a serious biological argument for the immutability of human aging.[6,7] This error clearly occurred because Olshansky is well known to be on the pessimistic side of the fence concerning the likely rate of biomedical (and hence demographic) progress in this century in postponing aging. It was only to be expected; one may thus question Olshansky's judgment in inviting it. Regardless, there is an urgent need for projections concerning future life spans that are based on serious, rather than rhetorical, scrutiny of plausible biomedical progress and society's response to it.

A PLAUSIBLE TIME LINE FOR DEVELOPING AND DISTRIBUTING DRAMATIC LIFE-EXTENSION THERAPIES

Four Life-Extension Milestones

The fact that we have made only modest progress hitherto in *slowing* aging (insofar as that can even be defined[8]) in mammals has led most gerontologists to feel that actually *reversing* mammalian age-related degeneration is too ambitious even to contemplate at this juncture. This has resulted in the virtual nonexistence of research on late-onset interventions to extend mammalian life span. However, as I have set out extensively elsewhere[9-11] (see TABLE 1), it may by much easier to repair the various types of accumulated molecular and cellular damage that eventually give rise to age-related frailty and diseases than to halve the rate of that accumulation without unacceptable side effects,

TABLE 1. Strategies for engineered negligible senescence: the "seven deadly things" that accumulate with age as side effects of metabolism and promising first-generation therapies to reverse or obviate that accumulation[a]

Category of lifespan-limiting damage	Feasible strategy to repair or obviate it
Cell death without matching replacement	Stem cell therapy, growth factors, exercise
Unwanted cells (e.g. visceral fat; senescent)	Cell surface marker–targeted cellular toxins
Oncogenic nuclear [epi]mutations	Somatic telomere elongation knockout ("WILT")
Mitochondrial mutations	Allotopic expression of 13 mtDNA-coded proteins
Extracellular protein/protein cross-links	Phenacyldimethylthiazolium chloride (ALT-711)
Extracellular aggregates (e.g., amyloid)	Immune-mediated phagocytosis
Intracellular aggregates (e.g., oxysterols)	Microbe-derived "xenohydrolases"

[a]for details, see Refs. 9–11.

particularly because such repair can be done without intervening in the processes by which the damage is laid down and thus without detailed knowledge of those processes.

This has led me to identify[12,13] three major milestones in the "future history" of life extension research and implementation:

1. *Robust mouse rejuvenation* (RMR): the reproducible trebling of the remaining life expectancy of genetically robust but wild-type *Mus musculus* with treatments begun in middle age. Quantitatively, it means using at least 50 mice of a strain with a life expectancy of 3 years, initiating treatment at the age of 2 years, and obtaining a mean age at death of 5 years. The extra two years must predominantly be ones of good health.

2. *Robust human rejuvenation* (RHR): doubling of the remaining life expectancy of humans with treatments begun in middle age, that is, the addition of roughly 30 years to the healthy and total life expectancy of humans who enter treatment in their 50s.

3. *Longevity escape velocity* (LEV): the point when improvements to the comprehensiveness and safety of human life-extension treatments are being made faster than people are aging: that is, when the remaining average life span of those who are receiving the latest therapies, and who are of the age that derives the most benefit from those therapies, begins to increase with time even though they are getting chronologically older.

4. *Actuarial escape velocity* (AEV): the point when the mortality rate of some cohort in the population under discussion (typically either global or national) begins to decline year by year as they get older. Cohorts that have exhibited a mortality rate above 20% in previous years are excluded.

Since the mortality rate at age N is roughly 10% greater than at age $N-1$ for the ages at which most people in the developed world die, this is equivalent to a 10% per year fall in age-specific mortality rates at some range of ages, which is a few times faster than the peak declines seen in the recent past (for example, infant mortality early in the 20th century).

An obvious feature of milestones (1) to (3) is that they will be achieved before they are shown to have been achieved. Milestone 1 will be demonstrated only a few years after the technology to implement it has been developed, but the corresponding lag for milestone 2 will be over half a century. Depending on one's criteria, milestone 3 may never be demonstrated, as the remaining life expectancy of those in a robust state will depend mainly on the unknown future rate of progress. Milestone 4, however, will become known to have been achieved more or less as soon as it is achieved. A transient decline in a cohort's mortality rate may occasionally be seen in the oldest old today, as a result of heterogeneity and small-number effects, so AEV must only refer to cohorts whose mortality rate has never risen high enough to be sensitive to such effects; the cutoff of 20% above is chosen for this purpose. In my view, the likeliest scenario is that AEV will be seen first in a cohort of age 80–90 years, who have benefited from life-extension therapies for 30–40 years and whose mortality rate has thereby peaked at that currently seen in the developed world at the age of 70 years or so.

Plausible Timeframes for Each Milestone

The timeframes I have predicted for RMR and RHR are, respectively:

1. RMR with focused funding of $100 million/year: estimate 2015, unlikely before 2012, very likely by 2020;
2. RMR with sluggish funding (comparable to current): estimate 2025, unlikely before 2020, very likely by 2040;
3. Lag between the attainment of RMR and of RHR: estimate 15 years, unlikely within 5 years, could take an arbitrarily long time.

These projections need not overly concern us here, however, because the question on which demographers have tended to take issue with me is that of the other two milestones enumerated above. Though they may be inclined to share the view of many biogerontologists that my timeframes for RMR and RHR are overoptimistic, they (mostly) recognize that which biogerontologists are right and which wrong remains to be seen. What exercises them are my assertions that:

I. LEV will probably be achieved at around the same time as RHR;
II. AEV will follow shortly thereafter.

Therefore, I will now describe in detail how I derive these predictions.

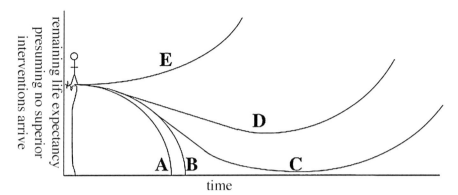

FIGURE 1. Actuarial escape velocity, explained by analogy with literal escape velocity. Remaining life expectancy follows a similar trajectory whether one walks off a cliff or merely ages: the timescales differ, but one's prognosis worsens with time. Mitigation of this (whether by upward jet propulsion or by rejuvenation therapies) merely postpones the outcome if too mild or begun too late, but sufficiently powerful intervention begun soon enough overcomes the force of gravity or aging and increasingly distances the individual from a sticky end. The plausible ages at the time first-generation rejuvenation therapies arrive of people following the respective trajectories are: A = 100, B = 80, C = 50, D = 30, E = 0. (Adapted with permission from de Grey.[12])

WHY LEV WILL PROBABLY ROUGHLY COINCIDE WITH RHR

Predictions here, illustrated in FIGURE 1, are based on the aforementioned rejuvenative character of these therapies, which by definition makes them inapplicable to those too young to have accumulated much age-related, pathogenic damage. Those who are already frail (FIG. 1, trajectories A and B) may not derive much benefit either, at least not from the first-generation rejuvenation therapies. Thus, the first beneficiaries will probably be those in middle age, 55 years say, with about 30 years still to live in the absence of rejuvenation therapies. Suppose these therapies achieve RHR as defined above, setting back frailty and death by at least 30 years. During those 30 years, the previously 55-year-old beneficiaries of those therapies will exhibit a mortality rate less than just before the therapies were first begun. Other things being equal, by the time they reach 85 years this group's mortality rate will have returned to that at pretreatment level and will then continue to rise, much as would have occurred without the therapies (but at a chronologically older age).

But other things will not be equal, because by then there will have been improvements to the treatments, which will have depressed this cohort's mortality rate. How much will it have been depressed? The most reliable measure is precedent from other technologies, whether medical or otherwise, during periods when they were amenable to cumulative, incremental improvements rather than requiring fundamental breakthroughs (as these therapies can be

TABLE 2. Major milestones in the history of powered flight

Milestone	Date
First attempt at flight	Prehistoric
First powered flight	1903
First transatlantic flight	1927
First commercial jetliner	1949
First supersonic airliner	1969

NOTE: Each milestone was barely imaginable at the time the previous one was achieved. The chronological intervals would be quite similar for many other technologies. It seems that while fundamental breakthroughs take unpredictably long, incremental advances (when driven by sufficient market pressure) occur at a rather uniform rate. This gives cause for optimism that RHR will suffice to achieve LEV.

anticipated to be in this phase). TABLE 2 illustrates the rate at which our prowess at powered flight advanced following the Wright brothers' initial achievement; each milestone listed is far enough beyond the previous one as to be technologically unimaginable to the previous milestone's achievers. A remarkably similar rate of progress occurred in computing, in DNA sequencing, and in the combatting of infectious diseases, to name but three areas of advancement. Thus, the life extension afforded by RHR is very likely to suffice to put its beneficiaries beyond LEV. As the improvement in treatment increasingly outstrips the rate of aging (i.e., as we maintain a rate of improvement in excess of escape velocity), this group's mortality rate will fall back to that currently experienced at the age of 40 years or lower (FIG. 1, trajectory C).

Next let us consider the trajectory of someone 20 years younger, that is, 30 years when the first rejuvenation therapies arrive. Such people—again assuming access to nearly state-of-the-art treatments—will not be suitable subjects for those treatments until perhaps 10 years after they have arrived, and thus after they have been tested on older people and their major safety shortcomings thereby identified and addressed. Hence, following the sequence of events rehearsed for the older cohort, it is likely that they will not appreciably advance beyond the mortality rate of today's 50-year-olds at any point, and indeed will not for long exceed that of today's 40-year-olds (FIG. 1, trajectory D).

A similar degree of confidence can be attached to the lag between LEV and AEV. Here the argument concerns sociopolitical dynamics rather than technology. Our projections of how society will respond to the arrival of RMR and RHR are clearly speculation, but we can confidently expect the achievement of RMR to convince society that RHR is foreseeable. My view is that it will promptly become impossible to get elected except on a manifest commitment to a "Manhattan Project" to achieve RHR as quickly as the science allows. I call this phase the "War on Aging" by analogy with Nixon's "War on Cancer"—but in fact the latter was a misnomer, being merely a doubling or so of funding for cancer research. The War on Aging will be a real war, in that society will choose to make sacrifices hitherto seen only in wartime in order to end the "slaughter" as soon as possible;[14,15] the hypothetical concerns of bioconservatives[16,17] will be forgotten as rapidly as they were when *in vitro* fertilization was perfected. And since ending the slaughter means achieving AEV, not just LEV, society will have already made the decision to expedite AEV before RHR even arrives, by voting for the high taxes needed to train enough medical personnel, etc.

CONSEQUENCES FOR COHORT LIFE EXPECTANCY

What does this mean for the life expectancies of the cohorts illustrated by trajectories C and D? We can easily compute this by reference to today's mortality rates at various ages, together with assumptions concerning the aging-independent mortality rates that the cohorts can be expected to experience. The latter are of necessity highly speculative, but I feel sure that risk aversion will rise at individual and national levels, leading to an increasing rarity of death from accidents, homicide, or war, and then to a mortality rate from aging-independent causes, which somewhat exceeds the best achieved at any age for each such cause at present. An order-of-magnitude estimate of mortality from age-independent causes is thus in the region of 10^{-4} per year, leading to a life expectancy in the complete absence of age-related mortality in the high thousands of years. Note that this is not materially altered by infant mortality: just as today's life expectancy cannot be much increased by further inroads into the already low mortality rates of infants in the developed world,[18] so in a world in which the mortality rates of young adults are retained indefinitely, the difference between life expectancy assuming a mortality rate of 10^{-4} from birth and that assuming an infant (and childhood) mortality rate equal to today's is also small.

To estimate the mean age at death of the cohorts discussed above, therefore, we now consider today's mortality rates from age-dependent causes at the ages in question. The older cohort described above (FIG. 1, trajectory C) will spend a few to several decades with a mortality rate exceeding that of today's 50-year-olds, and maybe a majority of that time at a mortality rate over twice that. Much of this cohort will die in that period, leading to a projected life expectancy for the cohort in the low hundreds of years. The younger cohort (FIG. 1 trajectory D), on the other hand, is projected to have the mortality rate of today's 50-year-olds only briefly and to return to that of those under 40 years today, which they will maintain for the remainder of their adult life. Their mean age at death is thus projected to exceed 1,000 years and, given the considerations regarding aging-independent mortality outlined above, may well exceed 5,000 years. Even if the timeframe predictions noted above for RMR and RHR are overoptimistic by a factor of five, therefore, cohorts born toward the end of the 21st century may well have a life expectancy exceeding 5,000 years.[19]

EXTRAPOLAHOLIC CHALLENGES TO THE SCENARIO
DISCUSSED HERE

The sheer magnitude of the dislocation in life expectancy and related statistics described here has led some demographers to throw up their hands
and ridicule it without according it the rigorous scrutiny that they employ
elsewhere.

Perhaps the most ill-considered argument is based on the astronomical reduction of age-specific mortality rates that would be required to achieve four-digit
life expectancies if it occurred at the same rate at all ages, or else with the
same ratio of rates at different ages as has been seen in the past century.[2] Quite
plainly, no such scenario is being predicted, so this is a transparent straw man
to those familiar with life tables, Gompertz distributions, and the like and has
no effect other than to mislead less knowledgeable readers into viewing something as absurd for invalid reasons. It is irrelevant that no sustained change in
the Gompertz slope has been seen in human populations hitherto: we are no
more talking about the smooth continuation of past trends in mortality rates
than we would talk of contemporary transAtlantic travel being a continuation
of 19th century trends. In 1900, extrapolation of trends in the speed of ocean-
going liners over the previous century or two would have predicted that the
time taken to travel from London to Washington D.C. in 2004 would be at
least a couple of weeks. I happen to be writing this paragraph while in tran-
sit on just such a trip, which began three hours ago and will end four hours
hence.

Sociological concerns other than inequality of access are also relevant to
the transition from LEV to AEV, as others have noted.[20] However, here again
the conclusion that life-span increase rates will be severely limited is decid-
edly hasty. The United States is perhaps not the best current example of a
nation in which increased length of life has translated into a greater respect
for the value of life, but in Europe the abandonment of the death penalty
and the increasing restrictions on firearms ownership are conspicuous manifestations of a change in attitudes, perhaps also exemplified by that con-
tinent's avoidance of any wars for almost 60 years (a duration last seen in
Roman times[21]). Death from infectious diseases in a world in which life spans
are potentially unlimited is similarly prone to overestimation: the main reason they are such a threat today is the purely financial fact that vaccines
are not very profitable, something which (as noted above) will not be al-
lowed to influence the situation. Obesity, another major cause of death in
the developed world and especially in the United States,[22] will cease to be
a major risk factor for death, simply because treating it will be an intrinsic
part (and a rather simple and cheap part at that) of the rejuvenation therapy
itself.

A third challenge involves the distinction between intrinsic and extrinsic
mortality, with the former being considered as caused by aging and the latter

not. It has been noted for some time[18] that the complete elimination of all major age-related diseases would extend life span by only a couple of decades; hence, it is argued, a rise of even a century in life expectancy is utterly fanciful. Yet, various researchers have calculated (as noted earlier) that a life expectancy in the region of 1,000 years would result from the indefinite possession of a mortality rate seen in young teenagers in wealthy societies today. The apparent paradox is no paradox at all, as it arises only from the over-restrictive definition of "age-related diseases" to include only causes that end up on death certificates and rarely kill the young. Death from some major causes that can afflict the young (such as road accidents) are much more life-threatening to the elderly because they are frail—in other words, because of aging.

CONCLUSION

Ultimately, all the fits of knee-jerk incredulity just listed have the same basis: in general, demographers are simply unwilling to regard the scenario of successful intervention in aging as plausible in the first place, so when impelled to opine on the demographic scenarios that would result from such interventions they opine instead on scenarios in which aging still exists but less obviously so. These are straw-man arguments of the first order: demographers should avoid this temptation. They are as entitled as anyone to express their opinions concerning the likely rate of biomedical progress, but they do not truly fulfill their professional obligations to the society that trained and funds them if they apply their specialist skills to compute the demographic outcomes only of the biomedical scenarios that they favor and not of alternative scenarios predicted by nondemographers. By the time we know for certain whose biomedical predictions are correct, it will be too late to fully undo the policy errors resulting from erroneous assumptions made as a result of this incomplete provision of information to policy makers. Society therefore needs—and is entitled to expect—demographers to set their biomedical opinions to one side for long enough to advise society of the demographic consequences if those opinions are wrong.

This is even clearer when one recalls that demographers are precisely the group who best appreciate how acute will be the problems facing society in coming decades if population aging is not accompanied by biomedical advances of the magnitude of RHR. Hence, just as in the case of biogerontologists who shun debate on such matters,[23–25] it is particularly unfortunate that they risk delaying RHR, LEV, and AEV by overconfidently touting their impossibility and thus dissuading society from working toward them. Recently, Olshansky and colleagues published an article explicitly focused on the biological basis for their pessimism about extreme life extension;[26] whether or not one considers its logic biologically naïve, we should hope that its publication sets a trend.

REFERENCES

1. OEPPEN, J. & J.W. VAUPEL. 2002. Broken limits to life expectancy. Science **296:** 1029–1031.
2. OLSHANSKY, S.J., B.A. CARNES & A. DESESQUELLES. 2001. Prospects for human longevity. Science **291:** 1491–1492.
3. OLSHANSKY, S.J., B.A. CARNES & R.N. BUTLER. 2001. If humans were built to last. Sci. Am. **284:** 50–55.
4. OLSHANSKY, S.J., L. HAYFLICK & B.A. CARNES. 2002. No truth to the fountain of youth. Sci. Am. **286:** 92–95.
5. CARNES, B.A., S.J. OLSHANSKY & D. GRAHN. 1998. Confronting the boundaries of human longevity. Am. Sci. **86:** 52.
6. HO, A. 2001. Live to 125? In your dreams. Straits Times, March 10.
7. FAUBER, J. 2001. As life spans stretch, new thoughts arise on age-old issues of aging. Milwaukee Journal Sentinel April 13.
8. DE GREY, A.D.N.J. 2005. "The rate of aging": a counterproductively undefinable term. Rejuvenation Res. **8:** 77–78.
9. DE GREY, A.D.N.J., B.N. AMES, J.K. ANDERSEN, et al. 2002. Time to talk SENS: critiquing the immutability of human aging. Ann. N.Y. Acad. Sci. **959:** 452–462.
10. DE GREY, A.D.N.J. 2003. An engineer's approach to the development of real anti-aging medicine. Sci. Aging Knowledge Environ. **2003:** vp 1.
11. DE GREY, A.D.N.J. 2003. Challenging but essential targets for genuine anti-ageing drugs. Expert Opin. Ther. Targets **7:** 1–5.
12. DE GREY, A.D.N.J. 2004. Escape velocity: why the prospect of extreme human life extension matters now. PLoS Biol. **2:** 723–726.
13. DE GREY, A.D.N.J. 2005. Foreseeable and more distant rejuvenation therapies. In Aging Interventions and Therapies. S.I.S. Rattan, Ed.:379–395. World Scientific. Singapore.
14. CAPLAN, A. 2004. Arthur Caplan: interview by Vicki Glaser. Rejuvenation Res. **7:** 148–153.
15. PERRY, D. 2004. Someone's knocking on the laboratory door. Rejuvenation Res. **7:** 49–52.
16. HURLBUT, W.B. 2005. William Hurlbut: interview by Vicki Glaser. Rejuvenation Res. **8:** 110–122.
17. DE GREY, A.D.N.J. 2005. The ethical status of efforts to postpone aging: a reply to Hurlbut. Rejuvenation Res, **8:** 129–130.
18. OLSHANSKY, S.J., B.A. CARNES & C. CASSEL. 1990. In search of Methuselah: estimating the upper limits to human longevity. Science **250:** 634–640.
19. RICHEL, T. 2003. Will human life expectancy quadruple in the next hundred years? Sixty gerontologists say public debate on life extension is necessary. J. Anti-Aging Med. **6:** 309–314.
20. OLSHANSKY, S.J., B.A. CARNES, R.G. ROGERS, et al. 1997. Infectious diseases: new and ancient threats to world health. Popul. Bull. **52:** 1–52.
21. COOK, C., Ed. 1992. Pears Cyclopedia, 100th ed. Pelham Books. London, UK.
22. OLSHANSKY, S.J., D.J. PASSARO, R.C. HERSHOW, et al. 2005. A potential decline in life expectancy in the United States in the 21st century. N. Engl. J. Med. **352:** 1138–1145.
23. DE GREY, A.D.N.J. 2004. Biogerontologists' duty to discuss timescales publicly. Ann. N.Y. Acad. Sci. **1019:** 542–545.

24. DE GREY, A.D.N.J. 2005. Resistance to debate on how to postpone ageing is delaying progress and costing lives. EMBO Rep. **6:** S49–S53.
25. DE GREY, A.D.N.J. 2005. The SENS Challenge: $20,000 says the foreseeable defeat of aging is not laughable. Rejuvenation Res **8:** 207–210.
26. CARNES, B.A., S.J. OLSHANSKY & D. GRAHN. 2003. Biological evidence for limits to the duration of life. Biogerontology **4:** 31–45.

The Value of Life and the Value of Life Extension

STEVEN HORROBIN

School of Law, University of Edinburgh, Old College, Edinburgh, EH8 9YL, UK

ABSTRACT: Recent developments in aging research have added new urgency to the bioethical debate concerning life and death issues, the value of life, and the reasonable limits of medicine. This paper analyzes the basic structures of the liberal and conservative components of this debate, showing that there has hitherto been inadequate analysis on both sides concerning the nature and implications of the value of life, as well as, and as distinct from the value of life extension. Classic concepts of the intrinsic or extrinsic value of life are argued to be tangential or actually irrelevant to the value of life's continuance and so to the value of life extension. An analysis of personhood is proposed which focuses explicitly upon the value of life extension to persons. This analysis shows that persons may only intelligibly be understood as processes, for whom life extension is an inalienable and fundamental value. It is further proposed that, properly understood, such an analysis may significantly narrow the liberal/conservative divide in bioethics.

KEYWORDS: ethics; aging; life extension; longevity; bioethics; conservative; liberal; personhood; intrinsic value; instrumental value; autonomy; suicide; euthanasia; value of life; value of life extension; aging research

THE CONTINGENT AND THE ABSOLUTE IN HUMAN LIFE SPAN: A QUESTIONABLE DICHOTOMY

Interventions in exogenous facts have been capable since time immemorial of altering human life expectancy. Hitherto no human intervention, medical or otherwise, has been capable of altering basic endogenous facts about human aging. This has meant that the human life span itself, as a background aspect of the human condition, has remained unaltered, and indeed unalterable. Our maximum span has remained fixed at an outside possibility of around 120 years, independent of facts about nutrition, wealth, access to medical care, freedom from infectious diseases, or other factors accessible to human agency. Life span, then, has thus far had features that may be described as absolute.

Address for correspondence: Steven Horrobin, School of Law, University of Edinburgh, Old College, Edinburgh, EH8 9YL, U.K. Voice: +44 7769 973 602.
e-mail: s_horrobin@hotmail.com

Ann. N.Y. Acad. Sci. 1067: 94–105 (2006). © 2006 New York Academy of Sciences.
doi: 10.1196/annals.1354.012

In light of advances in our understanding of the mechanisms of aging and our increasing capacity to influence fundamental endogenous biology, driven primarily by advances in the genetic sciences, the time may now be approaching when we will have the capacity to render this previously *de facto* noncontingent absolute space of human life span contingent and accessible to human intervention.[1,2]

AN EMERGING FEATURE OF THE LIBERAL–CONSERVATIVE DIVIDE IN BIOETHICS: A SURPRISING CASE OF INVERSION

Hitherto, bioethical debate concerning life and death issues has focused upon those issues that fall within the scope of the classically contingent human life span: for example, suicide, euthanasia, and abortion. The emerging debate concerning the ethics of radical interventions in human basic biology, which may have the effect of fundamental extension in human life span, has resulted in what appears, *prima facie*, a surprising inversion in some traditional positions regarding the bioethics of the preservation of human or person-instantiated life, and its end in death.

Traditionally, those of a predominantly "conservative"[a3] ethical persuasion, who are likely to be representatives of organized religions, or else to accept in some way content-full canonical ethical schemas that hold to the universal objectivity of at least some ethical principles,[4] have been inclined to describe themselves as being "pro-life" in all decisions concerning the ending of life. Thus they have tended to be anti-abortion, anti-suicide, and anti-euthanasia.[4–6] Those of predominantly "liberal" ethical persuasion are likely to be secular and to reject canonical, content-full moral schemas as well as assertions of true objectivity in ethics, holding that moral judgments do not generally or at all refer to objective normative values and should rather fit the pragmatic social and subjective aspects of any particular or general situation. These liberal ethicists have been inclined to describe themselves as "pro-choice," focusing upon the value of autonomy to persons, and so tending to be (*ex hypothesi*) *conditionally* pro-abortion, pro-suicide, and pro-euthanasia.[7,8]

One might have expected that, in the face of (purportedly) new questions about whether or not human or person-instantiated life should be indefinitely extended, the prejudices or commitments would run on similar lines, with the conservatives in favor, in relative harmony with the liberals, who would favor, as elsewhere, autonomous individual choice on the matter.[9] Curiously, however, in the case of the conservatives, the reverse is in fact generally true:

[a]The use of the terms "conservative" and "liberal" here are admittedly problematic. They are used as shorthand for clarity within this short essay. However, they do usefully refer to broad groupings of bioethical conviction as described by S. Holland: "The fault line is between life's intrinsic value, the sanctity view and conservatism, on the one side, and the subjective and instrumental value of life, the quality view and liberalism, on the other."[3] p. 58.

faced with such a prospect, bioethical conservatives have sought strongly to condemn any such intervention.[10–14]

How comes it that with regard to the extension of basic human life span the conservatives' ethical shoe, so to speak, is on the other foot?

CONSERVATIVE INTERPRETATIONS OF THE VALUE OF LIFE

In the canonical schema from which classic and modern conservative positions regarding the value of life and attitudes to life and death issues generally arise, the values of the bodily and fleshly life have traditionally been held to be of secondary importance, worldly concerns that obscure and abstract away from the true and underlying value of existence: the life of the *soul* in its eternal relationship with the Divine.

Adherence to such a schema *alone* is obviously impractical and self-limiting, as it would be inimical to the maintenance of a functioning ethics of the bodily living world. Religious and socially conservative movements have therefore formulated various strategies to defend more "pro- (bodily) life" positions. These additional schemas for grounding the ethics of bodily life and death may generally be described as concepts of the sanctity of life.[8]

The Sanctity of Life and the Role of Prerogative

Essentially, on this view, "sanctity" implies "inviolability." There are two basic ways in which life may be held as "sacred" and so "inviolable": the intrinsic and the extrinsic. Intrinsic concepts of the sanctity of life are exemplified by such schemas as the Jain idea that *all* life is manifestation of embodied divinity and as such is sacred and inviolable. This schema and its cousins differs, therefore, from those which generally motivate conservative positions in life and death ethics, as they appear in the West, since it locates divine value *within* the bodily world.[b]

Despite the frequent use of the term "intrinsic" value by conservative and religious ethicists, the underlying value of which they generally speak is extrinsic in nature. According to the schema of the Abrahamic religions, and therefore that from which conservative ethical positions in the West have generally arisen, life is held to be inviolable not because it is sacred or valuable in and of itself, but rather because life is held to be a divine "gift."[8] Its sanctity is therefore extrinsic, being underwritten by the external authority of divinity. An understanding of the mechanics of this concept and its more secular cousins

---

[b]Such schemas suffer other equally vexing practical problems, however, such as the obvious difficulty of being committed to argue that the lives of individual bacteria or viruses may have real and intrinsic value, and the difficulty of determining how such a value may be balanced with the value of a *person's* life. Are they really commensurate, or even commensurable?

is key to understanding the motivations behind the curious "inversion," noted above.

Essentially, the doctrine is that life is a gift to the person who is alive, and the willful rejection of this gift (so, suicide) or else the taking under whatever circumstances of it away from another (so, murder and also abortion and euthanasia) are infringements of the divine *prerogatives*, which the giver (God) is held to retain over this gift.[c]

The inversion focuses upon the notion of *prerogative* in this schema of the value of life and an intuition concerning the implications of this as regards endogenous longevity. If it is the case that life itself is fundamentally a gift "designed" and "ordained" by God, then the fundamental circumstances that attend it, such as the endogenous span of the lives of humans, will be held to be similarly part of the ordained design, which is a frame of the gift itself, and so falls within divine prerogative.[d]

There are significant problems with this picture of life's value. The first problem is that, in the absence of a belief in or warrant for the *particular* concept of the divine that underwrites it, or in the presence of wholly secular convictions, this conception gives no grounds or explanation whatever for the value of bodily life.

Further, as David Hume pointed out,[15] if it is accounted that we may infringe God's prerogative by the *taking* of life and so altering the divine timing of death, we may apparently similarly infringe the divine prerogative by intervening to *save* a life as well, whether by exogenous or endogenous medical intervention, or indeed by any means whatever.

There is a nexus between arguments concerning the prerogative of humans versus the prerogative of God, and those concerning the prerogative of humans versus the province of the "natural," which is somehow held to be morally prime. The latter is commonly used as a fall-back position in an attempt to secularize what is essentially a religious schema.[e][16] That this is intuitively widely accepted is evidenced by the common acceptance of at least the sense of the notion that human interference, say, in the human genome, would constitute a clear case of "playing God" *as well* as being "against nature." In view of this we may clearly see why, in conservative canonical religious or content-full bioethics, this inversion takes place. What is fundamentally objected to is *not* that persons will enjoy more life. Rather, it is an expansion of the area of human contingent influence, and thus the prerogative that is so uncomfortable for this

---

[c]It is noteworthy that the retention of prerogatives by the "giver" here already abstracts away from any ordinary definition of "gift." Furthermore, the idea that a basic predicate of existence may be "given" to the one who then exists is philosophically dubious. If life is a gift, *to whom* is it a gift? How can *my* life be a gift *to me*?

[d]The idea that humans are made in the "image" of God, and also that death through aging arises from Original Sin form part of this schema. Further, this nexus of ideas is what fundamentally motivates the conservative view that *biological* humanity is co-extensive with personhood, and thus moral respect.

[e]Callahan and his followers, for example, use the "natural" in essence as a surrogate for the "ordained."

view. The supposedly "pro-life" positions are not, then, "pro-life" at all, *as the conservative opposition to radical life extension uncomfortably reveals*. Rather, they are "*anti-prerogative*" or "anti-choice" as regards human agency over fundamental biological predicates.

Among others, I have elsewhere rejected the idea that humans can intervene in nature in a way that is beyond the scope of and so harms the natural, and should therefore have limited prerogative so to intervene.[f][17–19] Essentially, the "natural" can only rationally be understood to be that set of things, which is within space and time, which obviously includes humans and the product of all human agency. Hume basically agrees with this and denies that we may infringe God's prerogative, since if extant at all, it is *pervasive* as nature itself and applies to all our possible acts.[15]

Furthermore, conservative ethicists commonly accept the reasonableness of the human prerogative to combat diseases both exogenous and endogenous, through both exogenous and endogenous means. In absence of a clear reason why exogenous interventions in human lifespan are fundamentally, and relevantly different from endogenous interventions, and why aging itself is distinct from its associated infirmities, a position that denies our prerogative to extend life by endogenous means appears seriously inconsistent. No such relevant clear reason may be found.[g][1,20]

INTRINSIC AND EXTRINSIC CONCEPTS OF THE VALUE OF LIFE AND THE VALUE OF LIFE EXTENSION: A CRITIQUE OF THE CONSERVATIVE POSITION

Usually, liberals engage in the kind of critique given above to reject conservative conceptions of life's value, but this may not be necessary. The important question to ask is: even if such a value may coherently be established, can *any* concept of the intrinsic or extrinsic value of life tell us anything about whether it is good that life should be *extended*? It would appear, *prima facie*, that they should and could. But an analysis of the situation will, perhaps surprisingly, reveal the opposite conclusion.

Both intrinsic and extrinsic concepts of the value of life, such as that of the Sanctity of Life, are *ex hypothesi* devoid of reference to the conditions or circumstances of life itself, as lived by the living. This being so, a life is held to have value *whatever* the subjective state or physical situation of a living being.[h] Life, in the intrinsic or extrinsic (conservative) view, then, is held to have an *absolute* value.

---

[f] Further, the claim that nature is morally prime commits the "naturalistic fallacy."

[g] The distinction here is between "aging" and "disease." But ask: can one die of healthy old age? If not, is there such thing as aging *without* disease? If not, what remains of the notion of aging, beyond mere chronological extension?

[h] It is chiefly this intuition that motivates conservative ethicists to assert the moral impropriety of ending the lives of embryos, as well as those in a persistent vegetative state etc. Assertions as

But if this is so, then it must mean that this value is, in essence, *bivalent*. It cannot be diminished or added to, and obtains *in whole* for as long as any living being is actually alive, *regardless* of the subjective states, values, or concerns of that being, and is annulled on death. On the intrinsic or extrinsic view, if a creature lives for one day, the value of its life is absolute and whole; if it lives 30 years its value is the same, etc. If this is so, then given that all biological organisms are mortal, and will inevitably die *at some point*, it appears to make *no difference whatever to the intrinsic or extrinsic value of life of these beings whether they die at one time, rather than at another.* The total value outcome is unchanged by more or less extension in time.

On this analysis it seems, then, that the only thing we can learn from such a concept of the value of life is whether or not it is good to have lived *at all.* It appears clear that if this analysis is accepted, we must abandon any idea that such a value of life is useful in evaluating questions with regard to life *extension.* Furthermore, those who hold to it may be seriously mistaken as to its implications, possibly to the extent that it cannot be used as a basis even for concepts of inviolability, since life-ending action itself, without reference to subjective or similarly conditional considerations, will merely be accounted to be an alteration of the *timing* of death, which is hereby shown to be irrelevant to this value!

Given that conservatives seem most concerned about cases of the ending of life, it appears clear that if they wish to assert that their concern here is not simply a matter of prerogative, what the conservatives really wish to underwrite is not the value of life, *per se*, but rather the value of life's *continuance.* It thus appears clear that, in holding to such principles to underwrite the value of life's continuance, they are barking up the wrong tree.

SUBJECTIVIST IDEAS OF VALUE: THE LIBERAL VIEW

Liberal concepts of the value of life begin by asking the question: what is value? The answer to this question, on the liberal view, is roughly that values are not part of the furniture of the universe in the manner that objects are.[21] Values have no objective ontological status, independent of subjective *valuers*, who are described as valuing agents. On the liberal interpretation of utilitarian ethics, for example, what is "good" is defined with respect to the subjective preferences of valuing agents. It remains, therefore, to identify what are the basic requirements for a being to qualify for the status of "valuing agent." Essentially, these requirements are held to be that a valuing agent, at a minimum, must possess the features of self-consciousness, autonomy, and rationality.[22] Beings that possess these three features are generally considered,

to the *potential* of life to develop sentient, self-conscious states self-evidently refers to subjective considerations that are beyond the scope of this value, and lie, instead, within the province of subjectivist (liberal) interpretations of life's value.

on the liberal view, to be persons. Thus while all valuing agents are persons, not all humans are necessarily persons, and not all persons are necessarily human.[i] Given these considerations, on the liberal view, the value of life is the value of life to *persons.*

OBJECTIVITY, SUBJECTIVITY, AND PERSONHOOD—THE DIVIDE REVISITED AND A PROBLEM WITH THE LIBERAL VIEW

The divide is not as great as it may *prima facie* appear. After all, the religious canonical picture holds that it is in fact a moral agent, God, who is the valuer of the entire universe and everything in it. He is thus the guarantor of objective value *in the universe,* but this value is in fact of a fundamentally *subjective* character: it depends upon the will and authority of God.[j] Further, the subjectivist picture is not as purely subjective as it may first appear. After all, there exists a *universal* requirement, in the subjectivist liberal view, that values are derived from persons, and that persons *must* possess certain basic requirements. The dignity and value of persons in the liberal view therefore have something of an objective quality.

What then is the fundamental character of the fault line between the two views? The problem is that liberals object to the warrant for and coherence of the supposedly objectivist conservative bases of value, (e.g., the existence, location, and authority of the underwriter of objectivity), whereas the conservatives object to the apparent *whimsicality* of the subjectivist liberal position.[k] The problem then lies in a matter, once again, of prerogative. The conservatives are suspicious of the liberals' insistence, above all, on the *strength* of the principle of autonomy in their conception of value. Many liberals do in fact insist upon the idea that autonomous subjective preferences can themselves determine or influence the status of the apparently otherwise objective value of persons. An example would be the common liberal insistence upon the moral propriety of physician-assisted suicide, if sufficient autonomous force of preference is brought to bear.

The problem is that this insistence on an essentially limitless scope for autonomy, impinging as it does even upon the supposedly universal value of persons,

---

[i]On this view, an example of a human non-person would be an anencephalic baby, or one born with all organs and other physical structures intact, often including a brain-stem, but without any "higher" brain structures, such as cortex, that are necessary for consciousness. Examples of non-human persons might arguably be: chimpanzees and gorillas; bioengineered persons who are so far divergent from biological humans that they can no longer qualify as such (because, for example, breeding species barriers have arisen); intelligent extraterrestrials; or, indeed, God, should One exist!

[j]This will not, of course, apply to purely naturalistic interpretations of objective value.

[k]Of course, in the canonical view, the value of life is explicitly subject to the whim of the deity, hence the insistence upon "trust" in and fear of God.

suggests that values are indeed *fundamentally* subjective and determined, at base, solely by the subjective preferences of individual persons.[1]

In addition, if there is any merit in the concept of the universality of the value of persons as being the source of all subjective value, then, *on its own*, such a value would remain of an intrinsic and categoric nature. The above analysis of the lack of role that any intrinsic value in underpinning or explaining the value of continued existence shows that, in default of a subjective *endorsement* of the value of continuing life, this value really does evaporate, and so is whimsical in nature.

This is a serious difficulty for the liberal position, for if the value of life's continuance genuinely does rely solely upon the continued existence of an *instrumental* value of living according solely to the subjective preferences of persons, then it is indeed a whimsical value, and as such seems a dangerously poor candidate for so dignified a role. The question remains, then: how to resolve this issue? An analysis that leads both to the recognition of an indivisible link between the categoric and subjective aspects of the value of persons, together with a weakening of the view that a person's autonomous will can in reality have the effect of removing instrumental value from continued existence for that person, would appear to resolve this issue, and would constitute an extremely solid basis for the assertion of a fundamental value of continued life for persons. If such an analysis were successful, it would appear to obviate the whimsicality of this value, about which the conservatives are so concerned. In so doing, it may significantly narrow the gulf that currently bedevils bioethics.

A PROPOSED AMENDMENT TO THE LIBERAL VIEW: PERSONHOOD AS *PROCESS* AND THE VALUE OF LIFE EXTENSION

The classic liberal picture of value, based in the value of personhood, is incomplete. While it may be accepted that self-consciousness, autonomy, and rationality are necessary for personhood and for valuing activity to take place, they are insufficient. There is a further requirement that has often been neglected: the requirement for *significant* extension of the person in *time*.[23] A being that possesses all of these three attributes but has no extension in time does not exist, and is therefore not a *real* person. But can a being that has these attributes and that exists for merely *some* time be accounted to be a person? Imagine a being with these attributes that exists for merely a nanosecond. It appears intuitively that such a being cannot be accounted to be a person. This is because what it is to be a person is not merely to be possessed of these

---

[1]The force and function of *collective* preference ultimately arises from individual preferences and so is held *ceteris paribus* for the purposes of this article.

attributes and to exist, *but also to use* these attributes to engage in valuing activity in the world. A being that cannot do so by virtue of having insufficient temporal *scope* cannot be accounted as fully *being* a valuing agent and is not, therefore, a person.

For beings to be accorded the dignity of personhood, they must possess sufficient scope in time to take part in the *process* of valuing. Thus personhood may be seen to be necessarily a *process*, rather than simply a categorical state. This process of personhood is composed of desires, wishes, hopes, preferences, thoughts, plans, actions, experiences, emotions, memories, etc. These and the *temporally extended* interchanges between them are both necessary for and *indivisible from* valuing activity, *and thus the existence of persons*, and together they constitute the value of *living*.[17]

The value of *living*, then, is an instrumental *as well* as a categoric value and so is an *inalienable* value for persons. Neither aspect of this value may be separated from the other, as they are *co-dependent*.

But what can this analysis tell us about the value of *continued* life? The present and backward-directed elements of the process of being a person, such as experience and memory, have *necessary* forward-looking counterparts: hopes, desires, plans, etc. Hoping, desiring, and planning are intrinsically future-directed. Hoping for, desiring, or planning our past is meaningless or futile. Without the constant interchange between the future, present, and past elements of the process of being a person we should be fixed, and frozen, ourselves objectified and unable to fulfill, or even possess, an autonomous *will*, much less formulate rational values, designs, and desires, let alone actualize them. Our rationality, should we still possess it, would sit idle, since a desire to use it, even to analyze the past, is a desire that extends toward the future. Our autonomy would thus be stripped of meaning or potency. The process of valuing and thus being a person would cease, and the *continuance* of being itself would thereby be stripped of its value. Should we lose these future-directed elements of ourselves, then, we would no longer be persons, *and living would have no value*. Further, the desire for future goods is *driven* by the forward-looking aspect of personhood, which in turn represents a *categorical* desire[24] and is not contingent upon there being *particular* goods or objects that are presently identified by a person. The fundamental future-directed element of the process of personhood, this categorical desire, *presupposes the value of the continuation of a person into the future*.

From this view, then, there is then no point in time at which the continuation of a *person's* life may be said not to be valuable, since these forward-directed elements are necessary to the process of being a person. As such, the process of being a person is intrinsically open-ended.

In this way, it would appear that there can be no arbitrary upper limit on the good of the extension of life to a person. There is no point at which being a person does not involve the future-directed elements and their involvement in the process of interchange with the present and past elements. An attempt to set or discover such a general limit would appear to involve a misunderstanding of the nature of the process itself. That we may know some facts about human biology, which suggest that we indeed have an end in store, and even how far in the future that end is likely to be, in no way impinges upon the intrinsic nature of the future-directed elements that are fundamental to the process of being a person. These point toward the ever-distant horizon of the possible, *irrespective* of actual personal circumstances, such as, say, a terminal disease.[25]

If no general limit can arbitrarily be set or discovered, could one be set by a person upon themselves? That my desires, hopes, and plans may fix upon particular objectives does not in itself suggest that I can easily, or at all, fix these elements of myself purely upon and contained within some set of particular objectives, so that the categorical desire itself ends with the completion of this set. No matter what I specifically plan for, desire, or hope for, it seems that these aspects of my psychology overflow the limits of their particular objects without any particular act of will on my part. Furthermore, *willing* these aspects of ourselves to be contained within a fixed, time-limited framework would seem to be impossible. I may seek to direct or curtail my first-order desires (those that simply "I desire") with my second-order desires (those by which "I desire that I do or do not desire"),[26] but that a second-order desire to have *no* desires should be effective would seem impossibly self-defeating. For such a desire *is itself a future-directed desire*, and so arises from the inalienable categoric desire, which is a fundamental part of the process that itself enables the autonomous will to exist. We cannot *effectively* will ourselves not to be a person, while also being one, since that will *itself requires us to be a person*. Try to imagine a person setting a particular date beyond which she will be free of *all* desires. Such a picture strikes one as absurd. Further, if it is acknowledged that a person, in any particular moment of the extended process of their personhood, is rarely or never conscious of *all* the particular desires they themselves possess, much less the general and categoric desire that gives rise to them, this observation becomes greatly stronger. So it does not seem reasonable that a person may even set a limit to the good of *their own* future extension in time.

So long as we are persons, therefore, life extension will be a value without limitation.

CONCLUSION

Neither classical conservative nor standard liberal pictures of value can successfully underwrite a value of life extension, or the continuing life of persons. The personhood as process view, however, both explains and demonstrates the inalienable quality of this value. Further, it shows how personal autonomy does not extend to the reflexive denial of personhood, and so it cannot extend to the denial of the value of a person's own continued life, much less that of another.

This, then, provides a profound objection to the ethical propriety of suicide, based in a liberal subjectivist schema, as well as establishing a value of continued life for persons, which is far more stable than that which has generally formed the basis of liberal bioethical conceptions of value. This analysis may therefore substantially obviate the concern as to whimsicality, which has perhaps justifiably underwritten much of the suspicion that bioethical conservatives have harbored toward the liberal view.

REFERENCES

1. KIRKWOOD, T. 2001. Time of Our Lives: The Science of Human Aging. Oxford University Press. Oxford.
2. RATTAN, S. Ed. 2005. Aging Interventions and Therapies. World Scientific Publishing. Singapore.
3. HOLLAND, S. 2003. Bioethics: A Philosophical Introduction. Polity Press. Cambridge.
4. CALLAHAN, D. & C.S. CAMPBELL, Eds. 1990. Theology, Religious Traditions, and Bioethics. Hastings Center Rep. 1990 Jul–Aug; **20:** S1.
5. BERNARDIN, JOSEPH, CARDINAL. 1988. Euthanasia: ethical and legal challenge. Origins **18:** 52–1.
6. KASS, L.R. & N. LUND. 1996. Physician-assisted suicide, medical ethics, and the future of the medical profession. Duquesne Law Rev. **35:** 395–425.
7. GLOVER, J. 1977. Causing Death and Saving Life. Penguin Books. Harmondsworth, UK.
8. KUHSE, H. 1987. The Sanctity-of-Life Doctrine in Medicine: A Critique. Clarendon Press. Oxford.
9. HARRIS, J. 2004. Immortal ethics. Ann. N.Y. Acad. Sci. **1019:** 527–534.
10. KASS, L.R. 2001. L'Chaim and its limits: why not immortality? First Things. **113:** 17–24.
11. KASS, L.R., Chair. 2003. Ageless bodies. *In* Beyond Therapy: A Report of the President's Council on Bioethics. PCBE, Washington DC, pp. 157–201.
12. CALLAHAN, D. 1995. What Kind of Life? The Limits of Medical Progress. Georgetown University Press. Washington, DC.
13. FUKUYAMA, F. 2002. Our Posthuman Future: Consequences of the Biotechnology Revolution. Farrar, Straus, & Giroux, New York, NY.
14. MEILANDER, G. 2002. Genes as resources. Hedgehog Review **4:** 66–79.
15. HUME, D. 1978. On Suicide. *In* Ethical Issues in Death and Dying. T. L. Beauchamp & S. Perlin Eds.: 105–110. Prentice-Hall, Englewood Cliffs, NJ.
16. CALLAHAN, D. 1987. Setting Limits: Medical Goals in an Aging Society. Simon & Schuster Inc. New York, NY.
17. HORROBIN, S. 2005. The ethics of aging intervention and life-extension. *In* Aging Interventions and Therapies. S. Rattan Ed. World Scientific Publishing, Singapore.
18. MILL, J.S. 1998. On nature. *In* Three Essays on Religion: Nature, the Utility of Religion, Theism. Prometheus Books. New York, NY.
19. MILLAR, A. 1988. Following nature. Philos. Quart. **38:** 165–185.
20. CAPLAN, A. 2004. An unnatural process: why it is not inherently wrong to seek a cure for aging. *In* The Fountain of Youth: Cultural, Scientific, and Ethical

Perspectives on a Biomedical Goal. S.G. Post & R.H. Binstock, Eds. Oxford University Press. Oxford.

21. MACKIE, J.L. 1990. Ethics: Inventing Right and Wrong. Penguin. London.
22. FAN, R. 2000. Can we have a general conception of personhood in bioethics? *In* The Moral Status of Persons. Perspectives in Bioethics. G.K. Becker Ed.: Rodopi: Amsterdam/Atlanta, GA.
23. HEIDEGGER, M. 2004. Dasein and temporality. *In* Being and Time. Blackwell. Oxford, pp. 274–278.
24. WILLIAMS, B. 1973. The Makropulos case: reflections on the tedium of immortality. *In* Problems of the Self. Cambridge University Press. Cambridge, esp. pp. 86–100.
25. NAGEL, T. 1970. Death. *In* Mortal Questions. Cambridge University Press. Cambridge, pp. 1–10.
26. FRANKFURT, H. 1982. Freedom of the will and the concept of a person. *In* Free Will. Oxford Readings in Philosophy. G. Watson Ed.: 81–95. Oxford University Press, Oxford.

OXPHOS Supercomplexes

Respiration and Life-Span Control in the Aging Model *Podospora anserina*

FRANK KRAUSE,[a] CHRISTIAN Q. SCHECKHUBER,[b]
ALEXANDRA WERNER,[b] SASCHA REXROTH,[a]
NICOLE H. REIFSCHNEIDER,[a] NORBERT A. DENCHER,[a]
AND HEINZ D. OSIEWACZ[b]

[a]*Physical Biochemistry, Department of Chemistry, Darmstadt University
of Technology, Petersenstraße 22, D-64287 Darmstadt, Germany*

[b]*Botanical Institute, Johann Wolfgang Goethe-University,
Marie-Curie-Strasse 9, D-60439 Frankfurt am Main, Germany*

ABSTRACT: Recent biochemical evidence has indicated the existence of respiratory supercomplexes as well as ATP synthase oligomers in the inner mitochondrial membrane of different eukaryotes. We have studied the organization of the respiratory chain of a wild-type strain and of two long-lived mutants of the filamentous fungus *Podospora anserina*. This aging model is able to respire by either the standard or the alternative pathway. In the latter, electrons are directly transferred from ubiquinol to the alternative oxidase (AOX) and thus bypass complexes III and IV. We showed that the two pathways are composed of distinct respiratory supercomplexes. These data are of significance for the understanding of both respiratory pathways as well as of life-span control and aging.

KEYWORDS: aging; alternative oxidase; blue-native electrophoresis; colorless-native electrophoresis; complex I; complex III; cytochrome oxidase; mitochondria; oxidative phosphorylation; respirasome; supercomplex

INTRODUCTION

The inner mitochondrial membrane of eukaryotes as well as the plasma membrane of bacteria contain the four major respiratory complexes I (NADH:ubiquinone oxidoreductase), II (succinate:ubiquinone oxidoreductase), III (ubiquinol:cytochrome c oxidoreductase), and IV (cytochrome c

Address for correspondence: Frank Krause, Physical Biochemistry, Department of Chemistry, Darmstadt University of Technology, Petersenstraße 22, D-64287 Darmstadt, Germany. Voice: +49 6151/165376; fax: +49 6151/164171.
 e-mail: f_krause@pop.tu-darmstadt.de
 www.tu-darmstadt.de/fb/ch/Fachgebiete/BC/AKDencher/index_en.html

Ann. N.Y. Acad. Sci. 1067: 106–115 (2006). © 2006 New York Academy of Sciences.
 doi: 10.1196/annals.1354.013

oxidase, also referred to as COX) of the standard respiratory chain and the F_OF_1-ATP synthase (complex V) cooperatively performing oxidative phosphorylation (OXPHOS), which is responsible for most of the cellular ATP generation.[1] Apart from the standard respiratory chain, plants, some fungi, and protozoa contain alternative respiratory enzymes.[2,3]

Contrary to the prevailing opinion,[4] the "respirasome model" was introduced based on the results by blue-native (BN)-PAGE of efficiently but mildly solubilized bovine heart mitochondria leading to the separation of high yields of stoichiometric respiratory supercomplexes.[5,6] It postulates the quantitative assembly of the mammalian respiratory complexes I, III, and IV into two different supercomplexes ($I_1III_2IV_4$ and III_2IV_4), occurring in a 2:1 ratio, as building blocks of a large supramolecular network in agreement with the stoichiometry of complexes I, III, and IV in bovine heart mitochondria determined to be 1:3:6.[1,6] Indeed, by analyzing digitonin-solubilized mitochondria isolated from fresh bovine heart, with a particular gentle colorless-native (CN)-PAGE, nearly all of the complexes I, III, and IV could be found as supercomplexes.[7]

By means of corresponding approaches, respiratory supercomplexes of identical and/or different compositions, like those in bovine heart mitochondria, were detected in mitochondria of other mammals,[7,8] *Saccharomyces cerevisiae* lacking complex I,[5,9] higher plants[10–13] as well as in bacteria.[14] Concomitantly, significant amounts of dimeric[5–10,12,15,16] or even higher oligomeric ATP synthases[7,16] could be separated.

Of major functional significance to respiratory supercomplexes, an enzymatic advantage, in particular substrate chanelling, was proposed.[5] This is plausible since these supercomplexes represent assemblies of sequential enzymes but substrate challenging is difficult to prove experimentally.[17] Notwithstanding, inhibitor-titration studies indicated that complexes II, III, and IV in yeast[18] and complexes I and III, but not complex IV, in bovine heart mitochondria[19] represent functional units. Another pivotal function of respiratory supercomplexes appears to be stabilization of the individual complexes.[8,14,20,21] ATP synthase oligomerization was demonstrated to be crucially involved in the formation of cristae.[16,22]

Because of its central bioenergetic role, impairments of the OXPHOS machinery lead to severe diseases and are thought to be causatively involved in aging. The latter is conceptualized in the "mitochondrial theory of aging."[23] A paradigm of an organism in which mitochondria play an etiological role in aging is the filamentous fungus *Podospora anserina*. In contrast to almost all other fungi that are capable of infinite growth, all examined wild-type strains of *P. anserina* exhibit a characteristic "senescence syndrome."[24] After prolonged vegetative propagation, the growth rate of the culture decreases and the pigmentation of the mycelium changes. Finally, the filamentous "cells" of the mycelium, the hyphae, die at their tips. These features and the fact that a number of mutants were selected in which the life span is significantly increased led to extensive investigations aimed at understanding the molecular basis of aging in this model system.[25] The life span of *P. anserina* is determined by environmental factors (e.g., growth temperature, nutrition) and by both nuclear as well as extranuclear genetic traits. The most significant insight into the molecular mechanisms involved in life-span control of *P. anserina* is derived from the characterization of different long-lived mutants. Interestingly, some mutants are characterized by impairments of the standard respiratory chain at complex IV. They respire via an alternative oxidase (AOX), which circumvents the electron transport to complexes III and IV and directly transfers electrons from ubiquinol to oxygen.[25] It was demonstrated that respiration via this pathway leads to a reduction in ROS generation.[26] In addition, in such strains the mtDNA was found to be stabilized.[26–30]

Here, we present major results of a recent biochemical study of mitochondrial proteins from juvenile cultures of a wild-type strain (only COX respiration) as well as mutants ex1 (only AOX respiration) and grisea (both COX and AOX respiration) with emphasis on the characterization of the OXPHOS apparatus.[31]

RESULTS AND DISCUSSION

Distinct Respiratory Supercomplexes in Wild-Type and Ex1 Mitochondria

We separated by BN-PAGE proteins from mitochondria of a wild-type strain and of the immortal mutant ex1, which lacks assembled COX on account of the deletion of a mitochondrial gene encoding an essential COX subunit, each solubilized with various digitonin/protein ratios of 2–8 g/g. These conditions enabled near quantitative extraction of the five OXPHOS complexes (FIG. 1). Overall, the pattern of OXPHOS complexes and their supercomplexes of wild-type mitochondria was similar to that of bovine heart mitochondria, whereas ex1 mitochondria displayed significantly lesser amounts of high molecular weight species (FIG. 1). Subsequently, the native protein complexes in the first-dimension BN gel were dissociated during a second-dimension SDS-PAGE, leading to the migration of single subunits according to their apparent mass in a vertical line below their position in the first-dimension BN-PAGE and thus allowing the identification of the OXPHOS complexes.[31] In the wild-type mitochondria, most of the complexes I and III were found assembled together in three supercomplexes, each with a single copy of monomeric complex I and dimeric complex III as well as 0–2 copies of complex IV (FIG. 1, a–c). The most abundant supercomplex with an apparent molecular mass of $\sim$1,700 kDa was b ($I_1III_2IV_1$). As in the case of mammalian mitochondria,[5] the stability of supercomplexes was hardly affected by the digitonin/protein ratio, at least until 8 g/g. Importantly, the separated supercomplexes a–c were enzymatically active, as demonstrated by in-gel staining of NADH-dehydrogenase and cytochrome c oxidase activities according to their content of complex I and IV.[31]

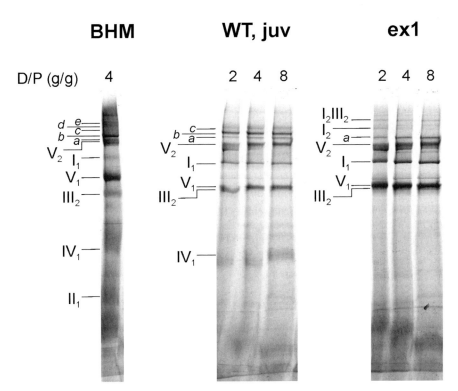

FIGURE 1. Distinct OXPHOS supercomplexes in mitochondria of *P. anserina* wild-types and of COX-free mutant ex1, respectively. BN-PAGE of digitonin extracts of juvenile wild-type s mitochondria (*WT, juv*) and mutant ex1 mitochondria, each solubilized with different detergent/protein ratios of 2–8 g/g, which are indicated on top of the lanes. Digitonin-solubilized bovine heart mitochondria (BHM) served as the mass standard (individual complexes I–V (130–1,000 kDa) and supercomplexes *a–e* (I$_1$III$_2$IV$_{0-4}$, 1,500–2,300 kDa). In wild-type mitochondria, three major supercomplexes *a–c* (I$_1$III$_2$IV$_{0-2}$) containing 0–2 copies of complex IV were separated. Contrary to that, ex1 mitochondria displayed predominantly monomeric complex I and dimeric complex III, but, specifically, dimeric complex I (I$_2$) and the supercomplex I$_2$III$_2$, which is apparently composed of dimeric complexes I and III, were found as a small fraction. Notably, the distinct interaction patterns of complexes I and III were found, although the ratio of ATP synthase dimers and monomers was essentially the same in both cases.

Contrary to that, ex1 mitochondria displayed predominantly individual complexes I and III. Nevertheless, besides I$_1$III$_2$ two novel supercomplexes (i.e., dimeric complex I (I$_2$) and I$_2$III$_2$ apparently composed of dimeric complexes I and III) were found as a small fraction, all exhibiting NADH dehydrogenase in-gel activity.[31] Notably, the distinct interaction patterns of complexes I and III were observed, although the ratio of ATP synthase dimers and monomers was essentially the same in wild-type and ex1 mitochondria. Dimeric ATP synthases (V_2) amount to $\geq 50\%$ of the total detected ATP synthase, and the remainder represents monomeric ATP synthase. This is comparable to the situation in mitochondria of yeast[5,15] and different mammalian organs[7] under the same conditions.

The OXPHOS Complex Interaction Patterns of COX- and AOX-Dependent Respiration are not Confined to Specific Strains

To examine whether the supramolecular organization of both respiratory pathways are general characteristics not confined to specific strains, we investigated the nuclear grisea mutant, which respires simultaneously via both pathways. The mutant phenotype of this strain is the result of a loss-of-function mutation in the nuclear gene coding for the copper-dependent transcription factor GRISEA.[32] Because GRISEA controls the expression of gene coding for the high-affinity copper transporter PaCTR3,[33] the grisea mutant is characterized by severely reduced intracellular copper levels and, consequently, a significant reduction of the copper-dependent COX. However, the mutant phenotype can be rescued to wild-type characteristics by supplementation of the growth medium with high amounts of copper.[34,35] Under these conditions, copper uptake occurs presumably via a low-affinity system and is efficient enough to restore the COX-dependent respiration and all other wild-type-specific features. We analyzed copper-deficient mutant grisea mitochondria each from independent juvenile cultures grown either under standard conditions or with the addition of 250 μM $CuSO_4$ to the growth medium. In fact, the interaction patterns of COX and AOX respiratory pathways and particularly their distinct supercomplexes found in wild-type and ex1 mitochondria (b, c, or I_2, I_2III_2, respectively) were also revealed in the grisea mutant by BN-PAGE/2D-SDS-PAGE.[31]

CN-PAGE Analysis Increases the Yields of Preserved Digitonin-Solubilized Supercomplexes

A striking difference revealed by BN-PAGE analysis was that the specific supercomplexes of the AOX pathway were significantly less abundant than those of the COX pathway. This may be the result of a reduced stability of the supercomplexes in the AOX pathway during BN-PAGE conditions. Indeed, the dissociative properties of anionic Coomassie Blue dye employed during BN-PAGE are known, which can disrupt labile subunits or weak interactions between protein complexes.[7,36,37] For this reason, we analyzed digitonin extracts of *P. anserina* mitochondria by the more gentle colorless-native PAGE (CN-PAGE) during which no Coomassie Blue dye is used.[38]

CN-PAGE supplemented with either 0.01% digitonin or 0.01% Triton X-100 revealed that in ex1 mitochondria, complex I–III interactions as well as

I–I interactions are also significant by increasing the yields of respective supercomplexes.[31] Taking together all the results, we concluded that dimeric complex I with bound complex III represents a major component of the AOX-dependent respiratory pathway in *P. anserina*.[31]

The COX and AOX Respiratory Pathways Might be Segregated from Each Other in the Inner Membrane

The enzymatically active supercomplex I_2III_2 of the AOX pathway is clearly not an assembly remnant of respirasome supercomplexes composed of complexes I, III, and IV left by the absence of complex IV, in which case only the supercomplex *a* (I_1III_2) would occur. Furthermore, it is unlikely that dimeric complex I is an erroneously formed species in the membrane. In fact, the other four OXPHOS complexes are known to form stable dimers or oligomers and it is reasonable that the dimeric complex I might provide a compact core for efficient substrate access and subsequent electron transfer to AOX. Indeed, we found a high NADH:ubiquinone oxidoreductase rate (complex I) as well as an unfavored NADH:cytochrome *c* reductase rate (complex I + III) of unsolubilized ex1 mitochondria in contrast to wild-type mitochondria,[31] which may indicate such a role. Apparently, there are two subpopulations of complexes I and III that are biochemically distinguishable by detergent treatment and subsequent native electrophoresis as well as enzymatic analysis. This finding suggests that both subpopulations of complexes I and III in the two pathways reside amid different lipid environments, which may be rather dispersive or form more extended membrane areas. Still missing is experimental evidence of whether AOX exclusively interacts with the distinct supercomplexes of the AOX pathway for electron transfer, which would mean a true segregation of COX and AOX pathways. In line with the respirasome model,[5,6] we proposed calling the distinct supramolecular organization of both fungal respiratory chains "COX-respirasome" and "AOX respiratory unit," respectively.[31]

Complex III seems to be Required for Assembly/Stability of Complex I

The demonstration that complex III is an abundant protein complex and at least partially bound to complex I in strains exclusively respiring via AOX is an intriguing finding, because assembly of itself as well as its supercomplexes with complex I is a sophisticated and energy-consuming process. Evidently, this respiratory protein complex has important and probably essential nonrespiratory functions. The AOX-dependent respiration is pivotally dependent on complex I to generate the electrochemical proton gradient across the inner mitochondrial membrane to drive ATP synthesis and other essential processes. In fact, recent reports have accumulated substantial evidence that mammalian and bacterial complex III is essential for assembly/stability of complex I,[8,14,20,21] which seems also to be one major function of complex III, besides other conceivable functions, in *P. anserina*.[31]

Respiration and Longevity in the Filamentous Fungus P. anserina

The proposal of a distinct supramolecular organization of COX and AOX respiratory pathways provides a unique basis to explain earlier findings, suggesting a crucial impact of respiration on the onset of senescence in the filamentous fungus *P. anserina*.[26–30,35] Long-lived strains with completely different genetic backgrounds like mutants ex1 and grisea were found to respire entirely or predominantly via AOX because of a lack or severe deficiency of COX, respectively. In two strains, a significantly lower production of mitochondrial reactive oxygen species than in the wild-type strain was demonstrated.[26] Interestingly, the plant AOX was also shown to reduce mitochondrial free radical production.[39] It appears that all of the events, which impair specifically the assembly/stability of complex IV (COX), lead to the induction of the AOX respiratory unit as a back-up system for performing obligatory aerobic metabolism. The accurate stoichiometry of respiratory complexes as well as their supramolecular arrangement (i.e., the type and number of supercomplexes and the fraction of free individual complexes) determine the overall throughput rates of the respiratory chain. Accordingly, the proper functioning of the AOX is supposed to be dependent on the specific composition of the AOX respiratory unit, e.g., the occurrence of dimeric complex I. Therefore, an exclusive overexpression of the AOX is expected to lead to features of the respective strains deviating from those of COX-deficient strains. Indeed, it was shown that transgenic expression of AOX in wild-type strains of *P. anserina* did not reduce reactive oxygen species production and exhibited no phenotypical differences compared with the wild type.[40] Furthermore, a significant overexpression of AOX in the COX-deficient cox5::BLE mutant led to simultaneous increase in ATP production and ROS formation, resulting in rescued female fertility and a significantly reduced life span.[40] We concluded that the precisely controlled formation of the AOX respiratory unit as a sustainable respiratory machinery in concert with the downregulation of the COX respirasome is responsible for the life-span extension in a number of long-lived *P. anserina* strains.[31]

OUTLOOK

The existence of respiratory supercomplexes as well as ATP synthase oligomers in the inner mitochondrial membrane is hitherto far from being generally accepted and even the respective studies, of which not all can be cited here, are not yet known to most scientists. Nevertheless, the next important step beyond the biochemical evidence to scrutinize the architecture of OXPHOS supercomplexes has just begun by providing electron microscopic images of single particles from such isolated assemblies.[41,42,43]

It is clear that the supramolecular organization of the OXPHOS machinery is of key importance to understanding the physiological function of mitochondrial respiration and its role in the aging process. Thus, the investigation of OXPHOS supercomplexes in a variety of model organisms from fungi to mammals—as a task of the new EU-funded consortium MiMage, the "integrated project on the role of mitochondria in conserved mechanisms in aging"[44]—is expected to result in a deeper understanding of the link between respiration and longevity at the molecular level.

REFERENCES

1. HATEFI, Y. 1985. The mitochondrial electron transport and oxidative phosphorylation system. Annu. Rev. Biochem. **54:** 1015–1069.
2. MOORE, A.L., M.S. ALBURY, P.G. CRICHTON, *et al.* 2002. Function of the alternative oxidase: is it still a scavenger? Trends Plant Sci. **7:** 478–481.
3. RASMUSSON, A.G., K.L. SOOLE & T.E. ELTHON. 2004. Alternative NAD(P)H dehydrogenases of plant mitochondria. Annu. Rev. Plant Biol. **55:** 23–39.
4. HACKENBROCK, C.R., B. CHAZOTTE & S.S. GUPTE. 1986. The random collision model and a critical assessment of diffusion and collision in mitochondrial electron transport. J. Bioenerg. Biomembr. **18:** 331–368.
5. SCHÄGGER, H. & K. PFEIFFER. 2000. Supercomplexes in the respiratory chains of yeast and mammalian mitochondria. EMBO J. **19:** 1777–1783.
6. SCHÄGGER, H. & K. PFEIFFER. 2001. The ratio of oxidative phosphorylation complexes I-V in bovine heart mitochondria and the composition of respiratory chain supercomplexes. J. Biol. Chem. **276:** 37861–37867.
7. KRAUSE, F., N.H. REIFSCHNEIDER, S. GOTO, *et al.* 2005. Active oligomeric ATP synthases in mammalian mitochondria. Biochem. Biophys. Res. Commun. **329:** 583–590.
8. SCHÄGGER, H., R. DE COO, M.F. BAUER, *et al.* 2004. Significance of respirasomes for the assembly/stability of human respiratory chain complex I. J. Biol. Chem. **279:** 36349–36353.
9. CRUCIAT, C.M., S. BRUNNER, F. BAUMANN, *et al.* 2000. The cytochrome bc_1 and cytochrome *c* oxidase complexes associate to form a single supracomplex in yeast mitochondria. J. Biol. Chem. **275:** 18093–18098.
10. EUBEL, H., L. JÄNSCH & H.P. BRAUN. 2003. New insights into the respiratory chain of plant mitochondria. Supercomplexes and a unique composition of complex II. Plant Physiol. **133:** 274–286.
11. EUBEL, H., J. HEINEMEYER & H.P. BRAUN. 2004. Identification and characterization of respirasomes in potato mitochondria. Plant Physiol. **134:** 1450–1459.
12. KRAUSE, F., N.H. REIFSCHNEIDER, D. VOCKE, *et al.* 2004. "Respirasome"-like supercomplexes in green leaf mitochondria of spinach. J. Biol. Chem. **279:** 48369–48375.

13. PINEAU, B., C. MATHIEU, C. GÉRARD-HIRNE, *et al.* 2005. Targeting the NAD7 subunit to mitochondria restores a functional complex I and a wild type phenotype in the *Nicotiana sylvestris* CMS II mutant lacking nad7. J. Biol. Chem. **280:** 25994–26001.
14. STROH, A., O. ANDERKA, K. PFEIFFER, *et al.* 2004. Assembly of respiratory complexes I, III, and IV into NADH oxidase supercomplex stabilizes complex I in *Paracoccus denitrificans.* J. Biol. Chem. **279:** 5000–5007.
15. ARNOLD, I., K. PFEIFFER, W. NEUPERT, *et al.* 1998. Yeast mitochondrial F_1F_O-ATP synthase exists as a dimer: identification of three dimer-specific subunits. EMBO J. **17:** 7170–7178.
16. PAUMARD, P., J. VAILLIER, B. COULARY, *et al.* 2002. The ATP synthase is involved in generating mitochondrial cristae morphology. EMBO J. **21:** 221–230.
17. SPIVEY, H.O. & J. OVADI. 1999. Substrate channeling. Methods **19:** 306–321.
18. BOUMANS, H., L.A. GRIVELL & J. BERDEN. 1998. The respiratory chain in yeast behaves as a single functional unit. J. Biol. Chem. **273:** 4872–4877.
19. BIANCHI, C., M.L. GENOVA, G. PARENTI CASTELLI, *et al.* 2004. The mitochondrial respiratory chain is partially organized in a supercomplex assembly: kinetic evidence using flux control analysis. J. Biol. Chem. **279:** 36562–36569.
20. SCHÄGGER, H. 2002. Respiratory chain supercomplexes of mitochondria and bacteria. Biochim. Biophys. Acta **1555:** 154–159.
21. ACÍN-PERÉZ, R., M.P. BAYONA-BAFALUY, P. FERNÁNDEZ-SILVA, *et al.* 2004. Respiratory complex III is required to maintain complex I in mammalian mitochondria. Mol. Cell **13:** 805–815.
22. GAVIN, P.D., M. PRESCOTT, S.E. LUFF, *et al.* 2004. Cross-linking ATP synthase complexes *in vivo* eliminates mitochondrial cristae. J. Cell Sci. **117:** 2333–2343.
23. FINKEL, T. & N.J. HOLBROOK. 2000. Oxidants, oxidative stress and the biology of ageing. Nature **408:** 239–247.
24. RIZET, G. 1953. Sur l'impossibilité d'obtenir la multiplication végétative ininterrompue et illimitée de l'Ascomycète *Podospora anserina.* C.R. Acad. Sci. **237:** 838–840.
25. OSIEWACZ, H.D. 2002. Genes, mitochondria and aging in filamentous fungi. Ageing Res. Rev. **1:** 425–442.
26. DUFOUR, E., J. BOULAY, V. RINCHEVAL, *et al.* 2000. A causal link between respiration and senescence in *Podospora anserina.* Proc. Natl. Acad. Sci. USA **97:** 4138–4143.
27. BORGHOUTS, C., E. KIMPEL & H.D. OSIEWACZ. 1997. Mitochondrial DNA rearrangements of *Podospora anserina* are under the control of the nuclear gene grisea. Proc. Natl. Acad. Sci. USA **94:** 10768–10773.
28. BORGHOUTS, C., S. KERSCHNER & H.D. OSIEWACZ. 2000. Copper-dependence of mitochondrial DNA rearrangements in *Podospora anserina.* Curr. Genet. **37:** 268–275.
29. SCHULTE, E., U. KÜCK & K. ESSER. 1988. Extrachromosomal mutants from *Podospora anserina*: permanent vegetative growth in spite of multiple recombination events in the mitochondrial genome. Mol. Gen. Genet. **211:** 342–349.
30. STUMPFERL, S.W., O. STEPHAN & H.D. OSIEWACZ. 2004. Impact of a disruption of a pathway delivering copper to mitochondria on *Podospora anserina* metabolism and life span. Eukaryot. Cell **3:** 200–211.
31. KRAUSE, F., C.Q. SCHECKHUBER, A. WERNER, *et al.* 2004. Supramolecular organization of cytochrome *c* oxidase- and alternative oxidase-dependent respiratory

chains in the filamentous fungus *Podospora anserina*. J. Biol. Chem. **279**: 26453–26461.

32. BORGHOUTS, C. & H.D. OSIEWACZ. 1998. GRISEA, a copper-modulated transcription factor from *Podospora anserina* involved in senescence and morphogenesis, is an ortholog of MAC1 in *Saccharomyces cerevisiae*. Mol. Gen. Genet. **260**: 492–502.

33. BORGHOUTS, C., C.Q. SCHECKHUBER, O. STEPHAN, *et al.* 2002. Copper homeostasis and aging in the fungal model system *Podospora anserina*: differential expression of *PaCtr3* encoding a copper transporter. Int. J. Biochem. Cell Biol. **34**: 1355–1371.

34. MARBACH, K., J. FERNANDEZ-LARREA & U. STAHL. 1994. Reversion of a long-living, undifferentiated mutant of *Podospora anserina* by copper. Curr. Genet. **26**: 184–186.

35. BORGHOUTS, C., A. WERNER, T. ELTHON, *et al.* 2001. Copper-modulated gene expression and senescence in the filamentous fungus *Podospora anserina*. Mol. Cell. Biol. **21**: 390–399.

36. NEFF, D. & N.A. Dencher. 1999. Purification of multisubunit membrane protein complexes: isolation of chloroplast F_OF_1-ATP synthase, CF_O and CF_1 by blue native electrophoresis. Biochem. Biophys. Res. Commun. **259**: 569–575.

37. PFEIFFER, K., V. GOHIL, R.A. STUART, *et al.* 2003. Cardiolipin stabilizes respiratory chain supercomplexes. J. Biol. Chem. **278**: 52873–52880.

38. SCHÄGGER, H., W.A. CRAMER & G. VON JAGOW. 1994. Analysis of molecular masses and oligomeric states of protein complexes by blue native electrophoresis and isolation of membrane protein complexes by two-dimensional native electrophoresis. Anal. Biochem. **217**: 220–230.

39. MAXWELL, D.P., Y. WANG & L. MCINTOSH. 1999. The alternative oxidase lowers mitochondrial reactive oxygen production in plant cells. Proc. Natl. Acad. Sci. USA **96**: 8271–8276.

40. LORIN, S., E. DUFOUR, J. BOULAY, *et al.* 2001. Overexpression of the alternative oxidase restores senescence and fertility in a long-lived respiration-deficient mutant of *Podospora anserina*. Mol. Microbiol. **42**: 1259–1267.

41. DUDKINA, N.V., H. EUBEL, W. KEEGSTRA, *et al.* 2005. Structure of a mitochondrial supercomplex formed by respiratory-chain complexes I and III. Proc. Natl. Acad. Sci. USA **102**: 3225–3229.

42. MINAURO-SANMIGUEL, F., S. WILKENS & J.J. GARCIA. 2005. Structure of dimeric mitochondrial ATP synthase: novel F_O bridging features and the structural basis of mitochondrial cristae biogenesis. Proc. Natl. Acad. Sci. USA **102**: 12356–12358.

43. SCHÄFER, E., H. SEELERT, N.H. REIFSCHNEIDER, *et al.* 2006. Architecture of active mammalian respiratory chain supercomplexes. J. Mol. Biol. In press.

44. SCHECKHUBER, C.Q. & H.D. OSIEWACZ. 2005. MiMage: a Pan-European project on the role of mitochondria in aging. Sci. Aging Knowledge Environ. **20**: pe14.

Unraveling Age-Dependent Variation of the Mitochondrial Proteome

NORBERT A. DENCHER,[a] SATARO GOTO,[b]
NICOLE H. REIFSCHNEIDER,[a] MICHIRU SUGAWA,[c]
AND FRANK KRAUSE[a]

[a]Physical Biochemistry, Department of Chemistry, Darmstadt University
of Technology, D-64287 Darmstadt, Germany

[b]Department of Biochemistry, Faculty of Pharmaceutical Sciences,
Toho University, Funabashi, Japan

[c]Charité – University Medicine Berlin, Department of Psychiatry,
Clinical Neurobiology, D-14050 Berlin, Germany

ABSTRACT: Blue-native and colorless-native gel electrophoresis combined with subsequent 2D-SDS-PAGE and MALDI mass spectrometry
are successfully applied for understanding the role of mitochondria in
cellular dysfunction, aging, and cellular death. The partial mitochondrial proteome maps of various tissues (liver, brain, kidney, heart, and
skeletal muscle) obtained from rat serve now as a database for the elucida-
tion of age-dependent changes, including alterations in protein–protein
interactions as well as in posttranslational modifications.

KEYWORDS: aging; mitochondria; membrane proteins; native electrophoresis; proteome

INTRODUCTION

Examination of age-dependent variation in the protein profile of organelles,
cells, and even the entire organism is currently a promising approach to elucidate the cause of aging and of age-related diseases. With this approach,
mechanisms of aging that are conserved in most species will be identified. We
study the role of mitochondria in aging and life-span control in various evolutionarily distant model organisms such as fungi and mammals. Mitochondria
are severely affected during aging and most probably trigger key steps in the
aging process.

Address for correspondence: Prof. Dr. Norbert A. Dencher, Physical Biochemistry, Department of
Chemistry, Darmstadt University of Technology, Petersenstr. 22, D-64287 Darmstadt, Germany. Voice:
+49-6151-165275; fax: +49-6151-164171.
  e-mail: nad@pop.tu-darmstadt.de
  www.tu-darmstadt.de/fb/ch/Fachgebiete/BC/AKDencher/index_en.html

Ann. N.Y. Acad. Sci. 1067: 116–119 (2006). © 2006 New York Academy of Sciences.
doi: 10.1196/annals.1354.014

Our main focus is the mitochondrial membrane system, especially the inner mitochondrial membrane with the respiratory chain complexes and other proteins specifically involved in life-span control and aging, such as the prohibitins. Variations of the mitochondrial proteome during aging are determined, emphasizing the composition, structure, and activity of membrane proteins and

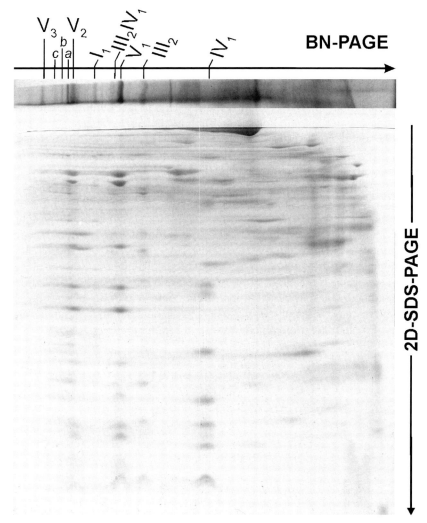

FIGURE 1. Native protein complexes and supercomplexes of digitonin-solubilized crude liver mitochondria isolated from a 10-month-old male rat (F344/DuCrj), as resolved by blue-native PAGE (BN-PAGE), and the corresponding protein profile of the individual subunits (2D-SDS-PAGE). Besides the ATP synthase monomer V_1, dimer V_2, and trimer V_3, the individual respiratory complexes I, IV, as well as III_2 dimer and the OXPHOS supercomplexes I_1III_2 (a), $I_1III_2IV_1$ (b), and $I_1III_2IV_2$ (c) are labeled in the first dimension.

their modulation by nutrition, oxidative stress, and exercise. By application of the blue-native (BN) PAGE[1–3] (FIG. 1) and especially of the even more gentle colorless-native (CN) PAGE in combination with MALDI-TOF mass spectrometry, the occurrence, architecture, and functional relevance of OXPHOS supercomplexes[4]—the natural assembly of the respiratory complexes I, III, IV, and V into supercomplexes such as $I_1III_2IV_{0-4}$[4] and the ATP synthase dimer V_2[4,5] as well as larger oligomers of V—are examined.[5] Analysis by MALDI-MS of tryptic peptide fragments provides a general approach that allows doubtless identification of the proteins. As analytical techniques BN- and CN-PAGE separate individual proteins, multisubunit membrane proteins, membrane protein supercomplexes as well as transiently interacting proteins in their native state.[6–8] Their functional activity can be tested directly in the gel[5,6] or upon electroelution out of the gel matrix. Upon electroelution, structural imaging of selected protein complexes such as the ATP synthase[9,10] and the OXPHOS supercomplexes I_1III_2 and $I_1III_2IV_1$[11] is feasible. It is important to note that in contrast to isoelectric focusing the efficiency of BN-PAGE is not affected by hydropathicity of individual proteins.[12]

One important aim is the establishment of a mitochondrial protein map covering both water-soluble and membrane proteins (e.g., OXPHOS-complexes, TCA-cycle, and fatty acid metabolism enzymes; FIG. 1) and exhibiting protein–protein interactions (FIG. 1) as well as posttranslational modifications. An additional focus is the interaction of free radicals, or reactive oxygen species such as hydrogen peroxide or peroxynitrite, and biological membranes, especially of energy-converting mitochondrial membranes, and age-dependent alterations of this interaction. Lipid peroxidation might contribute to the observed age-dependent increase in membrane viscosity[13] and could modulate assembly and stability of membrane protein complexes and supercomplexes.

ACKNOWLEDGMENTS

This work was supported by the EU FP6 MiMage (to N.A.D.).

REFERENCES

1. SCHÄGGER, H. & G. VON JAGOW. 1991. Blue native electrophoresis for isolation of membrane protein complexes in enzymatically active form. Anal. Biochem. **199:** 223–231.
2. NEFF, D. & N.A. DENCHER. 1999. Purification of multisubunit membrane protein complexes: isolation of chloroplast F_0F1-ATP-synthase, CF_0 and CF_1 by blue native electrophoresis. Biochem. Biophys. Res. Commun. **259:** 569–575.
3. POETSCH, A., D. NEFF, H. SEELERT, et al. 2000. Dye removal, catalytic activity and 2D-crystallization of chloroplast H^+-ATP synthase purified by blue native electrophoresis. Biochim. Biophys. Acta **1466:** 339–349.

4. SCHÄGGER, H. 2002. Respiratory chain supercomplexes of mitochondria and bacteria. Biochim. Biophys. Acta **1555:** 154–159.

5. KRAUSE, F., N.H. REIFSCHNEIDER, S. GOTO, *et al.* 2005. Active oligomeric ATP synthases in mammalian mitochondria. Biochem. Biophys. Res. Commun. **329:** 583–590.

6. KRAUSE, F., C.Q. SCHECKHUBER, A. WERNER, *et al.* 2004. Supramolecular organization of cytochrome c oxidase- and alternative oxidase-dependent respiratory chains in the filamentous fungus *Podospora anserina*. J. Biol. Chem. **279:** 26453–26461.

7. KRAUSE, F., N.H. REIFSCHNEIDER, D. VOCKE, *et al.* 2004. "Respirasome"-like supercomplexes in green leaves mitochondria of spinach. J. Biol. Chem. **279:** 48369–48376.

8. SCHÄGGER, H. 2001. Blue-native gels to isolate protein complexes from mitochondria. Methods Cell. Biol. **65:** 231–244.

9. SEELERT, H., A. POETSCH, N.A. DENCHER, *et al.* 2000. Proton-powered turbine of a plant motor. Nature **405:** 418–419.

10. SEELERT, H., N.A. DENCHER & D.J. MÜLLER. 2003. Fourteen protomers compose the oligomer III of the proton-rotor of spinach chloroplast ATP-synthase. J. Mol. Biol. **333:** 337–344.

11. SCHÄFER, E., H. SEELERT, N.H. REIFSCHNEIDER, *et al.* 2006. Architecture of mammalian respiratory chain supercomplexes. J. Mol. Biol. In press.

12. REXROTH, S., J.M.W. MEYER ZU TITTINGDORF, F. KRAUSE, *et al.* 2003. Thylakoid membrane at altered metabolic state: challenging the forgotten realms of the proteome. Electrophoresis **24:** 2814–2823.

13. SUGAWA, M., H. COPER, G. SCHULZE, *et al.* 1996. Impaired plasticity of neurons in aging: biochemical, biophysical, and behavioural studies. Ann. N. Y. Acad. Sci. **786:** 274–282.

Using *Caenorhabditis elegans* as a Model for Aging and Age-Related Diseases

ANDERS OLSEN, MAITHILI C. VANTIPALLI, AND GORDON J. LITHGOW

The Buck Institute, Novato, California 94945, USA

ABSTRACT: During the last three decades the soil nematode *C. elegans* has become a prominent model organism for studying aging. Initially research in the *C. elegans* aging field was focused on the genetics of aging and single gene mutations that dramatically increased the life span of the worm. Undoubtedly, the existence of such mutations is one of the main reasons for the popularity of the worm as model system for studying aging. However, today many different approaches are being used in the *C. elegans* aging field in addition to genetic manipulations that influence life span. For example, environmental manipulations such as caloric restriction and hormetic treatments, evolutionary studies, population studies, models of age-related diseases, and drug screening for compounds that extend life span are now being investigated using this nematode. This review will focus on the most recent developments in *C. elegans* aging research with the aim of illustrating the diversity of the field.

KEYWORDS: aging; stress; *C. elegans*; life span; drug screening

BASIC WORM AGING

Adult *C. elegans* worms are self-fertilizing hermaphrodites with a 3-day life cycle and a mean life span of approximately 18–20 days when cultured at 20°C. This nematode displays a number of age-related changes reminiscent of those observed in other organisms. With advancing age worms are less active, display uncoordinated movements, and eventually they stop moving. This appears to be the result of muscle degeneration rather than neuronal defects as the cellular integrity of the nervous system is preserved till very late in life.[1] Other age-related changes include accumulation of lipofuscin, dark pigments, presence of vacuole-like structures,[1] and increased levels of oxidized proteins.[2–4] It is worth noting that even in an isogenic population great variability in age-related changes between individual worms is observed, suggesting that stochastic factors play a role during nematode aging.[1]

Address for correspondence: Anders Olsen, The Buck Institute, 8001 Redwood Blvd., Novato, CA 94945, USA. Voice: 1-415-209-2091; fax: 1-415-209-2232.
  e-mail: aolsen@buckinstitute.org
  http://www.buckinstitute.org

Ann. N.Y. Acad. Sci. 1067: 120–128 (2006). © 2006 New York Academy of Sciences.
doi: 10.1196/annals.1354.015

GENETIC PATHWAYS INVOLVED IN *C. elegans* AGING

When nutrition is low or the population density is high, the worms activate an alternative developmental program that leads to the formation of the highly stress-resistant dauer larvae.[5–7] Many mutations that have an effect on dauer formation also influence longevity. Many of these mutations are found in the insulin/IGF-I signaling pathway.[8–13] Other genetic pathways determining life span in *C. elegans* include genes involved with caloric restriction,[14] genes involved with mitochondrial function,[15] and genes involved with lipophilic hormone signaling.[16–18] Mutations in the insulin/IGF-I signaling cascade are the best characterized and they cause large increases in the nematode life span.[8–13] Mutants in this pathway are often used as tools in aging experiments. In this respect, the key genes are: *daf-2, age-1,* and *daf-16. daf-2* encodes a homolog of the mammalian insulin/IGF-I receptor.[11] *age-1* encodes the catalytic p110 subunit of phosphoinositide-3-OH kinase (PI3K) found downstream of DAF-2.[19] Mutations in *age-1* and *daf-2* cause large increases in the nematode life span as well as enhanced stress resistance. DAF-16 encodes a homolog of the human FOXO forkhead transcription factor[20] and is required for all life span–extending mutations identified in this pathway.[21–23] Following stress or inactivation of the insulin/IGF-I signaling pathway, DAF-16 rapidly translocates to the nucleus.[24,25] The downstream targets of DAF-16 remain largely unknown although microarray analyses have identified several candidates.[26–28] One can predict that these genes must be involved in longevity and stress resistance and the other phenotypes displayed by mutants in the insulin/IGF-I signaling pathway. Over-expression of DAF-16 supports this view as elevated levels of DAF-16 result in slow growth and increase stress resistance and life span.[25] One DAF-16 target is the superoxide dismutase *sod-3* gene, whose promoter contains a putative DAF-16 binding site.[29] SOD-3 protein and mRNA levels are upregulated in insulin signaling mutants.[26,30] Another of the downstream targets, the small heat-shock protein *hsp-16*, will be discussed in more detail in the following sections.

LONG-LIVED *C. elegans* MUTANTS ARE RESISTANT TO STRESS

A mechanistic connection between stress resistance and longevity is well established in several different species but particularly in *C. elegans*. Most, if not all, long-lived mutants exhibit increased resistance to environmental stress, such as oxidative stress,[7,31] hypoxia,[32] heat shock,[33,34] UV irradiation,[35] and heavy metal stress.[36] A range of manipulations that enhances stress tolerance in *C. elegans* also results in longevity, for example, over-expression of the heat-shock proteins (HSPs) HSP-70[37] and HSP-16.[38] Multiple stressors, such as increased heat,[34] high oxygen,[39] and gamma irradiation[40] can induce a hormetic response in *C. elegans* and increase stress tolerance as well as extend life span. The insulin/IGF-I signaling pathway plays an important role in regulating nematode stress resistance. A number of stress response genes have been found to be upregulated in mutants from this pathway. For example, *age-1* mutant worms have elevated levels of the molecular chaperone HSP-16[41] as have *daf-2* mutants.[42] Furthermore, both *daf-2* and *age-1* mutants have higher expression levels of the metallothionein genes *mtl-1* and *mtl-2*.[36] Expression of some HSPs is regulated by a family of stress-regulated transcription factors, the heat-shock factors (HSFs).[43] In *C. elegans* there is only one heat-shock factor, *hsf-1,* and its inactivation reduces the life span of the nematode.[44-46]

LIFE-SPAN PREDICTION

Individual worms of an isogenic population display considerable variation in life span, paralleling the heterogeneity observed in physiological markers of aging.[1] Why is it that, given that all worms have the same genetic makeup and have been exposed to the same environment, some worms may die on day 14 while others die as late as on day 34? A recent study has attempted to answer this question.[47] A large population of worms were subjected to a sub-lethal heat shock to induce expression of *hsp-16* and were subsequently grouped based upon levels of HSP-16. The life span of these different groups was then measured. Worms with high levels of HSP-16 early in life were found to be significantly longer-lived and stress-resistant than worms with lower levels of HSP-16. Thus, levels of HSP-16 appear to reflect some physiological status that is linked to longevity. Although HSP-16 may only be one of the many proteins involved, it does provide a biomarker that early in life can be used to predict life span. It will be of interest to discover the targets of HSP-16.

SCREENS FOR LONGEVITY

Until recently, very few of the known age genes were in fact identified in screens for longevity. Rather, they have been identified through their function in other biological processes, for example, dauer formation, or in screens for life-span surrogate phenotypes such as stress resistance.[48-50] However, two whole genome RNAi screens for longevity have recently been conducted.[51,52] In combination, these two studies describe more than 100 novel genes that, when inactivated, extend life span. This is a staggering number that is in fact likely to increase owing to a number of reasons. First, RNAi is not effective for all genes. Second, the screens did not pull out any common genes, suggesting that neither screen was saturated. Third, the RNAi libraries used do not have complete genome coverage. Interestingly, most of the newly identified genes fall into already known aging pathways in *C. elegans*, mainly those involved with insulin signaling, caloric restriction, and endocrine pathways. It thus appears that many different genes may influence life span via a small number of conserved pathways. Understanding the mechanistic basis for the observed life-span increases remains a challenging task for the future.

There has also been considerable interest in identifying pharmacological agents that delay the aging process. Several compounds have been identified that significantly increase the nematode life span. One such compound is EUK-134, a synthetic superoxide/catalase mimetic, which probably extends the nematode life span by reducing oxidative stress.[53,54] The Sirtuin activator resveratrol is another compound that significantly increases the worm life span.[55] Caloric restriction may be the underlying mechanism, but resveratrol also has antioxidant capacity. The anticonvulsants ethosuximide, trimethadione, and 3,3-diethyl-2-pyrrolidinone dramatically increase the life span of *C. elegans* via an unknown mechanism.[56]

Compounds that extend the nematode life span may provide novel therapeutic targets for treatment of age-related diseases. However, the number of drugs identified is relatively small because only small targeted screens have been performed. It is thus timely to invest more effort in the discovery of such compounds via high-throughput screening (HTS). A variety of assays suitable for HTS for anti-aging compounds are being developed.[57,58] *C. elegans* provides a unique model system for high-throughput drug screening. Nematodes can be inexpensively cultured in large quantities and the relatively short life span of *C. elegans* makes it particularly attractive for anti-aging drug screening. Another advantage is that the effect of the drug can be tested directly in a whole organism. Thus, compounds that are toxic for development can be immediately eliminated. Once a drug has been identified the worm provides a good model system for identifying targets and mode of action. For example, RNAi and classical mutagenesis allow for screening to identify suppressors and enhancers of the discovered drugs. Furthermore, drugs are likely to identify targets that cannot be identified in RNAi screens—for example, genes in the nervous system that often are poor targets of RNAi[59] or genes that cause lethality when inactivated. Also as discussed in the following section several age-related diseases can be modeled in the worm and therefore identified drugs can easily be tested for their effect on age-related diseases. At the moment there are also limitations for using the worm in drugs, for example difficult drug delivery and lack of well-developed pharmacokinetics in the worm. However, it is likely that such obstacles will be resolved and dramatically improve the use of the worm in drug screening.

MODELS OF AGE-RELATED DISEASES

The *C. elegans* genome contains homologs of approximately two-thirds of all human disease genes.[60] Thus, the worm has become a popular organism for modeling human diseases,[61] including age-related diseases. To study Alzheimer's disease, transgenic animals were engineered to express human β-amyloid peptide (Aβ) and these worms form intracellular β-amyloid aggregates.[62,63] Parkinson's disease and degeneration of dopaminergic neurons can also be studied using transgenic nematodes.[64] Another very elegant example of disease modeling in the worm is the Huntington's disease model that addresses the effects of polyglutamine expansions.[65–68] Expression of a huntingtin fragment containing polyQ expansions leads to protein aggregate formation and neuronal dysfunction.[67] A strong correlation was found between age and number of aggregates.[65] Moreover, *age-1* mutants have a very significant delay in the onset of polyQ toxicity and appearance of protein aggregates. This could be explained by the fact that the *age-1* mutation increases life span in part by upregulating chaperone capacity, as discussed previously. Furthermore, more recently it was shown that resveratrol protects against polyglutamine cytotoxicity in the worm model of Huntington's disease.[69] The example of resveratrol nicely illustrates how *C. elegans* can be successfully used for drug screening as well as testing the relevance of a drug for age-related diseases. In the future, more disease models in the nematode combined with the use of *C. elegans* in drug screening will no doubt become much more widely used and provide greater insight to the aging process.

CONCLUSION

C. elegans has a strong tradition for being used in genetic approaches to understanding the aging process. However, today the worms are being used in a variety of other approaches, such as drug screening, disease modeling, and environmental manipulations. Collectively all these approaches are likely to provide a unique insight into the aging process.

REFERENCES

1. HERNDON, L.A., P.J. SCHMEISSNER, J.M. DUDARONEK, *et al.* 2002. Stochastic and genetic factors influence tissue-specific decline in ageing *C. elegans*. Nature **419:** 808–814.
2. ADACHI, H., Y. FUJIWARA & N. ISHII. 1998. Effects of oxygen on protein carbonyl and aging in *Caenorhabditis elegans* mutants with long (*age-1*) and short (*mev-1*) life spans. J. Gerontol. A. Biol. Sci. Med. Sci. **53A:** B240–B244.
3. NAKAMURA, A., K. YASUDA, H. ADACHI, *et al.* 1999. Vitellogenin-6 is a major carbonylated protein in aged nematode, *Caenorhabditis elegans*. Biochem. Biophys. Res. Commun. **264:** 580–583.
4. YASUDA, K., H. ADACHI, Y. FUJIWARA, *et al.* 1999. Protein carbonyl accumulation in aging dauer formation-defective (daf) mutants of *Caenorhabditis elegans*. J. Gerontol. A Biol. Sci. Med. Sci. **54:** B47–B51.

5. RIDDLE, D.L. & P.S. ALBERT. 1997. Genetic and environmental regulation of dauer larva development. *In* C. Elegans II. D.L. Riddle, T. Blumenthal, B.J. Meyer & J.R. Priess, Eds.: 739–768. CSHP. New York.

6. ANDERSON, G.L. 1978. Responses of dauer larvae of *Caenorhabditis elegans* (Nematoda: Rhabditidae) to thermal stress and oxygen deprivation. Can. J. Zool. **56:** 1786–1791.

7. LARSEN, P.L. 1993. Aging and resistance to oxidative damage in *Caenorhabditis elegans*. Proc. Natl. Acad. Sci. USA **90:** 8905–8909.

8. TISSENBAUM, H.A. & G. RUVKUN. 1998. An insulin-like signaling pathway affects both longevity and reproduction in *Caenorhabditis elegans*. Genetics **148:** 703–717.

9. OGG, S., S. PARADIS, S. GOTTLIEB, *et al.* 1997. The Fork head transcription factor DAF-16 transduces insulin-like metabolic and longevity signals in *C. elegans*. Nature **389:** 994–999.

10. MORRIS, J.Z., H.A. TISSENBAUM & G. RUVKUN. 1996. A phosphatidylinositol-3-OH kinase family member regulating longevity and diapause in *Caenorhabditis elegans*. Nature **382:** 536–539.

11. KIMURA, K.D., H.A. TISSENBAUM, Y. LIU, *et al.* 1997. *daf-2*, an insulin receptor-like gene that regulates longevity and diapause in *Caenorhabditis elegans*. Science **277:** 942–946.

12. DORMAN, J.B., B. ALBINDER, T. SHROYER, *et al.* 1995. The *age-1* and *daf-2* genes function in a common pathway to control the lifespan of *Caenorhabditis elegans*. Genetics **141:** 1399–1406.

13. LEE, R.Y., J. HENCH & G. RUVKUN. 2001. Regulation of *C. elegans* DAF-16 and its human ortholog FKHRL1 by the *daf-2* insulin-like signaling pathway. Curr. Biol. **11:** 1950–1957.

14. WALKER, G., K. HOUTHOOFD, J.R. VANFLETEREN, *et al.* 2005. Dietary restriction in *C. elegans*: from rate-of-living effects to nutrient sensing pathways. Mech. Ageing Dev. **126:** 929–937.

15. ANSON, R.M. & R.G. HANSFORD. 2004. Mitochondrial influence on aging rate in *Caenorhabditis elegans*. Aging Cell **3:** 29–34.

16. ANTEBI, A., W.H. YEH, D. TAIT, *et al.* 2000. *daf-12* encodes a nuclear receptor that regulates the dauer diapause and developmental age in *C. elegans*. Genes Dev. **14:** 1512–1527.

17. JIA, K., P.S. ALBERT & D.L. RIDDLE. 2002. DAF-9, a cytochrome P450 regulating *C. elegans* larval development and adult longevity. Development **129:** 221–231.

18. GERISCH, B., C. WEITZEL, C. KOBER-EISERMANN, *et al.* 2001. A hormonal signaling pathway influencing *C. elegans* metabolism, reproductive development, and life span. Dev. Cell **1:** 841–851.

19. MALONE, E.A., T. INOUE & J.H. THOMAS. 1996. Genetic analysis of the roles of *daf-28* and *age-1* in regulating *Caenorhabditis elegans* dauer formation. Genetics **143:** 1193–1205.

20. LIN, K., J.B. DORMAN, A. RODAN, *et al.* 1997. *daf-16*: An HNF-3/forkhead family member that can function to double the life-span of *Caenorhabditis elegans*. Science **278:** 1319–1322.

21. LARSEN, P.L., P.S. ALBERT & D.L. RIDDLE. 1995. Genes that regulate both development and longevity in *Caenorhabditis elegans*. Genetics **139:** 1567–1583.

22. KENYON, C., J. CHANG, E. GENSCH, *et al.* 1993. A *C. elegans* mutant that lives twice as long as wild type. Nature **366:** 461–464.

23. GOTTLIEB, S. & G. RUVKUN. 1994. *daf-2*, *daf-16* and *daf-23*: genetically interacting genes controlling Dauer formation in *Caenorhabditis elegans*. Genetics **137:** 107–120.

24. LIN, K., H. HSIN, N. LIBINA, *et al*. 2001. Regulation of the *Caenorhabditis elegans* longevity protein DAF-16 by insulin/IGF-1 and germline signaling. Nat. Genet. **28:** 139–145.

25. HENDERSON, S.T. & T.E. JOHNSON. 2001. *daf-16* integrates developmental and environmental inputs to mediate aging in the nematode *Caenorhabditis elegans*. Curr. Biol. **11:** 1975–1980.

26. MURPHY, C.T., S.A. MCCARROLL, C.I. BARGMANN, *et al*. 2003. Genes that act downstream of DAF-16 to influence the lifespan of *Caenorhabditis elegans*. Nature **424:** 277–283.

27. LEE, S.S., S. KENNEDY, A.C. TOLONEN, *et al*. 2003. DAF-16 target genes that control *C. elegans* life-span and metabolism. Science **300:** 644–647.

28. MCELWEE, J., K. BUBB & J.H. THOMAS. 2003. Transcriptional outputs of the *Caenorhabditis elegans* forkhead protein DAF-16. Aging Cell **2:** 111–121.

29. FURUYAMA, T., T. NAKAZAWA, I. NAKANO, *et al*. 2000. Identification of the differential distribution patterns of mRNAs and consensus binding sequences for mouse DAF-16 homologues. Biochem. J. **349:** 629–634.

30. HONDA, Y. & S. HONDA. 1999. The *daf-2* gene network for longevity regulates oxidative stress resistance and Mn-superoxide dismutase gene expression in *Caenorhabditis elegans*. FASEB J. **13:** 1385–1393.

31. VANFLETEREN, J.R. 1993. Oxidative stress and ageing in *Caenorhabditis elegans*. Biochem. J. **292:** 605–608.

32. SCOTT, B.A., M.S. AVIDAN & C.M. CROWDER. 2002. Regulation of hypoxic death in *C. elegans* by the insulin/IGF receptor homolog DAF-2. Science **296:** 2388–2391.

33. LITHGOW, G.J., T.M. WHITE, D.A. HINERFELD, *et al*. 1994. Thermotolerance of a long-lived mutant of *Caenorhabditis elegans*. J. Gerontol. **49:** B270–B276.

34. LITHGOW, G.J., T.M. WHITE, S. MELOV, *et al*. 1995. Thermotolerance and extended life-span conferred by single-gene mutations and induced by thermal stress. Proc. Natl. Acad. Sci. USA **92:** 7540–7544.

35. MURAKAMI, S. & T.E. JOHNSON. 1996. A genetic pathway conferring life extension and resistance to UV stress in *Caenorhabditis elegans*. Genetics **143:** 1207–1218.

36. BARSYTE, D., D.A. LOVEJOY & G.J. LITHGOW. 2001. Longevity and heavy metal resistance in *daf-2* and *age-1* long-lived mutants of *Caenorhabditis elegans*. FASEB J. **15:** 627–634.

37. YOKOYAMA, K., K. FUKUMOTO, T. MURAKAMI, *et al*. 2002. Extended longevity of *Caenorhabditis elegans* by knocking in extra copies of hsp70F, a homolog of *mot-2* (mortalin)/mthsp70/Grp75. FEBS Lett. **516:** 53–57.

38. WALKER, G.A. & G.J. LITHGOW. 2003. Lifespan determination in *C. elegans* by insulin-like regulation of a molecular chaperone. Aging Cell **2:** 131–139.

39. CYPSER, J.R. & T.E. JOHNSON. 2002. Multiple stressors in *Caenorhabditis elegans* induce stress hormesis and extended longevity. J. Gerontol. A Biol. Sci. Med. Sci. **57:** B109–B114.

40. JOHNSON, T.E. & P.S. HARTMAN. 1988. Radiation effects on life span in *Caenorhabditis elegans*. J. Gerontol. **43:** B137–B141.

41. WALKER, G.A., T.M. WHITE, G. MCCOLL, *et al*. 2001. Heat shock protein accumulation is upregulated in a long-lived mutant of *Caenorhabditis elegans*. J. Gerontol. A Biol. Sci. Med. Sci. **56:** B281–B287.

42. Hsu, A.L., C.T. Murphy & C. Kenyon. 2003. Regulation of aging and age-related disease by DAF-16 and heat-shock factor. Science **300:** 1142–1145.
43. Mathew, A. & R.I. Morimoto. 1998. Role of the heat-shock response in the life and death of proteins. Ann. N. Y. Acad Sci **851:** 99–111.
44. Garigan, D., A.L. Hsu, A.G. Fraser, *et al.* 2002. Genetic analysis of tissue aging in *Caenorhabditis elegans*: a role for heat-shock factor and bacterial proliferation. Genetics **161:** 1101–1112.
45. Walker, G.A., F.J. Thompson, A. Brawley, *et al.* 2003. Heat shock factor functions at the convergence of the stress response and developmental pathways in *Caenorhabditis elegans*. FASEB J. **17:** 1960–1962.
46. Hajdu-Cronin, Y.M., W.J. Chen & P.W. Sternberg. 2004. The L-type cyclin CYL-1 and the heat-shock-factor HSF-1 are required for heat-shock-induced protein expression in *Caenorhabditis elegans*. Genetics **168:** 1937–1949.
47. Rea, S.L., D. Wu, J.R. Cypser, *et al.* 2005. A stress-sensitive reporter predicts longevity in isogenic populations of *Caenorhabditis elegans*. Nat. Genet. **37:** 894–898.
48. Munoz, M.J. & D.L. Riddle. 2003. Positive selection of *Caenorhabditis elegans* mutants with increased stress resistance and longevity. Genetics **163:** 171–180.
49. Sampayo, J.N., N.L. Jenkins & G.J. Lithgow. 2000. Using stress resistance to isolate novel longevity mutations in *Caenorhabditis elegans*. Ann. N. Y. Acad. Sci. **908:** 324–326.
50. De, C.E., C.S. Hegi De & T.E. Johnson. 2004. Isolation of long-lived mutants in *Caenorhabditis elegans* using selection for resistance to juglone. Free Radic. Biol. Med. **37:** 139–145.
51. Hansen, M., A.L. Hsu, A. Dillin, *et al.* 2005. New genes tied to endocrine, metabolic, and dietary regulation of lifespan from a *Caenorhabditis elegans*. Genomic RNAi Screen PLoS. Genetics **1:** e17.
52. Hamilton, B., Y. Dong, M. Shindo, *et al.* 2005. A systematic RNAi screen for longevity genes in *C. elegans*. Genes Dev. **19:** 1544–1555.
53. Melov, S., J. Ravenscroft, S. Malik, *et al.* 2000. Extension of life-span with superoxide dismutase/catalase mimetics. Science **289:** 1567–1569.
54. Sampayo, J.N., A. Olsen & G.J. Lithgow. 2003. Oxidative stress in *Caenorhabditis elegans*: protective effects of superoxide dismutase/catalase mimetics. Aging Cell **2:** 319–326.
55. Wood, J.G., B. Rogina, S. Lavu, *et al.* 2004. Sirtuin activators mimic caloric restriction and delay ageing in metazoans. Nature **430:** 686–689.
56. Evason, K., C. Huang, I. Yamben, *et al.* 2005. Anticonvulsant medications extend worm life-span. Science **307:** 258–262.
57. Gill, M.S., A. Olsen, J.N. Sampayo & G.J. Lithgow. 2003. An automated high-throughput assay for survival in the nematode *Caenorhabditis elegans*. Free Radic. Biol. Med. **35:** 558–565.
58. Hertweck, M., T. Hoppe & R. Baumeister. 2003. *C. elegans*, a model for aging with high-throughput capacity. Exp. Gerontol. **38:** 345–346.
59. Maine, E.M. 2001. RNAi as a tool for understanding germline development in *Caenorhabditis elegans*: uses and cautions. Dev. Biol. **239:** 177–189.
60. Sonnhammer, E.L. & R. Durbin. 1997. Analysis of protein domain families in *Caenorhabditis elegans*. Genomics **46:** 200–216.
61. Baumeister, R. & L. Ge. 2002. The worm in us: *Caenorhabditis elegans* as a model of human disease. Trends Biotechnol. **20:** 147–148.

62. FAY, D.S., A. FLUET, C.J. JOHNSON, *et al*. 1998. In vivo aggregation of beta-amyloid peptide variants. J. Neurochem. **71:** 1616–1625.
63. LINK, C.D. & C.J. JOHNSON. 2002. Reporter transgenes for study of oxidant stress in *Caenorhabditis elegans*. Methods Enzymol. **353:** 497–505.
64. NASS, R., D.H. HALL, D.M. MILLER, III, *et al*. 2002. Neurotoxin-induced degeneration of dopamine neurons in *Caenorhabditis elegans*. Proc. Natl. Acad. Sci. USA **99:** 3264–3269.
65. MORLEY, J.F., H.R. BRIGNULL, J.J. WEYERS, *et al*. 2002. The threshold for polyglutamine-expansion protein aggregation and cellular toxicity is dynamic and influenced by aging in *Caenorhabditis elegans*. Proc. Natl. Acad. Sci. USA **99:** 10417–10422.
66. SATYAL, S.H., E. SCHMIDT, K. KITAGAWA, *et al*. 2000. Polyglutamine aggregates alter protein folding homeostasis in *Caenorhabditis elegans*. Proc. Natl. Acad. Sci. USA **97:** 5750–5755.
67. FABER, P.W., J.R. ALTER, M.E. MACDONALD, *et al*. 1999. Polyglutamine-mediated dysfunction and apoptotic death of a *Caenorhabditis elegans* sensory neuron. Proc. Natl. Acad. Sci. USA **96:** 179–184.
68. PARKER, J.A., J.B. CONNOLLY, C. WELLINGTON, *et al*. 2001. Expanded polyglutamines in *Caenorhabditis elegans* cause axonal abnormalities and severe dysfunction of PLM mechanosensory neurons without cell death. Proc. Natl. Acad. Sci. USA **98:** 13318–13323.
69. PARKER, J.A., M. ARANGO, S. ABDERRAHMANE, *et al*. 2005. Resveratrol rescues mutant polyglutamine cytotoxicity in nematode and mammalian neurons. Nat. Genet. **37:** 349–350.

Age-Dependent Decrease in Renal Glucocorticoid Receptor Function Is Reversed by Dietary Restriction in Mice

RAMESH SHARMA AND DEBIPREETA DUTTA

Department of Biochemistry, North Eastern Hill University, Shillong 793022, India

ABSTRACT: The effects of age and dietary restriction (alternate days of feeding for 3 months) on the concentration, activation, and DNase I digestion of nuclear-bound glucocorticoid receptors (GRs) in the kidney of male mice at two different ages (5 months as adult and 20 months as old) were investigated. A significant decrease (30%) in the concentration of renal GRs was observed in older *ad libitum* (AL)-fed mice as compared to the adult mice. Dietary restriction (DR) of older mice significantly increased (28%) the level of GRs as compared to the AL-fed control animals. The affinity of the receptor for the hormone remained the same for both AL- and DR-fed animals at both ages. Scatchard and slot blot analyses of the data confirmed the decreased level of renal GRs in older mice compared to the adult mice as well as an increased level of receptor in older DR mice. Activation studies of GRs by both salt and heat indicated a decreased (15–20%) activation of renal GRs in older animals compared to the adult mice in the AL-fed group. It was further observed that DR significantly enhanced (30%) the degree of both salt- and heat-dependent activation of GRs in older animals compared to the AL-fed animals of the age-matched group. DNase I digestion and extraction of nuclear-bound GR complexes showed a lower degree (26%) of extraction in older AL-fed animals compared to the adult animals. However, DR did not alter the pattern of digestibility of bound GR complexes. These above findings indicate that DR could reverse the decrease of GR function in older animals and may provide better adaptability of kidney in water and electrolyte balance.

KEYWORDS: renal glucocorticoid receptor; mice; aging; dietary restriction

Address for correspondence: Ramesh Sharma, Department of Biochemistry, North Eastern Hill University, Shillong 793022, India. Voice: +91-364-272-2113; fax: 91-364-255-0108.
e-mail: sharamesh@gmail.com

Ann. N.Y. Acad. Sci. 1067: 129–141 (2006). © 2006 New York Academy of Sciences.
doi: 10.1196/annals.1354.016

INTRODUCTION

One of the serious consequences of aging is the loss of the organism's ability to cope with a variety of stresses due to a failure of cellular homeostasis.[1] Glucocorticoids (GCs) play a pivotal role in regulating basal and stress-related homeostasis. These hormones influence a number of biological processes in different tissues, including the kidney, where they affect glomerular filtration rate, ion transport, and electrolyte balance.[2-4] Most of the cellular effects of glucocorticoids are mediated by binding to a 94-kDa intracellular protein, the glucocorticoid receptor (GR), predominantly localized in the cytoplasm. The GR belongs to a superfamily of ligand-activated transcription factors.[5] The domain structure of the GR consists of an amino terminal transactivation domain, a central Zn-finger domain, and a carboxy terminal ligand-binding domain. Glucocorticoids, upon binding to the GR, translocate into the nucleus through a process called activation and interact with specific DNA sequences known as glucocorticoid response elements (GREs), resulting in increased or decreased gene expression.[6,7]

Dietary restriction (DR) commonly refers to a lowering of calorie intake without a reduction in the micronutrients essential for normal growth and development.[8,9] After McCay's initial studies[10] on DR, various laboratories have shown that DR can significantly extend life span in different groups of animals.[11,12] Emerging data on primate studies suggest a similar effect of DR on nonhuman primates.[13] DR delays a variety of diseases such as renal disorders, neoplasias, autoimmune diseases, and diabetes in different experimental animals.[14] It retards various pathophysiological changes associated with aging,[12,15-17] reduces age-associated neurodegenerative disorders in rodents,[18,19] and is also known to have protective effects against several types of cancer through the inhibition of cell proliferation and the induction of apoptosis.[20,21] Currently, DR is the only experimental method to retard aging in laboratory animals, exhibiting an increase of both mean and maximum life span.[22] Some of the effects of DR, such as protection against insulin-dependent diabetes in rodents, impaired tissue growth and regeneration, neurological impairments, and reproductive senescence are parallel to the consequences of elevated levels of glucocorticoids. The anti-inflammatory and antineoplastic effects of DR are also consistent with the same effects of an elevated level of glucocorticoids.[23] The exact mechanism of glucocorticoid-dependent mediation of the above processes is not fully elucidated. However, the action of GCs depends on the level of their receptors and also on post-receptor events. Keeping in view that these studies may provide basic knowledge of the mechanism of action of GCs during late onset of DR, we have studied the effect of such a restriction on the GR level, its activation, and DNase I digestion of nuclear-bound GR in the kidney of old male mice. There has been a fruitful debate on the age of onset of DR in experimental animals[24] vis-à-vis its feasibility for human practices. Herein, we have shown that the decrease in renal glucocorticoid receptor function is reversed by DR even when performed in older animals.

MATERIALS AND METHODS

Animals and Diets

Swiss albino (Balb/c strain) male mice of two different age groups (5- and 20-months old), maintained under normal laboratory conditions, were used for experimentation. The animals were fed with a standard pellet diet (Amrut Laboratory, Pune, India) and water *ad libitum*. Old mice subjected to DR were fed on alternate days for a period of 3 months.[25,26] However, they had free access to water on all days.

Chemicals and Buffers

[1, 2, 4, 6, 7-^{3}H] dexamethasone, a synthetic glucocorticoid (specific activity 91 Ci/mmol), was purchased from Amersham, UK. Nonradioactive dexamethasone was from Sigma Chemical Co., USA. All the other chemicals used were of highest analytical grade. The radioactive counting (cpm) was carried out using a Wallac 1409 liquid scintillation counter having 68% efficiency for tritium. The buffers used were as follows: (A) 0.25 M sucrose/10 mM Tris–HCl, pH 7.5/1 mM EDTA/10 mM sodium molybdate/10% (v/v) glycerol/1 mM DL-dithiothreitol/10 mM NaCl; (B) 0.25 M sucrose/10 mM Tris–HCl, pH 7.6; (C) 0.25 M sucrose/10 mM Tris–HCl, pH 7.6/0.5% (v/v) Triton X-100; and (D) 0.25 M sucrose/10 mM Tris–HCl, pH 7.6/4.2 mM MgCl$_2$.

Cytosol Preparation and Glucocorticoid Receptor Assay

Glucocorticoid receptors were assayed in the kidney as described elsewhere.[3,27–30] The number of specific binding sites (fmol/mg protein) and the dissociation constants (K_d) were calculated according to the method of Scatchard.[31]

GR Slot Blot Analysis

Polyclonal anti-GR-AB, raised against amino acid sequence (SVFS-NGYSSPGMRPDVS) from the N-terminal region of the rat GR was a gift from Profs. N. Katunama and H. Kido, Japan. The experiment was performed on Bio-Rad Bio-Dot® SF Micro filtration apparatus following the instructions given in the user's manual and as done previously.[29,32]

Preparation of Activated GR Complexes

A 20% (w/v) homogenate of kidney was prepared in buffer B. It was centrifuged at $2,000 \times g$ for 10 min at $2°C$ to sediment the nuclei. The supernatant was then centrifuged at $40,000 \times g$ for 45 min at $2°C$ and to the clear cytosol [^{3}H]dexamethasone was added to a final concentration of 40 nM; bound hormone–receptor (H-R) complexes were separated by DCC (in buffer B) treatment. Aliquots of these complexes were then subjected to salt (20 mM Ca^{2+}) and heat ($25°C$) activation for 45 min to obtain activated complexes.[28,29,33] Aliquots of the cytosols were also kept at $0°C$ for 45 min to provide the unactivated receptor complexes as controls.

DNA Cellulose and Nuclear Binding Assays

The magnitude of activation of renal GR was studied using DNA cellulose and nuclear binding assays as described earlier.[3,28,29,34,35] The radioactivity bound in pellets was expressed as CPM/100 μg DNA.

DNase I Digestion Studies

DNase I digestion studies were performed on purified nuclei obtained from the kidney of AL- and DR-fed mice of both the age groups as detailed earlier.[28,29,36] The results were expressed as percentages of [^{3}H]dexamethasone-receptor complexes bound to nuclei. Controls were taken as 100% bound.

Protein and DNA Estimations

The protein content of the receptor preparation was measured according to the dye-binding method of Bradford,[37] using bovine serum albumin (BSA) as standard. The concentration of DNA in a purified nuclear suspension was determined by the method of Burton.[38] Data obtained from different sets of experiments were analyzed statistically. The level of significance (P value) between two sets of data was calculated according to Student's t-test.

RESULTS

A significant decrease in the body weight (23%; $P < 0.001$) was observed in old dietary-restricted mice compared to the AL-fed mice (data not shown), signifying the impact of DR on those animals.

Studies on the level of GR revealed a decreased (30%) receptor level in the kidney of older animals as compared to the adult animals, whereas, the dietary-restricted old animals showed a significant increase (28%) in the receptor concentration compared to the AL-fed counterparts (TABLE 1). Scatchard analyses

TABLE 1. Concentration and affinity of [^{3}H]dexamethasone–receptor in the kidney of adult, old, and old dietary-restricted male mice

Animals	Concentration (fmol/mg protein)	Affinity (nM)
Adult	111.2 ± 6.91	2.41 ± 0.03
Old	77.37 ± 6.27*	2.36 ± 0.11
Old-DR	99.50 ± 7.08**	2.46 ± 0.08

*Statistically significant ($P < 0.001$) with respect to adult mice.
**Statistically significant ($P < 0.001$) with respect to old mice.

of the data confirmed both the age-specific decrease of receptors in AL-fed mice, as well as the increase of receptors in DR animals compared to the AL-fed animals. Slopes of the plot did not exhibit any alteration in the affinity of the GR for its ligand in the two different age groups in the kidneys of DR-fed mice (FIG. 1). Slot blot analyses of the receptor preparation in both the age groups also confirmed the decreased level of GR in old mice, as well as an increased level of GR protein in old DR animals compared to the AL-fed animals (FIG. 2).

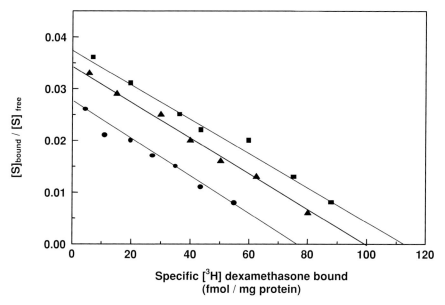

FIGURE 1. Scatchard plot of [^{3}H]dexamethasone binding in the kidney of adult (■), old (●), and old dietary-restricted (▲) male mice. Cytosols were incubated with 5–120 nM [^{3}H]dexamethasone ± 500-fold excess cold dexamethasone for 4 h at 0°C. Specific binding at each concentration was calculated by subtracting nonspecific binding from total binding, and the data obtained were analyzed by the Scatchard method. The slope of the curve gave the dissociation constant (K_d), and the intercept on the x-axis gave the maximum receptor binding sites. Each point is the mean of four separate experiments with 5–6 mice of each group.

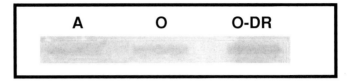

FIGURE 2. Slot blot analysis of kidney glucocorticoid receptor from adult (A), old (O), and old dietary-restricted (O-DR) male mice. Equal amount of kidney cytosol containing GR from each group of mice was applied onto each slot and processed for immunoblotting using anti-GR antibody and anti-rabbit IgG-HRP conjugate.

Salt- (20 mM Ca^{2+} at $0°C$ for 45 min) and temperature- ($25°C$ for 45 min) dependent activation of the GR was studied in the kidney of both adult and old mice using DNA cellulose and purified nuclear binding assays. Results indicated a lower activation of receptors (15–20%) in older animals compared to the adult animals. A higher level of activation by both salt and heat in older DR animals was observed compared to the AL-fed animals as judged by both the DNA cellulose (FIG. 3) and nuclear (FIG. 4) binding assays.

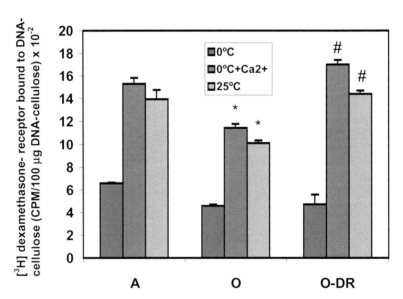

FIGURE 3. Specific binding of kidney [³H]dexamethasone–receptor complexes to DNA cellulose from the adult (A), old (O), and old dietary-restricted (O-DR) mice. Cytosols were prepared in buffer B and the hormone–receptor complexes obtained by incubating with 40 nM [³H]dexamethasone for 4 h at $0°C$. The hormone–receptor complexes were then subjected to Ca^{2+} (20 mM at $0°C$) and heat ($25°C$) activation for 45 min as against $0°C$ control. The results are mean ± standard deviation of four separate experiments with 5–6 mice of each group. *Statistically significant ($P < 0.05$) compared to the adult. #Statistically significant ($P < 0.001$) compared to the old mice.

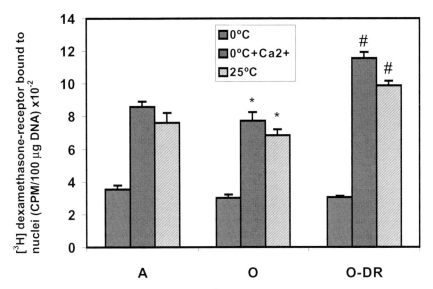

FIGURE 4. Specific binding of kidney [^{3}H]dexamethasone–receptor complexes to purified nuclei from the adult (A), old (O), and old dietary-restricted (O-DR) mice. The hormone–receptor complex preparations and activation conditions are the same as given in FIGURE. 3. Activated hormone–receptor complexes were incubated with purified nuclei instead of DNA cellulose. The results are mean ± standard deviation for four separate experiments with 5–6 mice of each group. *Statistically significant ($P < 0.05$) compared to the adult. #Statistically significant ($P < 0.001$) compared to the old mice.

DNase I digestion of bound GR from the kidney revealed a significantly higher (26%) extraction of nuclear-bound heat-activated [^{3}H]dexamethasone– receptor complexes from adults as compared to the old animals. However, no significant change in the magnitude of extraction was observed between old AL and DR animals (FIG. 5).

DISCUSSION

Aging is a progressive accumulation of changes that are associated with ever-increasing susceptibility to diseases and death. Investigators at a number of laboratories are striving to understand the mechanistic interactions between nutrition and aging.[39] Experiments have purportedly shown that DR provides a variety of protective mechanisms during aging.[8] Alterations in the adaptive responses to hormones and other biochemical stimuli, including a decreased ability to respond to stress, are characteristics of aged animals. The mechanisms controlling the adaptive responses to reduced calorie intake may involve a dynamic interplay of hormones that control energy balance, appetite, cell

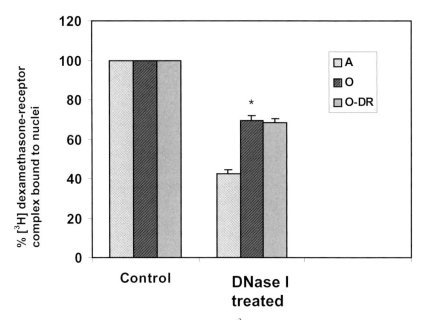

FIGURE 5. DNase I extractability of bound [^{3}H]dexamethasone–receptor complexes from the kidney nuclei of adult (A), old (O), and old dietary-restricted (O-DR) mice. Heat-activated, nuclear-bound hormone–receptor complexes were extracted using DNase I as per experimental protocols. The results are mean $\pm$ standard deviation of four separate experiments performed for each group. *Statistically significant ($P < 0.001$) compared to the adult.

proliferation and apoptosis, stress responses, inflammation, and repair systems.[23] All such effects in one way or another are regulated by glucocorticoids (GCs). GCs exert their cellular and molecular actions by binding to GRs, which ultimately modulate the expression of genes by a cascade of regulatory events.[4,40,41] GR concentration and properties change during aging and this decrease in receptor number has been observed in numerous tissues.[42–44] Herein, we have studied the long-term effect of DR on the endogenous level of GR, its activation, and digestion of nuclear-bound receptors by DNase I in the kidney of older animals. In our experimental schedule, we followed the 3-month dietary restriction regimen that gave the maximum stable change in GR expression. It was observed that 3-month DR significantly reduced the body weight of old mice. This observation of body weight reduction confirmed that the animals were indeed subjected to dietary restriction and that is consistent with earlier reports.[29,45]

Data on GR level suggest an overall decrease (30%) in the receptor level in the kidneys of old mice compared to the adult mice. The high level of receptors in the kidneys of the adult animals may be a contributory factor for the role of this hormone during the early growth and development of the organ.[2,3]

Decrease in the kidney GR level of old mice may impair renal functions, which may be one of the reasons for the reduced ability to maintain renal filtration rate and water and electrolyte homeostasis during old age.[28] Other reports also suggest a decrease in the GR level with aging in rat liver and kidney.[2,29,46] Lowered GR concentration is also observed in the presence of normal plasma GCs in aged humans. The reduction may indeed be an inherent part of the aging process.[47,48] Our data also exhibited an increase in the level of receptors in kidney during DR in old animals compared to the AL-fed animals. Such an increase in the receptor concentration may help the old animals control the GC-mediated responses during DR. GCs are known to influence glomerular filtration rate, ion transport, Na^+ uptake, and other metabolic functions in the kidney.[2,3,49,50] Higher level of GR in the kidney of older DR mice may help the animals to maintain electrolyte balance and a kidney filtration rate more efficiently, which would otherwise be affected by the aging process. Scatchard and slot blot analyses of the binding data confirmed the decreased level of receptor concentration with increasing age. However, slopes of the Scatchard plots did not reveal any change in the affinity of receptor for its ligand in the two different age groups. DR rodents are more resistant to a variety of stresses on account of increased production of stress proteins that may increase the resistance of cells.[51] In old animals, an elevated level of GR by dietary restriction might help to enhance different biological activities and quite likely provide better adaptability to the environment.[29]

Activation studies of GR were carried out in the kidney of old mice during dietary restriction to see any change in the magnitude of salt- (Ca^{2+} at $0°C$ for 45 min) and temperature- ($25°C$ for 45 min) dependent activation. A significant decrease (15–20%) was observed in the magnitude of activation in renal GR in old animals compared to the adult animals in the AL-fed mice. The differences in the endogenous modulators of GR functioning at two different phases of life span and/or alterations in the physicochemical properties of GRs might play a role in lowering the activation in older mice.[52] Low-temperature Ca^{2+}-dependent activation of the H–R complexes was more pronounced than temperature-mediated activation in the kidney of older animals. The exact mechanisms for this activation are not well understood. However, Ca^{2+} enhancement of nuclear and DNA cellulose binding of GR may be due to a direct interaction of Ca^{2+} with the receptor molecule and/or receptor-transforming factor(s), which results in a conformational change capable of exposing the DNA- and/or chromatin-binding domain.[2,53] Low-temperature Ca^{2+}-dependent activation was more pronounced when DNA cellulose rather than purified nuclei is used. This may be due to the open DNA binding sites in DNA cellulose compared with intact nuclei.[2] A greater activation (30%) of renal receptors was observed in old mice subjected to DR compared to the AL-fed mice. This increase in the receptor activation in aged DR animals may help them achieve better GC action at that stage of the life span.

The digestion and extraction of nuclear-bound GR by DNase I was studied in the kidney of adult, old, and old dietary-restricted mice in order to reveal the differences, if any, in the extraction of nuclear-bound receptors. Aging increases the compactness of chromatin and reduces its digestibility by DNase I.[54] DNase I cuts the DNA where it is maximally exposed and that depends on the degree of chromatin condensation. Our observation revealed a higher degree of extraction of nuclear-bound hormone–receptor complexes in the adult kidney as compared to the old, whereas DR did not show any effect on such extractability. It relates to the fact that there may not be any appreciable change in the organization of chromatin in DR animals compared to the AL-fed animals.[29] Our findings of reduced extractability by DNase I in aged animals corroborate with the observations of others who also reported reduced digestibility of chromatin by DNase I of the old rat brain compared to that of the young and the adult.[36,55]

In conclusion, our findings indicate a decreased level of GRs in the kidney of old mice and that long-term DR results in an increase in the GR level in those animals. DR also increases the magnitude of activation of GRs in older mice that is otherwise reduced. Hence, DR could be used to elevate the GR concentration in older animals whose receptor level is already reduced during that period of the life span. Furthermore, the higher magnitude of receptor activation in older DR mice could be an advantage to such animals for attaining better glucocorticoid-mediated renal responses and for adapting to stress in old age.[29]

ACKNOWLEDGMENTS

We are grateful to the Department of Science and Technology (DST), New Delhi (SP/SO/D-33/99) and to the North Eastern Hill University, Shillong for providing research facilities. D.D. thanks the DST for a Junior Research Fellowship.

REFERENCES

1. KIM, H.J., K.J. JUNG, B.P. YU, et al. 2002. Modulation of redox sensitive transcription factors by calorie restriction during aging. Mech. Ageing Dev. **123:** 1589–1595.
2. SHARMA, R. & P.S. TIMIRAS. 1988. Regulation of glucocorticoid receptors in kidney of immature and mature male rats. Int. J. Biochem. **20:** 141–145.
3. BORBHUIYA, M.A. & R. SHARMA. 1995. Postnatal changes in kidney glucocorticoid receptor of mice. Indian J. Biochem. Biophys. **32:** 125–129.
4. KINO, T., M.V. DEMARTINO, E. CHARMANDARI, et al. 2003. Tissue glucocorticoid resistance/hypersensitivity syndromes. J. Steroid Biochem. Mol. Biol. **85:** 457–467.

5. O'MALLEY, B.W., N.J. MCKENNA, J. XU, *et al*. 1999. Nuclear receptor coactivators: multiple enzymes, multiple complexes, multiple functions. J. Steroid Biochem. Mol. Biol. **69:** 3–12.

6. BARNES, P.J. 1998. Anti-inflammatory actions of glucocorticoids: molecular mechanism. Clin. Sci. (Lond) **94:** 557–572.

7. ADCOCK, I.M. 2000. Molecular mechanisms of glucocorticosteroid actions. Pulmon. Pharmacol. Therap. **13:** 115–126.

8. YU, B.P. 1996. Ageing and oxidative stress: modulation by dietary restriction. Free Radic. Biol. Med. **21:** 651–668.

9. SHARMA, R. 2004. Dietary restriction and its multifaceted effects. Curr. Sci. **87:** 1203–1210.

10. MCCAY, C.M., M.F. CROWELL & L.A. MAYNARD. 1935. The effect of retarded growth upon the length of life span and upon the ultimate body size. J. Nutr. **10:** 63–79.

11. RICHARDSON, A. 1985. The effect of age and nutrition on protein synthesis by cells and tissues from mammals. *In* Handbook of Nutrition in the Aged. W.R. Watson Ed.: 31–48. CRC Press, Boca Raton, FL.

12. WEINDRUCH, R. & R.L. WALFORD. 1988. The Retardation of Aging and Diseases by Dietary Restriction. Charles C Thomas, Springfield, IL.

13. ROTH, G.S., M.A. LANE, R. CABO, *et al*. 2004. The Roy Walford legacy: DR from molecules to mice to monkeys to man and onto mimetics. Exp. Gerontol. **39:** 897–902.

14. KOUBOVA, J. & L. GUARENTE. 2003. How does caloric restriction work? Genes Dev. **17:** 313–321.

15. MASARO, E.J. 1993. Dietary restriction and aging. J. Am. Geriatr. Soc. **41:** 994–999.

16. SOHAL, R. & R. WEINDRUCH. 1996. Oxidative stress, caloric restriction and aging. Science **273:** 59–66.

17. LEE, C.K., R. KLOPP, R., WEINDRUCH, *et al*. 1999. Gene expression profile of aging and its retardation by calorie restriction. Science **285:** 1390–1393.

18. DUAN, W. & M.P. MATTSON. 1999. Dietary restriction and 2-deoxyglucose administration improve behavioral outcome and reduce degeneration of dopaminergic neurons in models of Parkinson's disease. J. Neurosci. Res. **57:** 195–206.

19. ZHU, H., Q. GUO & M.P. MATTSON. 1999. Dietary restriction protects hippocampal neurons against the death promoting action of presenilin-1 mutation. Brain Res. **842:** 224–229.

20. JAMES, S. & L. MUSKHELISHVILI. 1994. Rates of apoptosis and proliferation vary with calorie intake and may influence incidence of spontaneous hepatoma in C57BL\6x C3H mice. Cancer Res. **54:** 5508–5510.

21. KRITCHOVSKY, D. 1997. Calorie restriction and experimental mammary carcinogenesis. Breast Cancer Res. Treat. **46:** 161–167.

22. YU, B.P. 2000. Dietary restriction and life-extension. *In* Aging Methods and Protocols. Y.A. Barnett & C.R. Bernett, Eds.: 353–359. Humana Press, Totowa.

23. LEAKY, J.E.A., L.T. FRAME & R.W. HART. 1998. Caloric restriction as a mechanism mediating resistance to environmental disease. Environ. Health Perspect. **106:** 313–324.

24. GOTO, S., R. TAKAHASHI, S. ARAKI, *et al*. 2002. Dietary restriction initiated in late adulthood can reverse age-related alterations of protein and protein metabolism. Ann. N.Y. Acad. Sci. **959:** 50–56.

25. MERRY, B.J. 1999. *In* Studies of Aging. H. Sternberg & P.S. Timiras, Eds.: 143–163. Springer-Verlag, Berlin.

26. NAGAI, M., R. TAKAHASHI & S. GOTO. 2002. Effect of dietary restriction beyond middle age: accumulation of altered protein degradation. Microsc. Res. Tech. **59:** 278–281.

27. KALIMI, M., S. GUPTA, J. HUBBARD, *et al.* 1983. Glucocorticoid receptors in adult and senescent rat liver. Endocrinology **112:** 341–347.

28. RANHOTRA, H.S. & R. SHARMA. 2001. Modulation of hepatic and renal glucocorticoid receptor during aging of mice. Biogerontology **2:** 248–251.

29. DUTTA, D. & R. SHARMA. 2004. Age-dependent dietary regulation of glucocorticoid receptors in the liver of mice. Biogerontology **5:** 177–184.

30. BEATO, M. & P. FIEGELSON. 1972. Glucocorticoid binding proteins of rat liver cytosol. I. Separation and identification of the binding proteins. J. Biol. Chem. **247:** 7890–7896.

31. SCATCHARD, G. 1949. The attractions of proteins for small molecules and ions. Ann. N.Y. Acad. Sci. **51:** 660–672.

32. DUTTA, D. & R. SHARMA. 2003. Regulation of hepatic glucocorticoid receptors in mice during dietary restriction. Horm. Metab. Res. **35:** 415–420.

33. SHARMA, R. & P.S. TIMIRAS. 1987. Age-dependent regulation of glucocorticoid receptor in the liver of male rats. Biochim. Biophys. Acta **930:** 237–243.

34. KALIMI, M., P. COLEMAN & P. FIEGELSON. 1975. The activated hepatic glucocorticoid receptor complex: its generation and properties. J. Biol. Chem. **250:** 1080–1086.

35. EBERHARDT, N.L., T. VALCANA & P.S. TIMIRAS. 1978. Triiodothyronine nuclear receptors: an in vitro comparison of the binding of triiodothyronine to nuclei of adult rat liver, cerebral hemisphere, and anterior pituitary. Endocrinology **102:** 556–561.

36. CHATURVEDI, M.M. & M.S. KANUNGO. 1983. Analysis of chromatin of the brain of young and old rats by micrococcal nuclease and DNase I. Biochem. Int. **6:** 357–363.

37. BRADFORD, M. 1976. A rapid and sensitive method for the quantitation of microgram quantities of protein using the principle of protein-dye binding. Anal. Biochem. **72:** 248–254.

38. BURTON, K. 1968. Determination of DNA concentration with diphenylamine. Meth. Enzymol. **12:** 163–166.

39. YU, B.P. & H.Y. CHUNG. 2001. Stress resistance by calorie restriction for longevity. Ann. N.Y. Acad. Sci. **928:** 39–47.

40. BIOLLA, A. & M. PALLARDY. 2000. Mode of actions of glucocorticoids. Presse Med. **29:** 215–223.

41. SCHAFF, M.J. & J.A. CIDLOWSKI. 2002. Molecular mechanisms of glucocorticoid action and resistance. Steroid Biochem. Mol. Biol. **83:** 37–48.

42. PETROVIC, J.S. & R.Z. MARKOVIC. 1975. Changes in cortisol binding to soluble receptor proteins in rat liver and thymus during development and aging. Dev. Biol. **45:** 176–182.

43. ROTH, G.S. & G.D. HESS. 1982. Changes in the mechanism of hormone and neurotransmitter action during aging: current status of the role of the receptor and post-receptor alterations. Mech. Ageing Dev. **20:** 175–194.

44. ARMANINI, D., M. SCALI, G. VITTADELLO, *et al.* 1993. Corticosteroid receptor and aging. J. Steroid. Biochem. Mol. Biol. **45:** 191–194.

45. LEE, J., P.J. HERMAN & M.P. MATTSON. 2000. Dietary restriction selectively decreases GR expression in the hippocampus and cerebral cortex of rats. Exp. Neurol. **166:** 435–441.

46. DJORDJOVIC-MARKOVIC, R., O. RADIC, V. JELIC, *et al.* 1999. Glucocorticoid receptors in aging rats. Exp. Gerontol. **34:** 971–982.
47. SAPOLSKY, R.M., M. ARMANINI, D. PACKAN, *et al.* 1987. Stress and glucocorticoids in aging. Endocr. Metab. Clin. **16:** 965–980.
48. ARMANINI, D., I. KARBOWIAK, M. SCALI, *et al.* 1992. Corticosteroid receptors and lymphocyte subsets in mononuclear leukocytes in aging. Am. J. Physiol. **262:** 464–466.
49. FANESTILL, D.D. & C. PARK. 1981. Steroid hormones and the kidney. Annu. Rev. Physiol. **43:** 637–649.
50. BERTRAM, C., A.R. TROWERN, W. COPIN, *et al.* 2001. The maternal diet during pregnancy programs altered expression of the glucocorticoid receptors and type 2 beta-hydroxysteroid dehydrogenase: potential molecular mechanism underlying the programming of hypertension *in utero*. Endocrinology **142:** 2841–2853.
51. WEINDRUCH, R., K.P. KEENAN, J.M. CARNEY, *et al.* 2001. Caloric restriction mimetics: metabolic interventions. J. Gerontol. **56A:** 20–33.
52. BODINE, P.V. & G. LITWACK. 1988. Evidence that the modulator of the glucocorticoid receptor complex is the endogenous molybdate factor. Proc. Natl. Acad. Sci. USA **85:** 1462–1466.
53. GRODY, W.W., W.J. SCHRADER & B.W. O'MALLEY. 1982. Activation, transformation and subunit structure of steroid hormone receptors. Endocr. Rev. **3:** 141–163.
54. KANUNGO, M.S. 1994. Genes and Aging. Cambridge University Press, Cambridge, UK.
55. CHAURASIA, P. & M.K. THAKUR. 1997. Nucleosomal organization of the rat satellite DNA-containing chromatin during aging. Mech. Ageing Dev. **95:** 63–70.

Investigation of Differentially Expressed Genes in the Ventricular Myocardium of Senescent Rats

AKIRA ISHIHATA[a] AND YUMI KATANO[b]

[a]*Department of Physiology I, Yamagata University School of Medicine, Yamagata 990-9585, Japan*

[b]*Division of Theoretical Nursing, Yamagata University School of Medicine, Yamagata 990-9585, Japan*

ABSTRACT: Aging alters a variety of physiological functions of the heart. The molecular basis of the age-related functional changes has not been fully understood. Differential gene expression provides the basis for many fundamental cellular processes associated with development and aging. The identification and cloning of genes whose expression is modulated by aging can be of importance for our better understanding of these age-related phenomena. In order to isolate and characterize gene products differentially expressed in senescent hearts, we applied a differential display method for screening those genes in rat ventricular myocardium. Total RNAs were isolated from 2-month-old (young) and 24-month-old rat (senescent) ventricles by the acid-guanidium-phenol-chloroform method. The first-strand synthesis of the cDNAs from each RNA was carried out with oligo-d(T) primers. The differential display screening was performed with three arbitrary primers and eight anchor primers, and the products were isolated on a 6% denaturing polyacrylamide gel. The bands showing differential expression were excised and subcloned into T-vector. We selected 19 upregulated clones and 66 downregulated clones in aged rat hearts. The differential expression of those candidate genes was confirmed by reverse Northern blot analysis. The selected genes were sequenced by dye-terminator methods. Among 31 clones, 15 clones were unknown. The known products included alpha-myosin heavy chain, cytochrome oxidase subunit, H^+-transporting ATP synthase F0 complex subunit c isoform 3 (ATP5G3), and Na^+-K^+-Cl^- cotransporter. The RT-PCR differential display method effectively identified genes differentially expressed in senescent hearts, and may be a useful tool for investigating factors responsible for age-related physiological changes.

KEYWORDS: aging; heart; rat; differential display

Address for correspondence: Akira Ishihata, M.D., Ph.D., Department of Physiology I, Yamagata University School of Medicine, 2-2-2, Iida-Nishi, Yamagata, 990-9585, Japan. Voice: +81-23-628-5214; fax: +81-23-628-5215.

e-mail: ishihata@med.id.yamagata-u.ac.jp

Ann. N.Y. Acad. Sci. 1067: 142–151 (2006). © 2006 New York Academy of Sciences.
doi: 10.1196/annals.1354.017

INTRODUCTION

It has been known that the physiological function of the heart is altered by aging. For example, aged hearts respond differently to sympathetic stimulation compared with young hearts. The positive inotropic effects of endothelin-1 is decreased by aging in the rat ventricles.[1] However, the molecular basis of these age-dependent functional changes has not been understood. Alteration in the expression of genes and its products in tissues or organs provides the basis for many fundamental cell physiological and pathophysiological changes associated with differentiation, development, cancer, degenerative diseases, and aging. The identification and cloning of genes whose expression is upregulated or downregulated may become an important step in further understanding these physiological/pathophysiological phenomena. The method for identifying those genes by differential display with RT-PCR was first reported by Zhang et al.[2] in 1996, and then the method was applied to studying the differential gene expression in normal and diseased conditions of various organs. In the heart, for example, differentially expressed genes following brief cardiac ischemia in pig were characterized,[3] and Li et al.[4] reported several genes of altered expression in the rat cardiac hypertropic models by using this technique.

In order to isolate and characterize gene products differentially expressed in aged heart, we applied the RT-PCR differential display method for screening those genes in rat ventricles. The present study showed that expression of several genes was shown to be altered by aging. They included several unknown genes in addition to genes already identified.

MATERIAL AND METHODS

Animals

In this study, 2-month-old and 24-month-old male Fischer 344 rats were obtained from Charles River Japan (Atsugi, Japan). Experiments were performed in accordance with the "Guide for Care and Use of Laboratory Animals" published by the U.S. National Institutes of Health (NIH Publication No. 85-23, revised 1996) and under the regulations of the Animal Care Committee of Yamagata University School of Medicine. Rats were anesthesized with diethylether and were sacrificed by cervical dislocation, and hearts were quickly removed and snap frozen in liquid nitrogen and stored at $-80°C$ until use.

Isolation of Messenger RNAs from Rat Ventricles

Total RNAs were isolated from 2-month-old and 24-month-old rat left ventricles by the acid-guanidium-phenol-chloroform method. Reverse transcription

TABLE 1. Primers used in differential display screening

	Anchored primers		
A	5′-AAG CTT TTT TTT TTT A-3′	B	5′-AAG CTT TTT TTT TTT C-3′
C	5′-AAG CTT TTT TTT TTT G-3′		
	Arbitrary primers		
R1	5′-AAG CTT GAT TGC C-3′	R2	5′-AAG CTT CGA CTG T-3′
R3	5′-AAG CTT TGG TCA G-3′	R4	5′-AAG CTT CTC AAC G-3′
R5	5′-AAG CTT AGT AGG C-3′	R6	5′-AAG CTT GCA CCA T-3′
R7	5′-AAG CTT AAC GAG G-3′	R8	AAG CTT TTA CCG C-3′

was done using 0.2 μg chromosomal DNA-free total RNA. The total RNA was mixed with RT buffer, 20 μM dNTP, and 0.2 μM of each anchored oligo-d(T) primer (TABLE 1). The mixture was heated to 65°C for 5 min, incubated at 37°C for 10 min. Next, MMLV-reverse transcriptase (1 μL) was added to each tube, and quickly mixed well before continuing incubation at 37°C for 50 min. Then, the tubes were heated to 75°C for 5 minutes to inactivate MMLV-reverse transcriptase without denaturing the mRNA/cDNA duplex to prevent initial mispriming by the arbitrary primer in the PCR reaction. Finally, the mixture was cooled on ice. The products of RT reaction were used for PCR reaction at the next step.

PCR

The PCR reaction was carried out in the mixture containing 1U of Taq DNA polymerase (Qiagen GmBH, Hilden, Germany), RT reaction mix (cDNA; 2 μL), anchored oligo-d(T) primer as used above (0.2 μM), each arbitrary primer (0.2 μM, TABLE 1), dNTP (2.5μM), and α-[^{33}P]dATP (2000 Ci/mmol, New England Nuclear, Boston, MA). After this mixture was overlayed with mineral oil, thermocycling was started (9700 thermocycler, Perkin-Elmer, Foster City, CA) (94°C for 15 s, 40°C for 2 min, 72°C for 30 s, 40 cycles) followed by 72°C for 5 min, and left at 4°C until use.

Six Percent Urea-Denaturing Polyacrylamide Gel Electrophoresis and Reamplification of the Genes of Interest

The PCR products (3.5 μL) mixed with loading dye were size-fractionated on 6% polyacrylamide gel containing 8 M urea. Electrophoresis was done at 40 W for 4 h at constant power. The gel was blotted onto a paper and dried at 80°C for 2.5 h, and exposed for 2 days. After developing the film, the differentially expressed bands of interest (>150 bp) were excised from the dried gel and purified.

Reamplification of the purified gene was done using the same primer set and PCR conditions described above except the dNTP concentration was at

20 μM instead of 2 μM and no isotopes were added. PCR products (30 μL) were run on a 1.5% agarose gel and stained with ethidium bromide. The remaining PCR samples were saved at −20°C for cloning: cDNAs were extracted by using QIAEX II, and cloned into a pBluescript KSII(+) T-vector, and used as cDNA probes.

Reverse Northern Blot Analysis

The recombinant plasmids were digested with Hind III to cut PCR products out. They were separated on 1.5% agarose gel in TAE buffer (100 V, 1 h) and extracted (QIAEX II). For the radiolabeling of first-strand cDNA by reverse transcription, the ReversePrime cDNA labeling kit (GeneHunter, Nashville, TN) was used. The labeled cDNA was used as probes to screen for the putative differentially expressed cDNA fragments isolated as above. This reverse Northern strategy allows us a large number of cDNA fragments of interest to be screened.[2] This technique facilitates the verification of differentially expressed cDNAs isolated by differential display, reduces the rate of false positives, and reduces the amount of RNA sample necessary for complete analysis. A pair of total RNA samples used for DD with same amount was labeled by reverse transcription with MMLV-RT. After gel filtration by the Sephadex G-50 column, equal amounts (cpm) from both young and aged cDNAs were used as probes to screen the cloned PCR fragments constructed above. Each amplified cDNA insert (30 μL) was mixed with 10 μL of 2N NaOH (with 2 mM EDTA), denatured at 95°C for 5 min, neutralized by adding 10 μL of 3 M sodium acetate (pH 5.0), and blotted onto duplicate Hybond N$^+$ membrane (Amersham, Arlington, IL) by using the slot-blot microfiltration system. The membranes were UV cross-linked and rinsed in 6×SSC (standard saline citrate) before hybridization.[5] After washing, membranes were dried and autoradiography was done.

Sequencing the Cloned Genes

Purified DNAs were sequenced by dye-terminator methods (ABI 310). The DNA sequences were compared on DNA sequence database by using BLAST or FASTA search program.[6]

Northern Blot Analysis

The selected genes were verified to be differentially expressed in the aged heart by using Northern blot analysis. Total RNA (20 μg) from left ventricles of young and aged rats was separated in a 1% agarose gel containing 2.2 M formaldehyde and transferred to a Hybond N$^+$ membrane. After the UV fixation of RNA onto the membrane, the filter was transferred to a solution of

0.5 M sodium acetate (pH 5.2) and 0.04% methylene blue for 5–10 minutes at room temperature to stain the RNA.[7] Prehybridization was carried out in 50% formamide, 6 × SSC (1 × SSC contains 0.15 M NaCl and 1.5 mM sodium citrate, pH 7.0), 2 × Denhardt's solution (0.1% Ficoll, 0.1% BSA, and 0.1% polyvinylpyrrolidone), 1% SDS, 10 mM sodium phosphate buffer, and 0.2 mg/mL denatured salmon sperm DNA for 4 h; then the membrane was hybridized with a ^{32}P-labeled probe for 16–24 h at 42°C. Membranes were washed and exposed to XAR-5 films (Kodak, Rochester, NY). The autoradiograms were quantified densitometrically. The 28S ribosomal RNA was used to normalize the differences in loaded and transferred RNA.

RESULTS AND DISCUSSION

Six Percent Urea-Denaturing Polyacrylamide Gel Electrophoresis

We compared the gene expression in the left ventricles of young (2 months old) and senescent (24 months old) rats. Typical examples of the differentially display gels are shown in FIGURE 1, where lanes 1 and 2 were obtained from senescent rat hearts and lanes 3 and 4 were obtained from young rat hearts. Most of the bands were unlikely to be of different densities. However, several bands were apparently differentially expressed. Arrowheads indicate the gene products we were interested in. Some of them were expressed more in young heart (arrowhead on right side), while others were upregulated in senescent rat (arrowhead on left side).

Reamplification of the Genes of Interest

To confirm that each gene was expressed more in the senescent rat ventricles, cDNA was purified from the band, reamplified, and used for reverse Northern blot analysis. The result of successful reamplification was shown in FIGURE 2. The reamplified PCR products were cloned into pBluescript KSII(+) T-vector, and reverse Northern analysis was done. FIGURE 3 shows the autoradiography of the reverse Northern blot analysis with slot-blot hybridization. These results

---

FIGURE 1. A typical differential display analysis of gene expression in left ventricular myocardium of young and senescent rats. The first two lanes in each gel are derived from aged rat hearts, and the second two lanes are of young hearts. *Arrowheads* to the right of each gel indicate that the products are more prominent in young rats and those to the left indicate the products of more prominent in aged hearts. Primers were indicated in the top of the figure. For example, A2 indicates that anchor primer was A and arbitrary primer was R2, as shown in TABLE 1. Age of the RNA sample was indicated in the top of each gel (A: aged, Y: young). Electrophoresis was carried out at 40 W for 4 h at constant power.

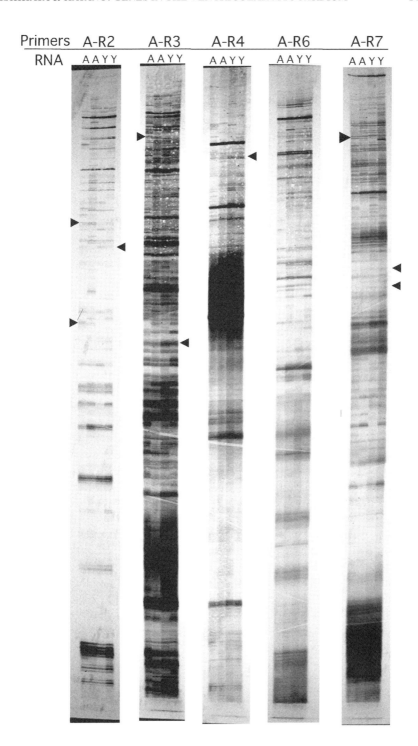

confirmed that the genes of A1, C1, C2, E2, F1, and G1 were more prominent in young heart, while B3, C3, D3, G3, and H3 were upregulated in aged heart.

Verification of the Differentially Expressed Genes in the Rat Heart by Northern Blot Analysis

Some genes were verified by conventional Northern blot analysis for their age-related changes in expression. FIGURE 4 shows that A1 and A12 expressions were downregulated in senescent rat heart. These differentially expressed genes were sequenced by using the dye-terminator method. By comparing with DNA database, A1 was revealed to be a part of H+ transporting ATP synthase F0 complex subunit c isoform 3 (ATP5G3) gene, and A12 was a part of the rat Na^+-K^+-Cl^- cotransporter.

Goyns et al.[8] (1998) reported that generally a relatively small number of PCR products (about 2% of the total number of PCR products observed) show age-related differences in all tissues. They demonstrated that in rat heart most of the PCR products were observed at similar levels in differential display gels, but one product appeared to be more prominent in the old hearts. That was revealed to be a part of the mitochondrial genome. They suggested that mito-chondrial sequences had been amplified on account of the anchored primer, priming the PCR reaction in both directions. In this study, we could detect several differentially displayed gene products in a polyacrylamide gel. ATP synthase is a key enzyme in oxidative phosphorylation and responsible for the production of most of the ATP in mammalian organisms. The absolute amounts of the transcripts of most subunits of rat H^+-ATP synthase exam-ined differed greatly in different tissues, showing the following hierarchy of tissue specificity: heart > kidney > brain, liver.[9] We demonstrated here that one of the ATP synthase subunits is downregulated in senescent heart. ATP synthase expression was reported to be decreased in the heart of those with chronic nicotine consumption,[10] while increased in the norepinephrine-infused hypertrophic heart.[4] These results suggest age-related changes in the energy metabolism in the heart. Another differentially expressed gene, confirmed in the present study, is Na^+-K^+-Cl^- cotransporter. It has been reported that bumetanide-sensitive Na^+-K^+-Cl^- cotransporter has a role in the positive in-otropic effect of ouabain in rat cardiac myocytes by increasing Na^+ influx into the cells.[11] We revealed here that the expression of Na^+-K^+-Cl^- cotransporter is downregulated in aged heart, suggesting that the myocardial dysfunction may be related, at least in part, to the decreased expression of the cotrans-porter. In general, it is not clear whether increase or decrease of expression of specific genes is a cause or an effect of age-related physiological changes. In addition, whether the alteration of gene expression in senescent heart is due to the decreased transcription or the instability of its mRNA, is unknown. How-ever, the identified genes in the present study were known to be physiologically

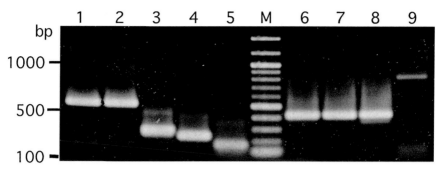

FIGURE 2. Reamplification of cDNAs excised from differential display gels by using the same primer set as the first time PCR. M: marker.

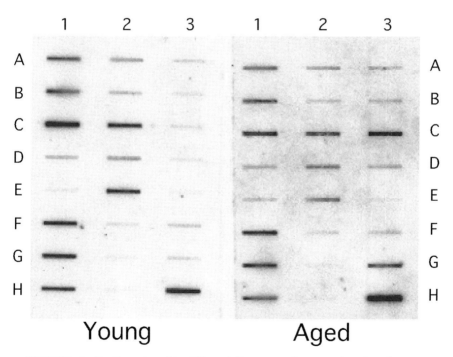

FIGURE 3. Confirmation of the differentially expressed gene products by using reverse Northern slot blot analysis. The selected PCR products were purified from differential display gels, reamplified by PCR, and cloned into pBlueScriptKS(+) vector. Equal amounts of inserts were spotted onto duplicate Hybond+ membranes by using slot-blot hybridization apparatus. Each membrane was hybridized with labeled cDNA (10^7 cpm) prepared from young heart total RNA (*left panel*) or that from aged heart RNA (*right panel*).

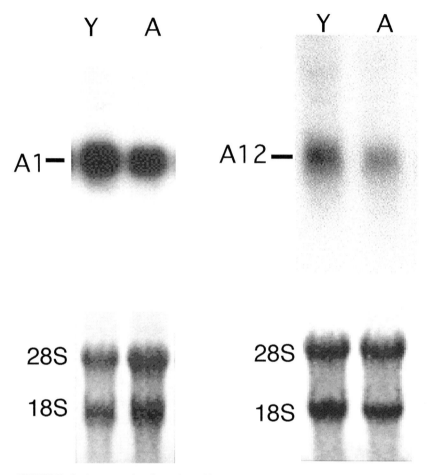

FIGURE 4. An example of Northern blot analysis. Expression of A1 and A12 genes was compared between young and senescent rat left ventricles. A1: H+ transporting ATP synthase F0 complex subunit c isoform 3 (ATP5G3), A12: Na^+-K^+-Cl^- cotransporter.

related to the cardiac function. Therefore, the differential display analysis of gene expression can be effectively used for studying the basis of age-related physiological changes in the heart.

ACKNOWLEDGMENTS

This study was supported by a Grant-in-Aid for Scientific Research (C) (No. 15590220 to Y.K., and No. 17590468 to A.I.) from the Ministry of Education, Science, Sports and Culture, Japan.

REFERENCES

1. KATANO, Y. *et al*. 1997. Age-related changes in the contractile response to endothelin-1 and in binding characteristics of the endothelin receptor in rat ventricular myocardium. *In* The Developing Heart. B. Qstadal *et al.* Eds.: 301–310. Lippincott-Raven. Philadelphia, PA.

2. ZHANG, H. *et al*. 1996. Differential screening of gene expression difference enriched by differential display. Nucleic Acids Res. **24:** 2454–2455.

3. KNOLL, R. *et al*. 1996. Characterization of differentially expressed genes following brief cardiac ischemia. Biochem. Biophys. Res. Commun. **221:** 402–407.

4. LI, P. *et al*. 2003. Gene expression profile of cardiomyocytes in hypertrophic heart induced by continuous norepinephrine infusion in the rats. Cell. Mol. Life Sci. **60:** 2200–2209.

5. AUSUBEL, F.M. *et al*. Ed. 1993. Current Protocols in Molecular Biology. Greene Publishing Associates, John Wiley & Sons, New York.

6. PEARSON, W.R. & D.J. LIPMAN. 1988. Improved tools for biological sequence comparison. Proc. Natl. Acad. Sci. USA **85:** 2444–2448.

7. HERRIN, D.L. & G.W. SCHMIDT. 1988. Rapid, reversible staining of Northern blots prior to hybridization. BioTechniques **6:** 196.

8. GOYNS, M.H. *et al*. 1998. Differential display analysis of gene expression indicates that age-related changes are restricted to a small cohort of genes. Mech. Ageing Dev. **101:** 73–90.

9. HIMEDA, T. *et al*. 2000. Synchronized transcriptional gene expression of H+-ATP synthase subunits in different tissues of Fischer 344 rats of different ages. Eur. J. Biochem. **267:** 6938–6942.

10. HU, D. *et al*. 2002. Altered profile of gene expression in rat hearts induced by chronic nicotine consumption. Biochem. Biophys. Res. Commun. **297:** 729–736.

11. PANET, R. *et al*. 1990. Role of the Na+/K+/Cl− transporter in the positive inotropic effect of ouabain in cardiac myocytes. J. Cell Physiol. **145:** 24–29.

Naïve T Cells in the Elderly

Are They Still There?

GERALD PFISTER,[a] DANIELA WEISKOPF,[a] LUTFAN LAZUARDI,[a]
RANIA D. KOVAIOU,[a] DANIEL P. CIOCA,[a] MICHAEL KELLER,[a]
BERND LORBEG,[b] WALTHER PARSON,[b] AND
BEATRIX GRUBECK-LOEBENSTEIN[a]

[a]Institute for Biomedical Aging Research, Austrian Academy of Sciences,
A-6020 Innsbruck, Austria

[b]Institute for Legal Medicine, Medical University of Innsbruck,
A-6020 Innsbruck, Austria

ABSTRACT: One of the most striking changes in the primary lymphoid
organs during human aging is the progressive involution of the thymus.
As a consequence, the rate of naïve T cell output dramatically declines
with age and the peripheral T cell pool shrinks. These changes lead to
increased incidence of severe infections and decreased protective effect of
vaccinations in the elderly. Little is, however, known of the composition
and function of the residual naïve T cell repertoire in elderly persons.
To evaluate the impact of aging on the naïve T cell pool, we investigated
the quantity, phenotype, function, composition, and senescence status
of CD45RA$^+$CD28$^+$ human T cells—a phenotype generally considered
as naïve cells—from both young and old healthy donors. We found a
significant decrease in the number of CD45RA$^+$CD28$^+$ T cells in the elderly, whereas the proliferative response of these cells is still unimpaired.
In addition to their reduced number, CD45RA$^+$CD28$^+$ T cells from old
donors display significantly shorter telomeres and have a restricted TCR
repertoire in nearly all 24 Vβ families. These findings let us conclude that
naïve T cells cannot be classified with conventional markers in old age.

KEYWORDS: aging; humans; immunosenescence; naïve T cells; TCR
clonality

INTRODUCTION

In the elderly the incidence of severe infections is high and the protective
effect of vaccinations is low. The major reason for this is thymic involution

Address for correspondence: Gerald Pfister, Institute for Biomedical Aging Research, Austrian
Academy of Sciences, Renwig 10, A-6020 Innsbruck, Austria. Voice: +43-(0)512-583919-14;
fax: +43-(0)512-583919-8.
 e-mail: gerald.pfister@oeaw.ac.at

Ann. N.Y. Acad. Sci. 1067: 152–157 (2006). © 2006 New York Academy of Sciences.
doi: 10.1196/annals.1354.018

leading to a dramatic decline of naïve T cell output and shrinkage of the peripheral T cell pool. So far, little is known of the composition and function of the residual naïve T cell repertoire in elderly persons. Theoretically, naïve T cells should proliferate well and contain a variety of cells of different antigen specificity as they have not yet been exposed to antigen and have not undergone clonal propagation. However, they may be subject to intrinsic aging processes and be damaged by environmental stress factors. The latter possibility seems to be supported by the fact that vaccination with neoantigen such as yellow fever–attenuated live virus has recently been shown to have insufficient efficacy and systemic side effects in the elderly.[1–3] In this study we evaluate the impact of aging on the naïve T cell pool by investigating the quantity, phenotype, function, composition, and the senescence status of purified $CD45RA^+CD28^+$ human T cells—a phenotype generally considered as naïve cells—from both young and old healthy donors.

MATERIAL AND METHODS

Heparinized blood samples were obtained from apparently healthy young (<35 years) and elderly (>65 years) persons, and peripheral blood mononuclear cells (PBMCs) were isolated as described elsewhere.[4] All participants gave informed written consent, and the study was approved by the local ethical committee. $CD4^+$ and $CD8^+$ $CD45RA^+CD28^+$ T cells were purified using a FACSVantage SE cell sorter (BD Biosciences, San Jose, CA) by appropriate gating and analyzed after staining with a panel of monoclonal fluorescent antibodies against CD3 (PE), CD4 (PE-Cy7), CD8 (PE-Cy7), CD45RA (FITC), and CD28 (APC). The isolated T cell populations were used for all experiments and had a purity between 95% and 99% (FIG. 1). TCR-mediated proliferation was induced by OKT-3 (30 ng/mL) or OKT-3 and IL-2 (20 ng/mL). Proliferation was determined by thymidine uptake after 5 days in the presence of irradiated autologous PBMCs at a density of 5×10^4 cells/well in 96-well plates. The telomere length of $CD4^+$ and $CD8^+$ $CD45RA^+CD28^+$ T cells was determined as recently described[5] and compared in cells from old and young donors. In brief, a fluorescent-labeled peptide nucleic acid (PNA) telomere probe was hybridized to telomeres for flow FISH analysis, and the tetraploid T cell lymphoblastic leukemia line 1301 was used as an internal standard for each telomere length measurement. To analyze the clonal composition regarding the TCR repertoire total RNA was extracted from purified $CD4^+$ and $CD8^+$ $CD45RA^+CD28^+$ T cells and reverse-transcribed. TCR Vβ transcripts were amplified by PCR with primers (MWG) specific for each of the human Vβ families and a specific primer for the constant region of the β chain and labeled with the fluorescent dye marker 6-FAM. An aliquot of the PCR product was analyzed on a CE 310 Genetic Analyzer (Perkin Elmer, Norwalk, CT). Analysis of the raw data was performed applying GeneScan

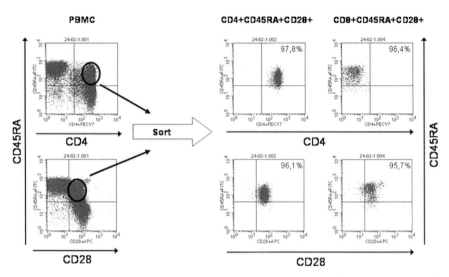

FIGURE 1. Representative dot plots of human CD4$^+$ and CD8$^+$ CD45RA$^+$CD28$^+$ T cells purified from PBMCs by FACS.

2.1 analysis software package (Applied Biosystems, Foster City, CA) using the Local Southern method for fragment size estimation.[4]

RESULTS

The proliferation of CD4$^+$ and CD8$^+$ CD45RA$^+$CD28$^+$ T cells from old donors is not impaired following mitogenic stimulation with PHA (data not shown). TCR-mediated proliferation after stimulation with OKT-3 is generally low in the cells from young donors. In addition, a higher and more variable proliferative response of CD45RA$^+$CD28$^+$ T cells from old donors in both the CD4$^+$ and CD8$^+$ subsets was observed (FIG. 2).

Regarding the TCR repertoire, CD45RA$^+$CD28$^+$ T cells from young donors show a polyclonal composition with a Gaussian distribution in almost all 24 human Vβ families, while CD45RA$^+$CD28$^+$ T cells from old donors display a clonal expansion in nearly all 24 Vβ families. On average, more than 95% of all 24 Vβ families in CD45RA$^+$CD28$^+$ T cells from young donors are polyclonal (diversity score I). In contrast, these cells are clonally restricted (diversity scores II and III) by almost 60% in the CD4$^+$ and 80% in the CD8$^+$ subset in the elderly (FIG. 3). Hence, the age-related clonal expansion regarding the TCR repertoire in CD45RA$^+$CD28$^+$ T cells is even more pronounced in the CD8$^+$ subset.

To evaluate the senescence status of the CD45RA$^+$CD28$^+$ T cells, we analyzed the telomere length in both CD4$^+$ and CD8$^+$ subsets from young and

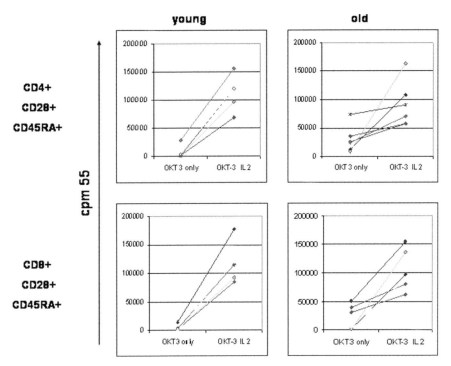

FIGURE 2. TCR-mediated proliferation of purified $CD4^+$ and $CD8^+CD45RA^+$ $CD28^+$ T cells from young and old donors after 5-day stimulation. Stimulation with OKT-3 leads to low proliferation in cells from young donors and higher and more variable proliferation in cells from old donors, whereas there is no different proliferative response after additional stimulation with IL-2.

elderly persons by flow FISH. The results indicate clearly shortened telomeres in the cells from old donors. Average telomere length of $CD45RA^+CD28^+$ T cells was reduced from 7.3 kb in the young to 4.9 kb in the elderly in the $CD4^+$, and from 6.9 kb to 4.5 kb in the $CD8^+$ subset.

DISCUSSION

During the process of aging, T lymphocytes are the most severely affected immune cells.[6,7] This is mainly due to the involution of the thymus, which starts soon after puberty and is almost complete by the age of 60 years.[8] Although all thymic T cell intermediates are still present and TCR gene rearrangement still occurs in the elderly, the rate of naïve T cell output from the thymus dramatically declines.[9] However, little is known about the composition and function of the naïve T cell populations during human aging. Our results show that although these cells are not impaired in their proliferative response to

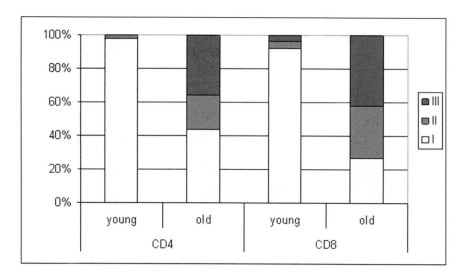

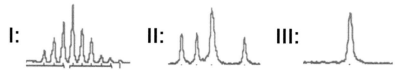

FIGURE 3. Diversity score of the TCR repertoire in purified $CD4^+$ and $CD8^+$ $CD45RA^+CD28^+$ T cells from young and old donors. More than 95% of all 24 Vβ families in $CD45RA^+CD28^+$ T cells from young donors are polyclonal (diversity score I), whereas these cells are clonally restricted (diversity scores II and III) in the elderly.

antigenic stimulation, their number is significantly reduced in the elderly. This is in accordance with data from the literature and gains a certain importance in the context of longevity. Some studies suggest that predictions on longevity can be based on the number of naïve T cells. Mice that have high numbers of $CD4^+$ naïve T cells and low numbers of $CD4^+$ and $CD8^+$ memory T cells lived longer, indicating that naïve T cell numbers may be used as a biomarker of aging that can predict longevity at middle age.[9,10]

In addition to their reduced number, $CD45RA^+CD28^+$ T cells display significantly shorter telomeres as a sign of cellular senescence and have a restricted TCR repertoire in all 24 Vβ families. Since naïve T cells by definition should not have been confronted with their specific antigen, they should consequently not have undergone substantial clonal expansion, and they should also have long telomeres.[11] Our results clearly show that this is not true for the investigated $CD45RA^+CD28^+$ T cells in both $CD4^+$ and $CD8^+$ subsets. Since this phenotype is generally considered as defining naïve T cells, we suggest being very cautious in defining naïve T cells in the elderly solely by a conventional phenotypic classification, and we propose to include functional aspects in the definition of such cells. Overall, we conclude that the investigated CD45RA$^+$CD28$^+$ T cell population has to be considered as not being naïve in the elderly, although their phenotype would indicate so. Therefore, naïve T cells cannot be classified with conventional markers in old age.

REFERENCES

1. MARTIN, M., T. TSAI, B. CROPP, *et al.* 2001. Fever and multisystem organ failure associated with 17D-204 yellow fever vaccination: a report of four cases. Lancet **358:** 98–104.
2. MARTIN, M., L.H. WELD, T.F. TSAI, *et al.* AND GEOSENTINEL YELLOW FEVER WORKING GROUP. 2001. Advanced age a risk factor for illness temporally associated with yellow fever vaccination. Emerg. Infect. Dis. **7:** 945–951.
3. KITCHENER, S. 2004. Viscerotropic and neurotropic disease following vaccination with the 17D yellow fever vaccine, ARILVAX®. Vaccine **22:** 2103–2105.
4. HERNDLER-BRANDSTETTER, D., S. SCHWAIGER, E. VEEL, *et al.* 2005. CD25 expressing CD8$^+$ T cells are potent memory cells in old age. J. Immunol. **175:** 1566–1574.
5. KOVAIOU, R., I. WEISKIRCHNER, M. KELLER, *et al.* 2005. Age-related differences in phenotype and function of CD4+ T cells are due to a phenotypic shift from naive to memory effector CD4+ T cells. Intl. Immunol. **17:** 1359–1366.
6. GLOBERSON, A. 1995. T lymphocytes and aging. Int. Arch. Allergy Immunol. **107:** 491–497.
7. PAWELEC, G., R.B. EFFROS, C. CARUSO, *et al.* 1999. T cells and aging. Front. Biosci. **4D:** 216–269.
8. GEORGE, A.J. & M.A. RITTER. 1996. Thymic involution with ageing: obsolescence or good housekeeping? Immunol. Today **17:** 267–272.
9. GRUBECK-LOEBENSTEIN, B. & G. WICK. 2002. The aging of the immune system. Adv. Immunol. **80:** 243–284.
10. MILLER, R.A. 2001. Biomarkers of aging: prediction of longevity by using age-sensitive T-cell subset determinations in a middle-aged, genetically heterogeneous mouse population. J. Gerontol. A. Biol. Sci. Med. Sci. **56:** B180–186.
11. WAGNER, M., B. HAMPEL, D. BERNHARD, *et al.* 2001. Replicative senescence of human endothelial cells in vitro involves G1 arrest, polyploidization and senescence-associated apoptosis. Exp. Gerontol. **36:** 1327–1347.

Brain Lipopigment Accumulation in Normal and Pathological Aging

DAN RIGA,[a] SORIN RIGA,[a] FLORIN HALALAU,[b] AND
FRANCISC SCHNEIDER[c]

[a]Department of Stress Research & Prophylaxis, "Al. Obregia" Clinical
Hospital of Psychiatry, RO-041914 Bucharest 8, Romania

[b]"V. Babes" National Institute of Pathology and Biomedical Sciences,
RO-050096 Bucharest 35, Romania

[c]Center for Applied Physiology and Molecular Biology, RO-310396 Arad,
Romania

ABSTRACT: A principal marker of brain vulnerability, stress, aging, and
related pathology is represented by lipopigments (LPs)—lipofuscin, and
ceroid. During ontogenesis, neuronal LP accumulations are significantly
correlated with important changes in nerve cell morphology and biochemistry. In the aged neurons, LPs are present in all cellular compartments. Moreover, neuronal LP accumulations coexist with glial LP storage, especially in microglia. Owing to their transporting properties, and
the migration capacity of microglia, glial cells deposit LP clusters in
pericapillary areas. Thus, LP conglomerates appear in the whole nervous tissue, creating specific patterns of LP architectonics. Direct interrelations, critical LP concentrations, which generate cascades of negative
subcellular events, and indirect impairment correlations determine characteristic neuropathologic aging profiles. These specific and associated
negative neuropathologic consequences of LP accumulation have multiple and detrimental impacts on neuron and glia homeostasis, ranging
from neuronal function to central nervous system physiology.

KEYWORDS: lipopigments; neurons; glial cells; neuropathology

INTRODUCTION

In the neurosciences, a multitude of studies, ranging from molecular and
subcellular levels to comparative neuroanatomy and neuropathology, and to
cognitive and behavioral sciences, have created the basis and opportunities

Address for correspondence: Dan Riga, Department of Stress Research & Prophylaxis, "Al. Obregia"
Clinical Hospital of Psychiatry, 10 Berceni Rd., Sector 4, RO-041914 Bucharest 8, Romania. Voice:
+40-21-334-3008; fax: +40-21-230-9579.
e-mail: d_s_riga@yahoo.com

Ann. N.Y. Acad. Sci. 1067: 158–163 (2006). © 2006 New York Academy of Sciences.
doi: 10.1196/annals.1354.019

to correlate parameters, processes, and phenomena. Moreover, the morphological ultradifferentiation and functional overspecialization of nervous tissue, compared with other tissue types, also impose the use of correlation methodologies in the neurosciences. In addition, the resultant data from correlation studies show new aspects and connections, and contribute to the better understanding of neurobiology and behavior in human beings.[1]

Therefore, ontogenesis, longevity, and normal and pathological brain aging, correlated with the factors that control, regulate, and disturb central nervous system (CNS) structure and function, open new paths of knowledge and intervention.[2] Systematic research in comparative zoology, comparative morphology, senescence of mammals, and biogerontology shows interesting connections, such as the following:

- relationships in mammals between the rate of aging (as deduced from maximum life span) and the size of the animal (body weight) and metabolic scales/rates;
- correlations in mammals between longevity and brain size/weight, as an absolute or relative (to body weight) value;[3]
- links between longer-lived species, with a slower rate in the accumulation of lipofuscin and increased resistance of brain to autooxidation, with increasing life span.

Brain senescence in humans is a complicated and heterogeneous process with high regional specificity and individuality. Therefore, important connections in normal and pathological aging of CNS can be pointed out between:

- neuronal density and different types of glial presence and reactivity;[1]
- brain lipopigments (LPs) in neurons and glia;[2]
- LPs in relationship with mitochondrial pathology (mtDNA mutations and giant mitochondria),[4] anabolic subcellular structures,[5] and lysosomal dysfunction;[3] and LPs and Alzheimer pathology (meganeurites, neurofibrillary tangles, and amyloid plaques).[6]

LPs IN THE BRAIN

The LPs lipofuscin and ceroid display almost identical biophysical, biochemical, and morphological characteristics and properties in their final steps.[7] By virtue of their implication and negative consequences on neuronal and glial physiology, LPs represent a main marker of brain vulnerability, stress, aging, and related pathology. LP accumulation in the brain has some important features:

- brain ubiquity: in all the central nervous system regions and zones, from cerebrum to spinal cord;

- presence in all the nervous tissue in whole cellular types,[8] from different kind of neurons to glia and endothelial cells;
- specific patterns of LP architectonics in close relation with senescence and age-related pathology;[6]
- LP accumulation in two stages: stage I—LPs increase in number, surface, volume, complexity, in both neurons and glial cells; stage II—LPs become constant in inflammatory degenerative nervous disorders (Alzheimer's and Parkinson's diseases, etc.).

In aged neurons, LP is present in all cellular compartments,[8] especially in perikaryon areas and dendrites, but also in axons and even in presynaptic components. Moreover, in neuroglia, from perineuronal glia to neuropil and pericapillary glia, LP storage is present in all cellular partitions:[8] gliosomas, glial arborizations, and capillary end-feet.

NEURONAL LP CORRELATES

As a time-dependent phenomenon, neuronal LP accumulations during ontogenesis, aging, and longevity constantly coexist and are significantly correlated with important negative synergistic metabolic and cell–subcellular events: modifications in neuron/glia index; changes of cyto-, pigmento-, and myelo-architectonics; alterations in the structure and function of subcellular systems.

In aging and aged-related neurodegenerative pathologic conditions, constant expansion of neuronal LPs is associated with neuronal loss and simultaneous increase in reactivity and number of neuroglial cells.[1,6,9,10] Glial activation, the canonical features of mammalian aging, and mediators of inflammatory and degenerative diseases in the brain, basically consist of astrocyte hyperactivity, fibrous phenotype, and microglial activation, increased expression of major histocompatibility complex (MHC) class II antigens, and increased levels of transforming growth factor-beta-1 mRNA (TGFβ-1), which are attenuated by caloric restriction.[9]

Neuronal LP conglomerates realize specific brain patterns of LP architectonics and modify neurono- and myelo-architectonics,[6] being correlated with a decrease in the surface/volume of neurosoma, dendritic aberrations, simplification and destruction, axonal enlargement to meganeurites,[3,6] considerable reduction of cortical myelin, and synaptic loss. Progressive neuronal LP storage is also associated with increase of oxidative stress,[11,12] decrease of the antioxidative defense,[11] accumulation of mtDNA mutations,[13] increased number of damaged, defective, impaired, and giant mitochondria with a low rate of degradation,[4] as well as decrease in the number and area of normal and functional healthy mitochondria.

Neuronal LPs and anabolic subcellular systems are in an inverse correlation with one another. The extension of LP clusters is connected with decrease of ribosomal RNA, total RNA, and water-soluble proteins, and consecutive diminution in the number and surface/volume of polyribosomes and rough endoplasmic reticulum.[5,14]

Neuronal LPs and catabolic subcellular systems show interesting correlations. For example, progressive LP accumulations and aggregations interact and are associated with proteasome instability and inhibition[15,16] and lysosome dysfunction,[3] deficient and poor function of cellular recycling systems, and finally with accumulations of water-insoluble proteins, oxidized proteins, advanced protein glycation/glycooxidation end-products, advanced lipid peroxidation end-products, as pluri-metabolic sources and compounds of subcellular garbage.[13,14]

LP storage interacts negatively with neuron structure and is constantly present and correlated with the appearance and development of cytoskeletal damage, as well as with amyloid deposit and amyloid-related pathologic conditions.[6,15]

GLIAL LP CORRELATES

Neuronal LP deposits coexist with large glial LP storage vacuoles in all types of glia. Thus, the glial paradox appears in brain aging and aged-related pathologic conditions. Neuroglia—mitotic cells, characterized by a moderate-to-high rate of divisions—are overloaded with two types of garbage: LP conglomerates, characteristic of neurons, and phagocytic-degraded neuronal apoptotic bodies. Microglial cells degrade oxidized extracellular proteins and neuronal apoptotic bodies,[17] subsequent sources of LPs. However, the large amounts of glial LPs (often up to 80–90% of the glioplasm) can also be explained by LP neurono-glial transfer.

Glial systems play an important role in collecting neuronal LPs. Owing to their transporting properties and the migratory capacity of microglia, glial cells deposit the LP clusters in pericapillary areas. These purged mechanisms can be activated and completed by neurometabolic, anti-oxidative, neurovascular, and nootropic therapy.[5,14]

BRAIN, AGING, AND ANTI-AGING INTERRELATIONSHIPS

Direct, causal interrelations and critical LP concentrations, which generate cascades of negative lifelong subcellular events, as well as indirect, associated impairment correlations, determine characteristic neuropathologic aging profiles. Specific and associated negative neuropathologic consequences of LP storage have multiple and detrimental impacts on neuronal and glial homeostasis, from neuronal function to brain physiology. Anti-homeostatic actions of oxidative stress (and implicitly LP accumulation and subcellular dysfunction) contribute to the maintenance and magnification of the brain aging cascade in an etio-pathogenic direction. Inversely, in a therapeutic direction, antioxidative medication, drugs for metabolic support/activation of brain homeostasis, and the adapting stimulation in hormesis[18] represent natural ways in anti-aging, rejuvenation, and prolongevity medicine.

REFERENCES

1. LANDFIELD, P.W., R.K. BASKIN & T.A. PITLER. 1981. Brain aging correlates: retardation by hormonal-pharmacological treatments. Science **214:** 581–584.
2. RIGA, D. & S. RIGA. 1998. Correlations between lipofuscin accumulation and aging neuropathology. Ann. N.Y. Acad. Sci. **854:** 495.
3. LYNCH, G. & X. BI. 2003. Lysosomes and brain aging in mammals. Neurochem. Res. **28:** 1725–1734.
4. BRUNK, U.T. & A. TERMAN. 2002. The mitochondrial-lysosomal axis theory of aging: accumulation of damage as a result of imperfect autophagocytosis. Eur. J. Biochem. **269:** 1996–2002.
5. RIGA, S. & D. RIGA. 1995. An antistress and antiaging neurometabolic therapy: accelerated lipo-fuscinolysis and stimulated anabolic regeneration by the Antagonic-Stress synergistic formula. Ann. N.Y. Acad. Sci. **771:** 535–550.
6. BRAAK, H. & E. BRAAK. 1988. Morphology of the human isocortex in young and aged individuals: qualitative and quantitative findings. *In* Histology and Histopathology of the Aging Brain. J. Ulrich, Ed.: 1–15. Karger. Basel.
7. PORTA, E.A. 1991. Advances in age pigment research. Arch. Gerontol. Geriatr. **12:** 303–320.
8. CERVÓS-NAVARRO, J. & H.-I. SARKANDER, Eds. 1983. Brain Aging: Neuropathology and Neuropharmacology. Raven Press. New York, NY.
9. FINCH, C.E., I. ROZOVSKY, D. STONE, *et al.* 1999. Glial activation during aging in the rat brain: gene expression and proliferative potential. *In* Molecular Biology of Aging. V. A. Bohr, B. F. C. Clark & T. Stevnsner, Eds.: 304–315. Alfred Benzon Symposium 44. Munksgaard, Copenhagen, DK.
10. GONZÁLES-SCARANO, F. & G. BALTUCH. 1999. Microglia as mediators of inflammatory and degenerative diseases. Annu. Rev. Neurosci. **22:** 219–240.
11. BECKMAN, K.B. & B.N. AMES. 1998. The free radical theory of aging matures. Physiol. Rev. **78:** 547–581.
12. FOSSLIEN, E. 2001. Mitochondrial medicine-molecular pathology of defective oxidative phosphorylation. Ann. Clin. Lab. Sci. **31:** 25–67.
13. TERMAN, A. & U.T. BRUNK. 2004. Aging as a catabolic malfunction. Int. J. Biochem. Cell Biol. **36:** 2365–2375.
14. RIGA, D., S. RIGA & F. SCHNEIDER. 2004. Regenerative medicine: Antagonic-Stress® therapy in distress and aging. I. Preclinical synthesis - 2003. Ann. N.Y. Acad. Sci. **1019:** 396–400.
15. GRUNE, T., T. JUNG, K. MERKER, *et al.* 2004. Decreased proteolysis caused by protein aggregates inclusion bodies, plaques, lipofuscin, ceroid, and "aggresomes" during oxidative stress, aging, and disease. Int. J. Biochem. Cell Biol. **36:** 2519–2530.
16. KECK, S., R. NITSCH, T. GRUNE, *et al.* 2003. Proteasome inhibition by paired helical filament-tau in brains of patients with Alzheimer's disease. J. Neurochem. **85:** 115–122.

17. STOLZING, A. & T. GRUNE. 2004. Neuronal apoptotic bodies: phagocytosis and degradation by primary microglial cells. FASEB J. **18:** 743–765.
18. RATTAN, S.I.S. 2005. Principles and practice of hormesis as an aging intervention. *In* Aging Interventions and Therapies. S.I.S. Rattan, Ed.: 365–377. World Scientific. Singapore.

Aging and Orchidectomy Modulate Expression of VEGF Receptors (Flt-1 and Flk-1) on Corpus Cavernosum of the Rat

DELMINDA NEVES,[a] JANETE SANTOS,[a] NUNO TOMADA,[b]
HENRIQUE ALMEIDA,[a] AND PEDRO VENDEIRA[a,b]

[a]Laboratory for Molecular Cell Biology of Faculty of Medicine of Porto,
4200-319 Porto, and IBMC of Universidade do Porto, Rua do Campo Alegre,
4150-180 Porto

[b]Department of Urology of S. João Central Hospital 4200-319 Porto, Portugal

ABSTRACT: Aging and hypogonadic states are known risk factors for erectile dysfunction (ED), contributing together to vascular damage of penile tissue. In the present study, VEGF-specific membrane receptor (VEGFR-1/Flt-1 and VEGFR-2/Flk-1) expression was studied by confocal immunofluorescence in the corpus cavernosum of control rats, rats aged 12 and 18 months, and orchidectomized Wistar rats (90 days of bilateral orchidectomy). Immunocytochemical results demonstrated VEGFR-2 expression restricted to the endothelium in both control and orchidectomized rats. Aged animals (12 and 18 months) presented enlarged vessels with intense VEGFR-2 endothelial staining. On the other hand, VEGFR-1 was demonstrated in smooth muscle fibers, particularly in those that surround vessel endothelium, the endothelial expression being very low in control and orchidectomized rats. However, in the aged rats, a shift resulting in a VEGFR-1 and VEGFR-2 co-localization in the endothelial cell was observed. The findings suggest an upregulation of VEGFR-1 in the corpora cavernosa during aging in the rat, which is evident from an increased expression by endothelial cells.

KEYWORDS: angiogenesis; erectile dysfunction; aging; orchidectomy; VEGF receptors

INTRODUCTION

Aging and hypogonadic states are known risk factors for erectile dysfunction (ED), a disease that affects more than 10% of the adult male population in

Address for correspondence: Delminda Neves, Laboratory for Molecular Cell Biology of Faculty of Medicine of Universidade do Porto, 4200-319 Porto, Portugal. Voice: 351225091468; fax: 351225510119.

e-mail: delmagal@med.up.pt

Ann. N.Y. Acad. Sci. 1067: 164–172 (2006). © 2006 New York Academy of Sciences.
doi: 10.1196/annals.1354.020

Europe. The incidence of cardiovascular disease also correlates closely with the prevalence of ED, which is considered to be an early signal of impending cardiovascular problems.[1] Vasculogenic ED, namely corporal veno-occlusive dysfunction, which occurs in two-thirds of the cases of ED, is caused by the impairment of the relaxation of the smooth muscle in the penile cavernosa associated with vascular insufficiency and structural alterations in the cavernous smooth muscle, nerves, and endothelium. The endothelium and angiogenesis have been a subject of much attention lately. Evidence for their important role in the establishment of erectile dysfunction led Goldstein to state, in a simple and lasting way, ED (erectile dysfunction) = ED (endothelium dysfunction).[2] Angiogenesis, a process by which new blood vessels are formed from preexisting ones, is thought to be regulated by the balance between angiogenesis inducers and inhibitors.[3] VEGF (vascular endothelial growth factor) is an endothelial cell-specific mitogen, a smooth muscle cell promoter of migration and proliferation,[4] and is the major vascular growth factor involved in physiologic and pathologic angiogenesis.[5] VEGF is essential for endothelial cell survival, and binds specifically to both tyrosine kinase membrane receptors, Flt-1 (fms-like tyrosine kinase-1 receptor) and KDR/Flk-1 (kinase insert domain-containing receptor).

In the present experimental study, corpus cavernosum was studied by immunofluorescence (IF) for VEGF-specific membrane receptors, (VEGFR-1 or Flt-1 and VEGR-2 or Flk-1) in normal, aged, and orchidectomized rats. Previous reports demonstrated Flt-1 and Flk-1 expression in cultured human cavernosal cells;[6] however, the role of VEGF receptors in penile vascularity, and the influence of aging and androgen depletion on its expression are still unknown. In this way, clarifying morphologic organization and angiogenic mechanisms in corpus cavernosum, will improve knowledge about the prevention and treatment of this pathologic condition.

MATERIALS AND METHODS

Wistar male rats obtained from the colony of the IBMC of UP were divided into four experimental groups ($n = 10$): Group I, control (young adults–2 months); Group II, orchidectomized (90 days of bilateral orchidectomy); Groups III and IV, aged rats, respectively, 12 and 18 months old. Rats were sacrificed by decapitation and penile fragments were obtained.

For the structural studies, some pieces were fixed in 10% buffered formaldehyde for 24 h and embedded in paraffin. Sections 4–6 μm thick were placed in 0.1% poly-L-lysine-covered (Sigma Diagnostics, St Louis, MO) microscopy slides for immunohistochemical detection of VEGF receptors. Detection of Flt-1 and Flk-1 was performed employing polyclonal antibodies, goat anti-Flt-1 (diluted to 1/200), and rabbit anti-Flk-1 (diluted to 1/500) (Santa Cruz Biotechnology), respectively. Immunoperoxidase staining was performed by means of an adequate secondary biotinylated antibody combined with a streptavidin-peroxidase complex (DakoCytomation) followed by hematoxylin *counterstaining*. Immunofluorescence detection of both VEGF receptors was also performed, employing a mix of secondary anti-goat antibodies conjugated with Alexa^{TM} 568 (red) and anti-rabbit conjugated with Alexa^{TM} 488 (green) both diluted to 1/100. Sections were observed in a confocal microscope (Bio-Rad).

For protein analysis, penile fragments were mechanically homogenized in an extraction buffer (Tris 50 nM pH 7.2, NaCl 0.1 M, EDTA 5 mM, Triton X-100 0.5%, PMSF 0.2%) for 20 minutes, and sonicated with five 10-s pulses at 10% power (Bandelin, Sonopuls HD2070). Total protein was quantified[7] and analyzed by SDS-PAGE[8] in 10% poly-acrylamide gel. The protein was transferred to a nitrocellulose membrane[9] (Schleicher & Schuell, pore 0.45 μm) and Western blot detection of VEGF, Flt-1 and FLk-1 was carried out with a monoclonal antibody anti-VEGF (R&D), and polyclonal antibodies were produced in rabbit for VEGF receptors (LabVision), respectively. Protein-specific bands were visualized by chemoluminescence. Serum testosterone was assayed by RIA employing a commercial kit (IBL-Hamburg).

RESULTS

Testosterone serum levels were measured in all experimental groups: control young rats (2 months) presented a mean value of 2.36 ng/mL (TABLE 1), and 12- and 18-month-old rats presented in average a value of 2.78 and 2.70 ng/mL, respectively (TABLE 1). After orchidectomy, serum testosterone levels decreased in all individuals to average levels of 0.02 ng/mL, which confirms androgen depletion in this animal group.

Immunohistochemical detection of VEGFR-2 in controls was restricted to the endothelium lining the major vessels of the rat penis or the corpus cavernosum sinusoidal trabeculae (FIG. 1A). This pattern could also be seen in orchidectomized rats (FIG. 1B); however, the overall expression was reduced on account of perceptible tissue atrophy. In older animals (12 and 18 months) penile vessels appeared enlarged, also presenting an intense Flk-1 endothelial staining (FIG. 1C and 1D, respectively).

TABLE 1. Serum testosterone

	Testosterone ng/mL
Control	2.36 ± 0.90
Orchidectomized	0.02 ± 0.01
Aged 12 months	2.78 ± 0.42
Aged 18 months	2.70 ± 0.52
$P < 0.01$	

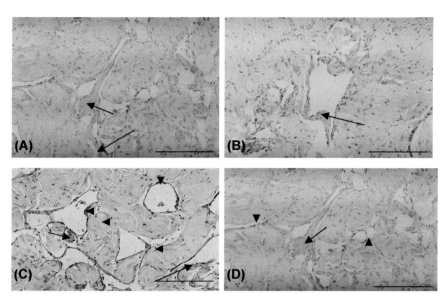

FIGURE 1. Flt-1 localization was demonstrated in smooth muscle cell (*arrows*) in control animals (**A**) and also in orchidectomized rats, which was observed through sparse endothelial staining (**B**). In aged rats (12 and 18 months) we observed a shift in VEGFR-1 expression, namely, an increase in endothelial localization (*arrowhead*) associated with a sparse expression in smooth muscle cell (**C** and **D**). Bar–50 μm.

Concerning VEGFR-1, we observed a scattered distribution of this peptide in the smooth muscle fibers in all experimental groups, particularly in those that surround vessel endothelium, the endothelial staining being very low in both control (FIG. 2A) and orchidectomized rats (FIG. 2B).

On the other hand, older rats showed an apparent shift in Flt-1 localization, this receptor being mainly localized in endothelial cells (FIG. 2C and 2D, respectively).

In fact, VEGFR-1 and VEGFR-2 co-localized in the endothelium of corpus cavernosum of 12- and 18-month-old rats (FIG. 3C and 3D), but failed to do so in the young (FIG. 3A) and orchidectomized rats (FIG. 3B).

Electrophoretic analysis of total proteins in the corpus cavernosum revealed multiple peptides; a 25-kDa protein band, which probably corresponds to VEGF was detected by Western blot with a specific antibody, and presented a crescent intensity in the fractions isolated from rats, whose age varied from 2 to 18 months (FIG. 4A). Western blot detection of Flt-1 demonstrated a 200-kDa band (FIG. 4B) with increased intensity in older rats (18 months), which corroborates the results obtained by immunocytochemistry (FIG. 2D). Flk-1 presented an apparent molecular weight of 180 kDa (FIG. 4C) which was expressed in all the protein fractions analyzed by Western blotting, decreasing in quantity in older animals, and particularly in orchidectomized rats (FIG. 4C).

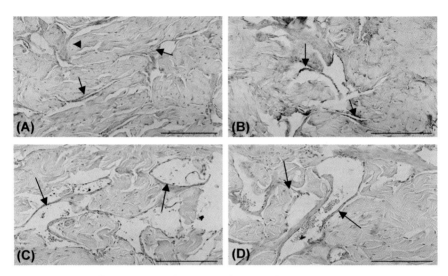

FIGURE 2. Flk-1 immunostaining was observed always in association with endothelium surrounding vessels (*arrows*) in control (**A**), orchidectomized (**B**), 12-month (**C**), and 18-month-old rats (**D**). Bar–50 μm.

DISCUSSION

Erectile function declines with aging, this correlation being well established in humans;[10] the prevalence of complete impotence varies on average from 5% to 15% in subjects between the ages of 40 and 70 years. A decline in ED was also demonstrated in the rat by *in vivo* and *in vitro* experiences.[11] The difficulty in assessing the pathophysiology of the decline of ED with aging usually lies in the intricate discrimination between aging effects and concomitant conditions such as smoking, alcoholism, hypertension, hypercholesterolemia, diabetes, and androgen decline. Previous work that employed animal models with controlled diet and favorable housing conditions demonstrated that aging by itself conduced to a general atrophy of the erectile tissue, affecting the corpora cavernosa compliance, with a slow kinetics of both erection and detumescence.[11]

Penile erection is a vascular event that is primarily regulated by the relaxation of the arterial and corporal smooth muscles, which play a major role in modulating penile blood flow during erection and detumescence.[12] Recent reports indicated a role for angiogenic growth factors such as VEGF in the modulation of rat penile vascularity.[4] This was supported by *in vivo* demonstration that the intracavernosal injection of VEGF, as well as adenovirus-mediated VEGF gene therapy,[13] lessened ED in aged rats.[14] VEGF, which can be considered the most potent angiogenic growth factor, and its receptors, were originally characterized in the endothelium, but

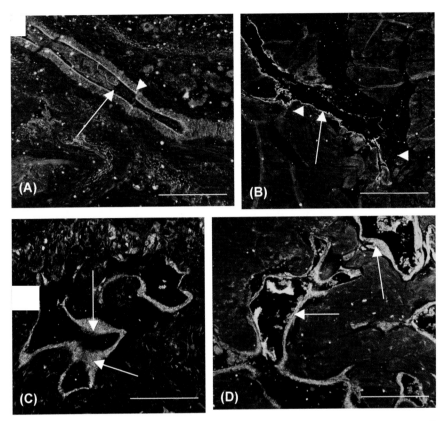

FIGURE 3. Double immunofluorescence detection of VEGF receptors VEGFR-1 (red) and VEGFR-2 (green). In control (**A**) and orchidectomized rats (**B**) a thin green endothelial staining (*arrow*) of VEGFR2 was observed, surrounded by smooth cell red staining (*arrowhead*). In older rats, 12 months (**C**) and 18 months (**D**) of age VEGFR-1 and VEGFR-2 expression co-localize at smooth muscle layer (*arrow*). Bar–100 μm.
Color available online only.

their presence was also demonstrated in human cavernosal smooth muscle cells.[6]

The aim of the present work was to characterize the expression of VEGF receptors 1 and 2 in the corpus cavernosum of rat during aging. To the best of our knowledge, this is the first time this kind of study has been performed in the aged rat. In order to evaluate the isolated action of androgen depletion on corpus cavernosum, orchidectomized rats were also studied.

In young adult rats, we found VEGFR-2 expression exclusively at the endothelium, while VEGFR-1 was detected predominantly at the perivascular smooth muscle. After orchidectomy we observed an apparent disorganized vascularization of corpus cavernosum, but with no significant change in the VEGF receptors' localization. In agreement with this result, the expression

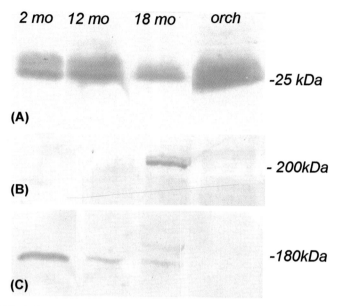

FIGURE 4. Western blotting detection of VEGF (**A**) with an apparent MW of 25 kDa showed that the VEGF band has higher intensity in 12- and 18-month-old rats (columns 12 mo and 18 mo) and orchidectomized rats (column orch) when compared with younger animals (column 2 mo). VEGFR-1 (**B**) was detected with an apparent MW of 200 kDa band that presents a higher intensity in older animals (column 18 mo). VEGFR-2 was detected with an apparent MW of 180 kDa and shows decreased intensity in older animals and also in orchidectomized rats.

of VEGF and Flt-1 by Western blotting demonstrated a similar profile in orchidectomized and control rats of the same age; Flk-1 expression was lower in orchidectomized rats. In this way, although the corpus cavernosum of the penis still remains an androgen-dependent organ even in the adult male,[15] testosterone deprivation apparently was not conducive to dramatic vascular damage or repression of vascular growth factors and specific receptors.

In older rats (12 and 18 months of age), whose vessels apparently enlarge and present a thicker layer of smooth muscle, our findings showed that VEGFR-1 and VEGFR-2 expression is modified. Our results allow us to conclude that during aging VEGF expression increases till 9 months (data not shown) and declines from 9 to 18 months in the rat; however, the total expression of VEGF was higher in 12- and 18-month-old rats than in young adults, which was clearly demonstrated by Western blotting. VEGFR-1 expression also increases with aging, the increased Flt-1 expression being clear in endothelial cells, which co-localize with Flk-1. In brief, our results suggest that VEGFR-1 and VEGFR-2 expression in aged rat corpus cavernosum is independent of an androgen-mediated pathway.

The exact role of VEGF receptors 1 and 2 in penile tissue is not known, nor is the way aging and androgen deprivation modulate vascular growth factors in corpus cavernosum angiogenesis. However, a clear understanding of the events that regulate penile tissue vascularity would aid in the identification of newer therapeutic approaches to improve tissue vascularity and blood flow to the penis.

ACKNOWLEDGMENTS

We thank Professor Carlos Reguenga for technical help with the protein image analysis system. Furthermore, we thank Dr. Isabel Gramaxo and Laboratório de Radioisótopos from Hospital de S. João-Porto for technical assistance.

REFERENCES

1. CHEITLIN, M.D. 2004. Erectile dysfunction: the earliest sign of generalized vascular disease? J. Am. Coll. Cardiol. **43**: 185–186.
2. GOLDSTEIN, I. 2003. The association of ED (erectile dysfunction) with ED (endothelium dysfunction). Int. J. Impot. Res. **15**: 229–230.
3. FOLKMAN, J. 1995. Angiogenesis in cancer, vascular, rheumatoid and other diseases. Nat. Med. **1**: 27–31.
4. LIU, X., C.-S. LIN, T. GRAZIOTTIN, *et al.* 2001. Vascular endothelial growth factor promotes proliferation and migration of cavernous smooth muscle cells. J. Urol. **166**: 354–360.
5. FERRARA, N. 2001. Role of vascular endothelial growth factoring regulation of physiological angiogenesis. Am. J. Physiol. Cell Physiol. **280**: C1358–C1366.
6. RAJASEKARAN, M., A. KASYAN, W. ALLILAIN, *et al.* 2002. Ex vivo expression of angiogenic growth factors and their receptors in human penile cavernosal cells. J. Androl. **24**: 85–90.
7. BRADFORD, M. 1976. A rapid and sensitive method for the quantitation of microgram quantities of protein utilizing the principle of protein-dye binding. Anal. Biochem. **72**: 248–254.
8. LAEMMLI, U.K. 1970. Cleavage of structural proteins during the assembly of the head of the bacteriophage T4. Nature **227**: 680–685.
9. TOWBIN, H., T. STAEHELIN & J. GORDON. 1979. Electrophoretic transfer of proteins from polyacrylamide gels to nitrocellulose sheets: procedure and some applications. Proc. Natl. Acad. Sci. USA **76**: 4350–4354.
10. FELDMAN, H.A., I. GOLDSTEIN, D.G. HATZICHRISTOU, *et al.* 1994. Impotence and its medical and psychosocial correlates: results of the Massachusetts Male Aging Study. J. Urol. **151**: 54–61.
11. CALABRÒ, A., G. ITALIANO, E.S. PESCATORI, *et al.* 1996. Physiological aging and penile erectile function: a study in the rat. Eur. Urol. **29**: 240–244.
12. CHRIST, G.J. 1995. The penis as a vascular organ: the importance of corporal smooth muscle tone in the control of erection. Urol. Clin. N. Am. **22**: 727–745.

13. ROGERS, R.S., T.M. GRAZIOTTIN, C.-S. LIN, *et al.* 2003. Intracavernosal vascular endothelial growth factor (VEGF) injection and adeno-associated virus-mediated VEGF gene therapy prevent and reverse venogenic erectile dysfunction in rats. Int. J. Impot. Res. **15:** 26–37.

14. PARK, K., K.Y. AHN, M.-K. KIM, *et al.* 2004. Intracavernosal injection of vascular endothelial growth factor improves erectile function in aged rats. Eur. Urol. **46:** 403–407.

15. SCHULTHEISS, D., R. BALDALYAN, A. PILATZ, *et al.* 2003. Androgen and estrogen receptors in the human corpus cavernosum penis: immunohistochemical and cell culture results. World J. Urol. **21:** 320–324.

Role of Angiotensin II and Endothelin-1 Receptors in Aging-Related Functional Changes in Rat Cardiovascular System

AKIRA ISHIHATA[a] AND YUMI KATANO[b]

[a]Department of Physiology I, and [b]Department of Theoretical Nursing and Pathophysiology, Yamagata University School of Medicine, Yamagata 990-9585, Japan

ABSTRACT: Angiotensin II (AII) and endothelin-1 (ET-1) are regarded as key players in the age-related changes in cardiovascular function. They are known to be involved in the pathogenesis of cardiac fibrosis and coronary vascular atherosclerosis. AII- and ET-induced vasoconstriction was augmented in coronary arteries of Langendorff-perfused heart from aged rats. In papillary muscles, ET-1-induced positive inotropic effect (PIE) was diminished by aging. On the other hand, both ET-1 and AII caused greater vasoconstriction in aged rat coronary arteries compared to those in the young rat. To further elucidate the mechanism of these age-dependent changes in cardiovascular effects of ET-1 and AII, we examined the expression of AII and ET-1 receptors in young (2-month-old) and aged (24-month-old) rats. Total RNA was isolated from left ventricles. For determination of the gene expression of AT_1 receptor and ET_A/ET_B receptor mRNA, competitive RT-PCR and Northern blot analysis were performed, respectively. $[^{125}I]ET-1$ receptor assay was carried out in left ventricular membrane fraction. AT_1-receptor, ET_A-, and ET_B-receptor mRNA were upregulated in the left ventricles of senescent rats compared with young ones. The affinity of ET-1-receptor was not changed, but receptor density was significantly increased in aged rats. Although the precise mechanism for the upregulation of AT_1 receptor and ET-1 receptor in the aged rat heart has not been clarified yet, these findings suggest that the activation of the renin–angiotensin system as well as ET receptor may be important for the physiological changes in aged hearts.

KEYWORDS: endothelin; receptor; gene expression; heart; angiotensin II; aging

Address for correspondence: Akira Ishihata, M.D., Ph.D., Department of Physiology I, Yamagata University School of Medicine, 2-2-2, Iida-Nishi, Yamagata 990-9585, Japan. Voice: +81-23-628-5214; fax: +81-23-628-5215.
e-mail: ishihata@med.id.yamagata-u.ac.jp

Ann. N.Y. Acad. Sci. 1067: 173–181 (2006). © 2006 New York Academy of Sciences.
doi: 10.1196/annals.1354.021

INTRODUCTION

Cardiac senescence alters responsiveness to vasoactive substances, and is closely related to cardiovascular remodeling. There is a variety of factors responsible for the age-related changes. Among them, both angiotensin II (AII) and endothelin-1 (ET-1) are considered key players. They are involved in the pathogenesis of cardiac fibrosis, hypertrophy, hypertension, and coronary vascular atherosclerosis.[1,2]

ET receptor exists in many tissues including cardiac muscles. There are two subtypes of the ET receptor, namely ET_A and ET_B receptor. In the heart, ET elicited a positive inotropic effect (PIE) as well as a hypertrophic effect. AII and its specific receptors also exist in the heart.[3] The receptors are AT_1 and AT_2, and AT_1 includes AT_{1a} and AT_{1b} receptors.[3] We previously showed that AII- and ET-induced vasoconstriction was augmented in coronary arteries of Langendorff-perfused aged rat hearts.[2,4] However, little is known about the mechanism of the age-related changes in the effect of ET and AII.

In order to elucidate the underlying mechanisms of age-dependent alteration in cardiovascular effects of ET-1 and AII, we investigated the changes in the gene expression of ET_A-, ET_B-, and AT_1 receptors as well as the binding characteristics of ET-receptors in young (2-month-old) and senescent (27-month-old) rats.

METHODS

Animals

In this study, 2–3-month-old and 24–27-month-old male Fischer 344 rats were obtained from Charles River Japan (Atsugi, Japan). Experiments were performed in accordance with the "Guide for Care and Use of Laboratory Animals" published by the U.S. National Institute of Health (NIH Publication No. 85-23, revised 1996) and under the regulations of the Animal Care Committee of Yamagata University School of Medicine. Rats were anesthetized with diethyl ether and were sacrificed by cervical dislocation, and hearts were quickly removed and snap-frozen in liquid nitrogen and stored at $-80°C$ until use.

Measurement of Cardiac Function in Isolated Papillary Muscle and Perfused Heart

Analysis of cardiac function was carried out in isolated papillary muscle and in Langendorff-perfused heart. Isolated papillary muscles were stimulated electrically at 1 Hz, and the developed tension was measured.[5] The concentration of calcium ion in the buffer solution was 1.25 mM. Isolated heart was perfused at a constant pressure (75 cm H_2O) by Langendorff's method at 37 $\pm$

$0.1°C.$[2] Acetylcholine (10, 30 pmol), ET-1, and AII (1 pmol) were injected into the coronary artery as a single bolus. Coronary flow (CF; mL/min), heart rate (HR), left ventricular pressure (LVP), and the first derivative of LVP (dP/dt) were measured.

Receptor Binding Assay

Ventricular muscle was homogenized by using a Polytron homogenizer. The membrane fraction of the ventricle was isolated as described previously.[6] The saturation binding assay of the receptor for ET-1 was carried out by using $[^{125}I]$-labeled ET-1. The data were analyzed by Scatchard plot analysis to obtain K_d (dissociation constant) value.

Northern Blot Analysis

For determination of the level of expression of ET_A- and ET_B-receptor mRNA, total RNA was isolated by the AGPC method. Total RNA from left ventricles (20 μg) was separated in a 1% agarose gel containing 2.2 M formaldehyde and transferred to a Hybond N^+ membrane. After the UV fixation of RNA onto the membrane, the filter was transferred to a solution of 0.5 M sodium acetate (pH 5.2) and 0.04% methylene blue for 5–10 min at room temperature to stain the RNA.[7] ET_A- and ET_B-receptor mRNA was detected with $[^{32}P]dCTP$-labeled probes to each mRNA. Prehybridization and hybridization were carried out as described previously.[3] After the membranes were washed, they were exposed to XAR-5 films, and the autoradiograms were quantified densitometrically. The 28S ribosomal RNA was used to normalize the differences in loaded and transferred RNA.

Competitive RT-PCR Analysis of AT_1 Receptor mRNA Expression

Reverse transcription and polymerase chain reaction (RT-PCR) were performed with subtype-specific oligonucleotide as primers. The competitor for the AT_{1A} and AT_{1B} receptor mRNA (deletion mutated ΔAT_{1A} and ΔAT_{1B}) was constructed as reported previously,[3] and the level of expression was quantified according to the ratio of $AT_{1A}/\Delta AT_{1A}$ or $AT_{1B}/\Delta AT_{1B}$.[3]

RESULTS

Influence of Aging on the ET-1-Induced Positive Inotropic Effect (PIE) in Rat Papillary Muscle

In experiments with isolated papillary muscles electrically stimulated at 1Hz, ET-1 concentration-dependently (0.3–30 nM) elicited PIE (25.4 ± 7.2%

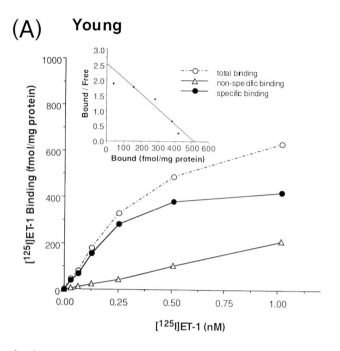

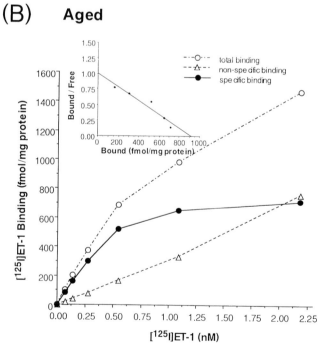

of the maximal response to isoproterenol in young rat, $n = 5$) in the presence of bupranolol (β-adrenergic receptor antagonist) in the young rat, but it scarcely affected the PIE in the aged rat (2.1% of the basal force, $n = 6$). The PIE was inhibited by FR-139317 (ET_A antagonist), but not by RES-701-1 (ET_B antagonist), indicating the involvement of the ET_A receptor in PIE. In Langendorff-perfused hearts from young rats, ET-1 concentration-dependently increased the dP/dt (145.8 ± 17.6% of basal value, $n = 6$), while ET-1 had little effect on the dP/dt in senescent rat hearts.

Influence of Aging on the Characteristics of Specific Receptors for ET-1

[^{125}I]ET-1 binding assay revealed that the maximal receptor binding (B_{max}) of ET-1 was significantly upregulated in aged rats. There was no significant difference in the affinity (K_d). FIGURE 1 shows the saturation binding curve of [^{125}I]ET-1 and the Scatchard plot. In young rat (2–3 months old), the K_d was 0.16 nM, and B_{max} was about 505.4 ± 29.4 fmol/mg protein ($n = 4$). In young adult rat (6 months old), B_{max} was 477 ± 43.8 fmol/mg protein ($n = 4$), which was similar to the B_{max} of young rat. In the senescent rat myocardium, the receptor B_{max} increased to 819.7 ± 80.8 fmol/mg protein ($n = 4$). However, the K_d value (0.30 ± 0.02) was not different from that of the young rat.

Influence of Aging on Gene Expression of ET-1 Receptors

The changes in gene expression of the ET receptor mRNA were determined by using Northern blot analysis (FIG. 2A). The sizes of ET_A mRNA were 4.2 kb and 5.2 kb. They represent alternative splicing of the same transcript. The size of ETB is 5 kb. In the rat, ET_A and ET_B mRNA are only 55% identical in the protein sequence. Densitometric analysis of Northern blot showed that expression of both ET_A- and ET_B-receptor mRNA significantly increased in aged rat to 10–20% (FIG. 2B). The ratio of ET_A and ET_B receptor mRNA was not changed, suggesting that the reduced responsiveness to ET-1 was not due to the relative increase in ET_B-receptor that may facilitate the production of NO in endothelial cells.

Influence of Aging on the Gene Expression of AII Receptors

FIGURE 3 shows the results of RT-PCR analysis of angiotensin AT_{1A} and AT_{1B} receptor mRNAs. The ratio of AT_{1A} to Δ AT_{1A} receptor mRNA was

---

FIGURE 1. [^{125}I]ET-1 saturation binding to the membrane fraction of ventricular myocardium from young (**A**) and aged (**B**) rats. The solid line indicates the specific binding of endothelin-1. *Insets* show Scatchard analysis of the binding experiments.

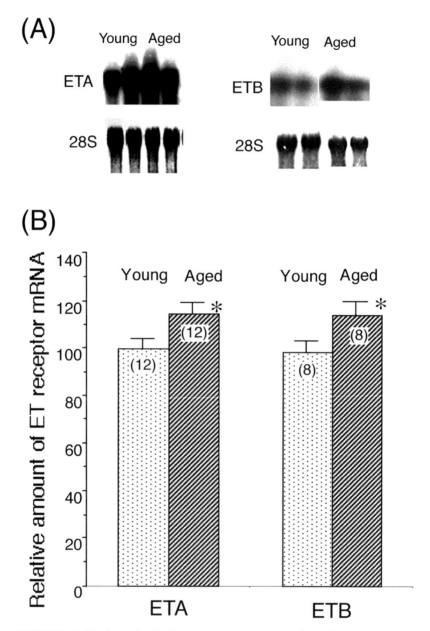

FIGURE 2. (**A**) Age-related changes in the gene expression of endothelin receptor mRNAs (ET$_A$ and ET$_B$ receptors) in the rat left ventricle determined by Northern blot analysis. (**B**) Densitometric analysis of ET$_A$ and ET$_B$ mRNA. Data are shown as mean ± SEM. The values are expressed as % of those in the young rat after normalization by the amount of 28S rRNA. Numbers in parentheses indicate the numbers of different animals used in each experiment. *$P < 0.05$ vs. young rat.

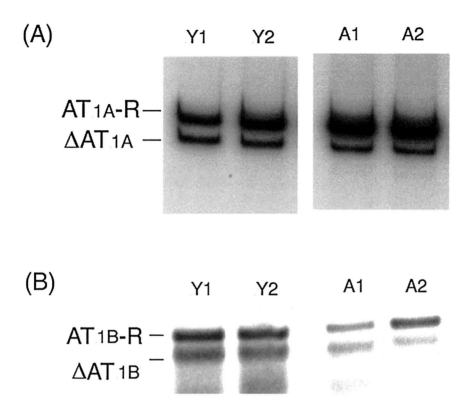

FIGURE 3. Age-related changes in the gene expression of angiotensin II receptor mRNAs (AT_{1A} and AT_{1B} receptors) in the rat left ventricle determined by competitive RT-PCR analysis. Total RNA from rat ventricles and deletion-mutated cRNA (ΔcRNA) for AT_{1A} or AT_{1B} as internal standards were amplified after reverse transcription. RT-PCR products were electrophoresed and analyzed densitometrically.

greater in the aged rat than the young rat, indicating the increased expression of AT_{1A} receptor mRNA in senescent hearts. AT_{1B} receptor mRNA was also upregulated in the aged rat hearts compared to young rats.

DISCUSSION

In the present study, we demonstrated that the cardiac inotropic response to ET-1 was attenuated in the aged rat myocardium, while the ET receptor (ET_A and ET_B) was upregulated in the senescent heart at the transcriptional level. The results of age-dependent alteration in ET-1-induced cardiac response are consistent with findings that the ET-induced increase in dP/dt was attenuated with age in perfused rat heart. The PIE of ET-1 was attenuated in the 6-month-old rat, but the B_{max} and K_d for ET-1 was not changed. On the other hand, the

ET receptor in senescent rat was significantly increased. These results suggest that increase in ET-1 receptor may occur after the inotropic effect of ET-1 was attenuated for a long time. Therefore, the increase in ET receptor could possibly be adaptive changes to reduced responsiveness to ET-1. In the aged myocardium, AT_1 receptor mRNA (AT_{1A} and AT_{1B}) was also increased. Kimbal et al.[8] reported that α_1-mediated inotropic effect and cardiac α_1-receptor density were diminished during aging in rats. Cardiac β-adrenoceptor is also decreased by aging.[9] On the other hand, we have shown here that ET-1 receptor was increased by aging.

In senescent hearts, the activation of the ET-1 signaling pathway as well as the renin–angiotensin system may be important for myocardial pathogenesis such as ischemic heart disease and cardiac hypertrophy. Expression of ET and AII receptors are known to be regulated by several pathologic conditions.[10,11] For example, in rats with ischemic heart failure caused by ligating the left coronary artery, left ventricular ET-1 mRNA levels correlated significantly with left ventricular end-diastolic pressure. Also, ET-1 receptor density increased and ET_A and ET_B receptor mRNA levels tended to increase after myocardial infarction. In coronary arteries, AII decreased the coronary flow both in young and aged rats. The coronary vasoconstriction was greater in aged rats than in young rats.[2] ET-1 also caused coronary vasoconstriction in a sustained manner. The effect was potentiated by aging.[4] One reason for these phenomena is the age-related decrease in the synthesis of NO,[2,4] but the increased expression of AT_1 and ET receptors may be involved in the strong vasoconstriction. Alternatively, these increased receptors may in turn cause cardiac hypertrophy and remodeling. Further studies are required to elucidate the mechanism and pathophysiologic relevance of the upregulation of ET and AII receptors with age.

ACKNOWLEDGMENTS

This study was supported by the Grant-in-Aid for Scientific Research (C) (No. 15590220 to Y.K. and No. 17590468 to A.I). from the Ministry of Education, Science, Sports and Culture, Japan.

REFERENCES

1. SCUBEITA, H.E. et al. 1990. Endothelin induction of inositol phospholipid hydrolysis, sarcomere assembly, and cardiac gene expression in ventricular myocytes: a paracrine mechanism for myocardial cell hypertrophy. J. Biol. Chem. **265:** 20555–20562.
2. ISHIHATA, A. et al. 1999. Differential modulation of nitric oxide and prostacyclin release in senescent rat heart stimulated by angiotensin II. Eur. J. Pharmacol. **382:** 19–26.

3. ISHIHATA, A. *et al*. 1998. Inhibition of the expression of the genes for angiotensin AT1 receptor by angiotensin II in the rat adrenal gland. Eur. J. Pharmacol. **350:** 129–139.

4. KATANO, Y. *et al*. 1993. Modification by aging of the coronary vascular response to endothelin-1 in the rat isolated perfused heart. Naunyn-Schmiedeberg's Arch. Pharmacol. **348:** 82–87.

5. ISHIHATA, A. *et al*. 1988. Enantiomers of dobutamine increase the force of contraction via beta adrenoceptors, but antagonize competitively the positive inotropic effect mediated by alpha-1 adrenoceptors in the rabbit ventricular myocardium. J. Pharmacol. Exp. Ther. **246:** 1080–1087.

6. ISHIHATA, A. *et al*. 1995. Species-related differences in inotropic effects of angiotensin II in mammalian ventricular muscle: receptors, subtypes and phosphoinositide hydrolysis. Br. J. Pharmacol. **114:** 447–453.

7. HERRIN, D.L. & G.W. SCHMIDT. 1988. Rapid, reversible staining of Northern blots prior to hybridization. BioTechniques **6:** 196.

8. KIMBAL, K.A. *et al*. 1991. Aging: changes in cardiac α_1-adrenoceptor responsiveness and expression. Eur. J. Pharmacol. **208:** 231–238.

9. KOJIMA, M. *et al*. 1990. Developmental changes in beta-adrenoceptors, muscarinic cholinoceptors and Ca^{2+} channels in rat ventricular muscles. Br. J. Pharmacol. **99:** 334–339.

10. LIU, J. *et al*. 1990. Ischemia and reperfusion increase ^{125}I-labeled endothelin-1 binding in rat cardiac membranes. Am. J. Physiol. **258:** H829–H835.

11. GU, X.H. *et al*. 1990. ^{125}I-labeled endothelin-1 binding to brain and cardiac membranes from normotensive and spontaneously hypertensive rats. Eur. J. Pharmacol. **177:** 205–209.

Mitochondria Damage Checkpoint, Aging, and Cancer

KESHAV K. SINGH

Department of Cancer Genetics, Cell and Virus Building, Room 247, Roswell Park Cancer Institute, Elm and Carlton Streets, Buffalo, New York 14263, USA

ABSTRACT: There is growing evidence supporting the progressing decline in mitochondrial function with age. Mitochondria are the major site of reactive oxygen species (ROS) production in the cell; therefore it is likely that progressive decline in mitochondrial function is due to the accumulation of oxidative damage with age. Despite this notion, a role for mitochondria in cellular senescence has been largely ignored. Our studies using mitochondrial gene knockout cells (ρ^0) from a variety of tissue types demonstrate that loss of mitochondrial function leads to cell cycle arrest, cellular senescence, and tumorigenic phenotype. In light of these and earlier studies we hypothesize the existence of a mitochondria damage checkpoint (*mitocheckpoint*) in human cells. *Mitocheckpoint* permits cells to arrest in the cell cycle in order to repair/restore mitochondrial function to the normal level. Upon overwhelming, persistent, or severe damage to mitochondria, *mitocheckpoint* machinery may allow cells to undergo senescence. Thus cellular senescence may function as another checkpoint before cells decide to initiate programmed cell death resulting in aging of tissues and organs. Alternatively, mutations occur in the mitochondrial and/or nuclear DNA, resulting in tumorigenesis.

KEYWORDS: mitochondria; apoptosis; tumorigenesis; cell mutation; cell senescence

INTRODUCTION

Mitochondria are multifunctional organelles that play a key role in free radical production, energy production, programmed cell death (apoptosis), thermogenesis, and calcium signaling.[1–3] Studies also demonstrate that mitochondria maintain the stability of the nuclear genome.[4–6] Mitochondrial biogenesis requires the coordinated expression of nuclear and mitochondrial DNA-encoded genes. Mitochondria contain approximately 1,000 proteins that are encoded by the nuclear genome. Only 13 proteins are encoded by the mitochondrial

Address for correspondence: Keshav K. Singh, Ph.D., Department of Cancer Genetics, Cell and Virus Building, Room 247, Roswell Park Cancer Institute, Elm and Carlton Streets, Buffalo, NY 14263, USA. Voice: 716-845-8017; fax: 716-845-1047.

e-mail: keshav.singh@roswellpark.org

Ann. N.Y. Acad. Sci. 1067: 182–190 (2006). © 2006 New York Academy of Sciences.
doi: 10.1196/annals.1354.022

genome. The mitochondrial DNA-encoded proteins constitute the essential subunits of electron transport. The mitochondrial genome also encodes 2 ribosomal RNA and 22 transfer RNAs. Aging dramatically increases the risk factors for cancer. A constant feature of aging and cancer is the accumulations of mutations in mtDNA and associated decline in mitochondrial function.[7] These observations suggest that mitochondrial DNA (mtDNA) mutations that accumulate during aging may have an impact on tumorigenesis. In this review we describe data obtained in our own and other laboratories in support of the argument that mtDNA exerts significant influence on both cellular aging and aging-associated diseases including cancer.

MtDNA MUTATION IS A COMMON FEATURE OF AGING TISSUES

As mitochondria perform oxidative phoshorylation to reduce oxygen to water by the addition of electrons they produce a significant amount of reactive oxygen species (ROS).[1,8] ROS produced in the mitochondria make the mtDNA extremely susceptible to damage and mutagenesis. This is because mtDNA contains no protective histones, is devoid of introns, and has limited DNA repair capacity.[1] Mitochondrial DNA mutations accumulate with age. The rate of somatic mutation in mtDNA is up to 20 times higher than that in nuclear DNA. This higher rate of mutation also appears to be due to the high-concentration ROS produced by oxidative phosphorylation operating in the mitochondria. Older people accumulate a variety of different mtDNA mutations including deletions, duplications, and point mutations in various tissues. These tissues include ovary,[9,10] skeletal muscle, myocardium, testis, adrenal gland, kidney, liver, lung, brain, and skin (FIG. 1, TABLE 1, reviewed in Wei and Lee,[11] and

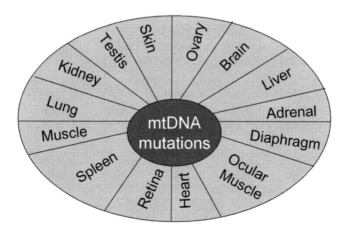

FIGURE 1. Aging-associated mtDNA mutations found in various tissues.

TABLE 1. Aging-associated mtDNA mutation in human tissues[a]

Mutation	Nucleotide position	Tissues
Deletions		
4977 bp	8483 to 13459	Liver, muscle, brain, heart, lung, spleen, testis, diaphragm, kidney, adrenal gland, hair follicle, skin, ovary, and retina
7436 bp	8649 to 16084	Heart, muscle, liver, and skin
6063 bp	7842 to 13904	Muscle and liver
3610 bp	1837 to 5446	Muscle
5827 bp	7993 to 13786	Muscle
6335 bp	8477 to 14811	Muscle
7635 bp	8440 to 16074	Muscle
8041 bp	8035 to 16075	Brain
Point mutations		
A3243G	3243	Muscle
A8344G	8344	Extraocular muscle
Duplications		
260 bp	−567/301	Muscle, skin and liver
200 bp	−493/301	Muscle and skin

[a]Table adapted from Wei and Lee. [11]

references therein). Recently, Trifunovic et al.[12] and Kujoth et al.[13] demonstrated that a homozygous knock-in mouse that expresses a proof-reading deficient version of polymerase γ shows increases in the levels of point mutation and in the amounts of mtDNA deletions. This mouse shows accelerated aging and an age-related disease phenotype, which provides further proof for the mitochondrial theory of aging proposed by Harman.[14]

In humans, the overall amount of mutant mtDNA is described to be low in various tissues as a whole in older individuals, but individual cells contain a high frequency of a single mutations, and different cells contain different mutant species.[15] It is believed that when a proportion of mutant mtDNA exceeds the threshold concentration, it then results in a mitochondrial OXPHOS defect. An OXPHOS defect may involve different respiratory chain complexes, including complex I, III, IV, and V. Of these, complex IV appears to be often affected and is easily detected by histochemical study in single cells.[15] Clonal expansion of mtDNA mutation may have a substantial effect on an OXPHOS function at cellular, tissue, and organ levels. One of the other possibilities is that mutant mtDNA in aging tissues may induce genetic instability in the nucleus, as reported by Rasmussen et al.[4] and Singh et al.[6] Mitochondria harboring mutant mtDNA can also be leaky and can activate endogenous endonucleases such as endonuclease G that reside inside the mitochondria and participate in caspase-independent pathway of DNA degradation during apoptosis. Activation of endonuclease G by mutant mitochondria may lead to nuclear genome instability. The degree of commitment to cell death by mutant mitochondria may decide whether cells complete the full apoptotic program or not. Incomplete mitochondrial commitment, termed *mitochondria interruptus*, can lead to activation of endonuclease G, resulting in nuclear genome instability. Execution of the full cell death program may be the cause of aging-associated neurodegenerative diseases. However, incomplete execution can result in accumulation of mutations induced by activation of endonucleases and tumorigenesis.

MtDNA MUTATION IS A COMMON FEATURE OF CANCER CELLS

Mutations in the mtDNA of primary tumors have been reported in virtually all forms of cancer examined to date.[2,3,6] MtDNA mutations in cancer cells include intragenic deletion, missense and chain-termination point mutations, and alterations of homoplasmic sequences that result in frame-shift mutations (reviewed in references[2,16,17] and references therein). Because each cell contains many mitochondria with multiple copies of mtDNA, it is possible that wild-type and mutant mtDNA can coexist in a state called heteroplasy. If only the wild-type or all mutant mtDNA is found in cells, it is described as homoplasic. FIGURE 2 provides a summary of organ sites where mtDNA mutations are reported to be present.[3] It is interesting to note that mutations in protein coding regions of mtDNA are homoplasic.[17] Recently, Carew and Huang[17] reported four main features of mtDNA mutations common to all tumor types: (1) the majority of the mutations are base substitutions; (2) mutations occur in all protein-coding mitochondrial genes; (3) the D-loop region is the most frequent site of somatic mutations across most tumor types; and (4) the presence of homoplasic mutant mtDNA in tumors suggests that they may play an

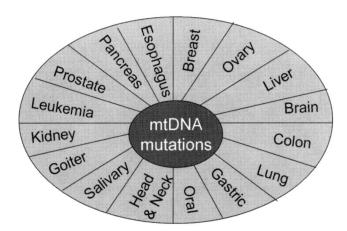

FIGURE 2. Mitochondrial mutations found in various tumors.

important role in the development of tumors. It is noteworthy that depletion of mtDNA is also reported in many kinds of cancer.[18,19]

CELLULAR SENESCENCE IN RESPONSE TO MITOCHONDRIAL DYSFUNCTION

Cellular senescence was first described by Hayflick in human fibroblasts.[20] Studies have revealed that senescence is largely due to loss of telomerase activity, resulting in the loss of telomeric DNA.[21] Telomeres consist of two components: (i) repetitive DNA sequence and (ii) the proteins, which cap the ends of linear chromosomes. Telomeres are essential for chromosomal integrity. Loss of telomeres results in genomic instability leading to the development of tumors. Our studies suggest that mitochondrial dysfunction leads to reduced telomerase activity and genomic instability in cultured cells.[6,22] Since a variety of tissues accumulate deleted mtDNA molecules during aging, we hypothesized that deletion of mtDNA may cause cellular senescence. We addressed this hypothesis by using a cell line completely devoid of mtDNA (ρ^0). Our studies demonstrated that mitochondrial genetic stress leads to cellular senescence. We measured various characteristics of cellular senescence in ρ^0 cells. We found that ρ^0 cells show increased senescence-associated β-galactosidase activity, accumulate increased level of lipofuscin, and show decreased telomerase activity.[23] We also demonstrated the increased expression of PAI-1, p16, p21, p27, and decreased expression of cyclin A and cyclin D1 in ρ^0 cells. We extended these studies in other ρ^0 derivatives such as those derived from breast carcinoma MDA-MB-435 ρ^0 cells. We found that the cellular senescence phenotype was a general feature associated with mitochondrial dysfunction in ρ^0 cells. These studies provide direct evidence that mitochondrial genetic stress leads to cellular aging and mtDNA mutations play a significant role in aging.

TUMORIGENICITY DUE TO MITOCHONDRIAL DYSFUNCTION

Using the ρ^0 approach, we addressed whether mitochondrial dysfunction leads to tumorigenic phenotype. We analyzed Matrigel migration and anchorage-independent growth of the ρ^0 cell line. We found that ρ^0 cells show transformed phenotype. We also demonstrated that the transfer of wild-type mitochondria resulted in the reversion of tumorigenic phenotype, which suggests a direct role for the mitochondrial genome in tumorigenesis. Furthermore, we showed that mitochondrial dysfunction leads to chromosomal instability (CIN), a hallmark of cancer cells. The identified CIN was also reported to be present in a variety of primary human tumors, suggesting that mitochondria-led nuclear mutations may be a causative factor in tumorigenesis. In addition, we found that redox factor 1 (Ref1, also known as Ape1 and Hap1) plays a key role in genomic instability. Ref1 expression was altered in a variety of tumors.[6] In combination, these studies suggest that mitochondria-to-nucleus retrograde redox regulation due to mitochondrial dysfunction may also contribute to tumorigenesis.[6]

MITOCHONDRIA DAMAGE CHECKPOINT IN AGING AND CANCER

I recently hypothesized the existence of a mitochondria damage checkpoint (*mitocheckpoint*) in eukaryotic cells that monitors and responds to spontaneous or induced damage to mitochondria.[24] The *mitocheckpoint* coordinates and maintains the proper balance between apoptotic and antiapoptotic signals. Upon damage to mitochondria, *mitocheckpoint* is activated to help repair damage to mitochondria, restore normal mitochondrial function, and avoid induction of mitochondria-defective cells. Thus *mitocheckpoint* allows cell cycle arrest and controls nuclear and mitochondrial gene expression to help repair the incurred damage (FIG. 3). Consistent with this hypothesis, our work and studies conducted in other laboratories have reported cell cycle arrest upon inhibition of mitochondrial function in human cells.[23,25] A highly coordinated cross-talk between mitochondria and the nucleus also exists in human cells.[2,3,6]

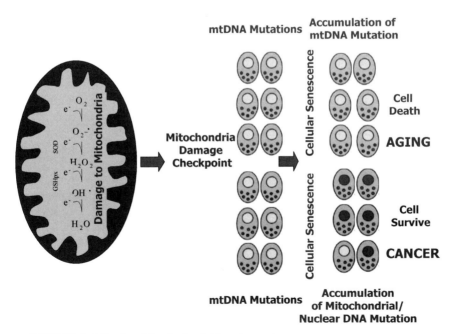

FIGURE 3. Mitochondria checkpoint in aging and cancer.

If mitochondria are severely damaged, such an event will trigger apoptosis, which in turn will trigger accelerated aging and aging-related diseases that are generally degenerative in nature, with an overall decline in tissue structure and function (FIG. 3). If damage to mitochondria is persistent and continues to accumulate with age and resulting in mtDNA mutations, it can lead to nuclear genome instability, which, in turn, can lead to cancer (FIG. 3). In support of this argument, we provide evidence that mitochondrial genetic defects in human cell culture and a model organism leads to impaired DNA repair, increased genomic instability, and increased cell survival.[4,5,6,22,26] A progressive decline in mitochondrial function is reported during aging. Interestingly, aging-related cancer reflects a gain-of-function disease. Thus accumulated nuclear genome mutations may help cells acquire new tumorigenic functions such as hyper-proliferation, migration, and invasive characteristics.

Recent studies suggest that cellular senescence may provide an important barrier to tumorigenesis. Cellular senescence limits the capacity to replicate, thus preventing the proliferation of cells. Senescence bypass appears to be an important step in the development of cancer.[27] Senescent cells typically show flat, vacuolated morphology, large size, senescence-associated β-galactosidase marker, reduced telomerase activity, and retinoblastoma hypophosphorylation. Our recent study suggests that mitochondrial gene knock-out in a variety of cell types leads to cellular senescence.[22] As expected, these mitochondrial gene knock-out cells also show many of the molecular markers of cellular senescence including increased senescence-associated β-galactosidase activity, reduced telomerase activity, and retinoblastoma hypophosporylation. I propose that mitochondrial damage-induced cellular senescence may act as an additional checkpoint mechanism that can function as a tumor suppressor[27] (FIG. 3). Recent studies conducted in various cell types provide *in vivo* evidence that senescence is a defining feature in premalignant tumors.[28–31] In summary, I suggest that damage to mitochondria can activate *mitocheckpoint*, leading to cell cycle arrest[22,24] that allows cells to repair and restore mitochondrial function. If damage to mitochondria is severe or persistent, *mitocheckpoint* may fail, which can lead to cellular senescence and consequently to programmed cell death (aging) or tumorigenesis due to the accumulation of mutations in mitochondrial and/or nuclear DNA (cancer). The *mitocheckpoint* mechanism may also involve mitochondria-to-nucleus retrograde redox regulation that can play an important role in aging and cancer.[23,24,32]

ACKNOWLEDGMENTS

I thank Ellen Sanders-Noonan for editing this manuscript. This study was supported by grants from the National Institutes of Health (RO1-097714) and the Breast Cancer Coalition of Rochester.

REFERENCES

1. SINGH, K.K. (Ed.) 1998. Mitochondrial DNA Mutations in Aging, Disease, and Cancer. Springer, New York.
2. MODICA-NAPOLITANO, J. & K.K. SINGH. 2002. Mitochondria as targets for detection and treatment of cancer. Expert Reviews in Molecular, Medicine. http://www-ermm.cbcu.cam.ac.uk/02004453h.htm.
3. MODICA-NAPOLITANO, J. & K.K. SINGH. 2004. Mitochondrial dysfunction in cancer. Mitochondrion **4:** 755–762.
4. RASMUSSEN, A.K., A. CHATTERJEE, L.J. RASMUSSEN, *et al.* 2003. Mitochondria-mediated nuclear mutator phenotype in *Saccharomyces cerevisiae*. Nucleic Acids Res. **31:** 3909–3917.
5. DELSITE, R.L., L.J. RASMUSSEN, A.K. RASMUSSEN, *et al.* 2003. Mitochondrial impairment is accompanied by impaired oxidative DNA repair in the nucleus. Mutagenesis **18:** 497–503.
6. SINGH, K.K., M. KULAWEIC, I. STILL, *et al.* 2005. Inter-genomic cross talk between mitochondria and the nucleus plays an important role in tumorigenesis. Gene **354:** 140–146.
7. SINGH, K.K. 2004. Mitochondrial dysfunction is a common phenotype in aging and cancer. Ann N.Y. Acad. Sci. **1019:** 260–264.
8. RICHTER, C., J.W. PARK & B.N. AMES. 1988. Normal oxidative damage to mitochondrial and nuclear DNA is extensive. Proc. Natl. Acad. Sci. USA **85:** 6465–6467.
9. SUGANUMA, N., T. KITAGAWA, A. NAWA, *et al.* 1993. Human ovarian aging and mitochondrial DNA deletion. Horm. Res. **39** (Suppl 1): 16–21.
10. KITAGAWA, T., N. SUGANUMA, A. NAWA, *et al.* 1993. Rapid accumulation of deleted mitochondrial deoxyribonucleic acid in postmenopausal ovaries. Biol. Reprod. **49:** 730–736.
11. WEI, Y.H. & H.C. LEE. 2002. Oxidative stress, mitochondrial DNA mutation, and impairment of antioxidant enzymes in aging. Exp. Biol. Med. **227:** 671–682.
12. TRIFUNOVIC, A., A. WREDENBERG, M. FALKENBERG, *et al.* 2004. Premature ageing in mice expressing defective mitochondrial DNA polymerase. Nature **429:** 417–423.
13. KUJOTH, G.C., A. HIONA, T.D. PUGH, *et al.* 2005. Mitochondrial DNA mutations, oxidative stress, and apoptosis in mammalian aging. Science **309:** 481–484.
14. HARMAN, D. 1972. The biologic clock: the mitochondria? J. Am. Geriatr. Soc. **20:** 145–147.
15. CHINNERY, P.F., D.C. SAMUELS, J. ELSON, *et al.* 2002. Accumulation of mitochondrial DNA mutations in ageing, cancer, and mitochondrial disease: is there a common mechanism? Lancet **360:** 1323–1325.
16. COPELAND, W.C., J.T. WACHSMAN, F.M. JOHNSON, *et al.* 2002. Mitochondrial DNA alterations in cancer. Cancer Invest. **20:** 557–569.
17. CAREW, J.S. & P. HUANG. 2002. Mitochondrial defects in cancer. Mol. Cancer **1:** 9.
18. LEE, H.C., P.H. YIN, J.C. LIN, *et al.* 2005. Mitochondrial, genome instability and mtDNA, depletion in human cancers. Ann. N.Y. Acad. Sci. **1042:** 109–122.
19. WU, C.W., P.H. YIN, W.Y. HUNG, *et al.* 2005. Mitochondrial DNA mutations and mitochondrial DNA depletion in gastric cancer. Genes Chrom. Cancer **44:** 19–28.
20. HAYFLICK, L. & P.S. MOORHEAD. 1961. The serial cultivation of human diploid cell strains. Exp. Cell Res. **25:** 585–621.

21. CAMPISI, J. 2005. Senescent cells, tumor suppression, and organismal aging: good citizens, bad neighbors. Cell **120:** 513–522.
22. PARK, S.Y., I. CHANG, S.W. KANG, *et al.* 2004. Resistance of mitochondrial DNA depleted cells against cell death: role of mitochondrial superoxide dismutase. J. Biol. Chem. **279:** 7512–7520.
23. PARK, S.Y., B. CHOI, H. CHEON, *et al.* 2004. Cellular aging of mitochondrial DNA-depleted cells. Biochem. Biophys. Res. Commun. **325:** 1399–1405.
24. SINGH, K.K. 2004. Mitochondria damage checkpoint in apoptosis and genome stability. FEMS Yeast Res. **2:** 127–132.
25. SWEET, S. & G. SINGH. 1995. Accumulation of human promyelocytic leukemic (HL-60) cells at two energetic cell cycle checkpoints. Cancer Res. **55:** 5164–5167.
26. SINGH, K.K., A.K. RASMUSSEN & L.J. RASMUSSEN. 2004. Genome wide analysis of signal transducers and regulators of mitochondrial dysfunction in *Saccharomyces cerevisiae*. Ann. N.Y. Acad. Sci. **1011:** 284–298.
27. DIMRI, G.P. 2005. What has senescence got to do with cancer? Cancer Cell **7:** 505–512.
28. SHARPLESS, N.E. & R.A. DEPINHO. 2005. Cancer: crime and punishment. Nature **436:** 636–637.
29. COLLADO, M., J. GIL, A. EFEYAN, *et al.* 2005. Tumour biology: senescence in premalignant tumours. Nature **436:** 642.
30. MICHALOGLOU, C., L.C. VREDEVELD, M.S. SOENGAS, *et al.* 2005. BRAFE600-associated senescence-like cell cycle arrest of human naevi. Nature **436:** 720–724.
31. CHEN, Z., L.C. TROTMAN, D. SHAFFER, *et al.* 2005. Crucial role of p53-dependent cellular senescence in suppression of Pten-deficient tumorigenesis. Nature **436:** 725–730.
32. DESOUKI, M.M., M. KULAWIEC, S. BANSAL, *et al.* 2005. Crosstalk, between mitochondria and superoxide generating NADPH oxidase in breast and ovarian tumors. Cancer Biol. Ther. **4:** 1367–1373.

DNA Damage by Free Radical Production by Aminoguanidine

GEORGE SUJI AND SUBRAMANIUM SIVAKAMI

Department of Life Sciences, University of Mumbai, Santacruz (E) Mumbai 400 098, India

ABSTRACT: Aminoguanidine (AG), a prototype therapeutic dicarbonyl scavenger, is the most potent drug available today to inhibit the formation of advanced glycation endproducts (AGEs) and to reverse glycation-mediated damage in normal aging. This paper examines the ability of AG to cause damage to supercoiled plasmid DNA in the presence of the transition metal, Fe^{+3}. Damage to DNA was dependent on the concentrations of both the transition metal and AG. We could detect hydroxyl radical as well as hydrogen peroxide during the incubation of AG with Fe^{+3}. Thus this finding further cautions against the indiscriminate use of AG in clinical prophylaxis in diabetes and questions its use as a therapeutic agent.

KEYWORDS: aminoguanidine; DNA damage; free radicals; prooxidant; diabetes mellitus

INTRODUCTION

Strategies to combat carbonyl stress exerted by the dicarbonyls involve use of therapeutic agents that can neutralize their toxicity and the damage caused by them to macromolecules. Many molecules have been identified as potential dicarbonyl-scavenging agents. Among them, the most well known is aminoguanidine (Pimagedine, AG), a hydrazine compound, and prototype dicarbonyl-scavenging agent. AG is a nucleophilic compound containing the hydrazine group $-NHNH_2$ and the dicarbonyl group $-NH-C$ $(=NH)$ NH_2.[1] AG scavenges dicarbonyls to form substituted 3-amino-1,2,4-triazines.[2] Since the first report of intervention to prevent formation of advanced glycation endproducts (AGE) by AG,[3] many studies both *in vitro* and *in vivo* have shown its ability to prevent long-term pathologic biomacromolecular changes associated with hyperglycemia.[3–5]

AG has been considered a nontoxic nucleophilic hydrazine ($LD_{50} = 1800$ mg/kg) in rodents.[6] However, undesirable pharmacological side effects

Address for correspondence: S. Sivakami, Department of Life Sciences, University of Mumbai, Santacruz (E) Mumbai 400 098, India. Voice: 91-22-2652-8847; fax: 91-22-2652-6053.
  e-mail: sivakami_s2000@yahoo.com

Ann. N.Y. Acad. Sci. 1067: 191–199 (2006). © 2006 New York Academy of Sciences.
doi: 10.1196/annals.1354.023

raise questions about its use as a therapeutic agent.[1] AG is known to produce hydrogen peroxide in a transition metal–catalyzed process, partially on account of its prior hydrolysis to semicarbazide and hydrazine.[7] Hydrazine is known to cause DNA damage in the presence of metal ions.[8] The rapid renal elimination of AG requires frequent administration to achieve the desired effect. It is therefore possible that prolonged exposure to these products may give rise to DNA damage. This prompted us to investigate the damage caused to DNA by AG and metal ion *in vitro*.

In this study, the cleavage to supercoiled plasmid DNA induced by AG in the presence of Fe^{+3} was investigated. This *in vitro* system is an extremely sensitive indicator of DNA damage.[8] The results presented here indicate that AG in the presence of transition metal ion Fe^{3+} may lead to oxidative damage to DNA through a mechanism that involves hydroxyl radicals.

METHODS

Analysis of DNA Damage

The pBR 322 plasmid DNA (0.5 μg) in 10 mM potassium phosphate buffer, pH 7.4, was incubated for 48 h at 37°C with AG in the presence and absence of Fe^{+3}. The reaction was stopped by freezing. Four microliters of loading buffer (0.25% bromophenol blue, 40% sucrose) were added and samples analyzed by electrophoresis in 0.8% agarose using TBE buffer (90 mM Tris, 90 mM boric acid, 2 mM EDTA, pH 8.0).[9] The gel was stained with ethidium bromide and photographed using a digital camera (powerShot G2, Canon, Japan).

Measurement of Hydroxyl Radical

Hydroxyl radicals were detected by measuring the hydroxylation of benzoic acid to fluorescent products (excitation 308 nm/emission 410 nm). Benzoic acid hydroxylation was quantified using salicyclic acid standard.[10]

Measurement of Superoxide Anion

The generation superoxide in the aerobic mixture was determined by cytochrome *c* reduction[11] in reaction mixtures containing AG with or without Fe^{+3}.

Measurement of H_2O_2

H_2O_2 was measured by the ferrous ion oxidation–xylenol orange (FOX1) assay.[12]

Replicates

Unless otherwise indicated, each result described in this paper is representative of at least three separate experiments.

RESULTS

Untreated plasmid DNA incubated for 48 h showed two bands corresponding to the supercoiled form (Form I) and nicked circular form (Form II) (FIG.1A). Damage resulted in the shift of the band from the supercoiled form to the nicked circular form (Form II). Although AG alone caused DNA damage (FIG. 1D, Lane 2), in the presence of Fe^{+3} AG completely degraded DNA, as indicated by the disappearance of (Form I) molecules and a concomitant increase in the nicked circular form (Form II) (FIG. 1A, lanes 3, 4, 5). The damage to DNA by AG alone may have been mediated by traces of contaminating transition metal ions. The effects of increasing concentrations of AG showed that DNA strand break increased on increasing the AG concentration (FIG.1A). This DNA strand breakage was inhibited by known hydroxyl scavengers like azide, sodium formate, and mannitol (FIG. 1C), suggesting the involvement of hydroxyl radical in the Fe^{+3}-mediated damage to DNA. The ability of hydrazine, a hydrolysis product of AG, to cause DNA damage at levels that can be formed in AG and metal was studied. Hydrazine did cause DNA damage though not to the same extent as that of AG (FIG.1D, lane 4) and the damage was not affected by the presence of metal ions (FIG.1D, lanes 3, 5). Thus it can be tentatively concluded that hydrazine alone is not the sole source of oxidants that cause damage in the AG and Fe^{+3} system.

As can be seen from FIGURE 2, the incubation of AG with Fe^{+3} for a period of 2 h resulted in the formation of H_2O_2, as detected by the FOX1 assay. This production of H_2O_2 was dependent on both the metal ion concentration as well as that of AG (FIG. 2). In the presence of purified bovine catalase (10 U), the formation of H_2O_2 was not detected. At the end of an incubation period of 2 h, 5 mM AG in the presence 100 μM $FeCl_3$ produced 0.53 μM H_2O_2. Thereafter, the formation of H_2O_2 increased, reaching a value of 3.81 μM H_2O_2 at 100 mM AG. At fixed concentrations of 50 mM AG and 10 μM $FeCl_3$, 0.34 μM of H_2O_2 was detected. Furthermore, the formation of H_2O_2 was curvilinear, reaching 2.82 μM of H_2O_2 at 80 μM $FeCl_3$.

Since AG is known to be an efficient dicarbonyl scavenger, the formation of H_2O_2 by AG and Fe^{+3} in the presence of methylglyoxal was studied. At a 1:1 ratio of AG and MG in the presence of Fe^{+3}, there was no detectable H_2O_2. AG is known to readily react with MG to form aminotriazine, which can be monitored by its characteristic absorption spectrum at 320 nm. The formation of the aminotriazine appears to be metal-independent.

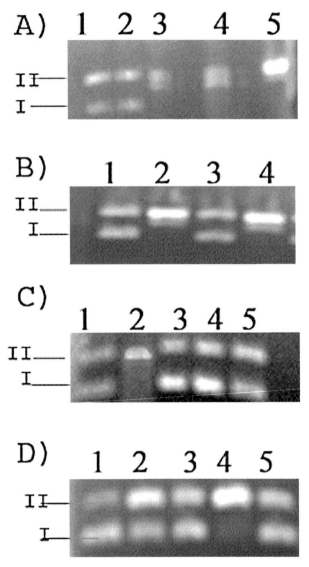

FIGURE 1. pBR322 (0.5 μg) was incubated with the following: **(A)** *lane* 1, DNA alone; *lane* 2, FeCl$_3$ (100 μM); *lane* 3, AG (1 mM) + FeCl$_3$ (100 μM); *lane* 4, AG (10 mM) + FeCl$_3$ (100 μM); *lane* 5, AG (100 mM) + FeCl$_3$ (100 μM). **(B)** *lane* 1, FeCl$_3$ (30 μM), *lane* 2, AG (1 mM) + FeCl$_3$ (30 μM); *lane* 3, FeCl$_3$ (60 μM); *lane* 4π AG (1 mM) + FeCl$_3$ (60 μM). **(C)** *lane* 1, DNA alone; *lane* 2, AG (1 mM) + FeCl$_3$ (30 μM); *lane* 3, AG (1 mM) + FeCl$_3$ (30 μM) + azide (250 mM); *lane* 4, AG (1 mM) + FeCl$_3$ (30 μM) + sodium formate (250 mM); lane 5, AG (1 mM) + FeCl$_3$ (30 μM) + mannitol (250 mM). **(D)** *lane* 1, DNA alone; *lane* 2, AG (1 mM); *lane* 3, hydrazine (5 μM); *lane* 4, AG (1 mM) + FeCl$_3$ (5 μM); *lane* 5, hydrazine (5 μM) + FeCl$_3$ (5 μM).

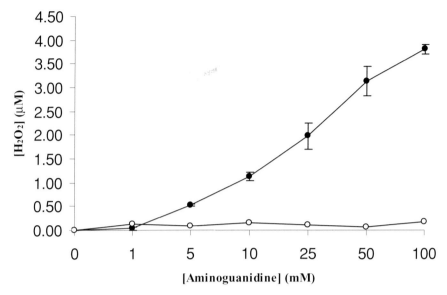

FIGURE 2. H_2O_2 production as a function of varying concentrations of AG in the absence and presence of 100 μM Fe^{+3} in potassium phosphate buffer (10 mM, pH 7.4) at 37°C for 2 h.

Monitoring of the benzoic acid hydroxylation to fluorescent products revealed the formation of hydroxyl radical in AG- and Fe^{+3}- system. The formation of hydroxyl radical was AG- and Fe^{+3}-dependent. At a lower concentration AG (1 mM) in the presence of Fe^{+3} produced higher amounts of hydroxyl radicals than at a higher concentration (100 mM) (FIG. 3). However, hydrazine showed a reverse trend—the formation of hydroxyl radical increased as the concentration of hydrazine was increased (FIG. 4). The production of hydroxyl radical by AG increased as the concentration of Fe^{+3} increased. The formation of hydroxyl radical by hydrazine decreased, while the concentration of Fe^{+3} increased.

To examine whether the superoxide radical was generated in the reaction system, cytochrome reduction assay was carried out. Superoxide could not be detected in incubation mixtures containing AG and Fe^{+3}. However, hydrazine, the hydrolytic product of AG, in the presence of Fe^{+3} was seen to generate the superoxide radical, the formation of which was also observed to be metal ion–dependent.

DISCUSSION

The prooxidant activity of AG has been well documented.[13,14] In this report, we have confirmed the prooxidant activity of AG and have shown, for the first

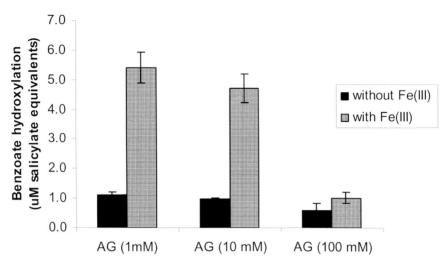

FIGURE 3. The generation of hydroxyl radical by various concentrations of AG in the absence and presence of $FeCl_3$ (50 µM) for 48 h is shown. AG was incubated with 1 mM benzoic acid, 100 mM potassium phosphate buffer (pH 7.4) at 37°C, with or without 50 µM ferric chloride. Generation of the fluorescent product of benzoic acid hydroxylation after 48 h is expressed as a salicylic acid equivalent.

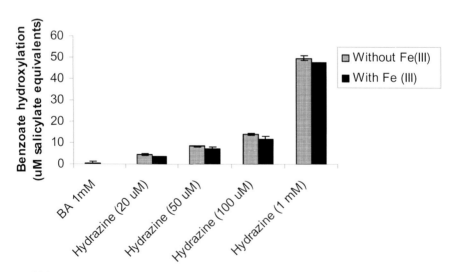

FIGURE 4. The generation of hydroxyl radical by various concentrations of hydrazine in the absence and presence of $FeCl_3$ (50 µM) for 48 h is shown. Various concentrations of hydrazine were incubated with 1 mM benzoic acid, 100 mM potassium phosphate buffer (pH 7.4) at 37°C, with or without 50 µM ferric chloride. Generation of the fluorescent product of benzoic acid hydroxylation after 48 h is expressed as salicylic acid equivalent.

time, AG-mediated structural damage to DNA in the presence of a transition metal like Fe^{+3}.

AG has been shown to generate H_2O_2 in the presence of metal ion. It decays to semicarbazide and finally to hydrazine by spontaneous hydrolysis. Hydrazine and semicarbazide have been shown to generate H_2O_2. However, hydrazine has a greater rate of H_2O_2 production than AG and semicarbazide. Reports suggest that hydrazine was present at a steady-state level of less than 0.02% of the AG concentration.[7] Thus a 1-mM solution of AG contained an upper limit of 0.5 μM hydrazine. Also, this level of hydrazine should contribute to 20% of total H_2O_2 derived from AG. The rest of the H_2O_2 in the incubation mixture may have been contributed by both semicarbazide and AG.[7] Damage to DNA by hydrazine at concentrations that can be formed in the AG and Fe systems reveal that damage to DNA by hydrazine alone was very minor when compared to that of AG.

It is interesting to note that in this study, during incubation of AG and MG in the presence of Fe^{+3}, H_2O_2 could not be detected, probably due to the fast kinetics of conversion of AG to triazine products. The reaction of MG with AG under physiological conditions produces isomeric triazine products, which do not require metal ions for their formation. Hence the metal-dependent formation of H_2O_2 is determined by the availability of unreacted AG, which has not been converted to triazine products.

In this study, although the formation of ·OH radical was shown, its formation was found to be dependent on AG and Fe^{+3} concentration. At a higher concentration of AG, the hydroxyl production was less, suggesting that at a higher concentration, AG acts directly as an antioxidant. The ·OH produced would then damage the DNA.

The formation of hydroxyl radical could not be measured by the well-established deoxyribose assay on account of the limitation of the assay as AG is known to react with malonaldehyde formed in the reaction mixture.[13] In this study DNA damage was also inhibited by hydroxyl radical scavengers azide, sodium formate, and mannitol, showing that Fe^{+3} produces hydroxyl ·OH, which causes DNA damage. The inability of catalase to protect against DNA damage may be due to inactivation of catalase by AG, as AG is known to inhibit catalase.[7]

During incubations of AG with $Fe^{+3,}$ the presence of the superoxide radical was not detected, but, with hydrazine and Fe^{+3}, the superoxide radical was detectable. Given that AG is a precursor of hydrazine, the reason for this discrepancy is not clear. It is possible that not enough of it is generated because of the very low levels of hydrazine formed from AG in vitro, but detectable superoxide is formed when commercial hydrazine is used at higher concentrations by the cytochrome assay.

Diabetes, evidence of an increase in the availability of redox active transition metals is suggested by reports of altered metal-handling capacity.[15] Elevated iron indices are more common in diabetic individuals.[16] Also, non-insulin-dependent diabetes mellitus is a common complication of diseases of iron overload such as hemochromatosis.[17] Thus, the implication of these observations must be considered in the context of the availability of redox active transition metals *in vivo*, as in the case of diabetes. The LD_{50} of AG in rodents is very high (1800 mg/kg), and plasma levels of about 13 mM have been reported after feeding in animals.[18] The maximum concentration of AG expected to be achieved in plasma *in vivo* at doses producing pharmacological effects associated with the prevention of diabetic complications (50 mg/kg of AG bicarbonate) is ~669 μM, given the distribution in total body water.[19] The IC_{50} value of AG for inhibition of early protein glycation by glucose is ~60 mM[1]. Although AG is kinetically competent to scavenge oxoaldehyde, the rapid elimination of AG (pharmacokinetic half-life 1.4 h) requires its frequent administration to achieve the desired effects.[1] Thus our studies show that AG can cause metal-dependent DNA damage *in vitro* at physiologically relevant concentrations. Although these studies have used an *in vitro* system, caution must be exercised in determining both dosage and duration of AG therapy. Also, further studies *in vivo* are needed to confirm the relevance of our studies to patients undergoing long-term treatment with AG.

REFERENCES

1. THORNALLEY, P.J. 2003. Use of aminoguanidine (Pimagedine) to prevent the formation of advanced glycation endproducts. Arch. Biochem. Biophys. **419:** 31–40.
2. HIRSCH, E.P. & M.S. FEATHER. 1992. The reaction of some dicarbonyl sugars with aminoguanidine. Carbohyd. Res. **232:** 125–130.
3. BROWNLEE, M., H. VLASSARA, A. KOONEY, *et al.* 1986. Aminoguanidine prevents diabetes-induced arterial wall protein cross-linking. Science **232:** 1629–1632.
4. REQUENA, J.R., P. VIDAL & J. CABEZAS-CERRATO. 1993. Aminoguanidine inhibits protein browning without extensive Amadori carbonyl blocking. Diabetes Res. Clin. Pract. **19:** 23–30.
5. HAMES, H., S. MARTIN, K. FEDERLIN, *et al.* 1991. Aminoguanidine inhibits the development of experimental diabetic retinopathy. Proc. Natl. Acad. Sci. USA **88:** 11555–11558.
6. EDELSTEIN, D. & M. BROWNLEE. 1992. Aminoguanidine ameliorates albuminuria in diabetic hypertensive rats. Diabetologia **35:** 96–97.
7. OU, P. & S.P. WOLFF. 1993. Aminoguanidine: a drug proposed for prophylaxis in diabetes inhibits catalase and generates hydrogen peroxide *in vitro*. Biochem. Pharmacol. **46:** 1139–1144.
8. SAGRIPANTI, J-L. & K.H. KRAEMERLL. 1969. Site-specific oxidative DNA damage at polyguanosines produced by copper plus hydrogen peroxide. J. Biol. Chem. **264:** 1729–1734.
9. KANG, J.H. 2003. Oxidative damage of DNA by the reaction of amino acid with methylglyoxal in the presence of Fe(III). Int. J. Biol. Macromol. **33:** 43–48.
10. HUNT, J.V., R.T. DEAN & S.P. WOLFF. 1988. Hydroxyl radical production and autoxidative glycosylation: glucose autoxidation as the cause of protein damage in

the experimental glycation model of diabetes mellitus and ageing. Biochem. J. **256:** 205–212.

11. BEAUCHAMP, C. & I. FRIDOVICH. 1971. Superoxide dismutase: improved assays and an assay applicable to acrylamide gels. Anal. Biochem. **44:** 276–287.

12. JIANG, Z.Y., A.C. WOOLLARD & S.P. WOLFF. 1990. Hydrogen peroxide production during experimental protein glycation. FEBS Lett. **268:** 69–71.

13. PHILIS-TSIMIKAS, A., S. PARTHASARATHY, S. PICARD, *et al.* 1994. Aminoguanidine has both pro-oxidant and antioxidant activity toward LDL. Arterioscler. Thromb. Vasc. Biol. **15:** 367–376.

14. SKAMARAUSKAS, J.T., A.G. MCKAY & J.V. HUNT. 1996. Aminoguanidine and its pro-oxidant effects on an experimental model of protein glycation. Free Radic. Biol. Med. **21:** 801–812.

15. CUTLER, P. 1989. Deferoxamine therapy in high-ferritin diabetes. Diabetes **38:** 1207–1210.

16. THOMAS, M.C., R.J. MACISAAC, C. TSALAMANDRIS, *et al.* 2004. Elevated iron indices in patients with diabetes. Diabet. Med. **21:** 798–802.

17. SALONEN, J.T., T-P. TUOMAINEN, K. NYYSSÖNEN, *et al.* 1998. Relation between iron stores and non-insulin dependent diabetes in men: case-control study. BMJ **317:** 727–730.

18. BAYLIN, S., Z. HORAKOVA & M.A. BEAVEN. 1975. Increase in food consumption and growth after treatment with aminoguanidine. Experientia **31:** 562–564.

19. LO, T.W., T. SELWOOD & P.J. THORNALLEY. 1994. The reaction of methylglyoxal with aminoguanidine under physiological conditions and prevention of methylglyoxal binding to plasma proteins. Biochem. Pharmacol. **48:** 1865–1870.

Effect of Lipid Restriction on Mitochondrial Free Radical Production and Oxidative DNA Damage

ALBERTO SANZ, PILAR CARO, JOSE GOMEZ SANCHEZ, AND GUSTAVO BARJA

Department of Animal Physiology II, Faculty of Biological Sciences, Complutense University, Madrid 28040, Spain

ABSTRACT: Many studies have shown that caloric restriction (40%) decreases mitochondrial reactive oxygen species (ROS) generation in rodents. Moreover, we have recently found that 7 weeks of 40% protein restriction without strong caloric restriction also decreases ROS production in rat liver. This is interesting since it has been reported that protein restriction can also extend longevity in rodents. In the present study we have investigated the possible role of dietary lipids in the effects of caloric restriction on mitochondrial oxidative stress. Using semipurified diets, the ingestion of lipids in male Wistar rats was decreased by 40% below controls, while the other dietary components were ingested at exactly the same level as in animals fed *ad libitum*. After 7 weeks of treatment the liver mitochondria of lipid-restricted animals showed significant increases in oxygen consumption with complex I-linked substrates (pyruvate/malate and glutamate/malate). Neither mitochondrial H_2O_2 production nor oxidative damage to mitochondrial or nuclear DNA was modified in lipid-restricted animals. Oxidative damage to mitochondrial DNA was one order of magnitude higher than that of nuclear DNA in both dietary groups. These results deny a role for lipids and reinforce the possible role of dietary proteins as being responsible for the decrease in mitochondrial ROS production and DNA damage in caloric restriction.

KEYWORDS: lipid; dietary restriction; free radicals; mitochondria; DNA damage; aging

INTRODUCTION

The oxygen free radical mitochondrial theory of aging is currently receiving considerable support both from comparative and experimental studies.[1,2] It

Address for correspondence: Dr. G. Barja, Departamento de Fisiología Animal-II, Facultad de Ciencias Biológicas, Universidad Complutense, c/Antonio Novais-2, Madrid 28040, Spain. Voice: 34-91-3944919; fax: 34-91-3944935.

e-mail:gbarja@bio.ucm.es

Ann. N.Y. Acad. Sci. 1067: 200–209 (2006). © 2006 New York Academy of Sciences.
doi: 10.1196/annals.1354.024

is well known that caloric restriction (CR) slows down the rate of aging of laboratory rodents and other animals.[3] However, the fundamental mechanisms underlying the effects of CR on aging and longevity are still uncertain.

Many studies have shown that CR decreases mitochondrial free radical production and oxidative damage to mitochondrial DNA in rodent tissues.[4] Low levels of these two characteristics are also constitutively exhibited by long-lived species when compared to short-lived species.[5] These results offer a plausible mechanism by which CR could slow down the rate of aging by decreasing oxidative damage and long-term accumulation of mutations in mitochondrial DNA.[2] However, it has not been investigated whether the decreases in mitochondrial production of reactive oxygen species (ROS) and oxidative DNA damage during CR are due to the reduction in calories themselves or to specific dietary components.

Although a general consensus was reached in the last decade that the life extension effect of CR is related to the reduction in calories themselves, variations in the proportions of the main dietary components can also modulate longevity.[6–8] We have thus initiated a series of studies to clarify the possible effect of restriction of those dietary components on mitochondrial oxidative stress. A report on the effect of protein restriction has been recently published.[9]

In the present investigation we study whether the restriction of dietary lipids can be responsible at least in part for the two main effects of CR related to oxidative stress described above. We have used a dietary protocol in which lipid ingestion is decreased, while the intake of proteins, carbohydrates, and other dietary components is maintained at the same level as in control animals. This avoids confusing the effects of lipid restriction with those of increasing the percentage of other dietary components.

We have previously shown that CR decreases mitochondrial ROS production and oxidative DNA damage in the liver,[10] heart,[11] and brain[12] of Wistar rats. However, while the detection of these decreases usually needs long-term restriction in other tissues,[13] in the liver the effect is quicker and can be detected after only 7 weeks of treatment.[10] We have thus selected this rat organ for the present study of lipid restriction because it allows performing the experiment (which needs the use of semipurified diets) in a much shorter time.

MATERIALS AND METHODS

Fourteen male Wistar rats of 250 g of body weight were obtained from Iffa-Creddo (Lyon, France) and were caged individually and maintained in a 12:12 (light:dark) cycle at $22 \pm 2°C$. Control animals were fed *ad libitum* the semipurified American Institute of Nutrition diet AIN-93G: 39.7486% cornstarch, dextrinized cornstarch 13.20%, sucrose 10.00%, soy protein 20.00%, soybean oil 7.00%, alphacel (nonnutritive bulk) 5%, mineral mix 3.5%, vitamin mix 1.0%, L-cysteine 0.3%, choline bitartrate 0.25%, and *tert*-butyl-hydroquinone 0.0014%. The diet given to the lipid-restricted animals was a modified AIN-93G diet. Its fat content was reduced while its content in carbohydrates, proteins, fat, and in all the rest of its components was appropriately increased. Its composition was: cornstarch 40.77156%, dextrinized cornstarch 13.61%, sucrose 10.31%, soy protein 20.62%, soybean oil 4.33%, alphacel 5.15%, mineral mix 3.61%, vitamin mix 1.03%, L-cysteine 0.309%, choline bitartrate 0.258%, and *tert*-butyl-hydroquinone 0.00144%. This diet was given each day to the lipid-restricted animals in an amount equal to 97% of the food eaten by the controls. The final result is that lipid-restricted animals ingested daily 40% fewer lipids than the controls, while the total amount of carbohydrates, fat, and the rest of dietary components eaten was the same in control and lipid-restricted animals. With this procedure, lipid-restricted animals ingested 6.7% fewer calories than the controls. The mean body weight at the end of the dietary experiment did not show significant differences between control (403 ± 8 g) and lipid-restricted animals (394 ± 9 g). After 7 weeks of dietary treatment the animals were sacrificed by decapitation. The liver was immediately processed to isolate mitochondria in the cold (at $5°C$) by differential centrifugation as previously described,[10] while liver samples were stored at $-80°C$ for the assays of oxidative damage to DNAs. Mitochondrial protein was measured by the Biuret method. The final mitochondrial suspensions were maintained over ice and were immediately used for the measurements of oxygen consumption and H_2O_2 production. The rate of mitochondrial H_2O_2 production was assayed by fluorometry with the homovanillic-horseradish peroxidase method as described,[14] except that the stopping solution was 2.0 M glycine-NaOH containing 50 mM EDTA. Substrates were 2.5 mM pyruvate/2.5 mM malate, 2.5 mM glutamate/2.5 mM malate, or 5mM succinate $+ 2$ μM rotenone. For maximum rates of H_2O_2 production the following concentrations of respiratory chain inhibitors were used: 2 μM rotenone, 10 μM antimycin A, and 10 μM thenoyltrifluoroacetone (TTFA). Mitochondrial oxygen consumption was measured by polarography with a Clark oxygen electrode under similar conditions to H_2O_2 production measurements. The assays were performed in the absence (state 4—resting) and in the presence (state 3—phosphorylating) of 500 μM ADP.

Liver nuclear DNA (nDNA) was isolated by the method of Loft and Poulsen,[15] except that the initial homogenization buffer contained 5 mM EDTA. Mitochondrial DNA (mtDNA) was isolated by the method of Latorre *et al.*[16] adapted to mammals.[17] The isolated nDNA and mtDNA were digested to deoxynucleoside level and 8-oxo-7,8-dihydro-2′-deoxyguanosine (8-oxodG) and deoxyguanosine (dG) were analyzed by high-performance liquid chromatography (HPLC) with online electrochemical (coulometric) and ultraviolet detection, respectively.[11,15] Comparison of areas of 8-oxodG standards injected with and without simultaneous injection of dG standards ensured that no oxidation of dG occurred during the HPLC run. Comparisons between *ad libitum* and lipid-restricted groups were statistically analyzed with Student's

TABLE 1. Oxygen consumption (nanomoles O_2/min · mg protein) of liver mitochondria in lipid-restricted and control rats

Substrate		Control	Lipid-restricted
Pyr/mal	(state 4)	6.3 ± 0.8	$8.4 \pm 0.6^*$
	(state 3)	16.4 ± 0.9	18.6 ± 1.4
	(RCI)	2.8 ± 0.3	2.3 ± 0.1
Glu/mal	(state 4)	9.7 ± 1.1	$14.8 \pm 1.1^{**}$
	(state 3)	64.3 ± 5.8	$81.1 \pm 6.7^*$
	(RCI)	7.1 ± 0.7	5.6 ± 0.5
Succinate	(state 4)	26.0 ± 4.1	26.5 ± 1.1
	(state 3)	98.9 ± 7.6	110.2 ± 8.6
	(RCI)	4.4 ± 0.4	4.2 ± 0.3

Values are means $\pm$ SEM from 7 different animals. Pyr/mal = pyruvate/malate; Glu/mal = glutamate/malate. Mitochondrial oxygen consumption is measured in the absence (state 4) and in the presence (state 3) of ADP.
  * Significant difference between lipid-restricted and *ad libitum*-fed groups ($^*P < 0.05$; $^{**}P < 0.01$).

t-tests. The minimum level of statistical significance was set at $P < 0.05$ in all the analyses.

RESULTS

The rate of oxygen consumption of rat liver mitochondria in state 4 with the complex I-linked substrates pyruvate/malate was significantly higher in the lipid restricted than in the control group (TABLE 1). Oxygen consumption with the alternative complex I-linked substrates glutamate/malate was also significantly higher in lipid-restricted than in control mitochondria both in state 4 and state 3. When succinate (complex II-linked substrate) was used, however, no significant differences in mitochondrial oxygen consumption were found between dietary groups. The high values of the respiratory control index (RCI = state 3/state 4 oxygen consumption) both with complex II- (succinate) and complex I-linked (Glu/mal) substrates indicated the tight coupling of the isolated mitochondria in both dietary groups.

The basal rates of H_2O_2 production of liver mitochondria did not show significant differences between dietary groups with any substrate (Pyr/mal, Glu/mal, or succinate, TABLE 2). H_2O_2 production was also assayed in the presence of respiratory chain inhibitors (rotenone, antimycin A, or TTFA) to measure stimulated rates with the ROS-producing respiratory complexes being fully reduced. Again, no significant differences between dietary groups were found (TABLE 2).

Oxidative damage to mtDNA was around one order of magnitude higher in mtDNA than in nDNA in both dietary groups (FIG. 1). In agreement with the lack of differences in mitochondrial ROS generation, 8-oxodG was not

TABLE 2. Rates of H_2O_2 production (nanomoles H_2O_2/min · mg protein) of liver mitochondria in lipid-restricted and control rats in the absence and presence of respiratory chain inhibitors

	Control	Lipid-restricted
Pyr/mal	0.15 ± 0.04	0.20 ± 0.03
Glu/mal	0.75 ± 0.13	0.77 ± 0.10
Succinate	0.43 ± 0.06	0.52 ± 0.08
Pyr/mal + rotenone	0.73 ± 0.10	0.78 ± 0.10
Glu/mal + rotenone	1.25 ± 0.10	1.26 ± 0.10
Succinate + AA	2.57 ± 0.25	3.49 ± 0.42
Succinate + TTFA	0.28 ± 0.06	0.36 ± 0.05

Values are means ± SEM from 7 different animals. Pyr/mal = pyruvate/malate; Glu/mal = glutamate/malate. AA = antimycin A; TTFA = thenoyltrifluoroacetone.

No significant differences between lipid-restricted and *ad libitum*-fed groups were found.

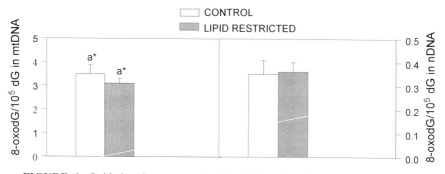

FIGURE 1. Oxidative damage to mitochondrial and nuclear DNA estimated as 8-oxodG in the liver of control and lipid-restricted animals. a*: significantly higher in mtDNA than in nDNA of the same dietary group. No significant differences due to lipid restriction were found.

significantly different between dietary groups in mtDNA, and the same was observed for nDNA (FIG. 1).

DISCUSSION

It is commonly believed that the anti-aging effect of CR is due to the decreased intake of calories rather than specific dietary components, although variations in the proportions of the main dietary constituents also seem to affect longevity.[6,7] Concerning the effects of protein restriction on aging, consideration of published studies performed in mammals shows that increases in longevity have been found much more commonly than no effects or decreases. Seven of eight published studies on rats or mice showed that protein restriction also increases maximum life span,[8,18–24] although the magnitude of the increase (around 20%) is usually lower than the one typically found in CR. These data suggest that protein restriction can be responsible for part of the life-prolonging effects of CR. This would also be consistent with the observation that methionine restriction increases the maximum life span of rats independently of energy restriction.[25,26] Caloric and protein restriction share many common effects in addition to life prolongation, including delays in puberty, decreases in growth rate, changes in metabolic rate, boosting of cell-mediated immunity, lowering of cholesterol, or decreases in preneoplastic lesions and tumors.[27] Low-protein diets also decrease IGF-1 levels and decelerate glomerulosclerosis in mice,[28] delay the occurrence of chronic nephropathy and cardiomyopathy in rats,[29] and protect rat liver against exposure to toxic chemicals.[30] A lower but significant life extension effect in protein than in CR would agree with the widely accepted notion that aging has multiple causes. CR could decrease aging rate through decreases in mitochondrial oxidative stress (like protein restriction) as well as through other mechanisms (e.g., by lowering insulin/IGF-1 signaling). Regarding the mechanism involved in the effects of protein restriction, it has recently been observed that this dietary manipulation decreases mitochondrial ROS production at complex I, lowers the percentage of total electron flow in the respiratory chain directed to ROS production, and decreases oxidative damage to mtDNA and nDNA (assayed as 8-oxodG) in rat liver mitochondria.[9] These changes also occur in CR in rat liver mitochondria.[4,10] Strikingly, the magnitude of these decreases is similar in both protein and caloric restriction, protein restriction perfectly mimicking CR regarding these effects. This suggests that restriction of protein intake can be responsible for the well-known decreases in mitochondrial ROS production and oxidative DNA damage that take place in CR.[4,5,10–13,31–35] The remaining effects of CR on aging rate could be related to decreases in other dietary components or in the calories themselves through different additional mechanisms.

What are the effects of lipid restriction on longevity? Many studies have discussed whether or not lipids are involved in CR effects, some supporting and some rejecting this idea based on different kinds of endpoint biochemical measurements and experiments.[36–39] But very few studies have directly tested the effect of lipid restriction on longevity. In a long-term study in Fisher 344 rats, increases in maximum and medium life span were found after 40% CR but not after 40% lipid restriction.[40] Another study also performed in Fisher rats did not find changes in longevity after lipid or mineral restriction without CR.[41] These and other studies led to the conclusion that restriction of calories, but not of fats, slows the primary aging process.[42] Thus, although available direct information is scarce and mainly limited to a particular rat strain, it seems safe to conclude that lipid restriction does not delay aging. If that is indeed the case, this will explain the lack of decrease in mitochondrial ROS production and then in oxidative DNA damage found in this investigation.

ROS production and oxidative DNA damage seems to correlate always with maximum longevity. They are lower in long-lived than in short-lived animals,[5] they decrease when maximum longevity increases after protein or caloric restriction,[4,5,9,10–13,31–35] and they do not change when maximum longevity is not modified (lipid restriction).

The lack of changes in ROS production, in spite of the increases in mitochondrial oxygen consumption observed in our investigation in lipid-restricted animals, is interesting. It confirms, in agreement with previous studies,[5,43,44] that mitochondrial ROS production is not necessarily proportional to aerobic metabolic rate. Instead, it is tightly regulated in cells and tissues independently of mitochondrial oxygen consumption. This is essential to avoid deleterious increases in oxidative stress when the rate of oxygen consumption increases, as in exercise,[43] after thyroid hormone-induced increases in metabolic rate,[44] or when strong differences in oxygen consumption between different animal species occur.[5] Regarding the reasons for the observed increase in oxygen consumption, they are presently unknown. However, mitochondrial beta-oxidation of fatty acid substrates is an important contributor to mitochondrial oxygen consumption and ATP production. The increased oxygen consumption of lipid-restricted animals can represent a compensation for the decrease in those lipid substrates. That putative compensation would increase rates of ATP production because the increase in oxygen consumption occurred not only in state 4, but also in the phosphorylating state 3. These increases were limited to measurements with complex I-linked substrates. This makes sense since most lipid catabolism-derived electrons enter the respiratory chain through complex I as NADH-reducing equivalents.

Finally, in agreement with the lack of changes in ROS production, no differences in DNA oxidative damage between lipid-restricted and control groups were observed. This is apparently in contrast with previous studies in humans or rats showing that high-fat diets can increase oxidative damage at least in nDNA. However, the amount of dietary fat used in those studies is in the range of 20–35%,[45,46] whereas we studied a much lower range, 7% fat in controls, and 4.2% fat in lipid-restricted rats. Thus, it seems that 8-oxodG levels are dependent on dietary fat content only at very high fat but not at low fat intakes.

In summary, 7 weeks of lipid restriction increases oxygen consumption of rat liver mitochondria without changing ROS production and DNA oxidative damage, whereas these last parameters are decreased after 7 weeks of protein or caloric restriction. These results suggest that those beneficial changes typically observed in CR rodents are not due to the restriction of lipids during CR. Instead, they further suggest that the restriction in dietary protein can be responsible for such anti-aging changes. Further studies concerning carbohydrate restriction are needed to establish that conclusion more firmly.

ACKNOWLEDGMENTS

This study was supported by Grant SAF 2002-01635 from the Spanish Ministry of Science and Technology to G. Barja. A. Sanz and P. Caro received a predoctoral fellowship from Complutense University and from the Spanish Ministry of Education and Science (FPI program), respectively.

REFERENCES

1. BECKMAN, K.B. & B.N. AMES. 1998. The free radical theory of aging matures. Physiol. Rev. **78:** 547–581.
2. BARJA, G. 2004. Free radicals and aging. Trends Neurosci. **27:** 595–600.
3. BARGER, J.L., R.L. WALFORD & R. WEINDRUCH. 2003. The retardation of aging by caloric restriction: its significance in the transgenic era. Exp. Gerontol. **38:** 1343–1351.
4. GREDILLA, G. & G. BARJA. 2005. The role of oxidative stress in relation to caloric restriction and longevity. Endocrinology **146:** 3713–3717.
5. BARJA, G. 2004. Aging in vertebrates and the effect of caloric restriction: a mitochondrial free radical production-DNA damage mechanism? Biol. Rev. **79:** 235–251.
6. MARK, M.C.M., K.M. REISER, R. HARRIS JR, *et al.* 1995. Source of dietary carbohydrate affects life span of Fischer 344 rats independent of caloric restriction. J. Gerontol. **50A:** B148–B154.
7. ARCHER, V.E. 2003. Does dietary sugar and fat influence longevity? Med. Hypotheses **60:** 924–929.
8. YU, B.P., E.J. MASORO & C.A. MCMAHAN. 1985. Nutritional influences on aging of Fischer 344 rats: I. Physical, metabolic, and longevity characteristics. J. Gerontol. **40:** 657–670.
9. SANZ, A., P. CARO & G. BARJA. 2004. Protein restriction without strong caloric restriction decreases mitochondrial oxygen radical production and oxidative DNA damage in rat liver. J. Bioenerg. Biomembr. **36:** 545–552.
10. GREDILLA, R., G. BARJA & M. LÓPEZ-TORRES. 2001. Effect of short-term caloric restriction on H_2O_2 production and oxidative DNA damage in rat liver mitochondria, and location of the free radical source. J. Bioenerg. Biomembr. **33:** 279–287.
11. GREDILLA, R., A. SANZ, M. LÓPEZ-TORRES, *et al.* 2001. Caloric restriction decreases mitochondrial free radical generation at Complex I and lowers oxidative damage to mitochondrial DNA in the rat heart. FASEB J. **15:** 1589–1591.
12. SANZ, A., P. CARO, J. IBAÑEZ, *et al.* 2005. Dietary restriction at old age lowers mitochondrial oxygen radical production and leak at complex I and oxidative DNA damage in rat brain. J. Bioenerg. Biomembr. **37:** 83–90.
13. GREDILLA, R., M. LÓPEZ-TORRES & G. BARJA. 2002. Effect of time of restriction on the decrease in mitochondrial H_2O_2 production and oxidative DNA damage in the heart of food restricted rats. Microsc. Res. Techn. **59:** 273–277.
14. BARJA, G. 2002. The quantitative measurement of H_2O_2 generation in isolated mitochondria. J. Bioenerg. Biomembr. **34:** 227–233.
15. LOFT, S. & H.E. POULSEN. 1999. Markers of oxidative damage to DNA: antioxidants and molecular damage. Method Enzymol. **300:** 166–184.

16. LATORRE, A., A. MOYA & A. AYALA. 1986. Evolution of mitochondrial DNA in *Drosophila suboscura*. Proc. Natl. Acad Sci. USA **83:** 8649–8653.

17. ASUNCIÓN, J.G., A. MILLAN, R. PLA, *et al.* 1996. Mitochondrial glutathione oxidation correlates with age-associated oxidative damage to mitochondrial DNA. FASEB J. **10:** 333–338.

18. BARROWS, C.H. JR. & G. KOKKONEN. 1975. Protein synthesis, development, growth and life span. Growth **39:** 525–533.

19. FERNANDES, G., E.J. YUNIS & R.A. GOOD. 1976. Influence of diet on survival of mice. Proc Natl. Acad. Sci. USA **73:** 1279–1283.

20. LETO, S., G.C. KOKKONEN & C.H. BARROWS, JR. 1976. Dietary protein, life-span, and biochemical variables in female mice. J. Gerontol. **31:** 144–148.

21. STOLTZNER, G. 1977. Effects of life-long dietary protein restriction on mortality, growth, organ weights, blood counts, liver aldolase and kidney catalase in Balb/C mice. Growth **41:** 337–348.

22. GOODRICK, C.L. 1978. Body weight increment and length of life: the effect of genetic constitution and dietary protein. J. Gerontol. **33:** 184–190.

23. DAVIS, T.A., C.W. BALES & R.E. BEAUCHENE. 1983. Differential effects of caloric and protein restriction in the aging rat. Exp. Gerontol. **18:** 427–435.

24. HORAKOVA, M., Z. DEYL, J. HAUSMANN, *et al.* 1988. The effect of low protein-high dextrin diet and subsequent food restriction upon life prolongation in Fischer 244 male rats. Mech. Ageing Dev. **45:** 1–7.

25. RICHIE, J.P. JR., Y. LEUTZINGER, S. PARTHASARATHY, *et al.* 1994. Methionine restriction increases blood glutathione and longevity in F344 rats. FASEB J. **8:** 1302–1307.

26. ZIMMERMAN, J.A., V. MALLOY, R. KRAJCIK, *et al.* 2003. Nutritional control of aging. Exp. Gerontol. **38:** 47–52.

27. YOUNGMAN, L.D., J-Y.K. PARK & B.N. AMES. 1992. Protein oxidation associated with aging is reduced by dietary restriction of protein or calories. Proc Natl. Acad. Sci. USA **89:** 9112–9116.

28. DOI, S.Q., S. RASAIAH, I. TACK, *et al.* 2001. Low-protein diet suppresses serum insulin-like growth factor-1 and decelerates the progression of growth hormone-induced glomerulosclerosis. Am. J. Nephrol. **21:** 331–339.

29. MAEDA, H., C.A. GLEISER, E.J. MASORO, *et al.* 1985. Nutritional influences on aging of Fischer 344 rats: II Pathology. J. Gerontol. **40:** 671–688.

30. RODRIGUES, M.A.M., M. SANCHEZ-NEGRETTE, M.S. MANTOVANI, *et al.* 1991. Liver response to low-hexachlorobenzene exposure in protein- or energy-restricted rats. Food Chem. Toxicol. **29:** 757–764.

31. DREW, B., S. PHANEUF, A. DIRKS, *et al.* 2003. Effects of aging and caloric restriction on mitochondrial energy production in gastrocnemius muscle and heart. Am. J. Physiol. **284:** R474–R480.

32. BEVILACQUA, L., J.J. RAMSEY, K. HAGOPIAN, *et al.* 2004. Effects of short- and medium-term calorie restriction on muscle mitochondrial proton leak and reactive oxygen species production. Am. J. Physiol. **286:** E852–E861.

33. JUDGE, S., A. JUDGE, T. GRUNE, *et al.* 2004. Short-term CR decreases cardiac mitochondrial oxidant production but increases carbonyl content. Am. J. Physiol. **286:** R254–R259.

34. LAMBERT, A.J. & B.J. MERRY. 2004. Effect of caloric restriction on mitochondrial reactive oxygen species production and bioenergetics: reversal by insulin. Am. J. Physiol. **286:** R71–R79.

35. RAMSEY, J.J., K. HAGOPIAN, T.M. KENNY, *et al.* 2004. Proton leak and hydrogen peroxide production in liver mitochondria from energy-restricted rats. Am. J. Physiol. **286:** E31–E40.
36. IKENO, Y., H.A. BERTRAND & J.T. HERLIHY. 1997. Effects of dietary restriction and exercise on the age-related pathology of the rat. Age **20:** 107–118.
37. MASORO, E.J. 2000. Caloric restriction and aging: an update. Exper. Gerontol. **35:** 299–305.
38. BARZILAI, N. & I. GABRIELY. 2001. The role of fat depletion in the biological benefits of caloric restriction. J. Nutr. **131:** 903S–906S.
39. MUURLING, M., M.C. JONG, R.P. MENSINK, *et al.* 2002. A low-fat diet has a higher potential than energy restriction to improve high-fat diet-induced insulin resistance in mice. Metabolism **51:** 695–701.
40. SHIMOKAWA, I., Y. HIGAMI, B.P. YU, *et al.* 1996. Influence of dietary components on occurrence of and mortality due to neoplasms in male F344 rats. Aging Clin. Exp. Res. **8:** 254–262.
41. IWASAKI, K., C.A. GLEISER, E.J. MASORO, *et al.* 1988. Influence of the restriction of individual dietary components on longevity and age-related disease of Fisher rats: the fat component and the mineral component. J. Gerontol. **43:** B13–B21.
42. MASORO, E.J. 1990. Assessment of nutritional components in prolongation of life and health by diet. Proc. Soc. Exp. Biol. Med. **193:** 31–34.
43. HERRERO, A. & G. BARJA. 1997. ADP regulation of mitochondrial free radical production is different with Complex I- or Complex II-linked substrates: implications for the exercise paradox and brain hypermetabolism. J. Bioenerg. Biomembr. **29:** 241–249.
44. LÓPEZ-TORRES, M., M. ROMERO & G. BARJA. 2000. Effect of thyroid hormones on mitochondrial oxygen free radical production and DNA oxidative damage in the rat heart. Mol. Cell. Endocrinol. **168:** 127–134.
45. DJURIC, Z. & D. KRITSCHEVSKY. 1993. Modulation of oxidative damage levels by dietary fat and calories. Mut. Res. **295:** 181–190.
46. LOFT, S., E.B. THORLING & H. POULSEN. 1998. High fat diet induced oxidative DNA damage estimated by 8-oxo-7,8-dihydro-2′-deoxyguanosine excretion in rats. Free Rad. Res. **29:** 595–600.

Establishment of H$_2$O$_2$-Induced Premature Senescence in Human Fibroblasts Concomitant with Increased Cellular Production of H$_2$O$_2$

STEPHANIE ZDANOV,[a] JOSE REMACLE,[a] AND OLIVIER TOUSSAINT[a,b]

[a]*Unit of Cellular Biochemistry and Biology, the University of Namur, FUNDP, Rue de Bruxelles, 61 B-5000 Namur, Belgium*

[b]*Straticell S.A, Rue Lecomte, 14 B-5000 Namur, Belgium*

ABSTRACT: Premature senescence of human fibroblasts is established after exposure to an acute sublethal concentration of H$_2$O$_2$. Overexpression of transforming growth factor-β1 (TGF-β1) was shown to be responsible for the appearance of the biomarkers of senescence in these conditions. Other studies have shown that incubation of human fibroblasts with TGF-β1 leads to overexpression of H$_2$O$_2$. In this work, we show an increased production of H$_2$O$_2$ by human fibroblasts as premature senescence is established after an initial exposure to H$_2$O$_2$.

KEYWORDS: senescence; oxidative stress; hydrogen peroxide; fibroblasts; transforming growth factor-β1 (TGF-β1)

INTRODUCTION

Cellular senescence limits the reproductive life span of cultured cells. During proliferation, telomeric DNA is lost with each round of replication and is thought to be the major pathway that limits the cell proliferation capacity because critically shortened telomeres activate the senescence process.[1] However, senescence-like phenotypes can be induced by DNA damaging agents[2] and oncogene overexpression.[3] Oxidative stress-induced premature senescence (SIPS) becomes established several days after single or repeated exposure of normal human diploid fibroblasts (HDFs) to subcytotoxic concentration of hydrogen peroxide (H$_2$O$_2$),[4] ethanol,[5] *tert*-hydroxyperoxide (*t*-BHP),[6,7] or UVB radiation.[8] Cells in stress-induced premature senescence (SIPS) remain alive for months. They display several features of replicative senescence-like

Address for correspondence: Dr. Olivier Toussaint, Unit of Cellular Biochemistry and Biology, the University of Namur, FUNDP, Rue de Bruxelles, 61 B-5000 Namur, Belgium. Voice: 0032-81-724132; fax: 0032-81-724135.

e-mail: olivier.toussaint@fundp.ac.be

Ann. N.Y. Acad. Sci. 1067: 210–216 (2006). © 2006 New York Academy of Sciences.
doi: 10.1196/annals.1354.025

typical cell morphology,[9] senescence-associated β-galactosidase activity (SA β-gal),[10] change in expression level of many genes, sharp decrease of the DNA synthesis, and an irreversible growth arrest in G1. The cyclin-dependent kinase inhibitor (CDKI) p21^{WAF-1} becomes overexpressed after exposure of HDFs to H$_2$O$_2$ at subcytotoxic concentration, which blocks the phosphorylation of retinoblastoma protein (Rb). Hypophosphorylated Rb is known to inactivate the transcription factor E$_2$F, which can no longer transactivate the promotor of the gene necessary to the S phase of the cell cycle.[11]

Although the mechanisms responsible for growth arrest are well known, very few studies were aimed at understanding how this growth arrest could be maintained for very long periods of time. In addition, the role of the classical p53-dependent pathway, a p38^{MAPK}-dependent mechanism, has been unveiled. Indeed, exposure to H$_2$O$_2$ leads to p38^{MAPK} activation, which in turn is indirectly responsible for the overexpression of TGF-β1 and increased secretion of TGF-β1. In addition, stimulation of HDFs with TGF-β1 triggers the appearance of biomarkers of SIPS as senescent morphology, SA β-gal activity, and overexpression of the mRNA of the senescence-associated genes as *fibronectin, osteonectin, apolipoprotein J, and SM22*. The neutralization of TGF-β1 or its receptor (TGF-β RII) using specific antibodies abrogates the stress-induced appearance of these biomarkers.[12,13] We also know that premature senescence induced by exposure to H$_2$O$_2$ at acute sublethal concentration is not dependent on critical telomere shortening.[14] It has been shown that the stimulation of IMR-90 HDFs with TGF-β1 induces a release of H$_2$O$_2$ through the activation of a plasma membrane NADH oxidase. Elevation in H$_2$O$_2$ release peaked at 16 h and gradually declined to undetectable levels at 48 h after TGF-β1 treatment.[15] These studies led to the hypothesis that a constant oxidative stress might be generated by a sustained overexpression and release of TGF-β1 after an initial exposure to H$_2$O$_2$. This would explain why cells in SIPS remain in a state of irreversible growth arrest. Here we show that, well after the initial exposure of IMR-90 HDFs to H$_2$O$_2$ at a concentration triggering SIPS, these cells increased their *de novo* production and release of H$_2$O$_2$ over a 72-h period after the initial exposure to H$_2$O$_2$. This overproduction could explain in part the appearance of SIPS and why Rb remains hypophosphorylated for a long term after stress, probably on account of sustained DNA damage.

MATERIALS AND METHODS

Cell Culture

Normal human fetal lung fibroblasts (IMR-90, European Cell Culture Collection, Salisbury, UK) were grown in a medium consisting of MEM (Gibco BRL, USA) supplemented with 10% fetal bovine serum (FBS). IMR-90 HDFs at 45–50% of *in vitro* proliferation life span were exposed for 2 h to 150 μM

H_2O_2 (Merck, Darmstadt, Germany) diluted in MEM + 10% FBS. The cells were rinsed with MEM and given fresh MEM + 10% FBS.

SA β-Gal Activity and [³H]-Thymidine Incorporation

At 48 h after the H_2O_2 stress, the cells were seeded in squared 35-mm culture dishes (BD Biosciences, Le Pont de Claix, France) at a density of 700 cells/cm². Senescence-associated β-galactosidase activity (SA β-gal) was determined 24 h later as described by Dimri *et al.*[10] The population of SA β-gal-positive cells was determined by counting 400 cells per dish. The proportion of cells positive for SA β-gal activity is given as a percentage of the total number of cells counted in each dish. The results were expressed as mean of triplicates ± SD.

At 24 h after the H_2O_2 stress, cells were seeded in 24-well plates (Corning, NY) at a density of 10,000 cells/well. 1μCi [³H]-thymidine (specific activity: 2 Ci/mmol, DuPont, NEN, Boston, MA) was added to the culture medium for a period of 48 h. The incorporated radioactivity was quantified by a scintillation counter (Packard Instrument Company, Meriden, CT). Results were expressed as mean values ± SD.

Measurement of H_2O_2 Release

H_2O_2 release from IMR-90 HDFs was assayed using a modification of a fluorimetric method developed earlier.[16] This method is based on the conversion of homovanillic acid to its fluorescent dimer in the presence of H_2O_2 and horseradish peroxidase (HRP). At each time point after exposure to H_2O_2, cells were first washed with phosphate-buffered saline, pH 7.4, and then incubated with a reaction mixture containing 5 units/mL HRP and 100 μM homovanillic acid in Hanks' balanced salt solution without phenol red, pH 7.4. This solution was then collected following a 1-h incubation, the pH was adjusted to 10.0 with 0.1 M glycine–NaOH buffer, and fluorescence was measured at excitation and emission wavelengths of 321 nm and 421 nm, respectively. The results were expressed as means ± SD with statistical Student's *t*-test.

RESULTS

Fetal lung IMR-90 HDFs were exposed to 150 μM H_2O_2 for 2 h, which represents subcytotoxic conditions[12] and triggers premature senescence. Indeed, at 3 days after the exposure to H_2O_2, the proportion of IMR-90 HDFs positive for SA β-gal activity was around 48% as compared with 18% in the control cells (FIG. 1A). The level of incorporation of [³H]-thymidine, between 48 h and 72 h after the stress, fell by 75% in IMR-90 HDFs exposed to H_2O_2 (FIG. 1B).

A.   B.

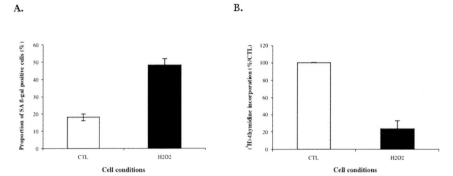

FIGURE 1. Effect of a single H_2O_2 stress on SA β-gal activity and incorporation of [^{3}H]-thymidine in IMR-90 HDFs. (**A**) Proportion of IMR-90 HDFs positive for SA β-galactosidase activity at 72 h after H_2O_2 stress. Results are given as mean ± SD of three independent experiments. White columns: control cells; black columns: cells after exposure to H_2O_2 at sublethal concentration. (**B**) Effect of H_2O_2 stress on the incorporation of [^{3}H]-thymidine. The results are expressed as a percentage of the values found in control cells at 72 h after H_2O_2 stress. The results are given as mean ± SD of three independent experiments. White columns: control cells; black columns: cells after exposure to H_2O_2 at sublethal concentration.

The rate of extracellular release of H_2O_2 was measured over a 72-h period after the initial exposure to H_2O_2. The release of H_2O_2 was also measured in control cells. The amount of H_2O_2 released by the stressed cells was expressed as a percentage of the amount of H_2O_2 released by the control cells at the same time after the stress. When compared with nontreated cells, a respective 1.3-, 1.5-, 1.4-, and 2.0-fold increase of *de novo* release of H_2O_2 by IMR-90 HDFs was obtained at 24, 44, 48, and 72 h, respectively, after stress (FIG. 2). These results demonstrate a release of H_2O_2 by IMR-90 HDFs after an initial exposure to H_2O_2 at a concentration which triggers premature senescence. Given the instability of H_2O_2 when diluted in complex buffers,[17] these results cannot be explained by a release of H_2O_2 to which the cells were initially exposed.

DISCUSSION

Well after the initial exposure of IMR-90 HDFs to a SIPS-inducing concentration of H_2O_2 we showed an increased *de novo* release of H_2O_2 over a 72-h period after the initial exposure to H_2O_2. In light of these results and those already obtained, we propose a simplified model to explain the establishment of hydrogen peroxide–induced premature senescence of human diploid fibroblasts (FIG. 3). After a few moments of exposure to H_2O_2, p38^{MAPK} becomes phosphorylated, which induces an overexpression of TGF-β1 through the activation of ATF-2. TGF-β1 secretion and TGF-β receptor II activation

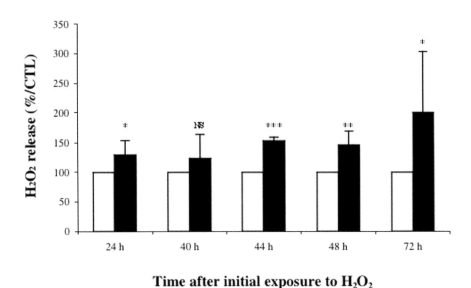

Time after initial exposure to H_2O_2

FIGURE 2. Quantification of H_2O_2 released in the culture medium by IMR-90 HDFs at various times after H_2O_2 subcytotoxic stress. The results are expressed as a percentage of the amount of H_2O_2 present in the control at each time after the stress. Results are given as mean ± SD of four independent experiments. Statistical analysis was carried out with the Student's t- test. ns, nonsignificant ($P > 0.05$); *, $0.05 > P > 0.01$; **, $0.01 > P > 0.001$; ***, $P < 0.001$. White columns: control cells; black columns: cells after initial exposure to H_2O_2 at sublethal concentration.

allow a sustained phosphorylation of p38^{MAPK} and ATF-2 : a regulatory loop is established between TGF-β1 overexpression and p38^{MAPK} phosphorylation. Cyclin-dependent kinase inhibitor p21^{WAF-1} is overexpressed on account of DNA damage, inhibiting the cyclin D-cyclin-dependent kinase 4 and 6 complexes' kinase activities, explaining in part why Rb becomes hypophosphorylated. In addition, cyclin-dependent kinase 2 is decreased at 72 h after stress,[18] also explaining in part why Rb becomes hypophosphorylated; and growth arrest occurs. At 24 h after stress, phosphorylated ATF-2 and hypophosphorylated Rb start to interact. This complex induces the appearance of biomarkers of senescence: senescence-like morphology, SA β-gal activity, and overexpression of the senescence-associated genes fibronectin, osteonectin, SM22, and apolipoprotein J.[12,13] In addition, TGF-β1 was shown to induce the overproduction of H_2O_2 in IMR-90 HDFs through the activation of a plasma membrane NADH oxidase,[15] thereby generating a constant oxidative stress, which likely explains the sustained activation of the p38^{MAPK} pathway as well as the overexpression of TGF-β1. This increased production of H_2O_2 could hypothetically lead to a sustained level of DNA damage.

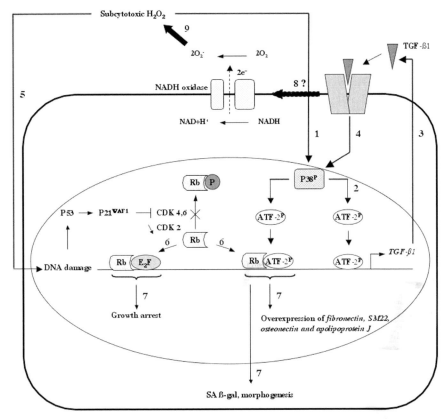

FIGURE 3. Integrative simplified model for the establishment of hydrogen-peroxide-induced premature senescence of human diploid fibroblasts. This model is based on a positive feedback loop engaged between the activation of the stress-activated protein kinase p38^{MAPK} and the overexpression of TGF-β1. The potential role of NADH oxidase in H$_2$O$_2$ production is outlined.

AKNOWLEDGMENTS

O. Toussaint is a research associate of the FNRS and S. Zdanov has a fellowship of the FRIA, Belgium.

REFERENCES

1. SHAY, J.W. & W.E. WRIGHT. 2000. Hayflick, his limit, and cellular ageing. Nat. Rev. Mol. Cell. Biol. **1:** 72–76.
2. VON ZGLINICKI, T., A. BURKLE & T.B. KIRKWOOD. 2001. Stress, DNA damage and ageing—an integrative approach. Exp. Gerontol. **36:** 1049–1062.

3. SERRANO, M. *et al*. 1997. Oncogenic ras provokes premature cell senescence associated with accumulation of p53 and p16INK4a. Cell **88:** 593–602.

4. CHEN, Q. & B.N. AMES. 1994. Senescence-like growth arrest induced by hydrogen peroxide in human diploid fibroblast F65 cells. Proc. Natl. Acad. Sci. USA **91:** 4130–4134.

5. PASCAL, T. *et al*. 2005. Comparison of replicative senescence and stress-induced premature senescence combining differential display and low-density DNA arrays. FEBS Lett. **579:** 3651–3659.

6. DUMONT, P. *et al*. 2000. Induction of replicative senescence biomarkers by sublethal oxidative stresses in normal human fibroblast. Free Radic. Biol. Med. **28:** 361–373.

7. TOUSSAINT, O., A. HOUBION & J. REMACLE. 1992. Aging as a multi-step process characterized by a lowering of entropy production leading the cell to a sequence of defined stages. II. Testing some predictions on aging human fibroblasts in culture. Mech. Ageing Dev. **65:** 65–83.

8. DEBACQ-CHAINIAUX, F. *et al*. 2005. Repeated exposure of human skin fibroblasts to UVB at subcytotoxic level triggers premature senescence through the TGF-beta1 signaling pathway. J. Cell Sci. **118:** 743–758.

9. BAYREUTHER, K. *et al*. 1988. Human skin fibroblasts in vitro differentiate along a terminal cell lineage. Proc. Natl. Acad. Sci. USA **85:** 5112–5116.

10. DIMRI, G.P. *et al*. 1995. A biomarker that identifies senescent human cells in culture and in aging skin in vivo. Proc. Natl. Acad. Sci. USA **92:** 9363–9367.

11. CHEN, Q.M. *et al*. 1998. Molecular analysis of H_2O_2-induced senescent-like growth arrest in normal human fibroblasts: p53 and Rb control G1 arrest but not cell replication. Biochem. J. **332**(Pt 1): 43–50.

12. FRIPPIAT, C. *et al*. 2001. Subcytotoxic H_2O_2 stress triggers a release of transforming growth factor-beta 1, which induces biomarkers of cellular senescence of human diploid fibroblasts. J. Biol. Chem. **276:** 2531–2537.

13. FRIPPIAT, C. *et al*. 2002. Signal transduction in H_2O_2-induced senescence-like phenotype in human diploid fibroblasts. Free Radic. Biol. Med. **33:** 1334–1346.

14. DUMONT, P. *et al*. 2001. Growth kinetics rather than stress accelerate telomere shortening in cultures of human diploid fibroblasts in oxidative stress-induced premature senescence. FEBS Lett. **502:** 109–112.

15. THANNICKAL, V.J. & B.L. FANBURG. 1995. Activation of an H_2O_2-generating NADH oxidase in human lung fibroblasts by transforming growth factor beta 1. J. Biol. Chem. **270:** 30334–30338.

16. RUCH, W., P.H. COOPER & M. BAGGIOLINI. 1983. Assay of H_2O_2 production by macrophages and neutrophils with homovanillic acid and horse-radish peroxidase. J. Immunol. Methods **63:** 347–357.

17. KNOOPS, B. *et al*. 1999. Cloning and characterization of AOEB166, a novel mammalian antioxidant enzyme of the peroxiredoxin family. J. Biol. Chem. **274:** 30451–30458.

18. FRIPPIAT, C., J. REMACLE & O. TOUSSAINT. 2003. Down-regulation and decreased activity of cyclin-dependent kinase 2 in H_2O_2-induced premature senescence. Int. J. Biochem. Cell Biol. **35:** 246–254.

CARF Regulates p19ARF-p53-p21WAF1 Senescence Pathway by Multiple Checkpoints

SUNIL C. KAUL, KAMRUL HASAN, AND RENU WADHWA

National Institute of Advanced Industrial Science & Technology (AIST), Central 4, 1-1-1 Higashi, Tsukuba, Ibaraki 305-8562, Japan

ABSTRACT: CARF was first cloned as a novel binding partner of ARF from a yeast-interactive screen. CARF and ARF colocalize in the perinucleolar region and have a collaborative function. In the nucleoplasm, CARF interacts with p53 and enhances its function. We demonstrate that p53 downregulates CARF in a negative feedback regulatory loop and may also involve p53 antagonist HDM2.

KEYWORDS: CARF (collaborator of ARF); ARF (alternative reading frame protein); p53; interaction; regulation

INTRODUCTION

The INK4a locus on chromosome 9p21 encodes two structurally distinct tumor suppressor proteins, p16INK4a and the alternative reading frame protein, ARF (p19ARF in mice and p14ARF in humans). Each of these proteins has a role in the senescence of primary cells, and activates the pathways for cell cycle control and tumor suppression. We had previously identified a novel collaborator of ARF, CARF, from a yeast-interactive screen using p19ARF as a bait. CARF is a nuclear protein that colocalizes and interacts with ARF in the perinucleolar region. It is coregulated with ARF and cooperates with it in activating p53. In the absence of ARF, CARF supports the p53 function directly. It binds to p53 in the nucleoplasm and activates its transcriptional activation function. It further extends its control on the p19ARF–p53–p21 pathway by interacting with a p53 antagonist, HDM2. Thus CARF interacts with the major components of the p19ARF–p53-HDM2–p21 pathway that is central to cellular senescence and is frequently altered in cancer.

Address for correspondence: Sunil C. Kaul, Ph.D., Gene Function Research Center, National Institute of Advanced Industrial Science & Technology (AIST), Central 4, 1-1-1 Higashi, Tsukuba, Ibaraki 305-8562, Japan. Voice: +81-29-861-6713; fax: +81-29-861-2900.
e-mail: s-kaul@aist.go.jp

Ann. N.Y. Acad. Sci. 1067: 217–219 (2006). © 2006 New York Academy of Sciences.
doi: 10.1196/annals.1354.026

RESULTS AND DISCUSSION

CARF was first isolated as an ARF-binding partner in a yeast-interactive screen using ARF as a bait.[1] It showed interactions with both mouse and human ARF proteins. cDNA encoding human CARF encoded a serine-rich (19%) protein of 563 amino acids with calculated molecular mass of 59.7 kDa. Human and mouse CARF proteins showed 84.2% homology and the CARF gene was assigned to human chromosome 4q35 between markers D4S415– D4S408 and mouse chromosome 8 C3-C4. Anti-CARF antibody raised against the recombinant protein detected CARF in the nucleus and was found to be excluded from the nucleolus. Double immunostaining for CARF and ARF revealed their colocalization in the perinucleolar region.[2] Whereas the cells compromised for CARF expression by RNA interference showed limited ARF function, an overexpression of CARF showed enhanced ARF function. On the basis of these findings CARF was assigned as a collaborator of ARF.[2] Similar experiments on the analysis of CARF binding partners revealed that CARF

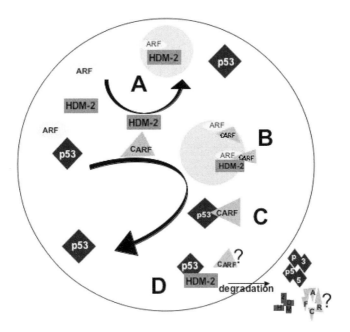

FIGURE 1. A model for the role of CARF in the ARF-p53 pathway: Nucleolar sequestration of HDM2 by ARF resulting in p53 activation (**A**); CARF-ARF interaction in the perinucleolar region resulting in an activation of ARF-mediated p53 function (**B**); CARF-p53 interaction in the nucleoplasm resulting in an activation of ARF-independent p53 function (**C**); and the possibility that the proteasome-mediated degradation pathway involving p53 and HDM2 may also involve CARF (**D**).

also interacts with p53 directly.[3] It localized with p53 in the nucleoplasm and enhances its function, most likely, by causing its stabilization.

In retrospect, p53 may cause degradation of CARF by a mechanism that may involve its binding with the p53 downstream regulator and antagonist HDM2 (Fig. 1).

The study has shown that CARF regulates the p53 pathway by direct interactions with ARF and p53 proteins.

REFERENCES

1. Wadhwa, R., T. Sugihara, M.K. Hasan, *et al.* 2003. A novel putative collaborator of p19ARF. Exp. Gerontol. **38:** 245–252.
2. Hasan, M.K., T. Yaguchi, T. Sugihara, *et al.* 2002. CARF is a novel protein that cooperates with mouse p19ARF (human p14ARF) in activating p53. J. Biol. Chem. **277:** 37765–37770.
3. Hasan, M.K., T. Yaguchi, Y. Minoda, *et al.* 2004. Alternative reading frame protein (ARF)-independent function of CARF (collaborator of ARF) involves its interactions with p53: evidence for a novel p53-activation pathway and its negative feedback control. Biochem. J. **380:** 605–610.

Structural and Functional Differences between Mouse Mot-1 and Mot-2 Proteins That Differ in Two Amino Acids

CUSTER C. DEOCARIS,[a,b] KAZUHIKO YAMASAKI,[a] SUNIL C. KAUL,[a] AND RENU WADHWA[a,b]

[a]*National Institute of Advanced Industrial Science & Technology (AIST), 1-1-1 Higashi, Tsukuba 305-8562, Japan*

[b]*Department of Chemistry and Biotechnology, School of Engineering, The University of Tokyo, Tokyo, 113-8656, Japan*

ABSTRACT: Chaperone functions mediated by the heat-shock protein (HSP) family constitute a fundamental mechanism that governs the life span of organisms. Here we investigated the chaperone activities of the mitochondrial HSP70 protein, mortalin, which is a heat-uninducible stress protein involved in immortalization and tumorigenesis. There are two mortalin alleles, mot-1 and mot-2, in mouse, encoding two distinct proteins. Whereas an overexpression of mot-1-induced senescence in NIH 3T3 cells, overexpression of mot-2 promoted their malignant properties. Here, we provide evidence that mot-1 possesses very low chaperone activity as compared to mot-2. A "lazy lid" hypothesis is proposed for their differential aging phenotypes.

KEYWORDS: heat shock protein 70; mortalin; alleles; chaperones; structure; differential functions

INTRODUCTION

Mortalin-1 and -2 (mot-1 and -2) are pancytoplasmically and perinuclearly distributed mitochondrial hsp70 proteins originally cloned from normal and immortal murine cells, respectively. Remarkably, the open reading frames of these two mortalins differ by only two amino acids, yet have contrasting biological activities (FIG. 1A).[1,2] Whereas mot-1 protein is distributed

Address for correspondence: Renu Wadhwa, Gene Function Research Center, National Institute of Advanced Industrial Science & Technology (AIST), Central 4, 1-1-1 Higashi, Tsukuba 305-8562, Japan. Voice: +81-29-861-9464; fax: +81-29-861-2900.
e-mail: renu-wadhwa@aist.go.jp

Ann. N.Y. Acad. Sci. 1067: 220–223 (2006). © 2006 New York Academy of Sciences.
doi: 10.1196/annals.1354.027

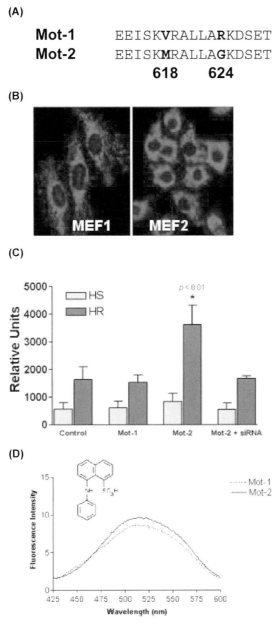

(A)

Mot-1   EEISK**V**RALLA**R**KDSET
Mot-2   EEISK**M**RALLA**G**KDSET
        618   **624**

(B)

MEF1   MEF2

(C)

(D)

FIGURE 1. Mouse mot-1 and mot-2 proteins are different structurally and functionally. (**A**) The two mortalin alleles differing only in two amino acids and (**B**) subcellular staining pattern of mot-1 and mot-2 proteins in mouse fibroblasts homozygous for mot-1 (MEF1) and mot-2 (MEF2). (**C**) *In vivo* luciferase refolding assay showing that mot-1 does not possess strong chaperone activity. (**D**) ANS fluorescence assay showing that mot-1 protein has less hydrophobic surface than mot-2 protein. Chaperone activity of mot-2 was neutralized by specific shRNA.

pancytoplasmically, mot-2 is perinuclear (FIG. 1B). Mot-1 when transfected to immortal NIH 3T3 cells conferred cellular senescence, whereas microinjection of its antibody reversibly stimulated cell division.[2] An overexpression of mot-2 invariably leads to malignant transformation in mouse immortal cells,[3] greater PDs enabling escape from senescence in *in vitro*-cultured human fibroblasts,[4] and life-span extension in *C. elegans*.[5] These pro-proliferative effects have been ascribed, in part, to the ability of mot-2 to inactivate wild-type p53[6,7] and interact with the Ras-Raf-MAPK signaling pathways.[8] In this study, we aim to understand from biophysical characteristics how the salient amino acid differences could lead to opposing biological functions of the two mortalin proteins.

THE STRONG AND WEAK CHAPERONES

In the present study, we investigated whether mot-1 and mot-2 proteins differ in their chaperone activities. We performed an *in vivo* chaperone assay by co-transfecting U2OS cells with the heat-sensitive firefly luciferase (PGL3) and mortalin expression constructs. After heat treatment (45°C, 30 min) and recovery (37°C, 4 h), we monitored refolding of luciferase by measuring its activity.

Heat-denatured luciferase was able to refold and gain significant activity in the presence of mot-2, but not mot-1 (FIG. 1C). We have also observed this weak chaperone activity of mot-1 in an *in vitro* chaperone assay that measures the degree of aggregation by light scattering after DTT treatment with insulin (data not shown). Consistent with the low chaperone activity of mot-1, we found that it has low hydrophobic surface as compared to mot-2 (FIG. 1D). The study has shown for the first time that mot-1 and mot-2 proteins have different structures and chaperone activities.

REFERENCES

1. WADHWA, R., S.C. KAUL, Y. IKAWA, *et al.* 1993. Identification of a novel member of mouse hsp70 family: its association with cellular mortal phenotype. J. Biol. Chem. **268:** 6615–6621.
2. WADHWA, R., S.C. KAUL, Y. SUGIMOTO, *et al.* 1993. Induction of cellular senescence by transfection of cytosolic mortalin cDNA in NIH 3T3 cells. J. Biol. Chem. **268:** 22239–22242.
3. KAUL, S.C., E.L. DUNCAN, A. ENGLEZOU, *et al.* 1998. Malignant transformation of NIH 3T3 cells by overexpression of mot-2 protein. Oncogene **17:** 907–911.
4. KAUL, S.C., R.R. REDDEL, T. SUGIHARA, *et al.* 2000. Inactivation of p53 and life span extension of human diploid fibroblasts by mot-2. FEBS Lett. **474:** 159–164.
5. YOKOYAMA, K., K. FUKUMOTO, T. MURAKAMI, *et al.* 2002. Extended longevity of *Caenorhabditis elegans* by knocking in extra copies of hsp70F, a homolog of mot-2 (mortalin)/mthsp70/Grp75. FEBS Lett. **516:** 53–57.

6. WADHWA, R., S. TAKANO, M. ROBERT, *et al.* 1998. Inactivation of tumor suppressor p53 by mot-2, a hsp70 family member. J. Biol. Chem. **273:** 29586–29591.
7. KAUL, S.C., S. TAKANO, R.R. REDDEL, *et al.* 2000. Transcriptional inactivation of p53 by deletions and single amino acid changes in mouse mot-1 protein. Biochem. Biophys. Res. Commun. **279:** 602–606.
8. WADHWA, R., T. YAGUCHI, K. TAIRA, *et al.* 2003. Mortalin-MPD (mevalonate pyrophosphate decarboxylase) interactions and their role in control of cellular proliferaction. Biochem. Biophys. Res. Commun. **302:** 735–742.

Proteasomal Oscillation during Mild Heat Shock in Aging Human Skin Fibroblasts

DAVID CHRISTIAN KRAFT,[a] CUSTER C. DEOCARIS,[b] AND
SURESH I. S. RATTAN[a]

[a]Laboratory of Cellular Aging, Danish Centre for Molecular Gerontology,
Department of Molecular Biology, University of Aarhus, Denmark

[b]Gene Function Research Center, National Institute of Advanced Industrial
Science and Technology (AIST), 1-1-1 Higashi, Tsukuba, Japan

ABSTRACT: Augmentation of proteasome machinery is emerging as a significant gerontomodulatory consequence of hormetic stimulation, such as mild heat stress. This study describes the phenomenon we term *hormetic proteasomal oscillation*, wherein mildly heat-stressed human fibroblasts (41°C, 1 h) display an adaptation response pattern in proteasome activity. Remarkably, such response appears to be diverse in severely heat-stressed or senescent fibroblasts. This proteasomal oscillation, as an innate cellular reaction to heat and aging, however, is independent of 20S proteasome protein levels and nuclear factor-E2-related factor 2 (Nrf2) transactivation.

KEYWORDS: proteasome; heat stress; fibroblast; hormesis; Nrf2; aging

INTRODUCTION

The proteasome is an essential protein quality-control mechanism responsible for the removal of abnormal or damaged proteins.[1] It is present in three forms with distinguishing functions: the 20S, the immuno-proteasome (20S + 11S), and the 26S (20S + 19S). The amount of the different forms of proteasome is dynamic relative to cell type, cell cycle, and physiologic environment.[2] Moreover, the proteasome is involved in signal transduction, cell cycle regulation, gene expression, apoptosis, and antigen presentation.[1] Hence, problems associated with proteasome function are bound to perturb cellular homeostasis and could lead to the accumulation of protein aggregates, deregulation of survival pathways, and senescence.[3]

Address for correspondence: Dr. Suresh I.S. Rattan, Department of Molecular Biology, University of Aarhus, Gustav Wieds Vej 10C, DK8000 Aarhus−C, Denmark. Voice: +45 8942 5034; fax: +45 8612 3178.

e-mail: rattan@mb.au.dk

Ann. N.Y. Acad. Sci. 1067: 224–227 (2006). © 2006 New York Academy of Sciences.
doi: 10.1196/annals.1354.028

Various stressors, such as heat, UV light, and oxidative agents, have been reported to inhibit proteasome function.[4–7] Imai *et al.*, however, have shown that this stress-associated decline in proteasome function is transient, and in fact, it was noted that proteasome activity even increases after exposure to heat shock.[5] The loss of 26S proteasome is the main reason for the downregulation of the proteasome activity, resulting in an increase in the relative amounts of the 20S proteasome.[5] After several hours, the level of the 20S proteasome is depressed as a result of the reassembly of 19S and 20S into the 26S proteasome.[5] From these findings, it has been proposed that the physical dynamics of the 19S regulatory units of the proteasome could lead to the oscillatory nature of proteasome activity. As this phenomenon has been elucidated in a yeast model and at nonphysiologic temperatures, we have investigated whether proteasome oscillation exists in normal human cells and within a hormetic framework.[9]

EXPERIMENTAL METHODS

Proteasome activity and Western analysis were performed as previously described.[10] Human adult skin fibroblast cells (ASF-2) were derived from the breast biopsy specimen of a consenting young healthy Danish woman (aged 28 years).

RESULTS AND DISCUSSION

After heat treatment of early-passage young ASF-2 cells at 41°C for 1 h, we describe the characteristic hormetic proteasomal oscillation as follows: phase I, the damage-response phase in which there is an initial decline of proteasome activity by 14%, remaining at low levels for 5 h; phase II, the hyperactivation phase in which there is a sudden burst of proteasome activity by about 25%; and phase III, the stabilization phase, in which there is gradual waning of proteasome activity until returning to the baseline levels in 2 h. Interestingly, the lag time prior to phase II was much extended when cells had become senescent and upon exposure to higher temperatures (FIG. 1A). Higher temperature caused proteasomal activity to decrease progressively during phase I (FIG. 1B). Proteasomal protein level was checked by measuring the level of the 20S α3 subunits, but there was no significant change found (data not shown). Furthermore, we also investigated the involvement of the transcription factor Nrf2, which is known to induce several proteasomal genes in response to oxidative stress, but no induction of Nrf2 was found in heat-shock-treated cells (data not shown).[11]

Consistent with the reported findings from mouse and yeast models, observations in human fibroblasts imply that the proteasomal oscillation as a heat stress response may be conserved.[5,6] In addition, preliminary data from our laboratory from *D. melanogaster* also confirm the proteasomal oscillation notion (data not shown).

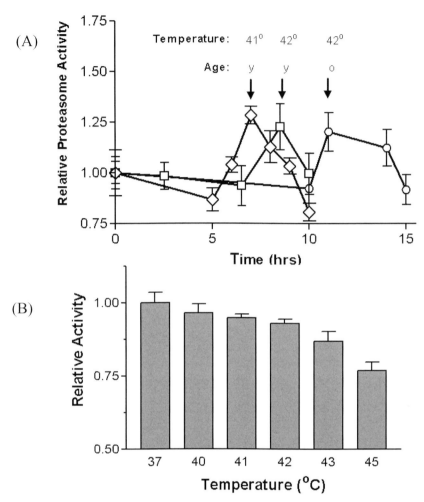

FIGURE 1. Chymotrypsin-like proteasome activity of ASF-2 cells. (**A**) Proteasome levels were measured within 15 h after heat shock (at 41 and 42°C) in young (Y) and old (O) cells, as indicated. (**B**) The effect of different temperatures on proteasome activity after 5 h post-heat treatment. Proteasome activity was measured as arbitrary fluorescence units of 7-amido-4-methylcoumarin (AMC) per mg protein per min liberated from the test substrate suc-LLVY-AMC.

More importantly, the data presented here show that such oscillation is induced at hormetically favorable temperatures. We surmise that this apparent downregulation of proteasomal activity may likely be a regulatory event more than a result of direct thermodynamic damage inflicted on the proteasome subunits. Bose *et al.* implicate the stress signaling pathways in altering the phosphorylation status of the proteasome that could lead to the detachment/ reattachment of the 29S cap.[12] Further investigations into the role of stress kinases in proteasome regulation during hormetic stress are under way. Understanding its regulatory pathways is important in manipulating the proteasome machinery for developing new anti-aging strategies and treatment of protein conformational disorders such as Alzheimer's disease.

ACKNOWLEDGMENTS

The authors thank the Gene Function Research Laboratory, National Institute for Advanced Industrial Science and Technology (AIST) for travel and research fellowship to David Christian Kraft. The Laboratory of Cellular Aging (University of Aarhus) is supported by research grants from the Danish Research Councils, Carlsberg Fund, Senetek PLC, and EU's Biomed Health Programmes.

REFERENCES

1. YANO, M. *et al.* 2005. Chaperone activities of the 26S and 20S proteasome. Curr. Protein Pept. Sci. **6:** 197–203.
2. BAJOREK, M., D. FINLEY & M.H. GLICKMAN. 2003. Proteasome disassembly and downregulation is correlated with viability during stationary phase. Curr. Biol. **13:** 1140–1144.
3. CHONDROGIANNI, N. *et al.* 2003. Central role of the proteasome in senescence and survival of human fibroblasts: induction of a senescence-like phenotype upon its inhibition and resistance to stress upon its activation. J. Biol. Chem. **278:** 28026–28037.
4. BULTEAU, A.L. *et al.* 2002. Impairment of proteasome function upon UVA- and UVB-irradiation of human keratinocytes. Free Radic. Biol. Med. **32:** 1157–1170.
5. IMAI, J. *et al.* 2003. The molecular chaperone Hsp90 plays a role in the assembly and maintenance of the 26S proteasome. EMBO J. **22:** 3557–3567.
6. KUCKELKORN, U. *et al.* 2000. The effect of heat shock on 20S/26S proteasomes. Biol. Chem. **381:** 1017–1023.
7. REINHECKEL, T. *et al.* 2000. Differential impairment of 20S and 26S proteasome activities in human hematopoietic K562 cells during oxidative stress. Arch. Biochem. Biophys. **377:** 65–68.
8. CARRARD, G. *et al.* 2003. Impact of ageing on proteasome structure and function in human lymphocytes. Int. J. Biochem. Cell Biol. **35:** 728–739.
9. RATTAN, S.I. *et al.* 2004. Slowing down aging from within: mechanistic aspects of anti-aging hormetic effects of mild heat stress on human cells. Acta. Biochim. Pol. **51:** 481–492.
10. BEEDHOLM, R., B.F. CLARK & S.I. RATTAN. 2004. Mild heat stress stimulates 20S proteasome and its 11S activator in human fibroblasts undergoing aging *in vitro*. Cell Stress. Chaperones **9:** 49–57.
11. KWAK, M.K. *et al.* 2003. Antioxidants enhance mammalian proteasome expression through the Keap1-Nrf2 signaling pathway. Mol. Cell Biol. **23:** 8786–8794.
12. BOSE, S. *et al.* 2004. Phosphorylation of 20S proteasome alpha subunit C8 (alpha7) stabilizes the 26S proteasome and plays a role in the regulation of proteasome complexes by gamma-interferon. Biochem. J. **378:** 177–184.

Apoptosis and Necrosis in Senescent Human Fibroblasts

SUSUMU OHSHIMA

Division of Morphological Science, Biomedical Research Center, Saitama Medical School, 38, Morohongo, Iruma, Saitama, 350-0495, Japan

ABSTRACT: To study the role of cell death in the aging process, cell death during spontaneous cellular senescence *in vitro* was examined with normal human fibroblasts. A small subset of the senescent cells showed aberrant morphology such as remarkable nuclear fragmentation or multiple micronuclei, and such cells often showed positive reactions with antibody to phosphorylated pRb. Cells showing caspase activation and binding of Annexin V, which indicate apoptotic change, increased in the senescent phase in flow cytometry analysis. Propidium iodide–positive cells, however, also increased with passaging. The results suggest that both apoptosis and necrosis are involved in cell death of senescent human fibroblasts.

KEYWORDS: senescence; apoptosis; necrosis; fibroblast

INTRODUCTION

Recent studies suggest that apoptosis is involved in the aging process of various tissues such as those of the nervous and immune systems.[1–3] Cell loss by apoptosis has been linked to the age-related decline of physiological functions or age-related disorders such as Alzheimer's disease or autoimmune diseases. However, *in vitro* studies of age-associated cell death are limited and the role of apoptosis in the aging process is poorly understood. For example, it has been reported that senescent human fibroblasts are resistant to some apoptotic stimuli,[4] while other investigators have found that senescent human fibroblasts undergo apoptosis in response to different apoptotic stimuli.[5] Another study reported that senescent human endothelial cells are relatively prone to undergoing spontaneous apoptosis compared to senescent human fibroblasts under the same conditions.[6] In a previous report, I presented some data suggesting that a small subset of human fibroblasts undergoes spontaneous apoptosis during stress-induced premature senescence and replicative senescence.[7] In this

Address for correspondence: Susumu Ohshima, Division of Morphological Science, Biomedical Research Center, Saitama Medical School, 38, Morohongo, Iruma, Saitama, 350-0495, Japan. Voice: 81-49-276-1448; fax: 81-49-276-1424.

e-mail: sohshima@saitama-med.ac.jp

Ann. N.Y. Acad. Sci. 1067: 228–234 (2006). © 2006 New York Academy of Sciences.
doi: 10.1196/annals.1354.029

study, cell death in spontaneously senescent human fibroblasts was further examined.

MATERIALS AND METHODS

Normal human fibroblasts designated HUC-F2 were obtained from RIKEN BioResource Center (Tsukuba, Japan) and grown in minimum essential medium with alpha modification (Sigma-Aldrich, St. Louis, MO) supplemented with heat-inactivated 10% fetal bovine serum. Cells were subcultured twice a week before they reached confluence and were maintained at medium-to-subconfluent density during the experimental period. Senescence-associated β-galactosidase of the cells cultured on dishes was histochemically detected with the Senescence Detection Kit (BioVision Mountain View, CA). For morphological observation, cells cultured on dishes or glass slides were fixed with methanol, stained with acridine orange, and then observed with fluorescent microscopy. For immnofluorescent detection of phosphorylated retinoblastoma protein (pRb), cells on glass slides were fixed with 80% methanol, permeabilized with 0.25% Triton-X, and incubated with antiphosphorylated pRb antibody (Santa Cruz Biotechnology, Santa Cruz, CA) followed by a fluorescein-conjugated secondary antibody. To detect caspase activation, cells were harvested with trypsin and stained with CaspGLOW™ Fluorescein Caspase Staining Kit (BioVision) for pan-caspase, caspase-3, -8, and -9, for flow cytometric analysis. To analyze annexin V binding, which detects transfer of phosphatidylserine to the outside of the membrane, cells were harvested with trypsin and stained with Annexin V-FITC Apoptosis Detection Kit (BioVision) for flow cytometer analysis. In some experiments, cells cultured on dishes or glass slides were stained for caspase activation and annexin V binding with the same kit as those used for flow cytometry analysis and observed by fluorescent microscopy.

RESULTS

Expression of Senescent Phenotype

The population doubling time (PDT) of HUC-F2 cells sharply increased after the 20th passage—a population doubling level (PDL) of about 40. Cell growth was arrested by the 23rd passage (about 44 PDL). More than 90% of the growth-arrested cells showed typical senescent phenotypes such as enlarged size or expression of β-galactosidase.

Change in Nuclear Morphology

A small subset of the senescent human fibroblasts showed aberrant nuclear morphology such as remarkable fragmentation or formation of multiple

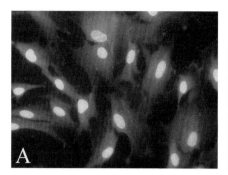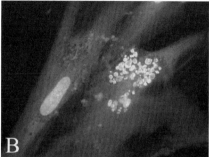

FIGURE 1. Acridine orange–stained human fibroblasts HUC-F2. Young proliferating cells in 14th passage (**A**) and senescent cells showing fragmented nuclei in 23rd passage (**B**).

micronuclei (FIG. 1). The mean percentage of cells showing such nuclear change increased from 0.6% in the growing phase (before the 19th passage) to 2.7% in the senescent phase (from the 19th passage).

Detection of Phosphorylated (Ser 807/811) pRb

When cells were labeled with antiphosphorylated (serine 807/811) pRb antibody, the cytoplasm of some aberrant cells with fragmented nuclei as well as normal mitotic cells showed positive reactions (FIG. 2). Such aberrant cells with phosphorylated pRb often showed a morphologic pattern suggesting that cells were in a stage immediately after mitosis and that nuclear fragmentation had taken place when cells underwent mitosis.

Activation of Caspases

In flow cytometry analysis, the cells in the senescent phase showed increased percentages of caspase (pan-caspase)-activated cells (FIG. 3). Significant differences in the activation of three caspase species (caspase-3, 8, and 9) were not observed. The percentages of propidium iodide–positive cells also increased with passaging (FIG. 4). When cells cultured on dishes or glass slides were stained *in situ* and observed with fluorescent microscopy, some cells with round shape showed positive staining.

Change in Membrane Lipid (Annexin V Binding)

In flow cytometry analysis, the cells in the senescent phase showed increased percentages of the FITC-Annexin V–positive cells (FIG. 5), which indicates

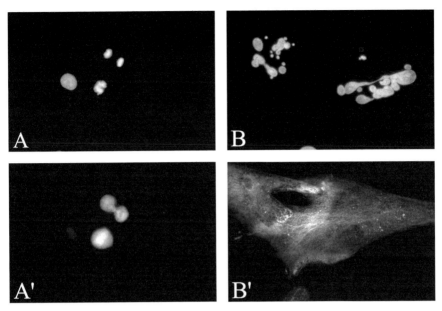

FIGURE 2. Images of nuclei stained with propidium iodide (*upper panels*) and localization of phosphorylated pRb (Ser 807/811) in the same cells (*lower panels*). In normal mitotic cells (**A** and **A′**), phosphorylated pRbs localize on condensed chromosomes and structures suggestive of mitotic spindles. In aberrant cells with fragmented nuclei (**B** and **B′**), phosphorylated pRb localizes with fibrous structures in the cytoplasm.

an early apoptotic change. When cells on dishes were stained *in situ*, apoptotic cells showing a round shape with FITC-Annexin V–positive surface and necrotic cells with PI-positive nucleus could be distinguished.

DISCUSSION

The results in this study suggest that a small subset of normal human fibroblasts undergo apoptosis concomitantly with cellular senescence *in vitro*. However, activation of caspases or increased binding of annexin V did not necessarily coincide with fragmentation of nuclei when observed with fluorescent microscopy. It is not clear whether these discrepancies indicate chronological changes of apoptosis or reflect changes from different phenomena in senescent cells. Positive reactions with antibody to phosphorylated pRb in some cells with fragmented nuclei suggest that nuclear fragmentation had taken place when the cells underwent mitosis. Recent studies show that the inactivation of pRb induces apoptosis in senescent cells.[8,9] Therefore, nuclear fragmentation in senescent fibroblasts might represent apoptosis in cells with compromised pRb function. There is another possibility, however, that the nuclear

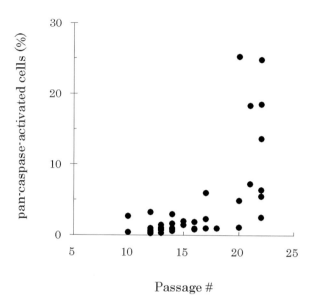

FIGURE 3. Frequencies of caspase-activated human fibroblasts. Harvested cells were stained with fluorescein-labeled pan-caspase inhibitor (FITC-VAD-FMK) and analyzed with a flow cytometer. Percentages of fluorescein-positive cells from dot-plot analysis were plotted against passage numbers.

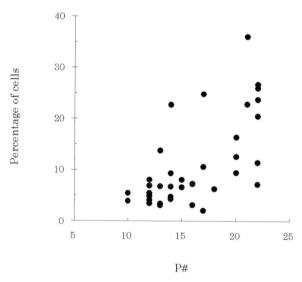

FIGURE 4. Frequencies of propidium iodide–positive human fibroblasts. Percentages of propidium iodide–positive cells in caspase analysis were plotted against passage numbers.

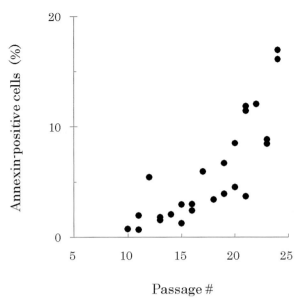

FIGURE 5. Frequencies of annexin V-positive human fibroblasts. Harvested cells were stained with fluorescein-labeled annexin V and analyzed with a flow cytometer. Percentages of fluorescein-positive cells from dot plot analysis were plotted against passage numbers.

fragmentation in senescent fibroblasts results from abnormal segregation of chromosomes caused by mitotic spindle failure, because lagging chromosomes with abnormally segregated nuclei could be recognized occasionally in cells with phosphorylated pRb. Some reports suggest that errors in the mitotic machinery of dividing cells and the inactivation of G2/M checkpoints may be involved in the aging process.[10,11] More detailed examinations regarding pathogenesis of nuclear fragmentation in senescent human fibroblasts are necessary. Even if the nuclear fragmentation observed in this study does not represent apoptosis, it is nevertheless certain that a small subset of human fibroblasts undergo apoptosis with senescence because activation of caspases and increased binding of annexin V of the cells were evident in the senescent phase. In addition, PI-positive cells, which indicate necrosis, also increased with passaging. These results suggest that both apoptosis and necrosis are involved in the cell death of senescent human fibroblasts *in vitro.* The significance of both types of cell death in the aging process is not clear and more advanced research is necessary.

REFERENCES

1. WARNER, H.R. 1999. Apoptosis: a two-edged sword in aging. Ann. N.Y. Acad. Sci. **887:** 1–11.

2. HIGAMI, Y. & I. SHIMOKAWA. 2000. Apoptosis in the aging process. Cell Tissue Res. **301:** 125–132.
3. ZHANG, J.H., Y. ZHANG & B. HERMAN. 2003. Caspases, apoptosis and aging. Ageing Res. Rev. **2:** 357–366.
4. WANG, E. 1995. Senescent human fibroblasts resist programmed cell death, and failure to suppress bcl2 is involved. Cancer Res. **55:** 2284–2292.
5. DEJESUS, V., I. RIOS, C. DAVIS, *et al.* 2002. Induction of apoptosis in human replicative senescent fibroblasts. Exp. Cell Res. **274:** 92–99.
6. WAGNER, M., B. HAMPEL, D. BERNHARD, *et al.* 2001. Replicative senescence of human endothelial cells in vitro involves G1 arrest, polyploidization and senescence-associated apoptosis. Exp. Gerontol. **36:** 1327–1347.
7. OHSHIMA, S. 2004. Apoptosis in stress-induced and spontaneously senescent human fibroblasts. Biochem. Biophys. Res. Commun. **324:** 241–246.
8. HUANG, Y. *et al.* 2004. Down-regulation of p21^{WAF1} promotes apoptosis in senescent human fibroblasts: involvement of retinoblastoma protein phosphorylation and delay of cellular aging. J. Cell Physiol. **201:** 483–491.
9. ALEXANDER, K., H-S. YANG & P. HINDS. 2003. pRb inactivation in senescent cells leads to an E2F-dependent apoptosis requiring p73. Molec. Cancer Res. **1:** 716–728.
10. LY, D.H., D.J. LOCKHART, R.A. LERNER & P.G. SCHULZ. 2000. Mitotic misregulation and human aging. Science **287:** 2486–2492.
11. MASON, D., T. JACKSON & A. LIN. 2004. Molecular signature of oncogenic ras-induced senescence. Oncogene **23:** 9238–9246.

Aging of Murine Mesenchymal Stem Cells

CHRISTINE FEHRER, GERHARD LASCHOBER, AND
GÜNTER LEPPERDINGER

*The Extracellular Matrix Research Group, Institute for Biomedical Aging
Research, Austrian Academy of Sciences, Rennweg 10 A-6020 Innsbruck, Austria*

ABSTRACT: Mesenchymal stem cells (MSCs) are able to differentiate into
distinct lineages such as adipo-, osteo-, and chondrocytes. MSCs were isolated from three mouse strains, which are short- (SAMP6, 9.7 months),
medium- (SAMR1, 16.3 months), or long-lived (C57BL/6, 28 months). We
investigated primary colony-forming units with regard to bone marrow
stroma and found differences that correlate with mean life expectancies of the particular genetic backgrounds. However, MSC derived from
the various mouse strains behaved equivalently *in vitro* with respect to
growth rate. By genomic means, we analyzed the cellular milieu *in vivo*
and found considerable differences among the various mouse strains.
This implies that, although individual MSCs show an equivalent differentiation potential *in vitro*, the primary stem cells are greatly influenced
by their molecular environment.

KEYWORDS: mesenchymal stem cell; niche; aging; senescence; *in vitro*
differentiation; array analysis; long-term culture

INTRODUCTION

Stem cells are believed to be involved in the continuous maintenance and repair of most tissue types. Stem cells are self-renewing entities while generating
multipotential progeny. Hence, this class of cells is of paramount importance for
an organism during infancy and adolescence as well as for cellular homeostasis during adulthood. Mesenchymal stem cells (MSCs) exhibit differentiation
into the adipo-, osteo-, and chondrogenic lineage and are therefore considered a
potential source for therapeutic applications in age-related diseases associated
with these tissue types.[1] MSCs have been successfully isolated from different
species including humans and mice.[2,3] However, murine MSCs (mMSCs) are
poorly characterized both *in vitro* and *in vivo*. In contrast to human MSCs,

Address for correspondence: Günter Lepperdinger, The Extracellular Matrix Research Group, Institute for Biomedical Aging Research, Austrian Academy of Sciences, Rennweg 10 A-6020 Innsbruck,
Austria. Voice: 0043 512 5839 1940; fax: 0043 512 5839 198.
  e-mail:guenter.lepperdinger@oeaw.ac.at

Ann. N.Y. Acad. Sci. 1067: 235–242 (2006). © 2006 New York Academy of Sciences.
doi: 10.1196/annals.1354.030

mMSCs are far more difficult to isolate and to expand in culture. Moreover, the precise characterization and distinct localization of MSCs in bone marrow are still unknown.[4]

We studied MSC aging in three mouse strains: a short-lived mouse strain, which is prone to accelerated senescence (SAMP6); the corresponding strain, which is resistant to senescence (SAMR1);[5] and as the particularly long-living strain, C57BL/6. From 6 months onward, SAMP6 mice were also found to show a higher incidences of osteoporosis and to increasingly develop marrow adiposity.[6] To date, no information is available on the number and quality of MSCs in these different mouse strains, nor is it known whether the mean life expectancy and the emergence of age-related diseases is influenced by the prosperity of MSCs.

We therefore isolated MSCs from these different mouse strains and characterized properties such as growth rates and the respective differentiation potentials *in vitro*. Furthermore, we also studied primary cultures of mouse bone marrow–adherent cells, which are believed to contain MSCs. Consequently, we also examined the expression profile of bone marrow of healthy young mice in order to learn whether the environment in which MSCs reside is different within those three mouse strains, and thus whether MSC prosperity would be influenced *in vivo* by exogenous parameters.

MATERIALS AND METHODS

Isolation and Expansion of mMSCs

C57BL/6J, SAMR1, and SAMP6 mice were obtained from Jackson Laboratories (Bar Harbor, ME), and Harland Ltd., (Oxon, UK). MSCs were isolated as described previously.[7] In detail, three female or male mice of each strain, 8–16 weeks old, were sacrificed by cervical dislocation. Connective tissue and muscle were carefully removed from tibia and femur, and in order to extract bone marrow, both ends of the long bones were clipped. The remaining fragments were inserted into a centrifuge tube and the cells were spun out at $400 \times g$ for 1 min. For counting in a hemocytometer, the cells were resuspended in complete isolation medium, CIM (RPMI 1640 supplemented with 9% horse serum, 9% fetal calf serum, 100 units/mL penicillin, 100 μg/mL streptomycin) and filtered through a 70-μM nylon mesh. Cells were plated at high density (1×10^6 cells/cm^2), which prevents growth of hematopoietic cells. After 24 h, the nonadherent cell population was removed by extensive washing with PBS before fresh medium was added. During the first three to four passages, cells were split at 1:3 ratios as they became confluent. At the fourth passage, colonies were further expanded in complete expansion medium (CEM), consisting of IMDM supplemented with 18% fetal calf serum, 100 units/mL penicillin, and

100 μg/mL streptomycin as low-density cultures (50 cells/cm^2). The rapidly growing cells were of fibroblastoid-like appearance. During initial phase, cells were passaged with the aid of ReagentPack Subculture Regents (Cambrex), and during expansion phase by incubation with 0.05% trypsin and 1mM EDTA for 3 min at 37°C. For long-term storage, cells were kept in liquid nitrogen (1−2 × 10^6 cells/mL in CEM supplemented with 30% fetal calf serum and 5% dimethylsulfoxide).

In Vitro Differentiation of mMSCs

Cells were plated at a density of 50 cells/cm^2 in 58 cm^2 dishes and grown for 3–4 days in CEM.[7] In order to induce osteogenic differentiation, the cultures were subsequently incubated in CEM supplemented with 20 mM β-glycerol phosphate, 1 nM dexamethasone, and 0.5 μM ascorbate-2-phosphate. The medium was changed twice per week for a period of 3 weeks. The cells were fixed with 4% *para*-formaldehyde solution for 10 min and stained with Alizarin Red, pH 4.1, for 20 min at room temperature.

For adipogenic differentiation, the cultures were incubated in CEM supplemented with 1 μM dexamethasone, 5 μg/mL insulin, 50 μM indomethacine, and 0.5 μM 3-*iso*-butyl-1-methylxanthine. The medium was changed twice per week for a period of 3 weeks. The cells were fixed with 4% *para*-formaldehyde solution for 10 min and stained with 0.5% Oil Red O in 85% propylene glycol for 20 min at room temperature.

Primary Culture of Murine Bone Marrow

Bone marrow isolates were plated in triplicate at a cell density of 5 × 10^5 cells/58 cm^2 on plastic (BD Biosciences) and grown for 3 weeks in CIM. Nonadherent cells were carefully removed by extensive washes with PBS. The media were changed twice a week. Colonies were fixed with 4% *para*-formaldehyde solution for 10 min and stained with 0.5% Crystal Violet in methanol at room temperature for 20 min. Colonies consisting of more than 10 cells were counted.

RNA Preparation and Array Analysis

RNA was isolated from bone marrow by homogenization in 4.2 M guanidinium thiocyanate, phenol extraction, and ethanol precipitation.[8] The resulting total RNA was further purified by LiCl precipitation (final concentration 4.5 M). Labeled cDNA was prepared with oligo(dT)-priming and [α-33P] dCTP. Nylon arrays (NIA mouse 9K set), a kind gift from Kevin Becker, Genome Center of the National Institute on Aging, Baltimore, MD, USA,[9] were hybridized for 48 h at 65°C (5× Denhardt's solution, 5 × SSC, 1% SDS), stringently washed, and exposed to Fuji Imaging Plates for 24–48 h. The plates were scanned by means of a Fuji BAS-1800-II reader and the images were processed using AIDA Image Analyzer 3.51 software (Raytest).

RESULTS AND DISCUSSION

Primary cultures derived from murine bone marrow-contain cells, that form colonies made of three distinct cell types, which are (i) large-flattened, (ii) star-shaped, and (iii) fibroblastoid-like cells.[10] During long-term culture together with passaging and replating for five times, fibroblastoid-like cells were enriched to homogeneity.[11] From this time point onward, the cells were kept in culture for more than 80 cumulative population doublings (FIG. 1A). The growth rate remained the same throughout culture, which is in contrast to what has been observed for human MSCs in culture.[12] Furthermore, cells did not show indications of *in vitro* senescence, which is to say that in any case, growth arrest and senescence-associated β-galactosidase were not detectable, although at high passages, colonies with aberrant morphology emerged (FIG. 1B). These long-term characteristics applied for C57BL/6 and both SAM strains.

In order to validate the multipotentiality of the putative stem cell–like cultures, differentiation could be induced *in vitro* into adipogenic and osteogenic lineages (FIG. 1B). At a low passage number, colonies readily differentiated. After long-term culture together with successive passaging, we observed that the rate of differentiation declined,[13] although the potential to differentiate into adipogenic and osteogenic progeny did not change.[14] Yet, no obvious differences were observed between cells derived from long- and short-lived mouse strains. We concluded that stem cell–like or progenitor cells that exhibited differentiation potential into various lineages could be derived from primary cultures of murine bone marrow. Moreover, these cells could proliferate in culture for many more generations than reported for fibroblasts and they maintained multipotentiality. By analogy to the published data, we thus call these cells mesenchymal stem cells. Yet irrespective of the genetic background of the mice from which these MSCs had been derived, they behaved equivalently with regard to the above-mentioned criteria.

Since MSCs are believed to descend from cells that grow in colonies within primary cultures of bone marrow, we carefully examined the plastic-adherent stromal fraction of the various mouse strains. Primary cells were plated at 9000 cells/cm^2 cell culture dish and were stained after 3 weeks with Crystal Violet. All colonies consisting of more than 10 cells were counted. More colonies in these primary cultures were found for C57BL/6 or SAMR1 mice, when compared to SAMP6 (FIG. 2A). This suggests that since cells show equivalent growth characteristics in culture later on, presumably, the extracellular microenvironment (that is, the MSC niche) appears instructive in order to harbor

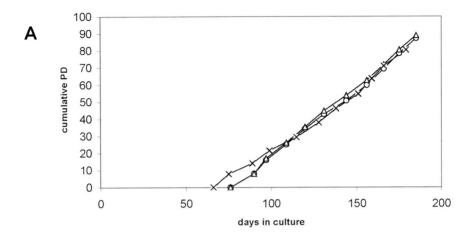

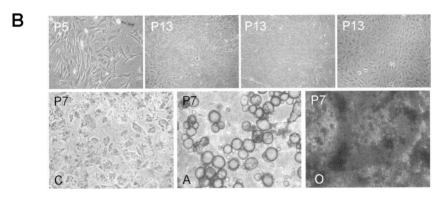

FIGURE 1. MSC morphology and proliferation rates. Growth of MSCs was only monitored from expansion phase onward, when cell culture showed homogenous characteristics. (**A**) Proliferation rates of MSCs derived from C57BL/6 (*crosses*), SAMR1 (*open triangles*), and SAMP6 (*open circles*) in long-term culture are shown. (**B**) *Upper panel* shows MSCs at passage 5; variant morphologies were apparent in cultures at passage 13. MSCs derived from C57BL/6 and cultured for approximately 50–60 population doublings were still capable of differentiating into distinct lineages at advanced passages (*lower panel*). (C) control; (A) adipogenesis (note accumulating lipid vesicles within enlarging cells), (O) osteogenesis; (observable as a tight meshwork of mineralized extracellular matrix).

a distinctive number of colony-forming cells within the bone marrow. Hence, although genetic variation did not appear to disturb the stem cell *per se*, the genetic background of the surrounding cells greatly determines the number of stem cell niches *in vivo.*[15]

MSCs appear to be quite rare within marrow. Moreover, stem cells are believed to reside in adult tissues in a solitary state; therefore, these cells are

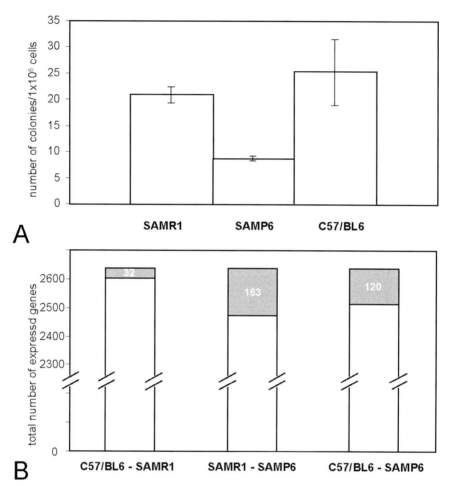

FIGURE 2. Primary cultures and expression profile of murine bone marrow. (**A**) Primary colony-forming units of total bone marrow cells from SAMR1, SAMP6, and C57BL/6 mice were determined per 1×10^6 total marrow cells. (**B**) Array analysis of total bone marrow cells was performed by using P-33-labeled cDNA of total bone marrow cells derived from SAMR1, SAMP6, and C57BL/6 mice to probe 9K mouse arrays, which were a gift from Kevin Becker, Genome Center of the National Institute on Aging. After image-processing and normalization of the results, signals above the background were further analyzed and genes that exhibited a greater than two-fold higher or lower expression level were considered to be differentially expressed (white numbers in gray columns).

entirely surrounded by "bone marrow cells," which thus determine the stem cell niche and presumably are also involved in stem cell and progenitor cell propagation. We therefore analyzed the expression profile of whole bone marrow of the three mouse strains by means of a 9K mouse array. Only greater than two-fold up- or downregulated genes were considered differentially expressed (FIG. 2B). Comparison of the expressed genes revealed a high resemblance of the expression profile of C57BL/6 and SAMR1, yet SAMP6 exhibited a moderately different gene expression, when compared to SAMR1 and C57BL/6.

CONCLUSION

MSCs derived from various mouse strains that under normal laboratory conditions exhibit different mean life expectancies behaved, after successive passaging, equivalently with regard to growth, altered morphology, and differentiation *in vitro*. By and large, the numbers of colony-forming cells extracted from bone marrow differ. Furthermore, in this compartment, where MSCs reside *in vivo,* array analysis of total bone marrow cells revealed differences in gene expression among the various mouse strains. We therefore conclude that MSCs are greatly influenced *in situ*, most likely because of differences generated by cells in the bone marrow other than MSCs.

ACKNOWLEDGMENTS

G.L. is an APART fellow of the Austrian Academy of Sciences and further supported by the Jubilee Fund of the Austrian National Bank as well as by the Austrian Science Fund, project S9309-B09. We are grateful to Brigitte Greiderer for excellent technical assistance and Stephan Reitinger for fruitful discussions and careful reading of the paper.

REFERENCES

1. GREGORY, C.A., D.J. PROCKOP & J.L. SPEES. 2005. Non-hematopoietic bone marrow stem cells: molecular control of expansion and differentiation. Exp. Cell Res. **306:** 330–335.
2. COLTER, D.C. *et al.* 2000. Rapid expansion of recycling stem cells in cultures of plastic-adherent cells from human bone marrow. Proc. Natl. Acad. Sci. USA **97:** 3213–3218.
3. PEREIRA, R.F. *et al.* 1995. Cultured adherent cells from marrow can serve as long-lasting precursor cells for bone, cartilage, and lung in irradiated mice. Proc. Natl. Acad. Sci. USA **92:** 4857–4861.
4. FEHRER, C. & G. LEPPERDINGER. 2005. Mesenchymal stem cells. Aging. Exp. Gerontol. **40:** 926–930.
5. TAKEDA, T., M. HOSOKAWA & K. HIGUCHI. 1997. Senescence-accelerated mouse (SAM): a novel murine model of senescence. Exp. Gerontol. **32:** 105–109.
6. CHEN, H. *et al.* 2004. Morphological study of the parathyroid gland and thyroid C cell in senescence-accelerated mouse (SAMP6), a murine model for senile osteoporosis. Tissue Cell **36:** 409–415.

7. PEISTER, A. *et al.* 2004. Adult stem cells from bone marrow (MSCs) isolated from different strains of inbred mice vary in surface epitopes, rates of proliferation, and differentiation potential. Blood **103:** 1662–1668.

8. CHOMCZYNSKI, P. & N. SACCHI. 1987. Single-step method of RNA isolation by acid guanidinium thiocyanate-phenol-chloroform extraction. Anal. Biochem. **162:** 156–159.

9. DONOVAN, D.M. & K.G. BECKER. 2002. Double round hybridization of membrane based cDNA arrays: improved background reduction and data replication. J. Neurosci. Methods **118:** 59–62.

10. MEIRELLES LDA, S. & N.B. NARDI. 2003. Murine marrow-derived mesenchymal stem cell: isolation, in vitro expansion, and characterization. Br. J. Haematol. **123:** 702–711.

11. TROPEL, P. *et al.* 2004. Isolation and characterisation of mesenchymal stem cells from adult mouse bone marrow. Exp. Cell Res. **295:** 395–406.

12. MATSUBARA, T. *et al.* 2004. A new technique to expand human mesenchymal stem cells using basement membrane extracellular matrix. Biochem. Biophys. Res. Commun. **313:** 503–508.

13. MURAGLIA, A., R. CANCEDDA & R. QUARTO. 2000. Clonal mesenchymal progenitors from human bone marrow differentiate in vitro according to a hierarchical model. J. Cell Sci. **113** (Pt 7): 1161–1166.

14. MULLER-SIEBURG, C.E. & E. DERYUGINA. 1995. The stromal cells' guide to the stem cell universe. Stem Cells **13:** 477–486.

15. LI, L. & T. XIE. 2005. Stem cell niche: structure and function. Annu. Rev. Cell. Dev. Biol.

Prevention of Accelerated Cell Aging in the Werner Syndrome

TERENCE DAVIS, MICHÈLE F. HAUGHTON, CHRISTOPHER J. JONES, AND DAVID KIPLING

Department of Pathology, School of Medicine, Cardiff University, Heath Park, Cardiff CF14 4XN, UK

ABSTRACT: In the Werner syndrome (WS) fibroblasts have an increased life span and growth rate when treated with the p38 inhibitor SB203580. Additionally, the cellular morphology reverts to that seen in young normal fibroblasts. The p38 pathway is activated in young WS cells, associated with high levels of p21^WAF1 leading to cell cycle arrest, and is suppressed by SB203580. As these changes are also seen in telomerized WS cells, these data show that the growth problems seen in WS cells, and perhaps the accelerated *in vivo* aging, are due to a *telomere-independent premature senescence* mechanism. The suppression of this mechanism by SB203580 treatment suggests a route whereby WS may be amenable to therapeutic intervention.

KEYWORDS: actin stress fibers; p21^WAF1; p38 MAPK; p53; SB203580; senescence; telomeres; telomerase; Werner syndrome

INTRODUCTION

The Werner syndrome (WS) is a rare genetic disorder in which patients show the premature onset of many clinical features of old age.[1,2] The median life expectancy is 47 years, with myocardial infarction or mesenchymal neoplasms as the major causes of death. With some exceptions, such as the absence of central nervous system degeneration, WS provides a stunning mimicry of normal aging and is widely used as a model disease to investigate the mechanisms underlying normal human aging.[1]

The molecular mechanism of WS appears to be related to accelerated cell aging. Cultured cells from normal individuals divide a limited number of times before they enter a growth-arrest state termed replicative cellular senescence.[3] This is postulated to contribute to normal human aging and is accelerated in WS, the fibroblasts from WS patients having a dramatically reduced cellular

Address for correspondence: Terence Davis, Department of Pathology, Henry Wellcome Building, School of Medicine, Cardiff University, Heath Park, Cardiff CF14 4XN, Wales, UK. Voice: +44-29-2074 3398; fax: +44-29-2074 4276.

e-mail: davist2@cardiff.ac.uk

Ann. N.Y. Acad. Sci. 1067: 243–247 (2006). © 2006 New York Academy of Sciences.
doi: 10.1196/annals.1354.031

life span.[4] This shortened life span is argued as a cause of the accelerated aging seen in WS individuals,[1,2] and the pathways leading to replicative senescence appear to be conserved in old WS fibroblasts.[5,6]

However, WS fibroblasts show several characteristics of cells growing under conditions of stress (e.g., slow growth rates and an elongated cell cycle) and WS may not be simply accelerated normal cell aging. Cells growing under stressful conditions are often enlarged with prominent F-actin stress fibers,[7] and many young WS cells resemble fibroblasts that have undergone stress-induced premature senescence (SIPS). SIPS results from the activation of p38 MAPK and the use of the p38 selective inhibitor SB203580 essentially prevents the accelerated aging seen in primary WS cells (FIG. 1A), showing that the accelerated aging is due to activation of an SB203580-suppressible pathway. p38 is activated in young WS cells with associated high levels of p21^{WAF1} and phospho-HSP27; thus young WS cells have actin stress fibers and show cell cycle arrest.[4] SB203580 treatment reduces the activated p38, p21^{WAF1}, and phospho-HSP27 levels. In contrast, control young MRC5 cells have low levels of activated p38 that increase as the cells age, and the p21^{WAF1} level is low in young and high in senescent MRC5 cells.[4,8]

Interestingly, SB203580-treated cells have stress fibers when they reach M1 despite low levels of phospho-HSP27.[4] However, normal and WS cells have elevated phospho-cofilin at M1 (FIG. 1E), which is known to induce stress fiber formation in fibroblasts.[9] This shows that several independent pathways are involved in stress fiber formation in fibroblasts. Phospho-cofilin is also elevated in young WS cells and appears to be suppressed with drug treatment. Thus, SB203580-treated young WS cells have low levels of both phospho-HSP27 and phospho-cofilin associated with low levels of F-actin stress fibers.

WS cells can be immortalized using ectopic expression of the catalytic sub-unit of human telomerase;[10] however, the telomerized WS cells retain the slow growth seen in primary WS cells. The growth rate for a typical telom-erized WS culture (AG03141.hTERT clone 8) is 0.31 ± 0.01 PD/day (FIG. 1B).[4] In the presence of SB203580 this rate significantly increases to 0.53 ± 0.02 PD/day, a rate not significantly different from that of telomerized HCA2 cells (0.55 ± 0.07 PD/day; $P > 0.65$). Upon drug removal the growth rate of AG03141.hTERT clone 8 reverts to that seen in untreated cells (0.30 ± 0.05 PD/day). By contrast, SB203580 treatment has no significant effect on the growth rate of telomerized HCA2 cells [0.58 PD/day (FIG. 1B)].

In addition to the slow-growth phenotype, the altered morphology seen in primary WS cells is still apparent in telomerized WS cells, and SB203580 treatment is successful in reverting this phenotype (FIG. 1D) to that seen in telomerized normal cells. The altered morphology of WS cells is associated with high levels of F-actin stress fibers[4] that are still apparent in the telomerized cells (FIG. 1C). As with the primary cells the level of stress fibers in SB203580-treated telomerized cells is low. By contrast, telomerized HCA2 cells have a morphology resembling that of young primary HCA2 cells with few stress fibers and this morphology is not altered by SB203580 treatment (not shown).

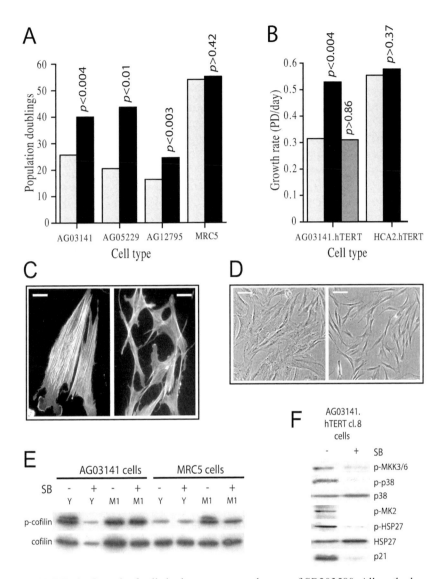

FIGURE 1. Growth of cells in the presence or absence of SB203580. All methods are as described.[4] (**A**) Replicative life span of WS (AG03141, AG05229, AG12795) and MRC5 cells. (**B**) Growth rates of telomerized WS and HCA2 cells. For growth rates: light gray bars = control; black bars = SB-treated; dark gray bar = growth rate after removal of SB203580, statistical significance is a two-tailed *t*-test. (**C**) Phalloidin staining and (**D**) phase-contrast of telomerized WS cells grown in the absence (*left panel*) and presence (*right panel*) of SB203580. Bar = 50 μm in (**C**) and 100 μm in (**D**). Immunoblot analysis of primary WS and MRC5 cells (Y = young, M1 = senescent) (**E**) and telomerized WS cells (**F**). Antibodies used for immunoblots: phospho-MKK3/6(S189/S207), phospho-p38(T180/Y182), p38, phospho-MK2(T334), phospho-HSP27(S82), HSP27, phospho-cofilin(S3), cofilin (cell signaling), p21 (6B6, Becton Dickinson).

That the p38 MAP kinase pathway is still activated despite the telomerized WS cells being immortalized is shown by the presence of phosphorylated forms of p38 and its activating kinase MKK3/6 (Fig. 1F). p38 activity leads to the activation of the downstream kinase MK2 (MAPKAP-K2), which in turn phosphorylates HSP27, leading to stress fiber formation. In addition, there is a high level of p21[WAF1] that should induce a degree of cell cycle arrest. Despite the high p21[WAF1] levels in the telomerized cells, this was a growing culture. As the immunoblot analysis measures an average level of p21[WAF1] for the whole cell population, it is possible that some of the cells had a high p21[WAF1] level and were growth-arrested, while the rest had low p21[WAF1] levels and were thus growing. This would provide an explanation for the slow growth rate of the culture. As expected, SB203580 treatment prevents the phosphorylation of MK2 and HSP27, inhibits stress fiber formation, and suppresses the level of p21[WAF1]. As is the case in young primary WS cells, SB203580 prevents the activation of p38 in telomerized WS cells, and in addition reduces the activation of MKK3/6 (Fig. 1F). These data suggest that the inducing signal in telomerized WS cells (and young WS cells) is distinct from the short-telomere-induced signal seen in old WS and MRC5 primary cells.[4]

CONCLUSIONS

Primary SB203580-treated WS fibroblasts have an increased replicative life span and growth rate compared to untreated cells. p38 is activated in young cells associated with high levels of p21[WAF1] that are suppressed in drug-treated cells. Moreover, p38 activation is still apparent in telomerized WS cells. These data using telomerized WS cells show that the growth problems are still present despite immortalization and telomere maintenance, and thus are most probably not due to major defects in telomere metabolism in WS cells.[11] Therefore, the shortened replicative life span seen in WS cells is due to the activation of a *telomere-independent* stress-induced pathway. As activation of this pathway is still apparent in hTERT-immortalized cells, these telomerized WS cells may be useful for investigating the pathways that lead to premature growth arrest in WS cells.

ACKNOWLEDGMENT

This work was funded by the BBSRC's Experimental Research on Aging Initiative.

REFERENCES

1. KIPLING, D. *et al.* 2004. What can progeroid syndromes tell us about human aging? Science **305**: 1426–1431.

2. MARTIN, G.M. *et al.* 1999. What geriatricians should know about the Werner syndrome. J. Am. Geriatr. Soc. **47:** 1136–1144.

3. HAYFLICK, L. & P.S. MOORHEAD. 1961. The serial cultivation of human diploid cell strains. Exp. Cell Res. **25:** 585–621.

4. DAVIS, T. *et al.* 2005. Prevention of accelerated cell aging in Werner Syndrome using a p38 MAP kinase inhibitor. J. Gerontol. A. Biol. Sci. Med. Sci. **60:** 1386–1393.

5. DAVIS, T. *et al.* 2004. Investigation of the signaling pathways involved in the proliferative lifespan barriers in Werner syndrome fibroblasts. Ann. N.Y. Acad. Sci. **1019:** 274–277.

6. DAVIS, T. *et al.* 2003. Telomere-based proliferative lifespan barriers in Werner-syndrome fibroblasts involve both p53-dependent and p53-independent mechanisms. J. Cell Sci. **116:** 1349–1357.

7. HUOT, J. *et al.* 1997. Oxidative stress-induced actin reorganization mediated by the p38 mitogen-activated protein kinase/heat shock protein 27 pathway in vascular endothelial cells. Circ. Res. **80:** 383–392.

8. DAVIS, T. *et al.* 2005. Replicative senescence in sheep fibroblasts is a p53 dependent process. Exp. Gerontol. **40:** 17–26.

9. PRITCHARD, C.A. *et al.* 2004. B-Raf acts via the ROCKII/LIMK/cofilin pathway to maintain actin stress fibers in fibroblasts. Mol. Cell Biol. **24:** 5937–5952.

10. WYLLIE, F.S. *et al.* 2000. Telomerase prevents the accelerated cell ageing of Werner syndrome fibroblasts. Nat. Genet. **24:** 16–17.

11. BAIRD, D.M. *et al.* 2004. Normal telomere erosion rates at the single cell level in Werner syndrome fibroblast cells. Hum. Mol. Genet. **13:** 1515–1524.

Oxidative Stress Induces Intralysosomal Accumulation of Alzheimer Amyloid β-Protein in Cultured Neuroblastoma Cells

LIN ZHENG,[a] KARIN ROBERG,[b] FREDRIK JERHAMMAR,[c] JAN MARCUSSON,[a] AND ALEXEI TERMAN[c]

[a]Division of Geriatric Medicine, Faculty of Health Sciences, Linköping University, Linköping, Sweden

[b]Division of Otorhinolaryngology, Faculty of Health Sciences, Linköping University, Linköping, Sweden

[c]Division of Experimental Pathology, Faculty of Health Sciences, Linköping University, Linköping, Sweden

ABSTRACT: Oxidative stress is considered important for the pathogenesis of Alzheimer's disease (AD), which is characterized by the formation of extracellular senile plaques, mainly composed of amyloid β-protein (Aβ). Aβ also accumulates within AD neurons and is believed to exert cellular toxicity through lysosomal labilization. We report that the exposure of human neuroblastoma cells to hyperoxia (40% vs. 8% ambient oxygen) induced the accumulation of large (over 1 μM) Aβ-containing lysosomes, which were not typical of control cells, showing a distinct localization of Aβ and lysosomal markers. An inhibitor of autophagy, 3-methyladenine, suppressed the effect of hyperoxia. The results suggest a link between the involvement of oxidative stress and lysosomes in AD.

KEYWORDS: Alzheimer disease; amyloid β-protein; autophagy; lysosomes; oxidative stress

INTRODUCTION

Alzheimer's disease (AD), the main cause of senile dementia, is a neurodegenerative disorder characterized by the formation of extraneuronal plaques, largely composed of amyloid β-protein (Aβ).[1] Aβ also has been found within neurons, and is believed to promote neuronal death, preceding senile plaque formation.[2] AD neurons are known to contain increased numbers of lysosomes,

Address for correspondence: Lin Zheng, Division of Geriatric Medicine, Faculty of Health Sciences, Linköping University, SE-58185 Linköping, Sweden. Voice: +46-13-222271; fax: +46-13-221529.
e-mail: linzh@inr.liu.se

Ann. N.Y. Acad. Sci. 1067: 248–251 (2006). © 2006 New York Academy of Sciences.
doi: 10.1196/annals.1354.032

suggesting their involvement in AD.[3] In addition to this point, Aβ has been shown to partially colocalize with neuronal lysosomes in transgenic mouse model of AD,[4] while in differentiated neuroblastoma cells lysosomes mediated the toxicity of Aβ added to the culture medium.[5,6] Another line of evidence implicates oxidative stress as an important contributor to AD pathogenesis.[7] It is, however, not clear whether the pathogenic role of oxidative stress in AD is dependent on the lysosomal system. To address this question, we studied the effect of oxidative stress on intracellular localization of Aβ42 (a more toxic form of the peptide than Aβ40) in differentiated neuroblastoma cells.

MATERIALS AND METHODS

Human SH-SY5Y neuroblastoma cells obtained from the American Type Culture Collection were differentiated in 10 μM all-*trans* retinoic acid for 14 days. Differentiated cells were plated at a density of 10^5 cells per cm^2 and maintained for 5 days either in OptiMEM1 medium (Gibco Paisley, UK) supplemented with 5% fetal bovine serum in 8% ambient oxygen (normoxia), or in serum-free OptiMEM under normoxia, or in serum-free OptiMEM under hyperoxia (40% ambient oxygen). Some cultures were simultaneously exposed to 5 mM 3-methyladenine for inhibition of autophagy. Formalin-fixed cells were double-immunostained for Aβ42 (rabbit anti-human antibodies, Chemicon Temecula, CA) and lysosomal-associated membrane protein 2 (LAMP-2, mouse anti-human antibodies, Southern Biotechnology, Birmingham, AL), or for Aβ42 and early endosomal marker rab5 (mouse anti-human antibodies, Pharmingen, SanDiego, CA). Secondary antibodies were Alexa Fluor 488-conjugated goat anti-rabbit and Alexa Fluor 595-conjugated goat anti-mouse IgG (both from Molecular Probes). For visualization of autophagy, cultures were processed for transmission electron microscopy.

RESULTS AND DISCUSSION

Neuroblastoma cells that were cultured under normoxia in the presence of serum contained small cytoplasmic Aβ42-positive granules, not colocalized with LAMP-2, a lysosomal and late endosomal marker (FIG. 1 A–C). Serum withdrawal (known to activate autophagy) resulted in the appearance of occasional large (over 1 μM in diameter) vacuoles, positive for both Aβ42 and LAMP-2 (not shown). The percentage of cells that contained such large vacuoles increased dramatically when serum withdrawal was combined with hyperoxia (17% vs. 0.7%). The Aβ42 and LAMP-2 positive vacuoles that occurred under hyperoxia were also larger than those found in normoxia. Aβ42 was usually seen in the interior of such vacuoles and was surrounded

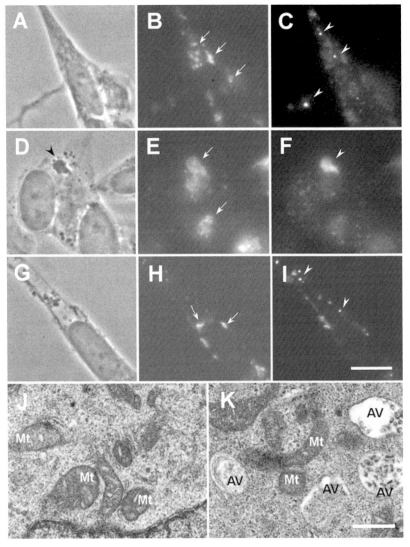

FIGURE 1. Autophagy of Aβ42 following oxidative stress. (A–I) SH-SY5Y neuroblastoma cells double-immunostained for LAMP-2 and Aβ42. (**A, D, G**) phase-contrast mode; (**B, E, H**) LAMP-2 immunoreactivity, red channel; (**C, F, I**) Aβ42 immunoreactivity, green channel. LAMP-2 (*white arrows*) and Aβ42 (*white arrowheads*) are not colocalized in cells cultured in the presence of serum under normoxia (**A–C**). Serum withdrawal combined with hyperoxia (**D–F**) induces the appearance of large vacuoles (*black arrowhead,* **D**) that are positive for both LAMP-2 and Aβ42, while 3-methyladenine inhibits this effect (**G–I**). (**J, K**) Electron micrographs of neuroblasoma cells maintained in the presence of serum under normoxia and without serum under hyperoxia, respectively. The number of autophagic vacuoles (AV) is dramatically increased in K versus J. Mt, mitochondria. Bars represent 10 and 0.5 μm for light and electron microscopy images, respectively.

by LAMP-2-positive membranes (FIG. 1 D–F). 3-Methyladenine prevented the formation of Aβ42-containing lysosomes/late endosomes (FIG. 1 G–I), suggesting that Aβ42 is autophagocytosed. The activation of autophagy in response to oxidative stress is confirmed by electron microscopy (FIG. 1 J, K). Rab5 was not colocalized with Aβ42 under any experimental condition (not shown), thus excluding the possibility that Aβ42 entered the lysosomal system through endocytosis. Our results suggest that oxidant-induced autophagy of Aβ followed by lysosomal-mediated Aβ toxicity to neurons[5,6] might represent a possible pathogenic mechanism of AD.

REFERENCES

1. MATTSON, M.P. 2004. Pathways towards and away from Alzheimer's disease. Nature **430:** 631–639.
2. GOURAS, G.K., J. TSAI, J. NASLUND, *et al.* 2000. Intraneuronal Abeta42 accumulation in human brain. Am. J. Pathol. **156:** 15–20.
3. NIXON, R.A., A.M. CATALDO & P.M. MATHEWS. 2000. The endosomal-lysosomal system of neurons in Alzheimer's disease pathogenesis: a review. Neurochem. Res. **25:** 1161–1172.
4. LANGUI, D., N. GIRARDOT, K.H. EL HACHIMI, *et al.* 2004. Subcellular topography of neuronal Abeta peptide in APPxPS1 transgenic mice. Am. J. Pathol. **165:** 1465–1477.
5. YANG, A.J., D. CHANDSWANGBHUVANA, L. MARGOL, *et al.* 1998. Loss of endosomal/lysosomal membrane impermeability is an early event in amyloid Abeta1-42 pathogenesis. J. Neurosci. Res. **52:** 691–698.
6. DITARANTO, K., T.L. TEKIRIAN & A.J. YANG. 2001. Lysosomal membrane damage in soluble Abeta-mediated cell death in Alzheimer's disease. Neurobiol. Dis. **8:** 19–31.
7. ZHU, X., A.K. RAINA, H.G. LEE, *et al.* 2004. Oxidative stress signalling in Alzheimer's disease. Brain Res. **1000:** 32–39.

The Genetics of Human Longevity

MIRIAM CAPRI,[a,b] STEFANO SALVIOLI,[a,b] FEDERICA SEVINI,[a,b] SILVANA VALENSIN,[a,b] LAURA CELANI,[a,b] DANIELA MONTI,[c] GRAHAM PAWELEC,[d] GIOVANNA DE BENEDICTIS,[e] EFSTATHIOS S. GONOS,[f] AND CLAUDIO FRANCESCHI[a,b,g]

[a]CIG, Interdepartmental Center "L.Galvani," University of Bologna, Bologna, Italy

[b]Department of Experimental Pathology, University of Bologna, Bologna, Italy

[c]Department of Experimental Oncology and Pathology, University of Firenze, Firenze, Italy

[d]Center for Medical Research, ZMF, University of Tübingen, Tübingen, Germany

[e]Department of Cell Biology, University of Calabria, Calabria, Italy

[f]Institute of Biological Research & Biotechnology, NHR Foundation, Athens, Greece

[g]INRCA, National Institute for Research on Aging, Ancona, Italy

ABSTRACT: Aging is due to a complex interaction of genetic, epigenetic, and environmental factors, but a strong genetic component appears to have an impact on survival to extreme ages. In order to identify "longevity genes" in humans, different strategies are now available. In our laboratory, we performed association studies on a variety of "candidate" polymorphisms in Italian centenarians. Many genes/polymorphisms gave negative results, while others showed a positive association with human longevity and a sometimes-positive association with unsuccessful aging (myocardial infarction, Alzheimer's disease, and type 2 diabetes). Results regarding genes involved in inflammation (IL-1 cluster, IL-6, IL-10, TNF-α, TGF-β, TLR-4, PPARγ), insulin/IGF-1 signaling pathway and lipid metabolism (apolipoproteins, CETP, PON1), and oxidative stress (p53, p66^{shc}) will be described. In addition, a strong role of the interaction between nuclear and mitochondrial genomes (mtDNA haplogroups and the C150T mutation) emerged from our findings. Thus, the genetics of human longevity appears to be quite peculiar in a context where antagonistic pleiotropy can play a major role and genes can have a different biological role at different ages.

Address for correspondence: Prof. Claudio Franceschi, M.D., CIG – Centro Interdipartimentale "L. Galvani," University of Bologna, Via S. Giacomo, 12, 40126 Bologna, Italy. Voice: +39 051 2094740; fax: +39 051 2094747.
e-mail: claudio.franceschi@unibo.it

Ann. N.Y. Acad. Sci. 1067: 252–263 (2006). © 2006 New York Academy of Sciences.
doi: 10.1196/annals.1354.033

KEYWORDS: IL-1 cluster; IL-6; IL-10; TNF-α; TGF-β; TLR-4; insulin/ IGF-1; apolipoproteins; CETP; PON1; p53, p66^{shc}; PPARγ; longevity genes

INTRODUCTION

The genetic trait plays a key role in survival to extreme ages. But which are the genes that, if modified or deregulated, have an impact on the life span? In order to answer this question different model systems have been used, such as *Saccharomyces cerevisiae*, *Caenorhabditis elegans*, *Drosophila melanogaster*, and *Mus musculus*. Nowadays, many data are available from these animal models, but in humans the situation is much more complex since human aging is due to interactions among genetic, epigenetic, environmental, and cultural factors. How is it possible to study adequately the longevity genes in this frame of interactions? At least five types of studies can be performed, with advantages and disadvantages for each one: (1) centenarians vs. young/old subjects; (2) very old sib pairs; (3) young/old twins; (4) families with very old members; and (5) longitudinal studies on cohorts of different ages. In addition, different strategies of genetic analysis can be applied, such as association studies on "candidate" genes, where the frequency of genetic variants is compared between young people and centenarians; genome scanning of the entire (or part) genome, without any *a priori* assumptions; and studies on genome regions having specific characteristics (e.g., high density of *Alu* sequence).

For many years, in our laboratory, association studies on different "candidate" genes have been performed by comparing Italian centenarians with young/old subjects, and the most important findings will be now described and are briefly summarized in FIGURE 1.

Inflammation and Immune-Response Genes

The *in silico* approach to understanding the cells' functional organization suggests a scale-free network and the presence of "hub" genes that could receive and direct the activity of many other genes.[1] Our recent data confirmed the topology of the network and suggest that some mediators of immune response, and specifically of inflammatory response, could be most responsible for "directive" interconnections inside the immune system.[2] This appears to be likely also in aging "remodeling." Indeed, it has been observed that a typical feature of the aging process is a general increase in plasma levels of and cell capability to produce proinflammatory cytokines.[3–8] This can lead to a chronic "proinflammatory" state, which promotes or exacerbates age-related pathological conditions (cardiovascular diseases, atherosclerosis, Alzheimer's

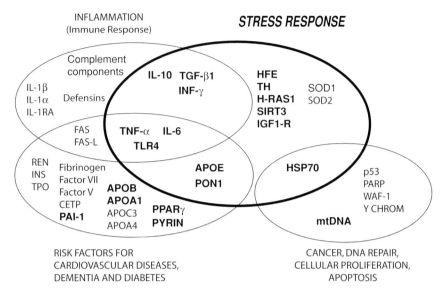

FIGURE 1. Candidate genes in association studies for human longevity. Different groups of genes were analyzed for their possible association with human longevity, but only the genes related to stress response were positively associated together with APOB, APOPA1, PAI-1, PPARγ PYRIN, and mitochondrial genome (mt DNA).

disease, arthrosis and arthritis, sarcopenia, and type 2 diabetes, among others). Large studies have demonstrated that high plasma levels of IL-6 are correlated with greater disability, morbidity, and mortality in the elderly.[9] Moreover, high levels of IL-6, IL-1β and C-reactive protein are significantly associated with poor physical performance and muscle strength in older persons.[10] Serum levels of TNF-α are considered a strong predictor of mortality in both 80-year-old people[11] and centenarians.[12] Thus, if a strong inflammatory response means higher risk of life-threatening diseases, longevity should be correlated with the capability to maintain an inflammatory response of low intensity. This has been partially confirmed by findings in centenarians, who are considered the best example of longevity. When we studied the polymorphism for a C to G transition at nucleotide −174 of the IL-6 gene promoter (−174 C/G locus), IL-6 production was increased in C− (GG genotype) but not in C+ (CC and CG genotypes) old subjects, and this phenomenon was significant only in males.[13] Moreover, we have recently found that the IL-6 −174 C/G polymorphism is an independent predictor of cardiovascular death after an acute coronary syndrome (ACS) in male patients. Data showed that ACS patients carrying the IL-6 −174 C− (GG) genotypes underwent a marked increase in 1-year follow-up mortality rate (HR = 3.89, 95% CI 1.71–8.86, $P = 0.001$), thus suggesting that the IL-6 −174 C/G polymorphism can be added to other clinical markers in order to identify a subgroup of elderly ACS male patients at a higher risk of death.[14]

Accordingly, in male centenarians the frequency of C− subjects was less than expected. Similar data on the decreased frequency of IL-6 −174 C− subjects in Irish octogenarian and nonagenarian subjects from the Belfast Elderly Longitudinal Free-living Ageing study have been recently reported.[15,16]

Indeed, we observed that plasma levels of an anti-inflammatory cytokine such as TGF-β are found to be increased in centenarians as compared to young people.[17] Another anti-inflammatory cytokine, IL-10, has a genetic polymorphism (−1082 G→A) that has been suggested to be correlated with high production of IL-10, and subjects carrying the −1082GG genotype are found to be more represented among centenarians[18] and to be less affected by diseases such as Alzheimer's disease.[19] Nevertheless, quite paradoxically, proinflammatory characteristics have also been documented in healthy centenarians.[20] It is thus evident that human longevity is at least in part determined by factors other than the capability to maintain an inflammatory response at low level of intensity. We addressed this point and hypothesized that *inflamm-aging*, a term coined by us to indicate a shift toward a proinflammatory profile at a systemic level[21] (despite being an inescapable result of long-lasting exposure to acute and chronic infections[22] and the consequent lifelong antigenic burden), by itself is not a sufficient condition to trigger age-related diseases and to reduce survival. We predicted that a second factor is necessary, including a genetic predisposition to the onset of specific age-related diseases (such as ApoE 4 polymorphism) and to strong inflammatory responses.[21,23]

Recently, another gene such as Toll-like receptor 4 (TLR-4) seems to be relevant for human longevity. It is a signaling receptor involved in innate immune defense, and its activity may be modulated by genetic polymorphisms. In atherosclerotic tissue, TLR-4 expression is markedly upregulated, and the inflammatory mediators produced by its activation exert various atherogenic effects. Recently, different TLR4 genotypes were evaluated in association with acute myocardial infarction (AMI) and with longevity. In particular, the Asp299Gly SNP was studied. G allele (Gly is the G allele) was less frequent in patients with acute myocardial infarction as compared to the general population, and in addition, was more frequent in the oldest old people, suggesting that it likely plays a role in longevity.[24] However, contradictory results are reported in the literature.[25]

Stress-Response Genes

Genes that counteract oxidative stress, such as the superoxide dismutase (SOD1 and SOD2) and paraxonase (PON1), are important "candidate" genes for longevity. Our study regarding SOD2 polymorphisms (T/C 401 nt) in 196 centenarians from northern and southern Italy did not reveal any age-dependent difference in the allelic or genotypic frequency.[26] PON1, a high-density lipoprotein (HDL)-associated esterase that hydrolyses lipoperoxides, could be a protective factor against oxidative modification of low-density lipoprotein (LDL) and may therefore play an important role in the prevention of the atherosclerotic process. Two polymorphisms have been extensively studied: a leucine (L allele) to methionine (M allele) substitution at codon 55, and a glutamine (A allele) to arginine (B allele) substitution at codon 192. These two amino acid changes have been examined in 579 people aged 20 to 65 years, and 308 centenarians. Results showed that the percentage of carriers of the B allele (B+ individuals) is higher in centenarians than in controls (0.539 vs. 0.447) and that among the B+ individuals this phenomenon is correlated to an increase of people carrying M allele at codon 55.[27] These results have been recently confirmed by an independent study performed on Irish octogenarians and nonagenarians.[28] Interestingly, the Leiden study[29] reported no significant effect of PON1 variability on mortality, leading to the hypothesis that this polymorphism does not have a major effect on the risk of fatal cardiovascular diseases at the population level, as recently confirmed in a large cohort study of British women.[30] However, PON1 variability at codon 192 appears to be a good marker of biological age in the elderly, being age indicators less numerous in B allele carriers.[31] Moreover, the combined analysis of the two polymorphisms (codon 192 and codon 55) in young, elderly, and centenarian subjects shows that the PON1 activity decreases significantly during aging; in detail, both B+ carriers and M− carriers have significantly higher PON1 activity, thus suggesting that paraoxonase activity contributes significantly to explaining the longevity phenotype.[32]

Insulin/IGF-1 Pathways

It has been observed in animal models that mutations in genes sharing similarities with human genes involved in the insulin/IGF-I signal transduction pathway can extend animal life span. Accordingly, studies in humans outlined that centenarians have preserved insulin responsiveness and low levels of serum IGF-I (reviewed in Ref. 33). The levels of IGF-I were also found to be affected by a polymorphism at IGF-I receptor and phosphoinositide 3-kinase genes.[34] Nevertheless, low levels of serum IGF-I have been correlated with greater disability and mortality in the elderly.[35] This apparent discrepancy is probably a case of antagonistic pleiotropy. Indeed, we showed that high levels of IGF-I contribute to maintaining the muscle mass and strength in the elderly, thus avoiding disability, but at the price of an increased incidence of cancer,[36] which likely takes advantage of high levels of growth factors such as IGF-I. On the other hand, low levels of IGF-I would protect against cancer growth thus favoring overall survival, but at the price of reduced muscle mass and increased disability. Moreover, it is to be noted that IGF-1 protection against muscle mass loss appears to depend on IL-6 levels.[37] Thus, if on the one hand the role of IGF-1 appears to be double-sided, on the other hand, high levels of IL-6 appear to be always detrimental for both longevity and disability.

Lower body mass index (BMI) means less muscle mass but also less adipose tissue. Can an efficient lipid metabolism favor longevity through the regulation of inflammatory responses? There is a large amount of evidence indicating that this is the case. Adipose tissue has long been considered as a mere store of lipids. Now, it appears to be an extremely active tissue at least from an endocrinological point of view, as it is considered one of the main sources of proinflammatory cytokines, such as IL-6, TNF-α, leptin, prostaglandins, C-reactive protein, plasminogen activator inhibitor-1 (PAI-1), angiotensinogen, and resistin (for a review, see Ref. 38). All these compounds are involved or suspected to play a role in atherosclerosis and vascular injury, insulin resistance, metabolic syndrome, and obesity-linked diabetes. Accumulation of fat tissue (obesity) and low-grade chronic inflammation are deeply connected; thus it is expected that in obese people inflamm-aging is much more evident than in lean people, and consequently lean people are expected to be, in general, less affected by inflammation-based diseases (therefore more long-living) than obese people. Furthermore, the study of the combined effect of peroxisome proliferator-activated receptor gamma (PPARγ) Pro/Ala, and interleukin-6 G174C gene variants showed that subjects carrying both PPARG and IL-6 gene variants (Ala+/C+) had a clearly more favorable profile of obesity-related risk factors than subjects with one variant, having lower BMI (22.8 ± 2.3 vs. 24.14 ± 1.9; $f = 5.31$; $P < 0.005$), insulin resistance (1.49 ± 0.70 vs. 2.13 ± 0.92; $f = 4.342$; $P = 0.038$), and triglyceride levels (79.15 ± 32.9 vs. 98 ± 6.73 mg/dL; $f = 3.120$; $P < 0.005$). These findings suggest that the effect of the two genetic variants on "obesity-related" factors is additive.[39]

These results suggest that the combined effect of PPARγ and IL-6 variants could have an important role in longevity, found in centenarians with low BMI and low insulin resistance.[40]

p53

p53 is important for its involvement not only in several molecular pathways (apoptosis, DNA repair, senescence, cell cycle arrest) and in antitumor activity but also in aging. Many p53 polymorphisms that displayed an association with different tumor types have been studied on more than 1,100 subjects from 20 up to 110 years of age. Surprisingly, no difference in the frequency of all these polymorphisms was found between young people and centenarians. Thus, apparently these polymorphisms do not seem to influence the possibility of reaching the extreme limits of life span,[41] but recently a study showed that variation in p53 gene at codon 72 (polymorphism encoding an arginine to proline amino acid substitution) affects old age survival and cancer mortality;

in particular Pro/Pro subjects have a 41% increased survival despite a 2.54-fold increase in proportional mortality from cancer.[42] Authors suggest that human p53 protects against cancer, but at the cost of longevity. These data are in contrast with those obtained in our previous studies;[41] it is to be noted that both the mean age and ethnicity of the studied populations were different and this can at least in part account for this discrepancy.

Moreover, this polymorphism at the 72 codon was found to influence the survival at 10 years of a subgroup of patients with mammary carcinoma[43] and it influences the susceptibility to undergo oxidative stress– or chemotherapeutic drugs–induced apoptosis (2-deoxy-D-ribose, cytosine arabinoside, doxorubicin, and camptothecin). In particular, the presence of proline allele is associated with lower susceptibility to apoptosis in comparison with its absence (arginine homozygotes), but this phenomenon is evident only in cells from elderly subjects and especially from centenarians.[44–46] These last results confirm the general hypothesis that the same allele could have different effects at different ages.

Apolipoproteins and mtDNA

A plethora of studies indicated that genes of apolipoproteins (APOE, APOB, APOA1, APOA4, APOC3) are involved in aging, longevity, and a number of age-related diseases. The ApoE4 allele is the most studied for longevity, with the most concordant results in the literature. This alllele is also associated with Alzheimer's disease and cardiovascular disease; it is considered as a sort of gold standard for the genetics of human longevity. Many studies on centenarians and young people confirmed that ApoE4 frequency is significantly lower in Italian centenarians (4.3%) in comparison with the control group (9.4%), confirming that the E4 variant plays a negative role in longevity. In the same studies, genotypic analysis of Alzheimer's patients was also performed, confirming that ApoE4 is increased in these patients (27%); thus the presence of at least one ApoE4 allele represents a high risk for Alzheimer's disease.[47] Anyway, the most interesting result in this work is related to the mitochondrial genome (mtDNA) and specifically to its polymorphic variants (haplogroups). Genotypic analysis of these germ-line variants of mtDNA revealed that the odds ratio for Alzheimer's disease varies in E4 subjects from 1 to 9, depending on the mtDNA haplogroup of the subject; in particular, K and U haplogroups seem to neutralize the harmful effect of E4 alleles. This suggests that the penetrance of the E4 allele strictly depends on the interaction (cross-talk) between mitochondrial and nuclear genomes.

Other data are concerned with VNTR-like polymorphisms (variable number of tandem repeats) of the ApoB gene. An age-related variation of the $3'$APOBVNTR genotypic pool (alleles: *Short, S,* <35 repeats; *Medium, M,* 35–39 repeats; *Long, L,* >39 repeats) with the homozygous *SS* genotype shows a convex frequency trajectory in a healthy aging population. This genotype was rare in centenarians, thus indicating that the *S* alleles are not favorable for longevity, while being common in adults, thus indicating a protective role at middle age.[48] Recently published data from the same group try to explain this kind of trajectory.[49] Moreover, the frequency of the longest variants was found to be significantly higher in centenarians in comparison with young people. Nevertheless, the same study performed using DNA from Danish centenarians did not confirm the data previously obtained for the Italian population, thus suggesting a more complex scenario of population genetics.[50]

A study on centenarians and young people from southern Italy showed no difference in allelic and genotypic polymorphisms of APOA4 and APOC3. On the contrary, the frequency of P allele of the APOA1 polymorphism (APOA1-msp1-RFLP, -75 nt from the transcription start site) is significantly increased in male centenarians.[51] It is interesting to note that this polymorphism is associated with a high serum level of LDL-C, which is a well-established risk factor for cardiovascular disease. This is not the first paradox found in centenarians: another example is given by the state of hypercoagulability[52] related to a high risk of thrombosis that is found in centenarians compared to the normal population.

In addition, when some years ago our group studied lipoprotein (a) (Lp(a)), and lipoprotein profile in subjects at different ages, results showed that Lp(a) serum levels did not vary with age. Remarkably, one-quarter of the studied centenarians had high Lp(a) serum levels, even though they never suffered from atherosclerosis-related diseases.[53] At variance with young and aged people, centenarians with high Lp(a) serum levels also had high plasma concentrations of the proinflammatory cytokine IL-6, suggesting that genetic control of the Lp(a) serum level may attenuate with age and that environmental factors such as chronic subclinical inflammatory processes may play a role.

Our recent study was focused on a common polymorphism (1405V) in exon 14 of the cholesteryl ester transfer protein (CETP) gene, which was found to be associated with healthy aging in Ashkenazi Jews,[54] but in a sample of 175 Italian centenarians and 189 controls, we did not confirm this association.[55] This result stresses the importance of replicating association studies on candidate genes on different populations in order to avoid false-positive results and to check the general value of the observation.

CONCLUSIONS

In conclusion, trying to answer the question of which genes could influence human longevity, it is possible to affirm that many functional polymorphisms/genes, and probably their interactions, could have this effect. In FIGURE 1 a scheme of the most important investigated genes is shown. In this figure, the genes that were positively associated with longevity appear to belong mostly to the group of stress-response genes together with some important genes such as APOB, APOA1, PAI-1 PPARγ, PYRIN, and mtDNA. Many of these genetic variants can influence the level of chronic inflammation, and thus the overall survival in the elderly. In addition, most of these genes could be "hub" genes that can shift and modify the activity of other genes (i.e., highly connected genes in critical metabolic pathways, such as stress response, inflammation, glucose and insulin metabolism, among others). Thus genomic functionality could be strictly associated with new epigenetic/genetic interactions due to the inflamm-aging microenvironment. Indeed, it is necessary to outline that the genetics of human longevity appears to be quite peculiar (a post-reproductive genetics) where antagonistic pleiotropy can play a major role and genes can have a different biological role at different ages.

However, it is necessary to replicate genetic studies in different populations, taking into account critical confounding variables, such as gender, ethnicity, and health status of the studied subjects. Moreover, it is important to outline again that studies with animal models could produce data that are not overlapping with humans. This is the case of p66[shc]. Knockout animals for this gene have an extended life span,[56] but we demonstrated that in centenarians p66[shc] is overexpressed,[57] thus suggesting that different and more complicated molecular pathways for human longevity are to be considered.

ACKNOWLEDGMENTS

This work has been supported by grants from the EU (European Union) 6th FP Project "GEHA—Genetics of Healthy Aging," "T-CIA – T-Cells Immunity and Aging," EU (Fondi Strutturali Obiettivo 2), the PRRIITT program of the Emilia-Romagna Region, MIUR (Italian Ministry of University) Programmi di Ricerca di Interesse Nazionale (PRIN) protocol 2003068355_002, and Fondo per gli Investimenti della Ricerca di Base (FIRB) protocols RBNE018AAP and RBNE018R89 to C.F.

REFERENCES

1. BARABASI, A.L. & Z.N., OLTVAI. 2004. Network biology: understanding the cell's functional organization. Nat. Rev. Genet. **5:** 101–113.
2. TIERI, P. *et al.* 2005. Quantifying the relevance of different mediators in the human immune cell network. Bioinformatics **21:** 1639–1643.
3. FAGIOLO, U. *et al.* 1993. Increased cytokine production in mononuclear cells of healthy elderly people. Eur. J. Immunol. **23:** 2375–2378.
4. DI IORIO, A. *et al.* 2003. Serum IL-1beta levels in health and disease: a population-based study. 'The InCHIANTI study'. Cytokine **22:** 198–205.
5. GERLI, R. *et al.* 2000. Chemokines, sTNF-Rs and sCD30 serum levels in healthy aged people and centenarians. Mech. Ageing Dev. **121:** 37–46.

6. WEI, J. *et al.* 1992. Increase of plasma IL-6 concentration with age in healthy subjects. Life Sci. **51:** 1953–1956.
7. ERSHLER, W.B. *et al.* 1993. Interleukin-6 and aging: blood levels and mononuclear cell production increase with advancing age and in vitro production is modifiable by dietary restriction. Lymphokine Cytokine Res. **12:** 225–230.
8. BRUUNSGAARD, H. *et al.* 1999. A high plasma concentration of TNF-alpha is associated with dementia in centenarians. J. Gerontol. A Biol. Sci. Med. Sci. **54:** M357–364.
9. FERRUCCI, L. *et al.* 1999. Serum IL-6 level and the development of disability in older persons J. Am. Geriatr. Soc. **47:** 639–646.
10. CESARI, M. *et al.* 2004. Inflammatory markers and physical performance in older persons: the InCHIANTI study. J. Gerontol. A Biol. Sci. Med. Sci. **59:** 242–248.
11. BRUUNSGAARD, H. *et al.* 2003. Predicting death from tumour necrosis factor-alpha and interleukin-6 in 80-year-old people. Clin. Exp. Immunol. **132:** 24–31.
12. BRUUNSGAARD, H. *et al.* 2003. Elevated levels of tumor necrosis factor alpha and mortality in centenarians. Am. J. Med. **115:** 278–283.
13. OLIVIERI, F. *et al.* 2002. −174 C/G locus affects in vitro/vivo IL-6 production during aging. Exp. Gerontol. **37:** 309–314.
14. ANTONICELLI, R. *et al.* 2005. The interleukin-6 −174 G>C promoter polymorphism is associated with a higher risk of death after an acute coronary syndrome in male elderly patients. Intl. J. Cardiol. **103:** 266–271.
15. REA, I.M. *et al.* 2003. Interleukin-6-gene C/G 174 polymorphism in nonagenarian and octogenarian subjects in the BELFAST study: reciprocal effects on IL-6, soluble IL-6 receptor and for IL-10 in serum and monocyte supernatants. Mech. Ageing Develop. **124:** 555–561.
16. ROSS, O.A. *et al.* 2003. Study of age-association with cytokine gene polymorphisms in an aged Irish population. Mech. Ageing Develop. **124:** 199–206.
17. CARRIERI, G. *et al.* 2004. The G/C915 polymorphism of transforming growth factor beta1 is associated with human longevity: a study in Italian centenarians. Aging Cell **3:** 443–448.
18. LIO, D. *et al.* 2002. Gender-specific association between −1082 IL-10 promoter polymorphism and longevity. Genes Immun. **3:** 30–33.
19. LIO, D. *et al.* 2003. Interleukin-10 promoter polymorphism in sporadic Alzheimer's disease. Genes Immun. **4:** 234–238.
20. BAGGIO, G. *et al.* 1998. Lipoprotein(a) and lipoprotein profile in healthy centenarians: a reappraisal of vascular risk factors. FASEB J. **12:** 433–437.
21. FRANCESCHI, C. *et al.* 2000. Inflamm-aging: an evolutionary perspective on immunosenescence. Ann. N. Y. Acad. Sci. **908:** 244–254.
22. GINALDI, L. *et al.* 2005. Chronic antigenic load and apoptosis in immunosenescence. Trends Immunol. **26:** 79–84.
23. FRANCESCHI, C. & M. BONAFÈ. 2003. Centenarians as a model for healthy aging. Biochem. Soc. Trans. **31:** 457–461.
24. BALISTRERI, C.R. *et al.* 2004. Role of Toll-like receptor 4 in acute myocardial infarction and longevity. JAMA **292:** 2339–2340.
25. SCHRÖDER, N.W.J. & R.R. SHUMANN. 2005. Single nucleotide polymorphisms of Toll-like receptors and susceptibility to infectious disease. Lancet Infect. Dis. **5:** 156–164.
26. DE BENEDICTIS, G. *et al.* 1998. Gene/longevity association studies at four autosomal loci (REN, THO, PARP, SOD2). Eur. J. Hum. Genet. **6:** 534–541.

27. BONAFÈ, M. *et al.* 2002. Genetic analysis of paraoxonase (PON1) locus reveals an increased frequency of Arg192 allele in centenarians. Eur. J. Hum. Genet. **10:** 292–296.

28. REA, I.M. *et al.* 2004. Paraoxonase polymorphisms PON1 192 and 55 and longevity in Italian centenarians and Irish nonagenarians. A pooled analysis. Exp. Gerontol. **39:** 629–635.

29. HEIJMANS, B.T. *et al.* 2000. Common paraoxonase gene variants, mortality risk and fatal cardiovascular events in elderly subjects. Atherosclerosis. **149:** 91–97.

30. LAWLOR, D.A. *et al.* 2004. The challenge of secondary prevention for coronary heart disease in older patients: findings from the British Women's Heart and Health Study and the British Regional Heart Study. Fam. Pract. **21:** 582–586.

31. XIA, Y. *et al.* 2003. Effect of six candidate genes on early aging in a French population. Aging Clin. Exp. Res. **15:** 111–116.

32. MARCHEGIANI, F. *et al.* 2006. Paraoxonase activity and genotype predispose to a successful aging. J. Gerontol. Ser. A Biol. Sci. Med. Sci. In press.

33. FRANCESCHI, C. *et al.* 2005. Genes involved in immune response/inflammation, IGF1/insulin pathway and response to oxidative stress play a major role in the genetics of human longevity: the lesson of centenarians. Mech. Ageing. Dev. **126:** 351–361.

34. BONAFÈ, M. *et al.* 2003. Polymorphic variants of insulin-like growth factor I (IGF-I) receptor and phosphoinositide 3-kinase genes affect IGF-I plasma levels and human longevity: cues for an evolutionarily conserved mechanism of life span control. J. Clin. Endocrinol. Metab. **88:** 3299–3304.

35. CAPPOLA, A.R. *et al.* 2003. Insulin-like growth factor I and interleukin-6 contribute synergistically to disability and mortality in older women. J. Clin. Endocrinol. Metab. **88:** 2019–2025.

36. POLLAK, M.N. *et al.* 2004. Insulin-like growth factors and neoplasia. Nat. Rev. Cancer **4:** 505–518.

37. BARBIERI, M. *et al.* 2003. Chronic inflammation and the effect of IGF-I on muscle strength and power in older persons. Am. J. Physiol. Endocrinol. Metab. **284:** E481–E487.

38. LAU, D.C. *et al.* 2005. Adipokines: molecular links between obesity and atheroslcerosis. Am. J. Physiol. Heart Circ. Physiol. **288:** H2031–H2041.

39. BARBIERI, M. *et al.* 2005. Role of interaction between variants in the PPARG and interleukin-6 genes on obesity related metabolic risk factors. Exp. Gerontol. **40:** 599–604.

40. PAOLISSO, G. *et al.* 2001. Low insulin resistance and preserved beta-cell function contribute to human longevity but are not associated with TH-INS genes. Exp Gerontol. **37:** 149–156.

41. BONAFÈ, M. *et al.* 1999. p53 variants predisposing to cancer are present in healthy centenarians. Am. J. Hum. Genet. **64:** 292–295.

42. VAN HEEMST, D. *et al.* and LONG LIFE STUDY GROUP. 2005. Variation in the human TP53 gene affects old age survival and cancer mortality. Exp. Gerontol. **40:** 11–15.

43. BONAFÈ, M. *et al.* 2003. Retention of the p53 codon 72 arginine allele is associated with a reduction of disease-free and overall survival in arginine/proline heterozygous breast cancer patients. Clin. Cancer Res. **9:** 4860–4864.

44. BONAFÈ, M. *et al.* 2002. p53 codon 72 genotype affects apoptosis by cytosine arabinoside in blood leukocytes. Biochem. Biophys. Res. Commun. **299:** 539–541.

45. BONAFÈ, M. *et al.* 2004. The different apoptotic potential of the p53 codon 72 alleles increases with age and modulates *in vivo* ischemia-induced cell death. Cell Death Differ. **11:** 962–973.

46. SALVIOLI, S. *et al.* 2005. p53 codon 72 alleles influence the response to anticancer drugs in cells from aged people by regulating the cell cycle inhibitor p21[WAF1]. Cell Cycle **4:** 1264–1271.

47. CARRIERI, G. *et al.* 2001. Mitochondrial DNA haplogroups and ApoE4 allele are non-independent variables in sporadic Alzheimer's disease. Hum. Genet. **108:** 194–198.

48. DE BENEDICTIS, G. *et al.* 1998. Age-related changes of the 3′APOB-VNTR genotype pool in ageing cohorts. Ann. Hum. Genet. **62**(Pt 2): 115–122.

49. GARASTO, S. *et al.* 2004. A study of the average effect of the 3′APOB-VNTR polymorphism on lipidemic parameters could explain why the short alleles (<35 repeats) are rare in centenarians. BMC Med. Genet. **5:** 3–9.

50. VARCASIA, O. *et al.* 2001. Replication studies in longevity: puzzling findings in Danish centenarians at the 3′ApoB-VNTR locus. Ann. Hum. Genet. **65**(Pt 4): 371–376.

51. GARASTO, S. *et al.* 2003. The study of ApoA1, ApoC3 and ApoA4 variability in healthy ageing people reveals another paradox in the oldest old subjects. Ann. Hum. Genet. **67:** 54–62.

52. COPPOLA, R. *et al.* 2003. Von Willebrand factor in Italian centenarians. Haematologica **88:** 39–43.

53. BAGGIO, G. *et al.* 1998. Lipoprotein(a) and lipoprotein profile in healthy centenarians: a reappraisal of vascular risk factors. FASEB J. **12:** 433–437.

54. BARZILAI, N. *et al.* 2003. Unique lipoprotein phenotype and genotype associated with exceptional longevity. JAMA **290:** 2030–2040.

55. CELLINI, E. *et al.* 2005. Cholesteryl ester transfer protein (CETP) I405V polymorphism and longevity in Italian centenarians. Mech. Ageing Dev. **126:** 826–828.

56. MIGLIACCIO, E. *et al.* 1999. The p66shc adaptor protein controls oxidative stress response and life span in mammals. Nature **402:** 309–313.

57. PANDOLFI, S. *et al.* 2005. p66(shc) is highly expressed in fibroblasts from centenarians. Mech. Ageing Dev. **126:** 839–844.

Search for Genetic Factors Associated with Susceptibility to Multiple Sclerosis

GIUSI IRMA FORTE,[a] PAOLO RAGONESE,[b] GIUSEPPE SALEMI,[b] LETIZIA SCOLA,[a] GIUSEPPINA CANDORE,[a] MARCO D'AMELIO,[b] ANTONIO CRIVELLO,[a] NORMA DI BENEDETTO,[b] DOMENICO NUZZO,[a] ANTONIO GIACALONE,[a] DOMENICO LIO,[a] AND CALOGERO CARUSO[a]

[a]Gruppo di Studio sull'Immunosenescenza, Sezione di Patologia Generale, Dipartimento di Biopatologia e Metodologie Biomediche, Università degli studi di Palermo, Palermo, Italy

[b]Dipartimento di Neurologia, Oftalmologia, Otorinolaringoiatria e Psichiatria, Università degli studi di Palermo, Palermo, Italy

ABSTRACT: Multiple sclerosis (MS) is a cell-mediated autoimmune disease characterized by type-1 cytokine production. Environmental and individual genetic background might influence this response particularly in cytokine gene polymorphisms. We evaluated whether polymorphisms of interleukin (IL)-10, IL-12, and tumor necrosis factor (TNF)-α genes, which might play a role in MS pathogenesis, are associated with MS susceptibility. Genotype frequencies for all the analyzed polymorphisms were not differently distributed between cases and controls. It is reasonable to suppose that the cytokine single-nucleotide polymorphisms (SNPs) studied must be considered against a larger genetic background involving other functional SNPs of Th1 regulator elements such as IL-21 and IL-23.

KEYWORDS: Multiple sclerosis; cytokine polymorphisms; SNP; IL-10; IL-12; TNF-α

INTRODUCTION

Multiple sclerosis (MS) is a chronic inflammatory–demyelinating disease characterized by multifocal damage of the central nervous system (CNS) caused presumably by an autoimmune process that induces demyelination, destruction of oligodendrocytes, and axonal injury.[1] Both environmental and genetic factors are involved in the development/progression of MS and several studies point to a complex inheritance involving interactions between

Address for correspondence: Prof. Domenico Lio, Chair of Clinical Pathology, Immunosenescence Study Group, General Pathology Section, Department of Pathobiology and Biomedical Methodologies, University of Palermo, Corso Tukory 211, 90134 Palermo, Italy. Voice: +39-091-655-5913; fax: +39-091-655-5933.
e-mail: dolio@unipa.it

Ann. N.Y. Acad. Sci. 1067: 264–269 (2006). © 2006 New York Academy of Sciences.
doi: 10.1196/annals.1354.034

combinations of loci that may influence the immune response.[2] Tissue damage is probably organized by a T helper 1 (Th1)–mediated autoimmune response against myelin-associated autoantigens.[3,4] These responses are influenced by the cytokine balance in relation to the type of antigenic stimulation and individual genetic background. Data in the literature on associations among cytokine polymorphisms and MS are extremely conflicting, being influenced by the type of approach (case-control or family studies) and end-point (association to susceptibility, to clinical outcome, or therapeutic response).[6–11] Intriguingly, the best evidence for the genes associated with MS susceptibility concerns variants of genes coding for molecules involved in the inflammatory reaction, such as IL-1β, IL-1R-antagonist.[6] In this paper we focus on the contemporaneous evaluation of single-nucleotide polymorphisms (SNPs) of anti-inflammatory interleukin (IL)-10[12] and proinflammatory IL-12 p40 (IL-12B)[13] and tumor necrosis factor (TNF-)-α genes,[14] which might play a role in MS susceptibility.

MATERIALS AND METHODS

DNA samples were collected from 91 patients affected by multiple sclerosis and 220 age- and sex-matched, healthy control subjects, from west Sicily. Written informed consent for enrolling in the study and for personal data management was obtained from all the subjects according to Italian laws.

The amplification refractory mutation system—polymerase chain reaction (ARMS-PCR) method was used in order to type control and patients with MS for −308GA SNP at promoter region of TNF-α and for −1082GA at promoter region of IL-10, as previously described.[15] The polymerase chain reaction–restriction fragment length polymorphism (PCR–RFLP) method described by Huang *et al.*[13] was applied for +1188AC SNP typing in the 3′UTR of IL-12B p40 subunit.

Genotype frequencies were evaluated by gene count. The data were tested for the goodness of fit between the observed and expected genotype values and their fit to the Hardy–Weinberg equilibrium. Contingency tables were constructed. Chi-square test with Yates adjustment was employed to determine the statistical significance of differences in percentages of homo- and heterozygous individuals for the single SNPs in patients and controls.

RESULTS

TABLE 1 shows genotype frequencies of, respectively, −308G→A TNF-α and −1082G→A IL-10 SNPs in patients and healthy subjects. The genotype, as well as allele frequency for all the analyzed polymorphisms, was not differently distributed between cases and controls. However, a nonsignificant trend of increased −308AA TNF-α genotype frequency was evidenced in the

TABLE 1. Genotype frequencies (%) of −308G→A promoter sequence polymorphisms at TNF- locus and −1082G→A promoter sequence polymorphism at IL-10 locus in MS-affected patients and in healthy controls (numbers of homozygous or heterozygous subjects are reported in parentheses)

		TNF-α −308			IL10 −1082		
	No.	GG	GA	AA	GG	GA	AA
Healthy controls	220	74.1 (163)	24.1 (53)	1.8 (4)	23.6 (52)	45.9 (101)	30.5 (67)
MS	91	70.3 (64)	26.4 (24)	3.3 (3)	19.8 (18)	48.4 (44)	31.8 (29)

TABLE 2. Genotype frequencies (%) of +1188C→A polymorphisms at IL12 p40 locus at 3′UTR sequence in MS-affected patients and in healthy controls (numbers of homozygous or heterozygous subjects are reported in parentheses)

		IL12B +1188		
	No.	AA	AC	CC
Healthy controls	74	59.0 (44)	38.0 (28)	3 (2)
MS	57	61.0 (35)	36.0 (21)	2 (1)

patients compared to the controls. In addition, the percentage of subjects contemporaneously homo- or heterozygous for −308A TNF-α and −1082A IL-10 promoter alleles (high TNF-α and low IL-10 producers) was increased among MS patients (25.3% vs. 18.2%), but the difference did not reach statistical significance (data not shown).

Finally, considering the role attributed to IL-12 in the pathogenesis of MS,[16] 57 of 91 MS patients and 74 of 220 control subjects were also typed for +1188 A→C (TABLE 2). The IL-12B genotype frequencies were not differently distributed between cases and controls.

DISCUSSION

Overwhelming evidence indicates that cytokines have been implicated widely in the immunopathogenesis of MS, but their exact role and how they are regulated in this disease remains controversial.

Th1 cytokines produced by activated autoreactive T cells, monocytes, and microglial cells have been found in MS lesions.[17] Moreover, inflammatory and regulatory cytokines produced by macrophages, including IL-1, IL-6, TNF-α, IL-10, and IL-12, are elevated in MS patients and these increased levels correlate with disease severity.[17,18]

A genetic tendency to develop a stronger Th1 response might involve some functional cytokine polymorphisms in the regulatory region, and be able to affect positively or negatively the mRNA transcription. Therefore, we have investigated the IL-10 −1082GA functional SNP, the TNF-α −308GA SNP, and the +1188 AC SNP in MS patients and in healthy controls from western

Sicily. It is known that homozygous carriers for −1082AA are IL-10-low producers; −308 AA TNF-α and IL12 +1188 AA are high producers. Thus, it is interesting to evaluate whether genetic background switched toward Th1 response affects the susceptibility to the disease.

Our data demonstrate that these SNPs are not associated with SM susceptibility. In fact, in spite of the role generally attributed to the genetic background, −1082AA IL-10, −308 AA TNF-α, and +1188 AA IL-12 genotypes, potentially able to facilitate a stronger type 1 response, are not overrepresented in our sample of Sicilian MS patients.

Our data are in agreement with several studies on other European populations. In a Norwegian population no correlation between IL-10 −1082GA SNP and the disease was found, but patients with low IL-10 expression haplotype showed a trend toward a worse clinical outcome.[6] In a U.K. Caucasian population, no associations were found for any IL-10 promoter polymorphisms with MS susceptibility nor with disease outcome.[7] Similar results were reported for −308 GA TNF-α SNP.[8–10] Therefore, it seems to be reasonable to definitively exclude −308 G/A TNF-α and −1082G/A, or their combined potentially risky genotypes, from playing any role in MS susceptibility in Caucasian populations.

Finally, literature data strongly suggest an implication of IL-12 p40 subunit in the pathogenesis of MS, considering in particular the positive role attributed to other Th1 cytokines as IL-23, which shares the subunit with IL-12 in MS.[16] Moreover, IL-12 and IL-23 play a critical role in the induction of murine experimental autoimmune encephalomyelitis.[19]

The role of +1188 AC IL-12 SNP in MS susceptibility is not well clarified. Our negative data are in agreement with those obtained in a TDT study on Irish and Belgian families,[20] while Van Veen *et al.* observed a positive correlation in a Dutch population-based study.[21]

The negative North–South trend in the incidence of the MS reveals that different environmental and genetic factors are involved in the development of MS.[22] On the other hand, evidence suggests that cytokine interplay is very complex and the delicate balance between different cytokines is more important than just a simple up- or downregulation of pro- or anti-inflammatory cytokines.[23]

Most likely the Th1 cytokine SNPs studied must be considered in a larger genetic background in which their influence is different in predisposition, severity, and outcome of the disease. Therefore, we will extend our research to other functional SNP- and IL-12-related Th1 regulator elements such as IL-21 and IL-23.

ACKNOWLEDGMENTS

This work was supported by grants from the Ministry of Education, University and Research to D.L., G.C.R., C.C., and G.C. G.I.F. A.C. and D.N. are

Ph.D. students in the Pathobiology Ph.D. course (directed by C.C.) of Palermo University and this work is in partial fulfillment of the requirement for the Ph.D.

REFERENCES

1. TRAPP, B.D. *et al.* 1998. Axonal transection in the lesions of multiple sclerosis. N. Engl. J. Med. **338:** 278–285.
2. CHIOCCHETTI, A. *et al.* 2005. Osteopontin gene haplotypes correlate with multiple sclerosis development and progression. J. Neuroimmunol. **163:** 172–178.
3. RAINE, C.S. 1994. The Dale E. McFarlin Memorial Lecture: the immunology of the multiple sclerosis lesion. Ann. Neurol. **36:** S61–S72.
4. STEINMAN, L. *et al.* 2002. Multiple sclerosis: deeper understanding of its pathogenesis reveals new targets for therapy. Annu. Rev. Neurosci. **25:** 491–505.
5. KANTARCI, O.H., M. DE ANDRADE & B.G. WEINSHENKER. 2002. Identifying disease modifying genes in multiple sclerosis. J. Neuroimmunol. **123:** 144–159.
6. MYHR, K.M. *et al.* 2002. Interleukin-10 promoter polymorphisms in patients with multiple sclerosis. J. Neurol. Sci. **202:** 93–97.
7. PICKARD, C. 1999. Interleukin-10 (IL10) promoter polymorphisms and multiple sclerosis. J. Neuroimmunol. **101:** 207–210.
8. FERNANDES FILHO, J.A. *et al.* 2002. TNF-alpha and -beta gene polymorphisms in multiple sclerosis: a highly significant role for determinants in the first intron of the TNF-beta gene. Autoimmunity **35:** 377–380.
9. ANLAR, B. *et al.* 2001. Tumor necrosis factor-alpha gene polymorphisms in children with multiple sclerosis. Neuropediatrics **32:** 214–216.
10. LUCOTTE, G., C. BATHELIER & G. MERCIER. 2000. TNF-alpha polymorphisms in multiple sclerosis: no association with −238 and −308 promoter alleles, but the microsatellite allele a11 is associated with the disease in French patients. Mult. Scler. **6:** 78–80.
11. PALACIO, L.G. *et al.* 2002. Multiple sclerosis in the tropics: genetic association to STR's loci spanning the HLA and TNF-. Mult. Scler. **8:** 249–255.
12. TURNER, D.M. *et al.* 1997. An investigation of polymorphism in the interleukin-10 gene promoter. Eur. J. Immunogenet. **24:** 1–8.
13. HUANG, D., M.R. CANCILLA & G. MORAHAN. 2000. Complete primary structure, chromosomal localisation, and definition of polymorphisms of the gene encoding the human interleukin-12 p40 subunit. Genes Immun. **1:** 515–520.
14. WILSON, A.G. *et al.* 1997. Effects of a polymorphism in the human tumor necrosis factor alpha promoter on transcriptional activation. Proc. Natl. Acad. Sci. USA **94:** 3195–3199.
15. LIO, D. *et al.* 2005. TNF-alpha, IFNgamma and IL-10 gene polymorphisms in a sample of Sicilian patients with coeliac disease. Dig. Liver Dis. **37:** 923–927.
16. GRAN, B., G.-X. ZHANG & A. ROSTAMI. 2004. Role of the IL-12/IL-23 system in the regulation of T-cell responses in central nervous system inflammatory demyelination. Crit. Rev. Immunol. **24:** 111–128.
17. FILION, L.G. *et al.* 2003. Monocyte-derived cytokines in multiple sclerosis. Clin. Exp. Immunol. **131:** 324–334.
18. SHI, F.-D. *et al.* 2000. IL-18 directs autoreactive T cells and promotes autodestruction in the central nervous system via induction of IFN-gamma by NK cells. J. Immunol. **165:** 3099–3104.

19. ZHANG, G.-X. *et al*. 2003. Role of IL-12 receptor 1 in regulation of T cell response by APC in experimental, autoimmune encephalomyelitis. J. Immunol. **171:** 4485–4492.
20. ALLOZA, I. *et al*. 2002. Interleukin-12 p40 polymorphism and susceptibility to multiple sclerosis. Ann. Neurol. **52:** 524–525.
21. VAN VEEN, T. *et al*. 2001. Interleukin-12p40 genotype plays a role in the susceptibility to multiple sclerosis. Ann. Neurol. **50:** 275.
22. DYMENT, D.A., G.C. EBERS & A.D. SADOVNICK. 2004. Genetics of multiple sclerosis. Lancet Neurol. **3:** 104–110.
23. CARUSO, C. *et al*. 2005. Inflammation and life-span. Science **307:** 208–209.

Opposite Role of Pro-Inflammatory Alleles in Acute Myocardial Infarction and Longevity

Results of Studies Performed in a Sicilian Population

GIUSEPPINA CANDORE,[a] CARMELA RITA BALISTRERI,[a]
MARIA PAOLA GRIMALDI,[a] FLORINDA LISTÌ,[a] SONYA VASTO,[a]
MARCO CARUSO,[b] GREGORIO CAIMI,[b] ENRICO HOFFMANN,[b]
GIUSEPPINA COLONNA-ROMANO,[a] DOMENICO LIO,[a]
GIUSEPPE PAOLISSO,[c] CLAUDIO FRANCESCHI,[d] AND
CALOGERO CARUSO[a]

[a]Gruppo di Studio sull' Immunosenescenza, Dipartimento di Biopatologia e
Metodologie Biomediche, Università di Palermo, Palermo, Italy

[b]Dipartimento di Medicina Interna, Malattie Cardiovascolari e Nefrourologiche,
Università di Palermo, Palermo, Italy

[c]Dipartimento di Medicina Geriatria e Malattie Metaboliche, II Università di
Napoli, Napoli, Italy

[d]Dipartimento di Patologia Sperimentale and Centro Interdipartimentale "L.
Galvani," Università di Bologna, Bologna and Istituto Nazionale di Riposo e
Cura per Anziani, Ancona, Italy

ABSTRACT: The major trait characterizing offspring in centenarians
is a reduction in the prevalence of cardiovascular disease. Because a
pro-inflammatory genotype seems to contribute significantly to the risk
of coronary heart disease, alleles associated with disease susceptibility
would not be included in the genetic background favoring longevity, as
suggested by our previous studies on inflammatory cytokines. To confirm
whether genotypes of inflammatory molecules play an opposite role in
atherosclerosis and longevity, we are studying the role of other proinflammatory alleles, such as pyrin and CCR5, in acute myocardial infarction
and longevity. The results support the hypothesis that the genetic background favoring cardiovascular diseases is detrimental to longevity. In
addition, they suggest that the centenarian genetic background may be

Address for correspondence: Calogero Caruso, M.D., Gruppo di Studio sull'Immunosenescenza,
Dipartimento di Biopatologia e Metodologie Biomediche, Corso Tukory 211, 90134 Palermo, Italy.
Voice: +39-09-1655-5911; fax: +39-09-1655-5933.
e-mail: marcoc@unipa.it

Ann. N.Y. Acad. Sci. 1067: 270–275 (2006). © 2006 New York Academy of Sciences.
doi: 10.1196/annals.1354.035

useful for investigating genetic key components of age-associated diseases that are characterized by a multifactorial etiology.

KEYWORDS: AMI; CCR5; inflammation; longevity; pyrin

INTRODUCTION

Individual changes in the type and intensity of immune response affecting life-span expectancy and aging seem to have a genetic component. Besides, a well-preserved immune function has been found in long-term-surviving exceptional individuals who reach the extreme age limits of human life. Centenarians seem to be genetically equipped for defeating major age-related diseases. They hold single nucleotide polymorphisms (SNPs) within the immune system genome, which seems to regulate immune-inflammatory responses associated with longevity. On the other hand, centenarians are characterized by marked delay or escape from age-associated diseases that, on average, cause mortality at earlier ages. Moreover, centenarian offspring have an increased likelihood of surviving to 100 years and show a reduced prevalence of age-associated diseases, such as cardiovascular disease and a lesser prevalence of cardiovascular risk factors. Therefore, genes involved in cardiovascular diseases may play an opposite role in human longevity. In addition, our recent findings suggest that different alleles of different cytokine genes coding for pro- or anti-inflammatory cytokines may affect individual life span expectancy by influencing the type and intensity of the immune-inflammatory responses against environmental stressors.[1-3]

Atherosclerosis and its complications contribute to a large percentage of morbidity and mortality in older people. Cardiovascular disease is the leading worldwide cause of morbidity and death. Inflammation is a key component of atherosclerosis, and genes coding for inflammatory or anti-inflammatory cytokines are therefore good candidates for the risk of developing atherosclerosis. Because genetic traits contribute significantly to the risk of coronary heart disease (CHD), a number of studies indicated that allelic variations in genes related to innate immunity may boost the risk of disease. Differences in the genetic regulation of immune-inflammatory processes might partially explain why some people, but not others, develop the disease and why some develop a greater inflammatory response than others. Accordingly, common gene polymorphisms regulating high inflammatory molecule production have been associated with atherosclerosis. Conversely, those associated with a positive control of inflammation might play a protective role against atherosclerosis.[4,5]

If pro-inflammatory genotypes significantly contribute to the risk of CHD, alleles associated with disease susceptibility should not be included in the genetic background favoring longevity. Hence, we hypothesized that genotypes of natural immunity might play an opposite role in atherosclerosis and longevity. In our previous reports, we have observed a significantly different distribution of anti-inflammatory interleukin (IL)-10 cytokine and pro-inflammatory tumor necrosis factor (TNF)-α genotypes among male controls, male centenarians, and male patients affected by acute myocardial infarction (AMI). The genotype high producer of IL-10 and the genotype low producer of TNF-α were significantly underrepresented in male AMI patients and overrepresented in centenarian men. In our judgment, this result strengthens the hypothesis that the genetic background protecting against cardiovascular disease is a relevant component of the longevity trait.[6,7] Trying to confirm our hypothesis, we are extending these data, by studying the role of other pro-inflammatory alleles in AMI and in longevous subjects in our homogeneous Sicilian population. In these studies, the Sicilian ethnicity of all subjects is confirmed by having all four grandparents born in Sicily; immigration and intermarriage have historically been rare. The diagnosis of AMI is based on typical electrocardiographic changes and increased serum activities of enzymes such as creatine kinase-MB, aspartate aminotransferase, and lactate dehydrogenase and confirmed by echocardiography and coronary angiography. To improve the power of our study, we select cases genetically loaded because they have an early AMI onset (<46 years).[8]

PRO-INFLAMMATORY ALLELES: THE CASE OF PYRIN

Pyrin is a basic protein of 781 amino acids encoded by MEFV gene, whose mutations are responsible for familial Mediterranean fever. Febrile attacks are characterized by a substantial influx of polymorphonuclear leukocytes into the affected tissues. The biological function of the wild protein is likely the regulation of inflammatory mediators and the stimulation of apoptosis. Therefore, mutations in the pyrin gene are liable to lead to leukocyte survival otherwise designed to follow the apoptotic pathway, increasing the inflammatory response.[9] To evaluate whether the anti-inflammatory allele of pyrin might contribute to the genetic background protection against cardiovascular diseases, and favoring longevity, we have analyzed the allelic frequency of Met694Val. Three cohorts of male subjects were chosen: young patients affected by AMI, age-matched controls, and oldest old subjects. Significant differences were observed in the frequency distribution of allele Met694Val among the three cohorts; in particular, the number of AMI patients showing the mutant allele was increased in comparison with young controls and oldest old subjects, who showed the lowest values. The results might be explained by the possible function of the mutated pyrin allele. By failing to downregulate the inflammatory response by monocytes,[9] it might influence inflammatory molecule secretion by increasing the risk of atherosclerotic complications in carriers.

PRO-INFLAMMATORY ALLELES: THE CASE OF CCR5

The CCR5 gene codes for a G protein–coupled chemokine receptor. Chemokines and their receptors form a regulatory network that controls the development, recruitment, and activation of leukocytes. In inflammatory tissues, macrophage inflammatory proteins 1α and 1β latch onto CCR5, leading monocytes to the correct site. The 32bp (Δ32) deletion of the CCR5 gene causes frame shift mutation at position 185, localized by the second extracellular loop of the receptor sequence, which stops protein maturation.[10] To evaluate whether the CCR5 genotype is a component of the genetic background protection against the AMI, we have genotyped for Δ32 AMI male patients, age- and gender-matched controls, and centenarian men. Significant differences were observed in the frequency of CCR5 genotypes among the three groups; in particular, the number of AMI patients positive for Δ32+ genotypes is decreased in comparison with both young and oldest old control subjects, who showed the highest frequency. This polymorphism, in the heterozygous state, seems to act by reducing to a half the receptor molecule number from the cell surface, which results in a decreased recruitment of monocyte/macrophage cells at the vascular wall.[10] Hence, carriers display a lower risk of atherosclerosis and a decreased risk of acute coronary events.

CONCLUSIONS

To gain insight into mechanisms of these reciprocal associations, the role of toll-like receptor (TLR)-4 may be paradigmatic. Macrophages express receptor molecules that recognize molecular patterns foreign to mammalian organisms but commonly found in pathogens, and are important in contributing to the inflammatory response. Along this first line of defense, TLRs recognize pathogen-associated molecular patterns. The transmembrane lipopolysaccaride receptor TLR4, which initiates the innate immune response to common gram-negative bacteria, activates the inflammatory cell via the NF-kB pathway by inducing the expression of a variety of cytokines and other molecules crucial to immune responses. TLR4 expression has been described in human atherosclerotic lesions and the inflammatory mediators produced through its activation seem to exert various atherogenic effects, which involves expression of adhesion molecules on endothelial cells, proliferation of smooth-muscle cells, activation of immune cells, stimulation of the acute-phase response, and matrix breakdown. TLR4 SNPs, known to attenuate receptor signaling, as ASP299GLY, seem to determine a minor risk of developing carotid atherosclerosis and less intima media thickness in the common carotid artery. Furthermore, the subjects with mutant genotype had lower levels of certain pro-inflammatory cytokines, acute-phase reactants, and soluble adhesion molecules.[11,12]

By studying three cohorts of male subjects—AMI patients, controls, and the oldest old—we have demonstrated that this SNP showed significantly lower frequency in AMI patients compared to controls, whereas the oldest old showed a higher frequency. Therefore, the TLR4 genotype, known to attenuate receptor signaling and therefore inflammatory responses, was found to be associated with the chance of reaching the extreme limit of human life span, whereas it was underrepresented in AMI patients.[13]

Epidemiologic studies and *in vitro* experiments suggest that the pathogenic burden, to which every individual has been exposed, may be linked to an increased risk of atherosclerosis and a worst prognosis of CHD.[11,12,14] Our data on TLR4 demonstrate that the presence of SNP with pro-inflammatory associations may fuel the inflammatory response by macrophages to gram-negative infection, promoting pro-inflammatory status and atheromatous plaque vulnerability. Conversely, people genetically predisposed to weak inflammatory activity have a lesser chance of developing CHD and, therefore, more chance of living longer.[14]

These results support our hypothesis that a genetic background favoring cardiovascular diseases is detrimental to longevity. In addition, centenarian genetic background studies may contribute to clarifying the role of key genetic components influencing age-associated diseases that are characterized by a multifactorial etiology.

Cardiovascular diseases are a late consequence of an evolutionary pro-inflammatory response programmed to resist infections in earlier life. Thus, genetic backgrounds promoting pro-inflammatory responses may play opposite roles in cardiovascular diseases and in longevity. Genetic polymorphisms responsible for a low inflammatory response might result in an increased chance of longer life span in an environment with a reduced pathogen burden, such as a modern-day health environment, which also permits obtaining a lower-grade survivable atherogenic inflammatory response.[15] What we have said occurs in men; further studies are necessary to validate this hypothesis in women.

ACKNOWLEDGMENTS

This work was supported by grants from the Ministry of Education, University and Research to D.L., G.C.R., C.C., and G.C. and the Ministry of Health (Markers genetici di sindrome coronarica acuta e valutazione della L-arginina nella prevenzione di eventi ischemici) to C.C. The collaboration between the "Gruppo di Studio sull'immunosenescenza" coordinated by Prof. C. Caruso and INRCA was enhanced by a cooperation contract (Longevity and Elderly Disability Biological Markers). C.R.B., S.V., F.L., and M.P.G. are Ph.D. students in the Pathobiology Ph.D. course (directed by C.C.) of Palermo University and this work is in partial fulfillment of the requirement for the Ph.D.

REFERENCES

1. TERRY, D.F. *et al*. 2003. Cardiovascular advantages among the offspring of centenarians. J. Gerontol. A Biol. Sci. Med. Sci. **58:** M425–431.
2. CARUSO, C. *et al*. 2005. Inflammation and life-span. Science **307:** 208–209.
3. FRANCESCHI, C. *et al*. 2005. Genes involved in immune response/inflammation, IGF1/insulin pathway and response to oxidative stress play a major role in the genetics of human longevity: the lesson of centenarians. Mech. Ageing Dev. **126:** 351–361.
4. LIBBY, P. *et al*. 2002. Inflammation and atherosclerosis. Circulation **105:** 1135–1143.
5. CANDORE, G. *et al*. 2006. Cytokine gene polymorphisms and atherosclerosis. *In* Cytokine Gene Polymorphisms in Multifactorial Conditions. K. Vandenbroeck, Ed.: CRC Press. Boca Raton, FL. In press.
6. LIO, D. *et al*. 2004. Opposite effects of IL-10 gene polymorphisms in cardiovascular diseases and in successful ageing: genetic background of male centenarians is protective against coronary heart disease. J. Med. Genet. **41:** 790–794.
7. CARUSO, C. *et al*. 2004. Genetic background of centenarians may be protective against cardiovascular disease. Immunology 2004, Proceedings of the International Immunology Congress, Canada, pp. 29–34. Mouduzzi. Bologna, Italy.
8. MARENBERG, M.E. *et al*. 1994. Genetic susceptibility to death from coronary heart disease in a study of twins. N. Engl. J. Med. **330:** 1041–1046.
9. MCDERMOTT, M.F. 2002. Genetic clues to understanding periodic fevers, and possible therapies. Trends Mol. Med. **8:** 550–553.
10. GONZALEZ, P. *et al.*, 2001. Genetic variation at the chemokine receptors CCR5/CCR2 in myocardial infarction. Genes Immun. **2:** 191–195.
11. ARROYO-ESPLIGUERO, R. *et al*. 2004. CD14 and toll-like receptor 4: a link between infection and acute coronary events? Heart **90:** 983–988.
12. SCHRODER, N.W. & R.R. SCHUMANN. 2005. Single nucleotide polymorphisms of Toll-like receptors and susceptibility to infectious disease. Lancet Infect. Dis. **5:** 156–164.
13. BALISTRERI, C.R. *et al*. 2004. Role of Toll-like receptor 4 in acute myocardial infarction and longevity. JAMA **292:** 2339–2340.
14. CANDORE, G. *et al*. 2006. Inflammation, longevity, and cardiovascular diseases: role of polymorphisms of TLR4. Ann. N.Y. Acad. Sci. **1067:** 282–287.
15. LICASTRO, F. *et al*. 2005. Innate immunity and inflammation in ageing: a key for understanding age-related diseases. Immun. Ageing **2:** 8.

Association between +1059G/C CRP Polymorphism and Acute Myocardial Infarction in a Cohort of Patients from Sicily

A Pilot Study

CARMELA RITA BALISTRERI,[a] SONYA VASTO,[a] FLORINDA LISTÌ,[a] MARIA PAOLA GRIMALDI,[a] DOMENICO LIO,[a] GIUSEPPINA COLONNA-ROMANO,[a] MARCO CARUSO,[b] GREGORIO CAIMI,[b] ENRICO HOFFMANN,[b] CALOGERO CARUSO,[a] AND GIUSEPPINA CANDORE[a]

[a]Gruppo di Studio sull' Immunosenescenza, Dipartimento di Biopatologia e Metodologie Biomediche, Università di Palermo, Palermo, Italy

[b]Dipartimento di Medicina Interna, Malattie Cardiovascolari e Nefrourologiche, Università di Palermo, Palermo, Italy

ABSTRACT: Inflammation plays a role in all the phases of atherosclerosis, and increased production of the acute-phase reactant, C-reactive protein (CRP), predicts future cardiovascular events. Furthermore, CRP has been claimed to play a role in the pathogenesis of atherosclerosis; therefore, CRP polymorphisms might be associated with acute myocardial infarction (AMI). We have analyzed male patients affected by AMI and healthy age-related male controls from Sicily for +1059G/C CRP single-nucleotide polymorphism (SNP). There was a significantly higher frequency of +1059C SNP ($P = 0.0008$; OR 3.86) in patients compared to controls. CRP serum levels were significantly higher in C+ healthy subjects rather than in C− subjects ($P = 0.0075$). The results of the present pilot case–control study performed in a homogeneous caucasoid population suggest that +1059C CRP gene SNP is associated with AMI. In any case, the results of the present study should add to the growing body of evidence on the role of pro-inflammatory genotypes in unsuccessful aging, determining susceptibility to immune-inflammatory diseases such as coronary heart disease.

KEYWORDS: acute myocardial infarction; CRP; immunogenetics; inflammation; SNP

Address for correspondence: Calogero Caruso, M.D., Gruppo di Studio sull'Immunosenescenza, Dipartimento di Biopatologia e Metodologie Biomediche, Corso Tukory 211, 90134 Palermo, Italy. Voice: +39-09-1655-5911; fax: +39-09-1655-5933.
e-mail: marcoc@unipa.it

Ann. N.Y. Acad. Sci. 1067: 276–281 (2006). © 2006 New York Academy of Sciences.
doi: 10.1196/annals.1354.036

INTRODUCTION

Current evidence supports a central role for inflammation in all phases of the atherosclerotic process—early atherogenesis, the progression of lesions, and the thrombotic complications.[1] The primary and earliest host response to inflammatory injury is the acute-phase response, a rapid adjustment in the blood concentration of acute-phase proteins, of which C-reactive protein (CRP) is the prototype.[2] Accordingly, in atherosclerosis elevation of acute-phase proteins clearly augments the risk for vascular event. Several population-based studies have demonstrated that baseline CRP levels predict future cardiovascular events.[1,3] Furthermore, CRP might be more than just an inflammation marker, playing a role in the pathogenesis of atherosclerosis by affecting disease progression. Evidence shows that CRP is present in atherosclerotic plaques, where it has been claimed to elicit potential pro-inflammatory and atherogenic outcomes. Among these effects we can find activation of complement, enhancement of monocyte recruitment into the arterial wall by inducing adhesion molecule expression, chemokine production, uptake of oxidized low-density lipoproteins (ox-LDL) by macrophages, and stimulation of tissue factor (TF) production by monocytes.[4-7]

Some polymorphisms have been described in CRP genes and several studies on the association between polymorphisms of the CRP gene and atherosclerosis suggest that variation of this molecule might be implicated in the prediction and pathogenesis of coronary heart disease (CHD).[8,9]

We therefore sought to determine the frequency of the recently described +1059G/C single nucleotide polymorphism (SNP) within exon 2 of the CRP gene[8] in a homogeneous cohort of 106 male patients and 120 age-related male controls from Sicily. The aim of this study was to assess the possible association with onset of acute myocardial infarction (AMI), and to improve the power of our analysis, we selected cases genetically loaded for having early-onset AMI (<46 years).[10]

MATERIALS AND METHODS

We have analyzed 106 young male patients (mean age: 41 years, age range: 20–46 years) admitted at the Cardiac Unit of Palermo University Hospital with a history of AMI, and 120 healthy male controls (mean age: 39 years, age range: 20–50 years) from Sicily. The controls were unrelated medical students and laboratory staff. The Sicilian ethnicity of all subjects was confirmed by having all four grandparents born in Sicily; immigration and intermarriage have historically been rare. The diagnosis of AMI was based on typical electrocardiographic changes and increased serum activities of enzymes such as creatine kinase-MB, aspartate aminotransferase, and lactate dehydrogenase, and confirmed by echocardiography and coronary angiography. The University

Hospital Ethics Committee approved the project and informed consent was obtained from each individual.

Blood specimens were collected in tripotassium EDTA sterile tubes, and DNA extracted and genotyped for +1059G/C CRP SNP according to published methods.[8] Twenty microliters of reaction mixtures containing DNA template, 1.5 U of TaqGold-DNA polymerase (PE BioSystem; Milan, Italy), deoxynucleotides at final concentration of 200 mM, 1 × reaction buffer (PE BioSystem), 5 μM of CRP-1059F, and CRP-1059R primers were used to perform the amplification. Polymerase chain reaction (PCR) cycling was performed at 95°C for 10 min and 30 cycles at 94°C for 30 s, 57°C for 30 s, and 72°C for 30 s, followed by a final extension of 10 min at 72°C. PCR products were analyzed by restriction fragment length polymorphism (RFLP) assay, in which the pattern coming from Mae III (Roche, Monza, Italy) restriction assay showed the presence of restriction sites leading, respectively, to two bands of 434 bp and 310 bp that identify 1059C allele and three bands of 310, 233, and 210 bp that identify the 1059G variant. The two patterns were revealed by electrophoresis on a 2% agarose gel and analyzed by a Kodak imaging analyzing system.

To measure CRP levels, different sera collected from healthy controls and frozen at −70°C were analyzed by a high-sensitivity ELISA kit (IBL, Hamburg, Germany). This assay is a solid-phase enzyme-linked immunoassorbent test based on the sandwich principle. The upper limit of the normal range lies between 5 and 8 μg/mL.

Genotypic and allele frequencies were evaluated by gene count and contingency tables (χ^2 test) constructed to determine statistical differences in SNP frequency of the two groups analyzed. The data were tested for goodness of fit between the observed and expected genotype values and their fit to the Hardy–Weinberg equilibrium (HWE) by χ^2 test. The strength of the statistical association was expressed by odds ratio (OR) and 95% confidence intervals (CI) with relative significance. Since the distribution of CRP was not normal, the statistical significance of CRP serum levels between C+ and C− controls was calculated by the Wilcoxon test.

RESULTS

TABLE 1 shows the genotype distribution and allele frequency for +1059G/C CRP SNPs in 106 young male patients (<46 years) and 120 age-related male controls from Sicily. Significant differences were observed in the frequency of CRP genotypes between controls and patients ($P = 0.007$); in particular, we found an increased number of patients with AMI positive for C+ (CC and CG) genotypes as compared to control subjects. According to the genotype data, there was a significantly higher prevalence of +1059C SNP (12.3% vs. 3.75%; $P = 0.001$) with an OR 3.59 (1.64–7.85 95% CI; $P = 0.0007$) in patients affected by AMI as compared to controls.

TABLE 1. Genotype distribution and allele frequency for +1059G/C CRP SNP in 106 young male patients (< 46 years) and 120 age-related male controls from Sicily

	GG	GC	CC	+1059G	+1059C
Patients	84 (79.3%)	18 (17%)	4 (3.7%)	186 (87.70%)	26 (12.30%)
Controls	112 (93.3%)	7 (5.8%)	1 (0.9%)	231 (96.25%)	9 (3.75%)

The distribution of genotypes was in HWE. Genotype and allele frequencies were significantly different between the two groups ($P = 0.007$ by χ^2 test, 3×2 tables, and, respectively, $P = 0.001$ by χ^2 test with Yate's correction). OR 3.59 (1.64–7.85 95% CI; $P = 0.0007$).

TABLE 2. CRP (γ/mL) serum values in 70 healthy Sicilians analyzed according to CRP genotype

Genotype	Median (25th–75th percentiles)
C+	4.5 (1.75–5.01)
C−	0.8 (0.62–2.10)

CRP serum levels were significantly higher in 6 C+ healthy subjects (CC plus CG) than in 64 C− healthy subjects (GG) ($P = 0.0075$ by Wilcoxon test).

AMI patients showed a positive familial history of CHD in 58% of cases, current smoking habits in 71% (ex plus current, 90%), history of type 2 diabetes in 17% of cases, history of obesity in 35%, and hypertension in 30%. Moreover, 64 and 45 of 106 patients displayed blood cholesterol levels and, respectively, triglyceride levels higher than 220 mg/dL and 160 mg/dL. No significant differences in genotype or allele frequencies were observed, by the stratification of these data, according to these risk factors' status. Thus, the role of +1059G/C SNP in AMI was seemingly not dependent on the above-mentioned risk factors.

TABLE 2 shows the serum CRP values in a small sample of healthy subjects according to genotype status. The upper limit of the normal range lies between 5 and 8 μg/mL. The CRP serum levels were significantly higher in C+ subjects (CC plus GC) than in C− subjects (GG) ($P = 0.0075$).

DISCUSSION

The results of the present case–control study performed in a homogeneous caucasoid population suggest that +1059C CRP gene SNP is associated with AMI. However, since the size and power of our study are very limited, our investigation should be considered a hypothesis-generating study, providing suggestive, although preliminary, evidence in favor of the association between the CRP genotype and AMI.

The association we have found is consistent with already published data related to the biology and etiology of atherosclerosis. In fact, CRP has been claimed to possess pro-atherogenic properties. CRP seems to activate endothelial cells to express adhesion molecules and chemokines as mono-cyte chemotactic protein 1. Furthermore, CRP may induce the secretion of interleukin-6 and endothelin-1 and decrease the expression and bioavailabil-ity of endothelial nitric oxide synthase in human endothelial cells. CRP also seems to elicit macrophages to express cytokine and TF and enhance ox-LDL uptake. Although these results need to be validated with the use of specific and selective inhibitors of CRP, we can put forward the idea that the CRP gene is a good candidate for being involved in the occurrence of AMI phenotype.[4–7]

Additionally, the SNP under study seemingly has functional effects on pro-tein production.[9] In fact, +1059 G/C SNP might influence CRP serum levels through linkage disequilibrium with a functional mutation in the CRP gene or with a nearby gene involved in CRP expression. The effect on serum levels differs among the different populations just studied on account of linkage dis-equilibrium in the different populations. Our preliminary observations suggest that in the Sicilian population, +1059 C SNP is associated with higher CRP serum level production. However, further studies are necessary because CRP, being a dynamic protein, with a 10,000-fold range, needs to be monitored re-peatedly and in larger cohorts of patients in order to perform an association study between genotypes.[2]

Association studies are influenced by the number of possible confounding factors, such as the total number of patients and controls and the homogene-ity of the population in terms of geographical origin among others. Artifacts might occur if the controls are not ethnically matched with the patients. We compared people belonging to the same homogeneous population from Sicily. We think therefore that, although based on a relatively reduced number of pa-tients and controls, our results might more reliable than studies performed on larger cohorts of patients from northern Europe and the United States that are ethnically matched referring to Caucasians in general.

On the other hand, even if the differences between patients and controls were highly significant with an OR of 3.59, only 22 out of 106 patients carried the +1059 C SNP. Therefore, the presence of the allele may be one of the factors genetically influencing the development of AMI and its role should be further investigated. However, since AMI is a multifactorial disease, any single mutation will only provide a small or modest contribution to the global risk, depending also on the interaction with a particular environment.[11]

Case–control studies with candidate genes have been widely used to study the role of polymorphisms in complex diseases. On the other hand, this approach has raised a lot of criticism that has been claimed to be usefully countered with an appeal to the principles of epidemiological investigation as discussed above.[12]

All in all, the results of the present study might add another piece to the growing body of evidence of the role of pro-inflammatory genotypes in un-successful aging, determining susceptibility to such immune-inflammatory diseases as CHD.[11,13–15]

ACKNOWLEDGMENTS

This work was supported by grants from the Ministry of Education, University and Research to D.L., G.C.R., C.C., and G.C. and the Ministry of Health (Markers genetici di sindrome coronarica acuta e valutazione della L-arginina nella prevenzione di eventi ischemici) to C.C. C.R.B., S.V., F.L., and M.P.G. are Ph.D. students in the Pathobiology Ph.D. course (directed by C.C.) of Palermo University and this work is in partial fulfillment of the requirement for the Ph.D.

REFERENCES

1. LIBBY, P. *et al.* 2002. Inflammation and atherosclerosis. Circulation **105:** 1135–1143.
2. PEPYS, M.B. & G.M. HIRSCHFIELD. 2003. C-reactive protein: a critical update. J. Clin. Invest. **111:** 1805–1812.
3. RIDKER, P.M. *et al.* 2002. Comparison of C-reactive protein and low-density lipoprotein cholesterol levels in the prediction of first cardiovascular events. N. Engl. J. Med. **347:** 1557–1565.
4. PASCERI, V. *et al.* 2001. Modulation of C-reactive protein mediated monocyte chemoattractant protein-1 induction in human endothelial cells by anti-atherosclerosis drugs. Circulation **103:** 2531–2534.
5. VERMA, S. *et al.* 2002. Endothelin antagonism and interleukin-6 inhibition attenuate proatherogenic effects of C-reactive protein. Circulation **105:** 1890–1896.
6. VENUGOPAL, S.K. *et al.* 2002. Demonstration that C-reactive protein decreases eNOS expression and bioactivity in human aortic endothelial cells. Circulation **106:** 1439–1441.
7. ZWAKA, T.P. *et al.* 2001. C-reactive protein mediated low density lipoprotein uptake by macrophages: implications for atherosclerosis. Circulation **103:** 1194–1197.
8. CAO, H. & R.A. HEGELE. 2000. Human C-reactive protein (CRP) 1059G/C polymorphism. J. Hum. Genet. **54:** 100–101.
9. EKLUND, C. *et al.* 2005. Epistatic effect of C-reactive protein (CRP) single nucleotide polymorphism (SNP) +1059 and interleukin-1B SNP +3954 on CRP concentration in healthy male blood donors. Int. J. Immunogenet. **32:** 229–232.
10. MARENBERG, M.E. *et al.* 1994. Genetic susceptibility to death from coronary heart disease in a study of twins. N. Engl. J. Med. **330:** 1041–1046.
11. CANDORE, G. *et al.* 2006. Cytokine gene polymorphisms and atherosclerosis. *In* Cytokine Gene Polymorphisms in Multifactorial Conditions. K. Vandenbroeck, Ed.: CRC Press. Boca Raton. In press.
12. TABOR, H.K. *et al.* 2002. Candidate-gene approach for studying complex genetic traits: practical considerations. Nat. Rev. Genet. **3:** 1–7.
13. LIO, D. *et al.* 2004. Opposite effects of IL-10 gene polymorphisms in cardiovascular diseases and in successful ageing: genetic background of male centenarians is prospettive against coronary heart disease. J. Med. Genet. **41:** 790–794.
14. BALISTRERI, C.R. *et al.* 2004. Role of Toll-like receptor 4 in acute myocardial infarction and longevity. JAMA **292:** 2339–2340.
15. CARUSO, C. *et al.* 2005. Inflammation and life-span. Science **307:** 208–209.

Inflammation, Longevity, and Cardiovascular Diseases

Role of Polymorphisms of TLR4

GIUSEPPINA CANDORE,[a] ALESSANDRA AQUINO,[a]
CARMELA RITA BALISTRERI,[a] MATTEO BULATI,[a]
DANIELE DI CARLO,[a] MARIA PAOLA GRIMALDI,[a] FLORINDA LISTÌ,[a]
VALENTINA ORLANDO,[a] SONYA VASTO,[a] MARCO CARUSO,[b]
GIUSEPPINA COLONNA-ROMANO,[a] DOMENICO LIO,[a] AND
CALOGERO CARUSO[a]

[a]Gruppo di Studio sull' Immunosenescenza, Dipartimento di Biopatologia e Metodologie Biomediche, Università di Palermo, Palermo, Italy

[b]Dipartimento di Medicina Interna, Malattie Cardiovascolari e Nefrourologiche, Università di Palermo, Palermo, Italy

ABSTRACT: The total burden of infection at various sites may affect the progression of atherosclerosis, the risk being modulated by host genotype. The role of lipopolysaccaride receptor TLR4 is paradigmatic. It initiates the innate immune response against gram-negative bacteria; and TLR4 polymorphisms, as ASP299GLY, suggested to attenuate receptor signaling, have been described. We demonstrated that TLR4 ASP299GLY polymorphism shows a significantly lower frequency in patients affected by myocardial infarction compared to controls, whereas centenarians show a higher frequency. Thus, people genetically predisposed to developing weak inflammatory activity, seem to have fewer chances of developing cardiovascular diseases (CVD) and, subsequently, live longer if they do not become affected by serious infectious diseases. These results are in agreement with our other data demonstrating how genetic background may exert the opposite effect with respect to inflammatory components in CVD and longevity. In the present report, to validate this hypothesis, the levels of interleukin (IL)-6, a pro-inflammatory cytokine involved in atherosclerosis and longevity, were determined by an enzyme-linked immuno-sorbent assay (ELISA) in supernatants from a whole blood assay after stimulation with subliminal doses of lipopolysaccaride (LPS) from Escherichia coli (E. coli). The samples, genotyped for the ASP299GLY polymorphism, were challenged with LPS for 4, 24, and 48 h. What we found was that Il-6 values were significantly lower in

Address for correspondence: Dr. Giuseppina Candore, Ph.D., Gruppo di Studio sull'Immunosenescenza, Dipartimento di Biopatologia e Metodologie Biomediche, Corso Tukory 211, 90134 Palermo, Italy. Voice: +39-09-1655-5932; fax: +39-09-1655-5933.
e-mail: gcandore@unipa.it

Ann. N.Y. Acad. Sci. 1067: 282–287 (2006). © 2006 New York Academy of Sciences.
doi: 10.1196/annals.1354.037

carriers bearing TLR4 mutation. Therefore, the pathogen burden, by interacting with host genotype, determines the type and intensity of the immune-inflammatory responses accountable for pro-inflammatory status, CVD, and unsuccessful aging. On the other hand, our present data seem to explain the inconclusive results obtained in case–control studies taking into account the role of functional IL-6 polymorphisms in successful and unsuccessful aging. In fact, IL6 levels seem to depend, in addition, on IL-6 polymorphisms and on innate immunity gene polymorphisms as well.

KEYWORDS: AMI; inflammation; interleukin-6; longevity; TLR4

INTRODUCTION

The total burden of infection at different sites may affect the progression of atherosclerosis, the risk being modulated by host genotype. The role of the lipopolysaccaride (LPS) Toll-like receptor (TLR)4 is paradigmatic. Macrophages express receptors that recognize molecular patterns foreign to mammalian organisms but commonly found in pathogens, and, at the same time, are important in contributing to the inflammatory response. In this first line of defense, TLRs recognize pathogen-associated molecular patterns. The transmembrane TLR4, which initiates the innate immune response to common gram-negative bacteria, activates the inflammatory cell via the NF-κB pathway by inducing the expression of a variety of cytokines and other molecules crucial to immune responses.[1–3]

TLR4 expression has been described in human atherosclerotic lesions and the inflammatory mediators produced through its activation seem to exert various atherogenic effects involving the expression of adhesion molecules on endothelial cells, proliferation of smooth-muscle cells, activation of immune cells, stimulation of the acute-phase response, and matrix breakdown. The ASP299GLY (+896A/G) TLR4 single nucleotide polymorphism (SNP), known to attenuate receptor signaling, seems to determine a minor risk of developing carotid atherosclerosis and lesser intima media thickness in the common carotid artery. Furthermore, the subjects with mutant genotype have been claimed to display lower levels of same pro-inflammatory cytokines, acute-phase reactants, and soluble adhesion molecules, although the results of *in vitro* stimulation are discordant.[1–5]

We demonstrated that ASP299GLY TLR4 polymorphism shows a significantly lower frequency in patients affected by acute myocardial infarction (AMI) compared to controls, whereas centenarians show a higher frequency.[4] Thus, people genetically predisposed to a weak inflammatory activity have fewer chances of developing cardiovascular diseases (CVD) and, therefore, without any serious infectious disease complication, have the chance of living longer. This is in agreement with our other data showing that genetic background controling inflammation might play an opposite role in CVD and in longevity.[6–8]

In the present report, to validate this hypothesis, the levels of interleukin (IL)-6, a pro-inflammatory cytokine involved in atherogenesis, AMI, and longevity,[9,10] were determined by ELISA in supernatants from +896 G+ and +896 G– cells after stimulation with LPS from *Escherichia coli* (*E. coli*).

METHODS

Sixteen healthy unrelated subjects, previously typed for ASP299GLY TLR4 SNP, were studied (age range 25–50 years, 8 females and 8 males). None of these subjects was affected by prolonged illness and at the time of study none was ill or under medication. Blood venous samples were withdrawn from the subjects under basal condition at 9.00 AM. Whole-blood assay was performed by challenging the cells, from eight subjects with the wild-type cells and eight subjects that were carriers of mutation, with subliminal doses of LPS (1 γ/mL) from *E. coli* (serotype 055:B5) (8 +896 G+ and 8 +896 G– samples) for 4, 24, and 48 h.[11] The supernatants, harvested after centrifugation, were stored at $-70°$C until the enzyme-linked immuno-sorbent assay (ELISA) test was performed. The IL-6 test ELISA was a commercially available kit (R&D System, Abingdon, Oxon, UK). All tests were performed according to the manufacturer's instructions. To standardize our results, reference preparations (recombinant human IL-6) were tested in all assays. Results were expressed as pg/mL. Detection limits in our laboratory were 1.6 pg/mL. Quantitative values given as mean $\pm$ SD were examined in positive and negative subjects using the Mann–Whitney test.

RESULTS AND DISCUSSION

FIGURE 1 shows that Il-6 levels were lower in carriers bearing TLR4 SNP, but because of the small number of samples examined, significance was attained only at 4 h ($P = 0.04$ by Mann–Whitney test). As discussed in the INTRODUCTION, carriers bearing the TLR4 mutant genotype displayed a reduced inflammatory response both *in vitro* and *ex vivo* and in clinical studies, although discordant results have been obtained.[2–5] However, by using a subliminal dose of LPS, we have been able to confirm previous reports on hyporesponsiveness of mutant TLR4 genotype. It might be relevant to note that, by using higher doses of LPS, carriers of both the genotypes showed exactly similar levels of IL-6 (data not shown).

Chronic infection by gram-negative microorganisms may contribute to the inflammatory component of atherosclerosis, and LPS exerts pro-atherogenic effects by contributing to low-density lipoprotein (LDL) oxidation and monocyte/macrophage activation.[1,12] A few genetic variants of TLR4 that affect

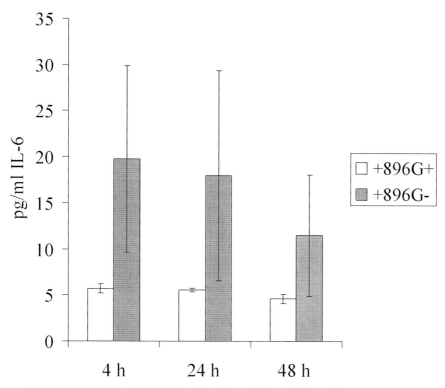

FIGURE 1. Il-6 levels (pg/mL) produced by cells from eight subjects with TLR4 wild-type and eight subjects that were carriers of mutation; these cells were stimulated for 4, 24, and 48 h in whole-blood assay, with subliminal doses of LPS (1 γ/mL). The significance was attained only at 4 h ($P = 0.04$ by Mann–Whitney test).

composition, structure, and function of the receptor have been identified. The Asp299Gly variant is biologically important, since it attenuates TLR4-mediated LPS signaling. Some studies have shown that subjects with the Asp299Gly TLR4 SNP have a lower risk of developing atherosclerosis and a decreased risk of acute coronary events independent of the standard coronary risk factors. However, discordant results have been reported. The causes of the discrepancies are not clear, but the inclusion criteria, the study populations, and the measured endpoint differed substantially among the studies. However, our recent results clearly support a role of TLR4 in AMI.[2–5] These results fit well with a recent study supporting a role of TLR4 in atherogenesis, and with the largest epidemiologic evaluation that showed lower levels of C-reactive protein with concomitant reduction in coronary artery disease risk in patients carrying the studied SNP.[13] These data suggest that the intensity of the genetically determined inflammatory response against pathogens might exert a major role in determining the magnitude of atherogenesis and subsequent clinical outcomes. Accordingly, in this preliminary study we have been able to demonstrate that this SNP strongly influences the *in vitro* response against LPS and carriers bearing TLR4 mutations produce a lesser amount of IL-6 than do wild-type carriers. Taking all this information together, it is tempting to consider TLR4 as the link between infection and the development of acute coronary events.[1–4,12]

On the other hand, these results might explain the inconclusive findings obtained in case–control studies on the role of functional IL-6 polymorphisms in successful and unsuccessful aging.[9,10] In particular, IL-6 has been suggested to play a key role in the pathogenesis of CHD through a combination of autocrine, paracrine, and endocrine mechanisms. Nevertheless, the role of the most common functional IL-6 SNP $-174C/G$ with respect to cardiovascular diseases is far from being clear. A number of studies reported clearly contradictory results with respect to the association of this SNP with cardiovascular risk or with other important parameters such as arterial responsiveness or CRP serum levels.[9] Discordant results have also been obtained by analyzing the converse association of this SNP with longevity.[10] The discordant results might be related to the fact that IL-6 serum levels are regulated also from innate immunity gene polymorphisms.

Finally, these data support the opinion that antagonistic pleiotropy plays a significant role in diseases and aging. The selection of genes with an enhanced inflammatory response against infection from earlier times may have switched to a maladaptive response in our modern environment, with its reduced pathogen load and improved control of severe infections by antibiotics.[3,8–10,14,15] In any case, all these data point out the strong relationship between infection, inflammation, genetics, and cardiovascular diseases.

ACKNOWLEDGMENTS

This work was supported by grants from the Ministry of Education, University and Research to D.L., G.C.R., C.C., and G.C. and the Ministry of Health (Markers genetici di sindrome coronarica acuta e valutazione della L-arginina nella prevenzione di eventi ischemici) to C.C. C.R.B., S.V., F.L., and M.P.G. are Ph.D. students in the Pathobiology Ph.D. course (directed by C.C.) of Palermo University and this work is in partial fulfillment of the requirement for the Ph.D. degree.

REFERENCES

1. ARROYO-ESPLIGUERO, R. *et al.* 2004. CD14 and toll-like receptor 4: a link between infection and acute coronary events? Heart **90:** 983–988.

2. SCHRODER, N.W. & R.R. SCHUMANN. 2005. Single nucleotide polymorphisms of Toll-like receptors and susceptibility to infectious disease. Lancet Infect. Dis. **5:** 156–164.
3. CANDORE, G. *et al*. 2006. Biology of longevity: role of the innate immune system. Rejuvenation Res. In press.
4. BALISTRERI, C.R. *et al*. 2004. Role of Toll-like receptor 4 in acute myocardial infarction and longevity. JAMA **292:** 2339–2340.
5. IMAHARA, S.D. *et al*. 2005. The TLR4 +896 polymorphism is not associated with lipopolysaccharide hypo-responsiveness in leukocytes. Genes Immun. **6:** 37–43.
6. LIO, D. *et al*. 2004. Opposite effects of IL-10 gene polymorphisms in cardiovascular diseases and in successful ageing: genetic background of male centenarians is prospective against coronary heart disease. J. Med. Genet. **41:** 790–794.
7. CARUSO, C. *et al*. 2004. Genetic background of centenarians may be protective against cardiovascular disease. Immunology 2004, Proceedings of the International Immunology Congress, Canada. pp. 29–34. Monduzzi. Bologna, Italy.
8. CARUSO, C. *et al*. 2005. Inflammation and life-span. Science **307:** 208–209.
9. CANDORE, G. *et al*. 2006. Cytokine gene polymorphisms and atherosclerosis. *In* Cytokine Gene Polymorphisms in Multifactorial Conditions. K. Vandenbroeck, Ed.: CRC Press. Boca Raton, FL.
10. REA, I.M. *et al*. 2006. Cytokine gene polymorphisms and longevity. *In* Cytokine Gene Polymorphisms in Multifactorial Conditions. K. Vandenbroeck, Ed.: CRC Press. Boca Raton, FL.
11. KRUGER, T. *et al*. 2004. *Ex vivo* induction of cytokines by mould components in whole blood of atopic and non-atopic volunteers. Cytokine **25:** 73–84.
12. STOLL, L.L. *et al*. 2004. Potential role of endotoxin as a proinflammatory mediator of atherosclerosis. Arterioscler. Thromb. Vasc. Biol. **24:** 2227–2236.
13. KOLEK, M.J. *et al*. 2003. Toll-like receptor 4 D299G polymorphism predicts lower risk of coronary artery diseases and diabetes. Circulation **108S:** Abstract 3476.
14. FRANCESCHI, C. *et al*. 2005. Genes involved in immune response/inflammation, IGF1/insulin pathway and response to oxidative stress play a major role in the genetics of human longevity: the lesson of centenarians. Mech. Ageing Dev. **126:** 351–361.
15. LICASTRO, F. *et al*. 2005. Innate immunity and inflammation in ageing: a key for understanding age-related diseases. Immun. Ageing **2:** 8. http://www.immunityageing.com/content/2/1/8.

Frequency of Polymorphisms of Signal Peptide of TGF-β1 and −1082G/A SNP at the Promoter Region of Il-10 Gene in Patients with Carotid Stenosis

ANTONIO CRIVELLO,[a] ANTONIO GIACALONE,[a] LETIZIA SCOLA,[a]
GIUSI IRMA FORTE,[a] DOMENICO NUZZO,[a] ROBERTINA GIACCONI,[b]
CATIA CIPRIANO,[b] GIUSEPPINA CANDORE,[a]
EUGENIO MOCCHEGIANI,[b] GIUSEPPINA COLONNA ROMANO,[a]
DOMENICO LIO,[a] AND CALOGERO CARUSO[a]

[a]Gruppo di Studio sull'Immunosenescenza, Sezione di Patologia Generale,
Dipartimento di Biopatologia e Metodologie Biomediche,
Università degli studi di Palermo, Palermo, Italy

[b]Sezione Nutrizione, Immunità ed Invecchiamento, Dipartimento di Ricerche
Immunologiche, IRCCS Istituto Nazionale Ricovero e Cura per gli Anziani
(INRCA) di Ancona, Ancona, Italy

ABSTRACT: The role of inflammation in atherosclerosis is well recognized. We have evaluated the allele frequencies of the +869T/C and +915G/C polymorphisms (SNPs) at the TGF-β1 gene and −1082G/A SNP at IL-10 promoter sequence, two well-known immunosuppressive and anti-inflammatory cytokines, in patients with carotid stenosis. Our data suggest a lack of association between these SNPs and the susceptibility to atherosclerosis although other reports have demonstrated this association. These results may be due to the pleiotropic effects of the cytokines and/or differences in haplotype combination that should be investigated to elucidate the role of TGF-β1 and IL-10 polymorphisms in atherosclerosis.

KEYWORDS: atherosclerosis; carotid stenosis; cytokine; SNP; IL-10; TGF-β1

INTRODUCTION

Atherosclerosis is considered an inflammatory response–mediated disease characterized by T helper 1 cells and monocyte recruitment in the arterial

Address for correspondence: Prof. Domenico Lio, Chair of Clinical Pathology, Immunosenescence Study Group, General Pathology Section, Department of Pathobiology and Biomedical Methodologies, University of Palermo, Corso Tukory 211, 90134 Palermo, Italy. Voice: +39-091-655-5913; fax: +39-091-655-5933.
e-mail: dolio@unipa.it

Ann. N.Y. Acad. Sci. 1067: 288–293 (2006). © 2006 New York Academy of Sciences.
doi: 10.1196/annals.1354.038

intima wall stimulated by the accumulation of oxidized lipoproteins. These cells secrete a variety of soluble factors including the pro-inflammatory cytokines, as interleukin (IL)-6, tumor necrosis factor-α, IL-1, and interferon-γ, which seem to be contributing to the formation and progression of lesions.[1] The outcome of the disease might, in theory, be positively influenced by the production of regulatory molecules as IL-10 and transforming growth factor (TGF-)-β1.[1] The TGF-β1 is a pleiotropic cytokine involved in the process of tissue remodeling, fibrosis, and angiogenesis.[2] A variety of experimental evidence, *in vivo* and *in vitro*, suggests, furthermore, an involvement of TGF-β1 in the stages of formation, progression, and break of atheromas.[3] In fact, TGF-β1 is a potent immunosuppressor[4] that is able to inhibit the synthesis of IL-6 from endothelial cells.[5] Moreover, other evidence suggests that TGF-β1 is able to induce the synthesis of IL-10,[6] to negatively regulate the expression of cellular adhesion molecules on endothelial cells,[7] and to inhibit the activity and expression of scavenger receptors and lipoprotein lipase.[8] On the other hand, this growth factor stimulates the synthesis of collagen from the vascular smooth cells, inhibiting contemporaneously the synthesis of metalloproteinase, contributing to the stability of plaque in the advanced stages of atherosclerosis.[9] *In vivo* experiments showed the anti-inflammatory effect of IL-10, in particular, that overexpression of this cytokine inhibits atherosclerosis in LDL receptor-deficient mice.[10] *In vitro* findings show that IL-10 downregulates the adhesion molecules on immune-competent cells and synthesis and function of metalloproteinases.[1] *In vivo* and *in vitro* studies demonstrated inter-individual variations in the production of TGF-β1 and IL-10,[11] suggesting possible genetic control over the expression and secretion of cytokine; particularly it is hypothesized that the functional polymorphisms in the promoter and codifying region of the genes play a central role.[12] In the human TGF-β1 gene, eight polymorphic sites have been identified, three of which are localized in the promoter region and the others localized in the codifying region.[13] In particular, polymorphisms of sequence at +869 and +915 nucleotides (codons 10 and 25 of signal peptide) of this cytokine are associated at an inter-individual variation in the levels of cytokine production.[11,12] The best documented of the polymorphisms localized at IL-10 locus is placed at −1082 from the start site of transcription and the G/A is able to affect cytokine production.[14] By studying a group of patients from central and northern Italy affected by carotid stenosis and a group of healthy control patients recruited in the same geographic area, we have evaluated the hypothesis that these genetic polymorphisms that are able to influence the production and function of TGF-β1 and IL-10 may play a role in the susceptibility to atherosclerosis.

MATERIALS AND METHODS

We analyzed the DNA from a group of patients with carotid stenosis living in the central and northern Italy ($n = 113$) who had carotid stenosis that was treated by endarterectomy. The patients were 60 to 85 years old (83 males and 30 females). One hundred and eighty-nine healthy old individuals matched for age and gender, who were recruited in the same geographic area, were also analyzed. The samples were collected at INRCA of Ancona. According to the Helsinki Declaration, informed consent was obtained from all patients involved in the study.

DNA samples were extracted by the salting-out technique. The +869T/C and +915G/C polymorphisms were analyzed by the sequence specific primer–polymerase chain reaction (SSP–PCR) method, employing two primers sense-specific for each allele (+869T, +869C, +915G, and +915C) and an antisense primer common to the two polymorphisms. PCRs were performed as described by Gewaltig et al.[13] −1082 G/A IL-10 promoter polymorphism was identified using SSP-PCR methodology as previously described.[15]

Genotype frequencies were evaluated by gene count. The data were tested for goodness of fit between the observed and expected genotype values and their fit to Hardy–Weinberg equilibrium. Contingency tables were constructed. A chi-square test with Yates adjustment was employed to determine the statistical significance of differences in percentages of homo- and heterozygous individuals for the single SNPs in patients and controls.

RESULTS AND DISCUSSION

TABLE 1 shows the results of IL-10 and TGF-β1 typing of patients and controls. The allele frequencies were not significantly different between the two groups that were analyzed. Moreover, no significant differences were observed considering genotype frequencies and stratifying data according to gender (data not shown).

The presence of a prolyn (+869C allele) in the codon 10 and/or an arginin (+915C allele) in position 25 of the amino acid sequence of TGF-β1 is related to increased functionality.[13] In spite of this functional relevance, our data, in

TABLE 1. IL-10 and TGF-β1 SNP allele frequencies in a group of patients affected by carotid stenosis[a]

	No. of alleles	IL-10 −1082G	IL-10 −1082A	TGF-β1 +869T	TGF-β1 +869C	TGF-β1 +915G	TGF-β1 +915C
Patients	226	0.451 (102)	0.549 (124)	0.456 (103)	0.544 (123)	0.885 (200)	0.115 (26)
Controls	378	0.449 (170)	0.551 (208)	0.458 (173)	0.542 (205)	0.910 (344)	0.090 (34)

Allele frequencies were found not significantly different between patient and control group by chi-square analysis. Not-significant differences were also observed considering genotype frequencies and stratifying data according to gender.
[a]The absolute number of genes counted is given in parentheses.

accord with those from other research groups, show that these polymorphisms are not associated with cardiovascular disease susceptibility,[16,17] although other reports have demonstrated this association.[18] Moreover, Grainger *et al.*[19] demonstrated a protective role on arterial walls, while an alternative role has been suggested by other studies that demonstrated the implication of this cytokine in pathological processes as vascular restenosis and thrombogenesis.[20,21] Different authors suggest that TGF-β1 is involved in the stabilization of plaque, proposing TGF-β1 as a possible therapeutic target in atherosclerosis.[9,22] Finally, other polymorphisms of the regulatory region of the TGF-β1 gene can participate in the regulation of cytokine synthesis so that, at the end, production might not depend on a single polymorphism but on the presence of "functional" haplotypes.

The $-1082G/A$ SNP is the most frequently investigated SNP at the IL-10 locus and its importance in IL-10 gene expression has been demonstrated by reporter gene assays. Higher IL-10 production seems to be associated with the $-1082G/G$ genotype. The IL-10 $-1082G/A$ polymorphism is highly predictive of cardiovascular events in dialysis patients, and our previous investigations have demonstrated that the IL-10 $-1082G/A$ polymorphism is a genetic marker for ischemic cardiovascular disease (myocardial infarction) risk.[15] On the other hand, according to data reported herein, other groups failed to identify an association between IL-10 polymorphisms and atherosclerosis-related diseases.[23,24] A possible explanation for these discrepancies might be that they are due to differences in the high polymorphism of the IL-10 gene.[25] Both SNPs and microsatellites that are able to affect the synthesis and production levels of the cytokine have been demonstrated in the IL-10 5′ flanking region and different extended haplotypes composed of SNP in the distal and proximal 5′ flanking region as well as by microsatellite alleles have been reported.[25] Therefore, to exclude the involvement of IL-10 polymorphisms in atherosclerosis, the role of IL-10 haplotypes should be investigated.

ACKNOWLEDGMENTS

This work was supported by grants from the Ministry of Education, University and Research, (local funding ex 60%) to D.L., G.C.R., C.C., and G.C. and the Ministry of Health (Markers genetici di sindrome coronarica acuta e valutazione della L-arginina nella prevenzione di eventi ischemici) to C.C. The collaboration with the "Gruppo di Studio sull'immunosenescenza," coordinated by Prof. C. Caruso and INRCA was enhanced by a cooperation contract (Longevity and elderly disability biological markers). A.C., G.I.F., and D.N. are Ph.D. students in the Pathobiology course (directed by C.C.) of Palermo University and this work is in partial fulfillment of the requirement for the Ph.D.

REFERENCES

1. OHSUZU, F. 2004. The roles of cytokines, inflammation and immunity in vascular diseases. J. Atheroscler. Thromb. **11:** 313–321.
2. COHEN, M.D., V. CIOCCA & R.A. PANETTIERI, JR. 1997. TGF–beta 1 modulates human airway smooth-muscle cell proliferation induced by mitogens. Am. J. Respir. Cell. Mol. Biol. **16:** 85–90.
3. GRAINGER, D.J., C.M. WITCHELL & J.C. METCALFE. 1995. Tamoxifen elevates transforming growth factor-beta and suppresses diet-induced formation of lipid lesions in mouse aorta. Nat. Med. **1:** 1067–1073.
4. DENNLER, S., M.J. GOUMANS & P. TEN DIJKE. 2002. Transforming growth factor beta signal transduction. J. Leukoc. Biol. **71:** 731–740.
5. CHEN, C.C. & A.M. MANNING. 1996. TGF–beta 1, IL-10 and IL-4 differentially modulate the cytokine-induced expression of IL-6 and IL-8 in human endothelial cells. Cytokine **8:** 58–65.
6. D'ORAZIO, T.J. & J.Y. NIEDERKORN. 1998. A novel role for TGF–beta and IL-10 in the induction of immune privilege. J. Immunol. **160:** 2089–2098.
7. DICHIARA, M.R. et al. 2000. Inhibition of E-selectin gene expression by transforming growth factor beta in endothelial cells involves coactivator integration of Smad and nuclear factor kappaB-mediated signals. J. Exp. Med. **192:** 695–704.
8. ARGMANN, C.A. et al. 2001. Transforming growth factor-beta1 inhibits macrophage cholesteryl ester accumulation induced by native and oxidized VLDL remnants. Arterioscler. Thromb. Vasc. Biol. **21:** 2011–2018.
9. MALLAT, Z. et al. 2001. Inhibition of transforming growth factor-beta signaling accelerates atherosclerosis and induces an unstable plaque phenotype in mice. Circ. Res. **89:** 930–934.
10. VON DER THUSEN, J.H. et al. 2001. Attenuation of atherogenesis by systemic and local adenovirus-mediated gene transfer of interleukin-10 in LDLr-/- mice. FASEB J. **15:** 2730–2732.
11. BIDWELL, J., L. KEEN, G. GALLAGHER, et al. 1999. Cytokine gene polymorphism in human disease: on-line databases. Genes Immun. **1:** 3–19.
12. HAUKIM, N. et al. 2002. Cytokine gene polymorphism in human disease: on-line databases, supplement 2. Genes Immun. **3:** 313–330.
13. GEWALTIG, J. et al. 2002. Association of polymorphisms of the transforming growth factor-beta1 gene with the rate of progression of HCV-induced liver fibrosis.Clin. Chim. Acta **316:** 83–94.
14. TURNER, D.M. et al. 1997. An investigation of polymorphism in the interleukin-10 gene promoter. Eur. J. Immunogenet. **24:** 1–8.
15. LIO, D. et al. 2004. Opposite effects of IL-10 common gene polymorphisms in cardiovascular diseases and in successful ageing: genetic background of male centenarians is protective against coronary heart disease. J. Med. Genet. **41:** 790–794.
16. SYRRIS, P. et al. 1998. Transforming growth factor-beta1 gene polymorphisms and coronary artery disease. Clin. Sci. (Lond.) **95:** 659–667.
17. WANG, X.L. et al. 1998. A common polymorphism of the transforming growth factor-beta1 gene and coronary artery disease. Clin. Sci. (Lond.) **95:** 745–746.
18. CAMBIEN, F. et al. 1996. Polymorphisms of the transforming growth factorbeta 1 gene in relation to myocardial infarction and blood pressure. The Etude

Cas-Temoin de l'Infarctus du Myocarde. (ECTIM) Study. Hypertension **28:** 881–887.

19. GRAINGER, D.J. *et al.* 2000. Dietary fat and reduced levels of TGF-beta1 act synergistically to promote activation of the vascular endothelium and formation of lipid lesions. J. Cell Sci. **113:** 2355–2361.

20. SCHULICK, A.H. *et al.* 1998. Overexpression of transforming growth factor beta1 in arterial endothelium causes hyperplasia, apoptosis, and cartilaginous metaplasia. Proc. Natl. Acad. Sci. USA **95:** 6983–6988.

21. OHJI, T. *et al.* 1995. Transforming growth factor beta 1 and beta 2 induce down-modulation of thrombomodulin in human umbilical vein endothelial cells. Thromb. Haemost. **73:** 812–818.

22. LUTGENS, E. & M.J. DAEMEN. 2001. Transforming growth factor-beta: a local or systemic mediator of plaque stability? Circ. Res. **89:** 853–855.

23. KOCH, W. *et al.* 2001. Interleukin-10 and tumor necrosis factor gene polymorphisms and risk of coronary artery disease and myocardial infarction. Atherosclerosis **159:** 137–144.

24. DONGER, C. *et al.* 2001. New polymorphisms in the interleukin-10 gene-relationships to myocardial infarction. Eur. J. Clin. Invest. **31:** 9–14.

25. KURREEMAN, F.A. *et al.* 2004. Transcription of the IL10 gene reveals allele-specific regulation at the mRNA level. Hum. Mol. Genet. **13:** 1755–1762.

Reduced Expression Levels of the Senescence Biomarker Clusterin/Apolipoprotein J in Lymphocytes from Healthy Centenarians

IOANNIS P. TROUGAKOS,[a] CHARIKLIA PETROPOULOU,[a,c]
CLAUDIO FRANCESCHI,[b,c] AND EFSTATHIOS S. GONOS[a]

[a]*Laboratory of Molecular & Cellular Ageing, Institute of Biological Research & Biotechnology, National Hellenic Research Foundation, 48 Vas. Constantinou Ave., Athens 11635, Greece*

[b]*Department of Experimental Pathology, University of Bologna, via San Giacomo 14, Bologna 40126, Italy*

[c]*These authors contributed equally to the work.*

ABSTRACT: Clusterin/apolipoprotein J (CLU) is a conserved, ubiquitously expressed secreted glycoprotein that has been implicated in several physiological processes and was found to accumulate in many severe physiological disturbances. We have previously shown that the CLU gene and protein are upregulated during replicative senescence, stress-induced premature senescence, *in vivo* aging, and in several age-related diseases. In this study we have examined the CLU gene relationship to human longevity. We recruited and further analyzed 96 blood samples from Italian and Greek healthy donors of different ages, including 49 centenarians. We found that although the CLU gene expression levels increase during aging, in the centenarians' samples CLU levels were lower than those found in old donors. We then investigated the possible existence of a genetic polymorphism related to longevity at the CLU structural locus. A neutral noncoding sequence variant was detected 35 nucleotides upstream from exon 6, which does not correlate, however, with the age of the donor. We conclude that CLU gene accumulation during *in vivo* aging does not directly relate to chronological age, but rather indicates increased levels of organismal stress due to a progressive failure of homeostasis and/or to prolonged exposure to a stressful environment.

KEYWORDS: aging; centenarians; clusterin/apolipoprotein J; lymphocytes; polymorphism

Address for correspondence: Efstathios S. Gonos, Laboratory of Molecular & Cellular Ageing, Institute of Biological Research & Biotechnology, National Hellenic Research Foundation, 48 Vas. Constantinou Ave., Athens 11635, Greece. Voice: +30-210-7273756; fax: +30-210-7273677.
e-mail: sgonos@eie.gr

Ann. N.Y. Acad. Sci. 1067: 294–300 (2006). © 2006 New York Academy of Sciences.
doi: 10.1196/annals.1354.039

INTRODUCTION

Clusterin/apolipoprotein J (CLU) is a conserved secreted glycoprotein of 449 amino acids that matures to a disulfide-linked heterodimeric protein form of ~70–80 kDa (reviewed in Ref. 16). Many diverse physiological functions have been attributed to CLU including cell–cell or cell–substratum interactions, membrane recycling, sperm maturation, lipid transportation, and tissue remodeling (reviewed in Ref. 7). In addition, it was recently proposed that CLU may also function as an extracellular chaperone that stabilizes stressed proteins in a folding-competent state (reviewed in Ref. 20). Another prominent feature of the CLU protein is its upregulation in many severe physiological disturbance states including tumor formation, kidney degenerative diseases, and several neurodegenerative conditions (for reviews see Refs. 1 and 16).

We have previously cloned CLU as a senescence-induced gene[4] and showed that CLU is upregulated during both replicative senescence and stress-induced premature senescence in human cells.[13] CLU also accumulates in human serum during *in vivo* aging as well as during several age-related diseases, including diabetes type II, myocardial infarction, and coronary heart disease.[17] Thus CLU is a biomarker of human aging and senescence. CLU has biological properties similer to these of apolipoprotein E (ApoE),[1] which has been previously associated with longevity.[14] Therefore, in this work, we have examined the relationship of the CLU gene to human longevity. Specifically, we assayed CLU gene expression levels in lymphocyte samples derived from healthy donors of different ages including centenarians and we investigated the possible existence of a genetic polymorphism related to longevity at the CLU gene's structural locus.

MATERIALS AND METHODS

Sample Collection

Heparinized whole blood samples or lymphocyte samples were collected from 96 Italian and Greek healthy donors of different ages by standard methods. The samples were grouped and named as young (age, 23–40 years; $n = 20$), old (age, 50–89 years; $n = 27$), and centenarian (age, 99–107 years; $n = 49$).

RNA Extraction and Semi-Quantitative RT-PCR Analysis

Total RNA was directly isolated from lymphocytes derived from 47 donors of different ages (young, $n = 9$; old; $n = 13$, centenarian, $n = 25$). RNA was reverse-transcribed and PCR amplified by standard methods. All target genes were co-amplified with β_2-microglobulin as an internal control.

CLU and β_2-microglobulin were amplified at 58°C for 25 cycles and fibronectin was amplified at 58°C for 20 cycles. Polymerase chain reaction primers for β_2-microglobulin have been described elsewhere.[12] CLU primers (forward; CGGGGTGAAACAGATAAAG, reverse; TGCGGTCACCATT CATCCA) and fibronectin primers (forward; CATTGCCTGTTCTGCTTC, reverse; TTGGGTGACTTTCCTACT) were originated by using the Oligo™ Version 4.0 for MacIntosh (Apple, Capertino, CA). Quantification analysis was carried out by using a Molecular Dynamics (Sunnyvale, CA) scanner and Image-Quant software.

Single-Strand Conformation Polymorphism (SSCP) Analysis

Genomic DNA was directly extracted from 3 mL of blood samples derived from 49 donors of different ages (young, $n = 11$; old, $n = 14$, centenarian, $n = 24$), by using the Wizard® Genomic DNA Purification System Kit (Promega Corporation, USA). Genomic DNA was subjected to PCR with upstream and downstream intronic primers flanking all nine coding exons of the CLU gene locus. All upstream and downstream primers were adapted from Tycko *et al.*,[18] apart from the reverse primer of exon 9 (5′-AGAGGACCCTCCAAGCGAT-3′). PCR amplification was carried out using 200 ng genomic DNA at 58°C for 30 cycles. PCR products were diluted 1:5 into 0.1% SDS/10 mM EDTA, heated to 65°C for 5 min, diluted 1:1 into a stop solution containing 95% formamide and 10 mM NaOH and finally heated to 94°C for 3–5 min. Denatured products were then loaded on a 0.5× Mutation Detection Enhancement gel solution and electrophoresis was carried out at 300 V at room temperature for 16–20 h. Single-strand DNA bands were visualized by silver staining and detected variants were further verified by direct sequencing analysis.

RESULTS AND DISCUSSION

Reduced CLU Gene Expression Levels in Centenarians

First, we assayed CLU gene expression levels in lymphocyte samples from donors of different ages including centenarians. As is evident in FIGURE 1A the expression levels of the CLU gene were found to increase during aging in accordance with previous findings.[17] Interestingly, the mean CLU gene expression levels were reduced in the samples derived from the centenarians as compared to elderly donors and were rather similar to those found in young donors. Preliminary analysis of skin fibroblast samples derived from donors of various ages including centenarians is in agreement with these data (not shown). To further verify these intriguing findings, we have also analyzed the expression levels of another established biomarker of senescence, namely

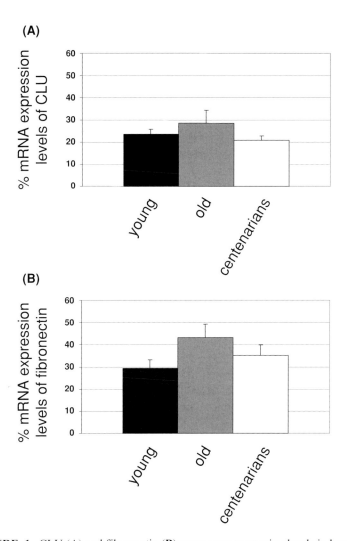

FIGURE 1. CLU (**A**) and fibronectin (**B**) mean gene expression levels in lymphocyte samples from young, old, and centenarian donors. Although the expression levels of both the CLU and fibronectin mRNAs increase from young to old donors, centenarians were found to have lower expression levels than those recorded in their old counterparts. Maximum detected CLU or fibronectin mRNA levels were arbitrarily set to 100%. Bars denote standard deviation (SD).

fibronectin.[8] As shown in FIGURE 1B, the mean fibronectin gene expression levels in centenarians were reduced as compared to the old donors, similar to the findings reported by the CLU gene expression analysis. It is well established that the expression of CLU is associated with both a wide variety of diseases (reviewed in Ref. 16), and "stress" conditions[9] including oxidative stress.[2,15,19]

As healthy centenarians represent the best example of successful aging, and various studies have shown that these individuals have escaped major age-associated diseases (reviewed in Refs. 3 and 5), we hypothesize that CLU accumulation during *in vivo* aging may indicate a direct response to a higher organismal oxidation state (or to general "accumulative stress"), a condition not necessarily present in centenarians.

Analysis of CLU Gene Sequence Variants in Relation to Longevity

Next, we search for CLU polymorphisms that may relate to longevity. Single-strand conformation polymorphism (SSCP) analysis in eight out of the nine exons of the CLU gene showed no alterations of single-strand conformations in all analyzed samples. However, SSCP analysis of exon 6 revealed two distinct migration patterns of the DNA bands indicative of a sequence variant (SV). Subsequent sequence analysis revealed that the detected variant presented a noncoding thymidine (T) deletion at the intron sequence, 35 nucleotides upstream from exon 6 (termed SV-6B). This polymorphism has not been described in previous studies concerning allelic ethnic variations of CLU. [6,11,18] The SV-6B was found in 8% of the samples analyzed; the remaining 92% of the samples did not present any nucleotide change, either in the coding sequence of exon 6 or in the intron sequence preceding or following exon 6 (termed SV-6A). The SV-6B distribution did not reveal any correlation with the age of the donor (TABLE 1) since it was evenly detected in all age groups.

To our knowledge these preliminary results represent the first screening for CLU alleles in relation to aging and longevity. One of the most striking observations regarding CLU is the breadth of its biological distribution and its high level of sequence homology (70–85%) among the various mammalian species cloned (reviewed in Ref. 16) The wide tissue distribution and species sequence conservation suggest that the protein performs a function of fundamental biological importance and thus if any functional CLU polymorphism exists it should be rare. In fact, although Tycko *et al.*[18] found seven CLU sequence variants (two of which altered the predicted amino acid sequence), none of these showed a consistent association with Alzheimer's disease. Similarly, the

TABLE 1. Age group distribution of the SV-6B found in the intron sequence of exon 6 of the CLU gene

Donor Groups	Age (years)	Number	Sex (M/F ratio)	6 A	6 B
	Subjects			SV	
Young	23–40	11	4/7	10 (91%)	1 (9%)
Old	50–89	14	6/8	12 (86%)	2 (14%)
Centenarians	99–107	24	6/18	23 (96%)	1 (4%)
Total		49	16/33	45 (92%)	4 (8%)

two-allele polymorphisms identified by Kamboh *et al.*[6] in populations with African ancestry showed no significant impact on the lipidemic profile of the examined participants. However, a recent study in the Japanese population identified 11 single nucleotide polymorphisms (SNPs) of CLU gene by direct sequencing, of which one was found to contribute to the serum lipid levels and the progression of carotid atherosclerosis in hypertensive Japanese females.[10] Thus these data cannot exclude a possible existence of a CLU allele that may be associated with longevity. Such a possibility should be confirmed by a broader population study.

In summary, this study provides evidence that CLU gene accumulation during *in vivo* aging does not directly correlate with chronological age, but rather it indicates increased levels of organismal stress due to progressive failure of homeostasis and/or prolonged exposure to a stressful environment. Given the important role of CLU in a variety of key biological processes, the reduced CLU levels detected in healthy centenarians may open up new directions for future biogerontological research.

ACKNOWLEDGMENTS

We would like to thank Drs. N. Chondrogianni, A. Dontas, C. Karageorgiou, and I. Sgouros for essential help during sample recruitment. The work described was supported by a European Union "Genetics of Healthy Aging (GEHA)" Grant (Contract No: LSH-CT-2004-503270) to E.S.G. and C.F., and by a European Union, Food/FP-6 "Zincage" grant (Contract No. FOOD-CT-2003-506850) to E.S.G.

REFERENCES

1. CALERO, M., A. ROSTAGNO, E. MATSUBARA, *et al.* 2000. Apolipoprotein J (clusterin) and Alzheimer's disease. Microsc. Res. Tech. **50:** 305–315.
2. DUMONT, P., F. CHAINIAUX, F. ELIAERS, *et al.* 2002. Overexpression of apolipoprotein J in human fibroblasts protects against cytotoxicity and premature senescence induced by ethanol and tert-butylhydroperoxide. Cell Stress, chaprones **7:** 23–35.
3. FRANCESCHI, C. & M. BONAFE. 2003. Centenarians as a model for healthy aging. Biochem. Soc. Trans. **31:** 457–461.
4. GONOS, E.S., A. DERVENTZI, M. KVEIBORG, *et al.* 1998. Cloning and identification of genes that associate with mammalian senescence. Exp. Cell Res. **240:** 66–74.
5. GONOS, E.S. 2000. Genetics of aging: lessons from centenarians. Exp. Gerontol. **35:** 15–21.
6. KAMBOH, M.I., J.A. HARMONY, B. SEPEHRNIA, *et al.* 1991. Genetic polymorphism of apolipoprotein J and its impact on quantitative lipid traits in normolipidemic subjects. Am. J. Hum. Genet. **49:** 1167–1173.

7. KOCH-BRANDT, C. & C. MORGANS. 1996. Clusterin: a role in cell survival in the face of apoptosis? Prog. Mol. Subcell. Biol. **16:** 130–149.

8. KUMAZAKI, T., R. WADHWA, S.C. KAUL, *et al.* 1997. Expression of endothelin, fibronectin, and mortalin as aging and mortality markers. Exp. Gerontol. **32:** 95–103.

9. MICHEL, D., G. CHATELAIN, S. NORTH, *et al.* 1997. Stress-induced transcription of the clusterin/apoJ gene. Biochem. J. **328:** 45–50.

10. MIWA, Y., S. TAKIUCHI, K. KAMIDE, *et al.* 2005. Insertion/deletion polymorphism in clusterin gene influences serum lipid levels and carotid intima-media thickness in hypertensive Japanese females. Biochem. Biophys. Res. Commun. **331:** 1587–1593.

11. NESTLERODE, C.S., C.H. BUNKER, D.K. SANGHERA, *et al.* 1999. Apolipoprotein J polymorphisms and serum HDL cholesterol levels in African blacks. Hum. Biol. **71:** 197–218.

12. NOONAN, K.E., C. BECK, T.A. HOLZMAYER, *et al.* 1990. Quantitative analysis of MDR-1 (multidrug resistance) gene expression in human tumors by polymerase chain reaction. Proc. Natl. Acad. Sci. USA. **87:** 7160–7164.

13. PETROPOULOU, C., I.P. TROUGAKOS, E. KOLETTAS, *et al.* 2001. Clusterin/apolipoprotein J is a novel biomarker of cellular senescence, that does not affect the proliferative capacity of human diploid fibroblasts. FEBS Lett. **509:** 287–297.

14. SCHÄCHTER, F., L. FAURE-DELANEF, F. GUÉNOT, *et al.* 1994. Genetic associations with human longevity at the APOE and ACE loci. Nat. Genet. **6:** 29–32.

15. SCHWOCHAU, G.B., K.A. NATH & M.E. ROSENBERG. 1998. Clusterin protects against oxidative stress *in vitro* through aggregative and nonaggregative properties. Kidney Int. **53:** 1647–1653.

16. TROUGAKOS, I.P. & E.S. GONOS. 2002. Clusterin/apolipoprotein J in human aging and cancer. Int. J. Biochem. Cell Biol. **34:** 1430–1448.

17. TROUGAKOS, I.P., M. POULAKOU, M. STATHATOS, *et al.* 2002. Serum levels of the senescence biomarker clusterin/apolipoprotein J increase significantly in diabetes type II and during development of coronary heart disease or at myocardial infarction. Exp. Gerontol. **37:** 1175–1187.

18. TYCKO, B., L. FENG, L. NGUYEN, *et al.* 1996. Polymorphisms in the human apolipoprotein-J/clusterin gene: ethnic variation and distribution in Alzheimer's disease. Hum. Genet. **98:** 430–436.

19. VIARD, I., P. WEHRLI, L. JORNOT, *et al.* 1999. Clusterin gene expression mediates resistance to apoptotic cell death induced by heat shock and oxidative stress. J. Invest. Dermatol. **112:** 290–296.

20. WILSON, M.R. & S.B. EASTERBROOK-SMITH. 2000. Clusterin is a secreted mammalian chaperone. Trends Biochem. Sci. **25:** 95–98.

Heat-Shock Protein 70 Genes and Human Longevity

A View from Denmark

RIPUDAMAN SINGH,[a] STEEN KØLVRAA,[b] PETER BROSS,[c]
KAARE CHRISTENSEN,[d] NIELS GREGERSEN,[c] QIHUA TAN,[e]
UFFE BIRK JENSEN,[a,h] HANS EIBERG,[f] AND
SURESH I. S. RATTAN[g]

[a]*Department of Human Genetics, University of Aarhus, Aarhus, Denmark*

[b]*Department of Clinical Genetics, Vejle Hospital, Vejle, Denmark*

[c]*Research Unit for Molecular Medicine, Aarhus University Hospital and Faculty of Health Sciences, Skejby Hospital, Aarhus, Denmark*

[d]*Institute of Public Health, University of Southern Denmark, Odense, Denmark*

[e]*Odense University Hospital, KKA, Department of Clinical Biochemistry and Genetics, Odense, Denmark*

[f]*Panum Institut, Copenhagen, Denmark*

[g]*Department of Molecular Biology, University of Aarhus, Aarhus, Denmark*

[h]*Department of Clinical Genetics, University of Aarhus, Aarhus, Denmark*

ABSTRACT: We have studied the association of three single nucleotide polymorphisms (SNPs) present in the three *HSP70* (heat-shock protein) genes on 6p21 with human longevity. The availability of biological samples from various population cohorts in Denmark has given us the opportunity to try novel methods of gene association with human longevity. A significant association of one haplotype with male longevity was observed. Furthermore, a significant difference in the survival of the carriers of the different genotypes in females was observed. We also found an age-dependant decline in the ability of peripheral blood mononuclear cells to respond to heat stress in terms of Hsp70 induction.

KEYWORDS: human longevity; aging; heat-shock proteins; heat-shock response; gene association; linkage disequilibrium

Address for correspondence: Ripudaman Singh, Department of Human Genetics, Bartholin Building, University of Aarhus, Aarhus C. Denmark. Voice: +45-8942-1682; fax: +45-8612-3173.
e-mail: singh@humgen.au.dk

Ann. N.Y. Acad. Sci. 1067: 301–308 (2006). © 2006 New York Academy of Sciences.
doi: 10.1196/annals.1354.040

INTRODUCTION

Human longevity is a multifactorial trait with both genetic and environmental factors playing an important role in its manifestation. Studies in twins on the genetic basis of human longevity indicated that approximately 25% of the observed differences in life expectancy are due to genetic variations.[1,2] The conventional approach for identifying longevity-determining genes has been by population-based association studies, where a group of long-lived individuals (LLIs) is compared to a group of young individuals for differences in the gene and genotype frequencies of candidate genes.[3] This approach, though common, has several limiting factors.[3]

HSP70 GENE AND HUMAN LONGEVITY

Heat-shock proteins (Hsps)[4] are ubiquitous, highly conserved proteins which are a part of the cellular safety and rescue mechanisms. At the cellular level all organisms respond to stress by synthesizing Hsps at the expense of other proteins. This phenomenon is called "heat-shock response" (HSR),[5] which protects cells from subsequent damage and aids them to counteract the effects of the stress. The capacity to respond rapidly to stress at the gene level determines the adaptive and, therefore, the survival capacity and longevity of the organism.[6] One way of indicating the relationship between human longevity and stress response is to demonstrate an association between single nucleotide polymorphisms (SNPs) in *Hsp* genes (*HSP*) and longevity[7,8] or parameters of human aging.[9]

Of all the various heat-shock proteins, Hsp70 is the most prominent and best characterized of the stress protein families. Hsp70 is a highly inducible and most actively synthesized protein in the cell upon heat shock. In humans there are 11 different isoforms of *HSP70* encoded by different genes located at dispersed loci. Three of the 11 isoforms of *HSP70* are localized within the major histocompatibility complex (MHC) class III region on chromosome 6p21.[10] These are intron-less *HSP70A1A (HSP70-1), HSP70A1B (HSP70-2),* and *HSP70A1L (HSP70-Hom)*[11] genes. They display a very high sequence similarity but differ in their regulation. We have studied the association of three SNPs, one in each MHC-linked *HSP70* gene, with human longevity, survival, and parameters of aging (TABLE 1).

CHOICE OF SUBJECTS AND METHODS

With the ever-increasing number of elderly persons in the population and in well-maintained health and population registries, [12,13] the availability of a unique set of biological samples for research from various well-established

TABLE 1. SNPs in HSP70 genes studied for their association with human longevity

SNP (position)	Marker	Nucleotide change
HSPA1A A>C (−110; 5′ flanking)	rs1008438	A to C transversion
HSPA1B A>G (1267 coding)	rs1061581	A to G transition
HSPA1L T>C (2437 coding)	rs2227956	T to C transition (Met to Thr substitution)[a]

[a] Variation may affect the substrate specificity and chaperone activity of the Hsp70.

TABLE 2. Different population cohorts in Denmark used for studying the association of HSP70 genes with human longevity

Population cohorts	Mean age at the time of sampling (in years)
Twins (LSADT)	75.6
Danish families (only parents)	40.8
1905 Cohort	92.8
Centenarians (DLCS)	—
Heat-shock response study	young = 22.6; middle-aged = 56.3

population databases, and from different age-related cohorts, in Denmark, provides a rare opportunity to perform novel population-based genetic association studies by mitigating many of the limiting factors [9,14–17] (TABLE 2).

For our research we have used DNA samples from 426 participants from the following groups:

(1) Longitudinal Study of Ageing Danish Twins (LSADT), which is the oldest twin registry in the world.[18] These twins, sampled in 1999, are between the ages of 70 and 91 years (mean age 75.6 years), and have been categorized according to the absence or presence of various age-related diseases and for various age-related parameters including scores of physical and cognitive tests.[19]

(2) One hundred fifty-seven DNA samples collected in 1998 from individuals born in 1905[13] have been used to perform survival analyses.

(3) Trio samples (mother, father, and child) from 42 Danish families[20,21] were used for molecular haplotyping.

(4) Sixty-two samples from the Danish Longitudinal Centenarian Study (DLCS) were also used. The DLCS is a clinical epidemiological survey of all persons living in Denmark who celebrated their 100th birthday during the period April 1, 1995 to May 31, 1996 (276 people).

The three SNPs in the three *HSP70* genes were genotyped using real-time polymerase chain reaction on the LightCycler system (Roche Applied Sciences), which allows monitoring of the amplification of the PCR product in real time, using fluorescent labeled oligonucleotide probes (TIB MOL-BIOL, Germany) and primers (DNA Technology A/S, Denmark) specific for each SNP (sequences of primers and probes can be provided on request).

For different population cohorts haplotypes were generated by using the computer program PHASE (Version 2.0.2), which implements a Bayesian statistical method for reconstructing haplotypes from population data.[22,23]

Pair-wise linkage Disequilibrium (LD) among the three markers was calculated using Java LINkage Disequilibrium Plotter (JLIN) (http//www.genepi.com.au/projects/jlin).

Blood samples were also collected from a group of young (mean age 22.6 years) and middle-aged individuals (mean age 56.3 years). Mononuclear cells (monocytes and lymphocytes) were isolated and then studied for age-related HSR after giving 1 h of heat shock for 42°C followed by 5 h of recovery. The amount of induced protein was quantified by using a flow cytometer.

RESULTS AND DISCUSSION

The gene and genotype frequency of the three SNPs was found to be in a Hardy–Weinberg equilibrium. In LSADT "Self-rated health" ($P = 0.0046$) and "Relative self-rated health" ($P = 0.018$), which represent an individual's overall sense of physical well-being and which have been shown to be both predictors of survival at older ages and better indicators of future survival than objectively measured health status, were associated with heterozygosity for $-110A > C$ polymorphism in the promoter region of *HSP70-1*.[9]

The molecular haplotype analyses on Danish family samples have revealed high LD among the three markers (TABLE 3). Pair-wise LD calculated among the three markers also showed a high LD ($D' = 1$) between the SNP at *HSPA1A* with the other two SNPs at *HSP70A1B* and *HSP70A1L* (FIG. 1). This information is very important when it comes to discovering genes that influence complex traits such as longevity.[24] On analyzing the frequency distribution of

TABLE 3. Comparison of haplotype frequencies in the family samples (only parents) generated by PHASE and from allele frequencies

Haplotypes[a]	Observed frequency (generated by PHASE)	Expected frequency (generated from allele frequency)
A-A-T	0.41	0.3
A-A-C	0.18	0.09
G-A-T	0.03	0.2
G-A-C	0.02	0.06
A-C-T	0	0.16
G-C-T	0.34	0.1
G-C-C	0	0.03
A-C-C	0	0.05

Chi-square = 171.457; df = 7; P value < 0.0001.
[a]The first position in the haplotypes is the marker at gene *HSPA1B*, second at *HSPA1A*, and third at *HSPA1L*.

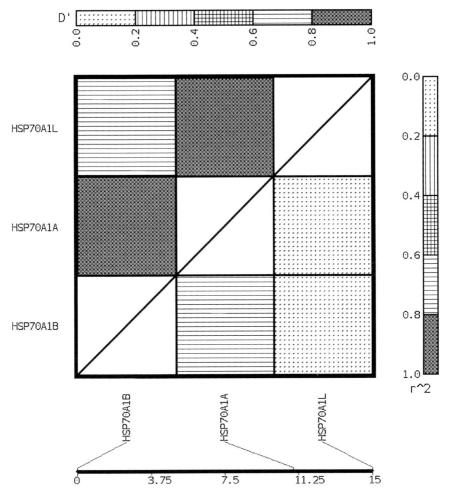

FIGURE 1. Pair-wise measurement of LD among the three *HSP70* gene markers. The figure shows two common ways of measuring LD, D′, and r^2. The distance shown among the markers is the relative distance, in kilobases, where position 0 corresponds to *HSP70A1B*.

haplotypes across different age groups from young individuals to centenarians we found a significant age-dependent increase in the frequency of one haplotype in males (Singh *et al.*, in preparation).

As mentioned above most of the genetic association studies on human longevity are performed in a case–control manner by comparing the gene/genotype frequencies between young and LLIs. This method, though widely used, has a shortcoming in that comparing the young with LLIs may give false-positive results, where the differences in the frequencies of the gene in study might just be owing to secular changes in population demographic and genetic parameters of the two groups and not necessarily age. To mitigate this factor, cohort studies, which focus on tracking the survival of a group of individuals born in the same time period, are appropriate alternatives. Our work on the cohort persons of Danish form in the year 1905 has provided us with the opportunity to perform such studies. We have seen a significant difference in the survival of the carriers of different genotypes. Female carriers of CC genotype of *HSP70A1A* survive better than the noncarriers (AA and AC) ($P = 0.005$). It was also observed that female carriers of GG genotype in *HSP70A1B* survive better than noncarriers ($P = 0.04$). (Singh *et al.*, in preparation).

We have also seen that peripheral blood mononuclear cells of young and middle-aged individuals respond differently to heat stress, confirming that in humans there is significant age-dependent attenuation in the ability to respond to stress (Singh *et al.*, in preparation). Also, in the young subjects a positive association was found between the *HSPA1L* (T2Y37C) polymorphism and HSR. CC carriers had significantly lower induction than TT carriers in both monocytes ($P = 0.015$) and lymphocytes ($P = 0.004$). This polymorphism, which is present in the coding region of the *HSPA1L* gene, can affect the chaperoning function of Hsp70.

Our results from the association of SNPs in three *HSP70* genes with human longevity, survival, and parameters of aging have reiterated our belief that the genes involved in cellular maintenance and repair mechanisms are indeed important candidates for deciphering the genetics of human longevity. Additionally, the availability of samples from different population cohorts in Denmark has provided us with the opportunity to perform novel studies by mitigating many confounding factors.

ACKNOWLEDGMENTS

We are thankful to Christian Knudsen for his technical support and to Mari Sild for her help in genotyping. We also thank the personnel of the Blood Bank, Skejby Sygehus. The studies received financial support from the Danish Center for Molecular Gerontology (DCMG), Danish Research Councils, and Novo Nordisk Fund.

REFERENCES

1. HERSKIND, A.M., M. MCGUE, N.V. HOLM, *et al.* 1996. The heritability of human longevity: a population-based study of 2872 Danish twin pairs born 1870–1900. Hum. Genet. **97**: 319–323.
2. TAN, Q.H., G. DE BENEDICTIS, A.I. YASHIN, *et al.* 2001. Measuring the genetic influence in modulating the human life span: gene-environment interaction and the sex-specific genetic effect. Biogerontology **2**: 141–153.

3. DE BENEDICTIS, G., Q. TAN, B. JEUNE, *et al.* 2001. Recent advances in human gene-longevity association studies. Mech. Ageing Dev. **122:** 909–920.

4. VERBEKE, P., J. FONAGER, B.F.C. CLARK, *et al.* 2001. Heat shock response and ageing: mechanisms and applications. Cell Biol. Int. **25:** 845–857.

5. VERBEKE, P., B.F.C. CLARK & S.I.S. RATTAN. 2001. Reduced levels of oxidized and glycoxidized proteins in human fibroblasts exposed to repeated mild heat shock during serial passaging in vitro. Free Radic. Biol. Med. **31:** 1593–1602.

6. RATTAN, S.I.S. 2004. Aging intervention, prevention, and therapy through hormesis. J. Gerontol. Series A-Biol. Sci. Med. Sci. **59:** 705–709.

7. ALTOMARE, K., V. GRECO, D. BELLIZZI, *et al.* 2003. The allele (A)(-110) in the promoter region of the HSP70-1 gene is unfavorable to longevity in women. Biogerontology **4:** 215–220.

8. ROSS, O.A., M.D. CURRAN, K.A. CRUM, *et al.* 2003. Increased frequency of the 2437T allele of the heat shock protein 70-Hom gene in an aged Irish population. Exp. Gerontol. **38:** 561–565.

9. SINGH, R., S. KOLVRAA, P. BROSS, *et al.* 2004. Association between low self-rated health and heterozygosity for $-110A > C$ polymorphism in the promoter region of HSP70-1 in aged Danish twins. Biogerontology **5:** 169–176.

10. GOATE, A.M., D.N. COOPER, C. HALL, *et al.* 1987. Localization of a human heat-shock Hsp-70 gene sequence to chromosome-6 and detection of 2 other loci by somatic-cell hybrid and restriction-fragment-length-polymorphism analysis. Hum. Genet. **75:** 123–128.

11. MILNER, C.M. & R.D. CAMPBELL. 1990. Structure and expression of the three MHC-linked HSP70 genes. Immunogenetics **32:** 242–251.

12. KYVIK, K.O., K. CHRISTENSEN, A. SKYTTHE, *et al.* 1996. The Danish twin register. Dan. Med. Bull. **43:** 467–470.

13. NYBO, H., D. GAIST, B. JEUNE, *et al.* 2001. The Danish 1905 cohort: a genetic-epidemiological nationwide survey. J. Aging Health **13:** 32–46.

14. SKYTTHE, A., K. KYVIK, N.V. HOLM, *et al.* 2002. The Danish twin registry: 127 birth cohorts of twins. Twin Res. **5:** 352–357.

15. MCGUE, M., J.W. VAUPEL, N. HOLM, *et al.* 1993. Longevity is moderately heritable in a sample of Danish twins born 1870–1880. J. Gerontol. **48:** B237–B244.

16. FREDERIKSEN, H. & K. CHRISTENSEN. 2003. The influence of genetic factors on physical functioning and exercise in second half of life. Scand. J. Med. Sci. Sports **13:** 9–18.

17. CHRISTENSEN, K., D. GAIST, J.W. VAUPEL, *et al.* 2002. Genetic contribution to rate of change in functional abilities among Danish twins aged 75 years or more. Am. J. Epidemiol. **155:** 132–139.

18. CHRISTENSEN, K., N.V. HOLM, M. MCGUE, *et al.* 1999. A Danish population-based twin study on general health in the elderly. J. Aging Health **11:** 49–64.

19. FREDERIKSEN, H., D. GAIST, H.C. PETERSEN, *et al.* 2002. Hand grip strength: a phenotype suitable for identifying genetic variants affecting mid- and late-life physical functioning. Genet. Epidemiol. **23:** 110–122.

20. EIBERG, H. & J. MOHR. 1981. Genetics of paraoxonase. Ann. Hum. Genet. **45:** 323–330.

21. MOHR, J. & H. EIBERG. 1977. Colton blood groups: indication of linkage with the Kidd (Jk) system as support for assignment to chromosome 7. Clin. Genet. **11:** 372–374.

22. STEPHENS, M., N.J. SMITH & P. DONNELLY. 2001. A new statistical method for haplotype reconstruction from population data. Am. J. Hum. Genet. **68:** 978–989.

23. STEPHENS, M. & P. DONNELLY. 2003. A comparison of Bayesian methods for haplotype reconstruction from population genotype data. Am. J. Hum. Genet. **73:** 1162–1169.

24. CARDON, L.R. & G.R. ABECASIS. 2003. Using haplotype blocks to map human complex trait loci. Trends Genet. **19:** 135–140.

Possible Associations between Successful Aging and Polymorphic Markers in the Werner Gene Region

MARI SILD,[a] CEMILE KOCA,[a] METTE H. BENDIXEN,[a]
HENRIK FREDERIKSEN,[b] MATT McGUE,[b] STEEN KØLVRAA,[a]
KAARE CHRISTENSEN,[b] AND BJØRN NEXØ[a]

[a]*Institute of Human Genetics, University of Aarhus, Aarhus, Denmark*

[b]*Institute of Public Health, University of Southern Denmark, Odense, Denmark*

ABSTRACT: Werner syndrome (WS) is an autosomal recessive segmental progeroid syndrome caused by mutations in the Werner (*WRN*) gene leading to the early onset of many (but not all) aspects of normal aging. To investigate whether the *WRN* gene affects the course of aging in non-Werner syndrome individuals, we performed association studies analyzing several single nucleotide polymorphisms (SNPs) in the *WRN* locus. We found certain close-set SNPs in the 5' flanking region and 5' UTR to be significantly associated with the cognitive functioning level in old age.

KEYWORDS: Werner syndrome; WRN; cognition; normal aging

Werner syndrome (WS) is a rare autosomal recessive disorder caused by mutations in the *WRN* gene.[1] Patients start developing premature aging symptoms such as graying of the hair, wrinkling of the skin, cataract, osteoporosis, and several age-related diseases after puberty and predominantly die before the age of 50 years.[2,3]

The exact molecular background of the WS remains vague, although the protein encoded by the *WRN* gene has been thoroughly investigated and found to exhibit helicase, DNA-dependent ATPase, and 3'-5' exonuclease activities.[3,4] WS is associated with significantly increased genomic instability and transcriptional deficiencies. Studies of the WRN protein also indicate that it plays a role in DNA repair.[4,5]

As mutations in one gene result in so many aging-like phenotypic changes, it has been hypothesized that minor differences in the *WRN* gene function-

Address for correspondence: Mari Sild, Institute of Human Genetics, The Bartholin Building, Wilhelm Meyers Allé 240, Aarhus University, DK-8000 Aarhus C, Denmark. Voice: +45 8942 1631; fax: +45 8612 3178.

e-mail: sild@humgen.au.dk

Ann. N.Y. Acad. Sci. 1067: 309–310 (2006). © 2006 New York Academy of Sciences.
doi: 10.1196/annals.1354.041

ing might contribute to the fact that the normal aging process differs among individuals.[6] To investigate this, we analyzed various SNPs in the *WRN* locus for possible associations with various indicators of normal aging, considering physical and cognitive factors as well as the occurrence of usual age-associated diseases. The DNA samples and personal data from 426 participants were obtained from the Danish Database of Ageing Twins (Longitudinal Study of Ageing Danish Twins) and genotyping was done with the Roche LightCycler real-time polymer chain reaction instrument.

To our surprise we found significant association values among the three SNPs in noncoding areas of the *WRN* gene (5′ UTR and 5′ flanking area) and a parameter of normal aging–cognitive functioning level as measured by a cognitive composite score.[7] The SNPs rs2251621, rs2725335, and rs2725338 demonstrated *P* values of 0.003, 0.004, and 0.001, respectively. Interestingly, mental impairment is not a typical WS feature.

In addition, three other SNPs (one in an exon) appeared to be associated with another parameter, "grip strength," with *P* values of 0.038, 0.005, and 0.003.

These SNPs might be located in or be in linkage disequilibrium with the yet undefined gene expression regulatory areas. We continue with haplotype studies and functional research.

REFERENCES

1. YU, C.E. *et al*. 1996. Positional cloning of the Werner's syndrome gene. Science **272:** 258–262.
2. EPSTEIN, O.J. *et al*. 1966. Werner's syndrome: a review of its symptomatology, natural history, pathologic factors, genetics and relationship to the natural aging process. Medicine **45:** 177–221.
3. BOHR, V.A. 2002. Human premature ageing syndromes and genomic instability. Mech. Ageing Dev. **123:** 987–993.
4. BOHR, V.A. *et al*. 2001. DNA repair and mutagenesis in Werner syndrome. Environ. Mol. Mutagen. **38:** 227–234.
5. BALAJEE, A.S. *et al*. 1999. The Werner syndrome protein is involved in RNA polymerase II transcription. Mol. Biol. Cell **10:** 2655–2668.
6. CASTRO, E. *et al*. 1999. Polymorphisms at the Werner locus: I. Newly identified polymorphisms, ethnic variability of 1367 Cys/Arg, and its stability in a population of Finnish centenarians. Am. J. Med. Genet. **82:** 399–403.
7. BENDIXEN, M.H. *et al*. 2004. A polymorphic marker in the first intron of the Werner gene associates with cognitive function in aged Danish twins. Exp. Gerontol. **39:** 1101–1107.

The Pattern of Chromosome-Specific Variations in Telomere Length in Humans Shows Signs of Heritability and Is Maintained through Life

J. GRAAKJAER,[a] J.A. LONDONO-VALLEJO,[b] K. CHRISTENSEN,[c] AND S. KØLVRAA[d]

[a] Institute of Human Genetics, University of Aarhus, Bartholin Building, Vilhelm Meyers Alle, Aarhus, Denmark

[b] UMR7147 CNRS-I, Curie-UPMC, Paris, France

[c] Section for Epidemiology, Institute of Public Health, University of Southern Denmark, Odense, Denmark

[d] Department of Clinical Genetics, Vejle Hospital, 7100 Vejle, Denmark

ABSTRACT: This paper characterizes the distribution of telomere length on individual chromosome arms in humans. By fluorescent *in situ* hybridization (FISH), followed by computer-assisted analysis of digital images, it is shown that the distribution of telomere length on individual chromosome arms is not random, but that humans have a common telomere profile. This profile exists in lymphocytes, amniocytes and fibroblasts, and seems to be conserved during life. A closer look at the overall pattern of the profile shows that the length of the telomeres in general follows the total chromosome length. In addition to the common profile, it is found that each person has specific characteristics, which are also conserved throughout life. Studying both twins and families we have obtained indications that these individual characteristics are at least partly inherited. Altogether, our results suggest that the length of individual telomeres might occasionally play a role in the heritability of life span.

KEYWORDS: telomere profile; heritability; human longevity; aging

INTRODUCTION

The genome in all higher organisms is organized in linear chromosomes. This poses a problem for the cell, since what would appear to be a double-stranded DNA break is present at each end of a chromosome. Such

Address for correspondence: Steen Kølvraa, Department of Clinical Genetics, Vejle Hospital, 7100 Vejle, Denmark. Voice: +4579406551; fax: +4579406871.
e-mail: stekol@vgs.vejleamt.dk

Ann. N.Y. Acad. Sci. 1067: 311–316 (2006). © 2006 New York Academy of Sciences.
doi: 10.1196/annals.1354.042

ends would normally signal cell cycle arrest. Higher organisms have solved this problem by developing specialized structures at each chromosome extremity that effectively hide those ends from the DNA quality-control system.[1] These structures, named telomeres, are composed of highly conserved DNA sequences and of a number of proteins which bind specifically to these sequences. The telomeric DNA, composed of 5–15 kb of tandem repeats of the sequence TTAGGG, is believed to form a loop, thereby hiding the free end.[2]

A special feature of telomeres is that the number of repeats diminishes progressively throughout life. This is mainly due to the "end replication problem" and to replication-related processing reactions, although oxidative DNA damage may also play a role.[3] It is believed that when telomeres are shortened below a certain limit, they loosen the loop structure (undergo "uncapping"), thereby exposing the free DNA end, and that this initiates cell cycle arrest, senescence, and ultimately cell death.[4]

In recent years a number of observations have indicated, that it is the shortest—or one of the shortest—telomere in the cell that activates the DNA damage-control pathway in connection with shortening telomeres.[5–7] We have therefore for some time studied the length of telomeres on individual chromosomes and have characterized both the telomere profile of human cells and the dynamics of this profile.

METHODS

For this study we used metaphase spreads from short-term cultures of primary human cells. We incorporated lymphocytes from individuals aged 20 to 105 years, including four monozygotic twin pairs and six dizygotic twin pairs aged 76 to 83 years. In addition, amniocytes from pregnancies at week 10, and fibroblasts from individuals aged 20 to 55 years were included. From all these cells we produced metaphase spreads by standard techniques.

The telomere length of individual chromosome ends was measured by FISH analysis, using a PNA probe, specific for telomeres as previously described.[8] Digitized images for each metaphase were collected and analyzed in a dedicated software package from DAKO, Denmark. From each sample 20 metaphases were analyzed.

For each metaphase telomere length values were either normalized using the formula

$$Z = (X)/\mu$$

where

Z = normalized telomere length value,
X = raw telomere length value,
μ = mean telomere length of all telomeres in the metaphase

or standardized using the formula

$$Z = (X - \mu)/\sigma$$

where

Z = standardized telomere length value,
X = raw telomere length value,
μ = mean telomere length of all telomeres in the metaphase, and
σ = standard deviation of all telomeres in the metaphase

These two procedures gave in general very similar distributions. The final telomere length value for a given chromosome end was then expressed as the mean of the values obtained from 20 metaphases.

In some analyses we wanted to be able to distinguish the two homologues in a set. This was achieved by doing FISH analysis of the metaphases already analyzed by telomere FISH, but this time using probes representing polymorphic subtelomeric sequences as previously described.[9]

RESULTS

A Telomere Profile Common to Humans

When we compared the distribution of telomere length on the total set of chromosomes among different cells in an individual, it was obvious that some chromosome ends always had short telomeres and some had long telomeres (FIG. 1), and when we obtained two blood samples from the same individual, analyzed 20 metaphases from each sample, calculated means, and plotted val-

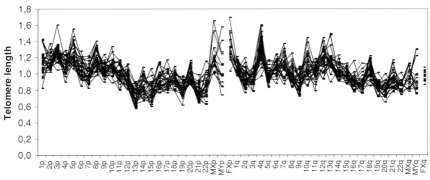

FIGURE 1. The chromosome-specific telomere length measured on lymphocyte cells from 20 individuals aged 76–83 years. Telomere length values have been normalized with regards to cell. Each line represents one individual.

ues for corresponding chromosome ends in a XY-plot, we always obtained high correlations (always over 0.75, $P < 0.001$).[8] This indicates that the person has a characteristic telomere profile, at least in lymphocytes. When we compared the profile among different individuals, we also obtained significant correlations, but somewhat lower than what we obtained between two samples from the same individual. This clearly suggests the existence both of a common profile in humans and of superimposed individual characteristics. A Friedman test performed on the data set from a number of individuals also confirmed the existence of a profile ($P < 0.00001$).[8] Furthermore, a telomere profile similar to the lymphocyte profile was found in other cell types as well. So far we have investigated fibroblasts, amniocytes, and mesenchymal stem cells.

A closer look at the profile revealed an overall pattern, where small chromosomes generally had small telomeres and large chromosomes had longer telomeres. If telomere length (both p and q) is plotted against chromosome size (in kbs), a correlation of 0.79 is obtained.[8]

Conservation of Profile throughout Life

Cells from individuals at different ages were also investigated. In this series, the telomere profile was determined in lymphocytes from individuals in the age span of 25 to 105 years. In general, we found a high degree of conservation of the profile with correlations to the combined, overall profile in the range of 0.7–0.9 in individuals up to 85 years of age. Only in centenarians did we find a certain degeneration of profile with correlations in the range of 0.5–0.6.[8]

Also, the conservation of individual characteristics in profile was investigated. This was done by analyzing the same homologue of a chromosome in 3 MZ twin pairs older than 75 years. These two chromosomes are both derived from the same chromosome in the fertilized egg, but has been replicated many times for more than 75 years in two different individuals. Their degree of similarity in telomere length thus is a measure of the ability of a chromosome to preserve its characteristics throughout life. For comparison, we also measured similarities between two homologues within the same individual and among individuals. The dissimilarity here represents the sum of differences between different copies of a chromosome in the population at conception and the differences developed through a person's life. In total 20 chromosome pairs in the MZ twins were informative for polymorphic markers and were included in the study, as were 22 chromosomes in the control groups. To our surprise we found the highest degree of similarity when looking at the same chromosome in two different MZ twins. By calculating variance components we found that only 22% of the total variance between different copies of a chromosome in the population occurs during life in the individual examined (as variation caused by replication-associated telomere erosion and oxidative damage) and the remaining 78% is due to preconception differences in telomere length of different copies of a chromosome.[9] In other words, the precision of the dynamics (lengthening and shortening reactions) of telomere metabolism throughout life is unexpectedly high.

Inheritance of Telomere Profile

Since the data indicated that the characteristics of an individual's profile (for example, the presence of an unusually short telomere) would be preserved throughout life, we finally wanted to investigate whether that profile could be transmitted from generation to generation. We did this by performing a classical twin study, comparing similarities in specific deviations from the common profile between twin members in MZ twins compared to DZ twins.[8] When deviations from the common profile were calculated and normalized, we consistently found that the similarity in profile, defined as correlation coefficients when plotting the two twins in a pair against each other, was higher in MZ twin pairs (0.5–0.8) than in DZ twin pairs (–0.1–0.4).[8] This much higher similarity in MZ twin pairs is compatible with the assumption that the telomere profile is transmitted to offspring. One should, however, be cautious with such a conclusion, since different fertilized eggs may have different profiles, simply because telomeres are dynamic structures and, in particular, are actively maintained in the germ cells. The high dissimilarity in DZ twin pairs could therefore be due to differences in telomere length profiles within the parent's gamete pool. We have, however, recently obtained results from direct comparisons between parents and offspring, indicating that telomere length profiles are in fact transmitted to offspring (unpublished).

DISCUSSION

In the present communication we have focused on investigations aimed at elucidating whether an unusually short telomere, present in a parent, can be transmitted and, if so, whether such a telomere will remain short, compared to other telomeres, throughout life in the offspring. Collectively, our data suggest that this is the case. We first demonstrated that the distribution of telomere length over the various chromosome ends in an individual is not random, but rather corresponds to a specific pattern, named the telomere profile. On top of this general human profile, each individual has his own personal deviations that are conserved throughout life. We have also obtained evidence that these personal characteristics in the profile are defined in the zygote and most probably inherited from the parents. This opens the possibility that if an individual receives an unusually short telomere at conception, this telomere will be among the shortest during this individual's life. At the moment when all telomeres have undergone progressive shortening, this particular telomere may uncap prematurely, triggering cell senescence or chromosome instability. At the level of the whole organism, this premature telomere uncapping may translate into a risk of early aging manifestations or increased cancer predisposition. Furthermore, since this unusually short telomere will be in all likelihood passed on as such to children, the increased risk of premature aging and cancer predisposition will also be transmitted to the offspring. We would like to suggest that inheritance of particularly short telomeres may very well be a factor in the well-established 25% heritability of life span in humans.

REFERENCES

1. ZAKIAN, V.A. 1995. Telomeres: beginning to understand the end. Science **270:** 1601–1607.
2. GRIFFITH, J.D., L. COMEAU, S. ROSENFIELD, *et al*. 1999. Mammalian telomeres end in a large duplex loop. Cell **97:** 503–514.
3. HARLEY, C.B. 1991. Telomere loss: mitotic clock or genetic time bomb? Mutat. Res. **256:** 271–282.
4. BLACKBURN, E.H., S. CHAN, J. CHANG, *et al*. 2000. Molecular manifestations and molecular determinants of telomere capping. Cold Spring Harbor Symp. Quant. Biol. **65:** 253–263.
5. HEMANN, M.T., M.A. STRONG, L.Y. HAO, *et al*. 2001. The shortest telomere, not average telomere length, is critical for cell viability and chromosome stability. Cell **107:** 67–77.
6. TAN, Z. 1999. Telomere shortening and the population size-dependency of life span of human cell culture: further implication for two proliferation-restricting telomeres. Exp. Gerontol. **34:** 831–842.
7. ZOU, Y., A. SFEIR, S.M. GRYAZNOV, *et al.* 2004. Does a sentinel or a subset of short telomeres determine replicative senescence? Mol. Biol. Cell **15:** 3709–3718.
8. GRAAKJAER, J., C. BISCHOFF, L. KORSHOLM, *et al*. 2003. The pattern of chromosome-specific variations in telomere length in humans is determined by inherited, telomere-near factors and is maintained throughout life. Mech. Ageing Dev. **124:** 629–640.
9. GRAAKJAER, J., L. PASCOE, H. DER-SARKISSIAN, *et al*. 2004. The relative lengths of individual telomeres are defined in the zygote and strictly maintained during life. Aging Cell. **3:** 97–102.

Identification of Genes Involved in Healthy Aging and Longevity

JENS WEIBEL, MORTEN DRÆBY SØRENSEN, AND PETER KRISTENSEN

Department of Molecular Biology, University of Aarhus, Aarhus, Denmark

ABSTRACT: Studies suggest that the region around microsatellite marker D4S1564 on chromosome 4 is in some way linked to longevity. As a part of the integrated European project Genetics of Healthy Aging (GeHA), we set out to investigate the genes found in this region using a proteomics approach. Here, we report the cloning of six candidate genes.

KEYWORDS: genetics; functional genomics; phage display; antibodies

INTRODUCTION

Longevity has a strong genetic component as has been shown in a multiplicity of organisms. A large body of evidence suggests that the intricate genetic pathways of metabolism and stress resistance are central for longevity. Moreover, it has been shown that longevity and healthy aging in humans are inherited phenotypes across multiple generations.

Prior studies have suggested that three genomic regions—on chromosome 4, D4S1564, on chromosome 11, 11.p15.5, and on chromosome 19, around apolipoprotein E (APOE)—are involved in aging and longevity. The present study is aimed at a characterization of some of the specific genes on chromosome 4 and the corresponding proteins to establish their possible influence on the aging process.

The chromosomal region D4S1564 covers 12 million base pairs and contains around 50 putative genes. Using bioinformatics we have selected candidate genes for further studies. The genes are cloned into expression vectors, allowing production of recombinant proteins, followed by generation of monoclonal antibodies by use of phage display technology. This will allow us to examine gene expression changes and protein localization changes during aging. This in turn can increase our understanding of some of the molecular and cellular mechanisms involved in the aging process and in age-related diseases;

Address for correspondence: Dr. Peter Kristensen, Department of Molecular Biology, University of Aarhus, Gustav Wieds Vej 10C, DK8000 Aarhus−C, Denmark. Voice: +45 8942 5032; fax: +45 8612 3178.
e-mail: pk@mb.au.dk

Ann. N.Y. Acad. Sci. 1067: 317–322 (2006). © 2006 New York Academy of Sciences.
doi: 10.1196/annals.1354.043

and might help to identify methods to reduce the age-related loss of cellular functions.

METHODS

Amplification of Genes

The oligonucleotides used to amplify the genes are listed in TABLE 1. The reactions were performed in 25 µL volumes containing 10 ng template, 10 pmol of each primer, 100 µM dNTPs, and 0.8 U of Taq polymerase (Sigma-Aldrich Brøndby, Denmark). Thermal profile: denaturation at 94°C for 5 min, addition of Taq pol, and 35 cycles of 1 min at 94°C, 1 min at 58°C, and 1min 30 sec at 72°C. Final extension is 10 min at 72°C. Reamplification of the polymerase chain reaction products was performed under similar conditions. The template cDNA is obtained from human brain and smooth skeletal muscle cDNA libraries (Matchmaker, Clontech, Mountain View, CA).

Cloning

The final PCR product was digested with NotI and NcoI restriction enzymes, ligated into vector pET11d, previously modified to contain a His-tag and c-myc tag at the C-terminal part of the fusion protein. The ligation mixture was electroporated into BL21 (DE3)pLysS electrocompetent cells and plated on TYE plates containing 100 µg/mL ampicillin +1% glucose and incubated at 37°C overnight.

Colony PCR

The oligonucleotides used to amplify the genes were T7 terminator and T7 promoter (Novagen). The reactions were performed in 25 µL volumes containing one colony picked with a toothpick from the cells containing the cloned vector, 10 pmol of each primer, 100 µM dNTPs, and 0.8 U of Taq polymerase (Sigma-Aldrich). Thermal profile: denaturation at 94°C for 5 min, addition of Taq pol, and 35 cycles of 1 min at 94°C, 1 min at 58°C, and 1min 30 sec at 72°C. Final extension is 10 min at 72°C.

Expression

Ten milliliters 2×TY media containing 1% glucose and 100 µg/mL ampicillin were inoculated with one colony and incubated overnight at 37°C with shaking (200 rpm). Then 5 mL of 2×TY containing 100 µg/mL ampicillin

TABLE 1. Forward and backward primer used in amplification of the genes indicated

Gene	Forward primer	Backward primer
C4orf17	ATGATGTGCGGCCGCCTACAGAAGAGTGGCTTTTATTTC	AGGAGATATACCATGGATGAAACCTCAACCCCCGAC
Bank1	TGATGATGTGCGGCCGCCTTAATGATCTTTCTTGCAACAGAAACC	TATACCATGGATGCTGCCAGCAGCGCCAGG
Cxxc4	GATGATGTGCGGCCGCTTAAAAGAACCATCGGAATGCTTCAG	TTTAAGAAGGAGATATACCATGGATGCACCACCG
MANBA	TGGTGATGATGATGTGCGGCCGCTCAGTAAAATATCTGTTA	AAGGAGATATACCATGGATGCGCCTCCACCTGCTCCTGCT
NOLA1	GGTGATGATGATGTGCGGCCGCTTAATGTCCTCTCCCTCT	GAAGGAGATATACCATGGATGTCTTTTCGAGGCGGAGGTC
PAPSS1	GTGATGATGATGTGCGGCCGCCTAAGCTTTCTCCAAGGAT	AAGGAGATATACCATGGATGCAGAGAGCAACCAATGTCAC
EMCN	ATGATGTGCGGCCGCTCAGTTCTTGGTTTTTCCTTGTGCAG	GAGATATACCATGGATGGAACTGCTTCAAGTGACCATTCT

NOTE: Gene names refer to the names assigned in GENBANK.

and 1% glucose was inoculated with 50 μL of the overnight culture and left to grow until OD ∼0.5. Expression was induced with 1 mM IPTG and was continued overnight at room temperature.

RESULTS AND DISCUSSION

The notion that human life span is influenced by genetic factors receives compelling support from a plethora of publications studying various species. The genetic factor of life expectancy is estimated to be around 25%[1,2] and for achieving extreme age even higher.[3] Studies suggest that healthy physical aging is under a significant degree of genetic influence, with heritability above 50%.[4] However, till today most genetic studies dealing with aging in humans are focused on linking individual disease genes to aging.

In a study from 2001, Puca *et al.* made a genome scan using 137 sibling pairs and found that three genomic regions could be involved in aging and longevity: on chromosome 4, around microsatellite marker D4S1564, on chromosome 11 at 11.p15.5, and on chromosome 19, around APOE.[5] Later the same investigators tried to identify a specific gene and gene variants by making a haplotype-based fine-mapping study of the interval around D4S1564 on chromosome 4.[6] They identified a haplotype marker within microsomal transfer protein (MTP) as a modifier of the human life span. This result, however, could not be verified by other groups, and thus the supposed association between MTP and longevity is still a matter of controversy.[7,8]

In May 2004, a large European project was initiated—the integrated project entitled Genetics of Healthy Aging (GeHA). The aim was to collect material from 2,800 sibling pairs from across Europe obtaining sufficient statistical power to allow stronger genetic conclusions to be drawn. After the material was collected and the genetic analysis performed, we set out to study some of the gene products or putative gene products around D4S1564.[5,9]

There are around 50 putative genes in the area and it was difficult to exclude any of the genes on the basis of functional considerations. In addition, it is possible that the polymorphism underlying the linkage was not within any of these 50 putative genes. Thus the selection of genes was based mainly on expression profiles within specific tissues as obtained from the database found at http://www.genecards.org/database. For a number of gene products in question, activity assays or antibodies already exist, thus enabling proteomics studies of the individual proteins with respect to aging. As a start, we have concentrated on the generation of antibodies against gene products or putative gene products for which no specific antibodies exist. This will allow simultaneous analysis of multiple proteins encoded by genes around D4S1564.

From the 50 putative genes we selected a total of 19 genes, of which six so far have been successfully cloned. The cloned genes are Bank1, Cxxc4, EMCN, MANBA, NOLA1, and PAPSS1.

BANK1 is a B cell scaffold protein with ankyrin repeats, one recently identified to be involved in B cell signaling. Cxxc4 is a WNT-signaling molecule associating with Dishevelled family proteins. EMCN (endomucin precursor) has been suggested to interfere with the assembly of focal adhesion complexes and inhibition of interaction between cells and the extracellular matrix. MANBA (mannosidase, beta A, lysosomal) is an exoglycosidase that cleaves the single beta-linked mannose residue from the nonreducing end of all N-linked glycoprotein oligosaccharides. NOLA1 (nucleolar protein family A, member 1) is part of a complex that is required for ribosome biogenesis and telomere maintenance. PAPSS1 (3'-phosphoadenosine 5'-phosphosulfate synthase 1) is a bifunctional enzyme with both ATP sulfurylase and APS kinase activity, which mediates two steps in the sulfate activation pathway, and is the sole source of sulfate in mammals (source: http://www.ebi.ac.uk/seqdb/UniProt.html).

The next step will be the generation of recombinant antibodies by phage display. This will allow a proteomic verification of expression level and cellular localization with regard to aging and help in elucidating the importance of the individual gene products.

CONCLUSION

In the chromosomal region D4S1564 around 50 putative genes were identified. Of these 19 were initially selected for further investigation based on the expression profiles in specific tissues and the absence of antibodies allowing proteomics studies. The ultimate aim will be to perform proteomics studies on most of the 50 putative genes within this chromosomal region.

At the moment we have successfully cloned six of the proteins and we are attempting to express them, although only the proteins Cxxc4 and BANK1 have been expressed so far. At the moment we are attempting to express the remainder of the six proteins and continuing the effort to clone the remaining 14 proteins. Following large-scale expression, phage antibody technology will be applied to generate antibody fragments, allowing proteomics analysis.

ACKNOWLEDGMENT

This work was supported by the Genetics of Healthy Aging project (EU Contract No. FP6-503270).

REFERENCES

1. GUDMUNDSSON, H., D.F. GUDBJARTSSON, M. FRIGGE, *et al.* 2000. Inheritance of human longevity in Iceland. Eur. J. Hum. Genet. **8:** 743–749.

2. PERLS, T. *et al.* 2000. Exceptional familial clustering for extreme longevity in humans. J. Am. Geriatr. Soc. **48:** 1483–1485.
3. PERLS, T., L. KUNKEL & A. PUCA. 2002. The genetics of aging. Curr. Opin. Genet. Dev. **12:** 362–369.
4. REED, T. & D.M. DICK. 2003. Heritability and validity of healthy physical aging (wellness) in elderly male twins. Twin Res. **6:** 227–234.
5. PUCA, A.A. *et al.* 2001. A genome-wide scan for linkage to human exceptional longevity identifies a locus on chromosome 4. Proc. Natl. Acad. Sci. USA **98:** 10505–10508.
6. GEESAMAN, B.J. *et al.* 2003. Haplotype-based identification of a microsomal transfer protein marker associated with the human lifespan. Proc. Natl. Acad. Sci. USA **100:** 14115–14120.
7. NEBEL, A. *et al.* 2005. No association between microsomal triglyceride transfer protein (MTP) haplotype and longevity in humans. Proc. Natl. Acad. Sci. USA **102:** 7906–7909.
8. BATHUM, L. *et al.* 2005. No evidence for an association between extreme longevity and microsomal transfer protein polymorphisms in a longitudinal study of 1651 nonagenarians. Eur. J. Hum. Genet. **13:** 1154–1158.
9. REED, T., D.M. DICK, S.K. UNIACKE, *et al.* 2004. Genome-wide scan for a healthy aging phenotype provides support for a locus near D4S1564 promoting healthy aging. J. Gerontol. A. Biol. Sci. Med. Sci. **59:** 227–232.

Prevention and Treatment of Skin Aging

JERRY L. McCULLOUGH AND KRISTEN M. KELLY

Department of Dermatology, University of California, Irvine, California, USA

ABSTRACT: Skin aging is a complex biological process that is a consequence of both intrinsic or genetically programmed aging that occurs with time, and extrinsic aging caused by environmental factors. The dramatic increase in the aging population and the psychosocial impact of skin aging has created a demand for effective interventions. The advances that have been made in the past 25 years in our understanding of the clinical, biochemical, and molecular changes associated with aging have led to the development of many different approaches to reduce, postpone, and in some cases, repair the untoward effects of intrinsic programmed aging and extrinsic environmental injury.

KEYWORDS: skin aging; anti-aging; photoaging; skin rejuvenation; photoprotection; sunscreen; antioxidant; cytokinin; cosmeceutical

INTRODUCTION

The skin is a unique organ that reflects the inevitable changes that occur in the body's aging process. In the 21st century, we now have an understanding of the factors that contribute to the pathogenesis of skin aging and consequently we can develop rational approaches to both prevent and treat the effects of this process.

Intrinsic Aging

Genetically programmed intrinsic aging (or chronological aging) causes structural and functional changes in all layers of the skin.[1] In the epidermis, there is a progressive decrease in the renewal rate of epidermal cells. Epidermal turnover, which in young adult skin takes about 28 days, requires 40–60 days in the elderly.[2] Slower turnover causes thinning of the epidermis that gives aged skin a translucent appearance. Diminished epidermal renewal also adversely affects skin barrier function and repair and cell exfoliation. In aged skin, the corneocytes tend to clump together on the surface, giving a

Address for correspondence: Jerry L. McCullough, Ph.D., Department of Dermatology, University of California, Irvine, Irvine, CA 92697-2400. Voice: 949-824-5516; fax: 949-824-5407.
  e-mail: jlmccull@uci.edu

Ann. N.Y. Acad. Sci. 1067: 323–331 (2006). © 2006 New York Academy of Sciences.
doi: 10.1196/annals.1354.044

rough, scaly appearance, and texture. Histologically, one of the most prominent changes with intrinsic aging is a flattening of the dermal–epidermal junction, which increases skin fragility and decreases transfer of nutrients between the two layers. In aged skin, there are fewer melanocytes populating the epidermis and decreased functional activity of the remaining melanocytes, resulting in dyschromic changes, such as mottled pigmentation, freckles, and lentigines. Because the skin is thinner and has fewer melanocytes, it is more susceptible to sunburn. Aging also affects the Langerhans cells, the immunocompetent cells in the epidermis. There is nearly a 50% decrease in the Langerhans cells in late adulthood.[3] This compromises the skin's level of immune surveillance and leads to a higher risk of skin cancer.

In the dermis, there is a decrease in the number of fibroblasts as well as synthesis of the fibroblast products collagen and elastin, resulting in skin wrinkling and loss of elasticity. Aging also results in considerable loss of dermal microvasculature, reducing blood supply to the skin and contributing to atrophy of the skin and its appendages. Loss of sebaceous glands in the dermis makes the skin dry due to reduced oil production.

Further, intrinsic aging causes a decrease in subdermal fat tissue. This loss of support contributes to wrinkling and sagging (laxity) of the skin. With less padding, skin is more susceptible to trauma and bruising. Decreased insulation also affects the body's ability to conserve heat.

Although intrinsic aging causes all the above-described structural changes, effects are mostly functional, with only minor impact on skin appearance, which can be summarized as generalized fine wrinkling, dryness, and thinning. It is also important to note that the genetic program of intrinsic aging differs per individual in terms of rate and severity of effect.

Extrinsic Aging

Extrinsic aging is superimposed on intrinsic aging and is caused by environmental factors such as ultraviolet damage, pollution, harsh weather, and cigarette smoke. Chronic sun exposure is the principal environmental cause of extrinsic skin aging and is responsible for the majority of age-related changes, including fine wrinkles, roughness, mottled hyperpigmentation, dilated blood vessels, and loss of skin tone. Acute effects of ultraviolet irradiation are inflammation, sunburn, pigmentation, epidermal hyperproliferation, and immune suppression.[4] Chronic effects are photoaging and photocarcinogenesis.[5] Shorter UVB (290–320 nm) wavelengths only penetrate to the epidermis. Longer UVA wavelengths penetrate deeper into the skin and are primarily responsible for clinical changes seen with photoaging. The UVA wavelength is split up into UVA1 (340–400 nm) and UVA2 (320–340 nm). It is the longer wavelength (UVA1) that causes the most photoaging.[6] The primary cause of skin damage by UVA light is oxidative stress. UVA is absorbed by chromophores present in skin (e.g., trans-urocanic acid), generating various reactive oxygen species (ROS)[7] that cause oxidative damage to nucleic acids, cellular proteins, and lipids. The ROS trigger a host of cytokine cascades that result in photoaging and photocarcinogenesis. One of the primary effects of UVA oxidative damage is ROS-induced synthesis of a series of matrix metal-loproteinases[8] that cause collagen degradation resulting in wrinkles.

PREVENTION OF SKIN AGING

While it is currently impossible to halt or reverse the genetic processes responsible for intrinsic aging, skin changes associated with extrinsic aging are largely preventable.

Photoprotection

Protection from ultraviolet light at any age reduces photoaging and decreases the risks of age-related skin diseases. Various photoprotective measures, including sun avoidance, wearing protective clothing, and use of sunscreen, retard the onset and slow the progression of photoaging.[9] Since approximately 80% of the skin's sun damage is thought to occur by the age of 18 years[10] (although it does not become apparent until years later), preventive measures should begin in early childhood. The use of sunscreens is the "gold standard" for protecting the skin from ultraviolet light. Clinical studies have well documented that regular use of a broad spectrum sunscreen can prevent not only sunburn, but also many skin-aging effects (e.g., wrinkles, pigmentary changes).[11] Sunscreens have also been shown to reduce actinic keratoses, solar elastosis, and squamous cell carcinoma.[12] The use of sunscreens and sun protection is important in association with implementation of skin-aging treatments, as the beneficial effects of skin rejuvenation measures will be minimized, or even cancelled if unprotected sun exposure continues to induce skin damage.

Sunscreen technology includes chemical or physical blockers that filter various UV wavelengths.[13] Early sunscreens used *para*-aminobenzoic acid (PABA) or PABA derivatives to protect from UVB. However, there was no protection against harmful UVA wavelengths and a significant incidence of contact sensitivity. Newer chemical sunscreen formulations use UVB protectors with lower allergenicity (aminobenzoates, cinnamates, salicylates, and benzophenones) in combination with chemicals such as oxybenzone that extend protection to UVA wavelengths. Physical sunscreens containing titanium dioxide or zinc oxide provide broad spectrum coverage that blocks or reflects UVA and UVB.

The sun protection factor (SPF) is the international standard for rating the effectiveness of sunscreens and is based solely on prevention of erythema (sunburn) induced by UVB.[14] There is no similar universal standard for UVA protection. The inadequacy of rating UVA protection has raised the concern that the use of a high SPF product may provide a false sense of protection (prevent sunburn), allowing individuals to spend greater time in the sun, without adequate UVA protection, particularly UVA-1.[15] Some manufacturers have introduced a star rating system, which defines the ratio of UVA relative to UVB protection.[16] When used in combination with the SPF rating, this gives a more complete picture of a sunscreen's overall performance for protecting the skin and preventing aging.

Antioxidants

Antioxidants provide yet another approach for the prevention and treatment of intrinsic and extrinsic skin aging. Free radicals play a pivotal role in the biological events that lead to the clinical manifestations of skin aging. Skin has an integrated endogenous antioxidant defense mechanism that scavenges free radicals and protects cells from damage.[17] Naturally occurring antioxidants are reduced in chronically aged skin and further reduced in photodamaged skin.[18] Various approaches have been used to supplement the levels of these antioxidants in the skin to enhance defense mechanisms. Oral supplementation has not been successful in augmenting skin antioxidant levels due to physiological processes including absorption, transport, and metabolism.[19] Studies have shown that antioxidants can be delivered percutaneously to directly supplement the skin's antioxidant reservoir. Topical vitamin C, when properly formulated, effectively penetrates the skin and enhances 20-fold endogenous cutaneous levels vitamin C.[20] Most studies evaluating antiaging effects of topical antioxidants have been done *in vitro* or in animal skin. Studies in pig skin demonstrated that the combination of topical vitamins C and E synergistically provide protection against UV-induced erythema and formation of sunburn cells and thymine dimers.[21,22] Although there are countless commercially available antiaging products that contain "antioxidants," only a few studies have been done to establish the efficacy of topical antioxidants in *in vivo* human skin for skin protection and rejuvenation.[23,24] Clinical studies with long-term follow-up are needed to establish the protective and therapeutic effects of topical antioxidants in skin aging.

REJUVENATION OF AGING SKIN

Topical Medications

The topical retinoid, tretinoin (all-*trans*-retinoic acid), was the first medically approved product for the treatment of photodamaged skin. Now, over a decade of basic and clinical studies document the beneficial clinical and histological effects of retinoids for the treatment of photodamaged[25,26] and intrinsically aged skin.[27] Clinically, topical retinoids are effective in minimizing fine lines and wrinkles and improving skin texture and mottled hyperpigmentation.[28] Tretinoin decreases fine wrinkles by increasing dermal collagen production via stimulation of synthesis,[29] reducing collagen degradation by inhibiting UV-induced matrix metalloproteinases,[30] and stimulating epidermal turnover, resulting in a thicker epidermis. Clinical changes are dose-dependent, with progressive improvement over a 6- to 12-month period, and slow regression once treatment is discontinued. The greatest obstacle to topical retinoid use is the high incidence of skin irritation, dryness, and the potential for increased photosensitivity.[31] New topical retinoids (e.g., tazarotene, adapalene) and novel formulations (e.g., microsponge) available in the last few years have fewer adverse effects and improved tolerance.[32,33]

Cosmetics and Cosmeceuticals

More than US$ 230 billion is spent annually worldwide on over-the-counter cosmetics and cosmeceuticals to improve the appearance of aging skin.[34] Antiaging cosmetics are touted to erase wrinkles and rejuvenate the skin. Most of these products serve only to camouflage wrinkles and moisturize the skin. Cosmeceuticals, a new category of antiaging products introduced in the 1990s, represent the fastest growing segment of the skin care market.[35] These antiaging products are not classified as prescription drugs or regulated by the Food and Drug Administration, but produce changes in skin structure or function. Examples include the alpha and beta hydroxy acids, which are generally found in over-the-counter preparations at relatively low concentrations (3–15%) and may be used to exfoliate the skin, increase cell turnover, and reduce fine wrinkles and mottled hyperpigmentation.[36]

Kinetin (N6-furfuryladenine) is a cosmeceutical used for the prevention and treatment of skin aging. It is a naturally occurring plant growth factor that retards senescence in plants[37] and has anti-aging effects on human adult skin fibroblasts in vitro.[38] Kinetin appears to be both a direct anti-oxidant[39] and a signaling molecule that stimulates pathways of the maintenance and repair in cells.[40] In a 52-week clinical study in 96 subjects with photodamaged facial skin, twice-daily application of kinetin lessened skin roughness (63%), mottled hyperpigmentation (32%), and fine wrinkles (17%), and also improved skin barrier function as measured by a decrease in transepidermal water loss.[41] Extended treatment with kinetin was well tolerated and did not cause irritation. Other cytokinins may also provide benefit for aging prevention, intervention, and therapy.[42]

The list of cosmeceuticals continues to grow and claims proliferate. It is important that scientific efforts be devoted to the rational development of anti-aging products and that clinical testing be done to substantiate claims.

Cosmetic Skin Rejuvenation Procedures

Topical agents alone provide some skin-aging prevention and treatment. However, combining use of topical compounds with one or several of the wide array of available cosmetic procedures can help maximize antiaging effects. Botulinum toxin, a purified neurotoxin, is one of the most popular procedures for temporary paralysis of select facial muscles and resultant diminution or elimination of unwanted lines in areas such as the glabella, periorbital, and perioral regions.[43,44] A multitude of injectable dermal fillers is available for diminishing skin atrophy and fine and deep rhytides.[45] Nonablative light-based procedures can be used to improve fine lines, and possibly skin tone.[46] Various skin resurfacing methods, including chemical peels,[47] dermabrasion,[48] and laser resurfacing[49] can been used to improve wrinkles, skin texture, and dyspigmentation. Cosmetic surgery produces the greatest improvement in wrinkles and skin laxity, but also has the highest associated risk and longest recovery period.

The current trend is to address skin aging before cosmetic surgery is required.[50] This is accomplished by combining available aging prevention and treatment options including daily sun protection and use of topical products, such as retinoids, kinetin, and moisturizers; regular-interval treatments (e.g., botulinum toxin, fillers, and nonablative light-based treatments); and only occasional major surgical procedures, as necessary. Youthful skin appearance can be preserved to some degree with less-invasive options, mitigating the need for cosmetic surgery. Implementation of skin protection and anti-aging treatment regimens should begin as early as possible and continue throughout life to counteract the effects of intrinsic and extrinsic skin aging. The future in the treatment of skin aging is bright and promises more effective preventive and therapeutic strategies.

REFERENCES

1. MONTAGNA, W. & K. CARLISLE. 1979. Structural changes in aging human skin. J. Invest. Dermatol. **73:** 47–53.
2. GROVE, G.L. & A.M. KLIGMAN. 1983. Age-associated changes in human epidermal cell renewal. J. Gerontol. **38:** 137–142.
3. GILCHREST, B.A., G.F. MURPHY & N.A. SOTER. 1982. Effect of chronologic aging and ultraviolet irradiation on Langerhans cells in human epidermis. J. Invest. Dermatol. **79:** 85–88.
4. COOPER, K.D., L. OBERHELMAN, T.A. HAMILTON, et al. 1992. UV exposure reduces immunization rates and promotes tolerance to epicutaneous antigens in humans: relationship to dose, CD1a-DR+ epidermal macrophage induction, and Langerhans cell depletion. Proc. Natl. Acad. Sci. USA **89:** 8497–8501.
5. MATSUMURA, Y. & H.N. ANANTHASWAMY. 2004. Toxic effects of ultraviolet radiation on the skin. Toxicol. Appl. Pharmacol. **195:** 298–308.

6. LAVKER, R.M., D.A. VERES, C.J. IRWIN, *et al.* 1995. Quantitative assessment of cumulative damage from repetitive exposures to suberythemogenic doses of UVA in human skin. Photochem. Photobiol. **62:** 348–352.

7. HANSON, K.M. & J.D. SIMON. 1998. Epidermal trans-urocanic acid and the UVA-induced photoaging of the skin. Proc. Natl. Acad. Sci. USA **95:** 10576–10578.

8. FISHER, G.J., H.C. CHOI, Z. BATA-CSORGO, *et al.* 2001. Ultraviolet irradiation increases matrix metalloproteinase-8 protein in human skin *in vivo*. J. Invest. Dermatol. **117:** 219–226.

9. KULLAVANIJAYA, P. & H.W. LIM. 2005. Photoprotection. J. Am. Acad. Dermatol. **52:** 937–958.

10. STERN, R.S., M.C. WEINSTEIN & S.G. BAKER. 1986. Risk reduction for non-melanoma skin cancer with childhood sunscreen use. Arch. Dermatol. **122:** 537–545.

11. GILCHREST, B.A. 1996. A review of skin ageing and its medical therapy. Br. J. Dermatol. **135:** 867–875.

12. NAYLOR, M.F. & K.C. FARMER. 1997. The case for sunscreens: a review of their use in preventing actinic damage and neoplasia. Arch. Dermatol. **133:** 1146–1154.

13. DEBUYS, H.V., S.B. LEVY, J.C. MURRAY, *et al.* 2000. Dermatologic aspects of cosmetics: modern approaches to photoprotection. Dermatol. Clin. **18:** 577–590.

14. COLE, C. 2001. Sunscreen protection in the ultraviolet A region: how to measure effectiveness. Photodermatol. Photoimmunol. Photomed. **17:** 2–10.

15. HAYWOOD, R., P. WARDMAN, R. SANDERS, *et al.* 2003. Sunscreens inadequately protect against UVA-induced free radicals in skin: implications for skin aging and melanoma? J. Invest. Dermatol. **121:** 862–868.

16. BOOTS. 2004. The Revised Guidelines to the Practical Measurement of UVA:UVB Ratios According to the Boots Star Rating System. The Boots Company. Nottingham, UK.

17. SHINDO, Y., E. WITT, D. HAN, *et al.* 1994. Enzymic and non-enzymic antioxidants in epidermis and dermis of human skin. J. Invest. Dermatol. **102:** 122–124.

18. RHIE, G., M.H. SHIN, J.Y. SEO, *et al.* 2001. Aging and photoaging-dependent changes of enzymic and nonenzymic antioxidants in the epidermis and dermis of human skin in vivo. J. Invest. Dermatol. **117:** 1212–1217.

19. WERNINGHAUS, K., M. MEYDANI, J. BHAWAN, *et al.* 1994. Evaluation of the photoprotective effect of oral vitamin E supplementation. Arch. Dermatol. **130:** 1257–1261.

20. PINNELL, S.R., H. YANG, M. ORMAR. *et al.* 2001. Topical L-ascorbic acid: peruitanerus absorption studies. Dermatol. Surg. **27:** 137–142.

21. DARR, D., S. DUNSTON, H. FAUST, *et al.* 1996. Effectiveness of antioxidants (vitamin C and E) with and without sunscreens as topical photoprotectants. Acta Derm. Venerol. **76:** 264–268.

22. LIN, J.Y., M.A. SELIM, C.R. SHEA, *et al.* 2003. UV photoprotection by combination topical antioxidants C and vitamin E. J. Am. Acad. Dermatol. **48:** 866–874.

23. FITZPATRICK, R.E. & E.F. ROSTAN. 2002. Double-blind, half-face study comparing topical vitamin C and vehicle for rejuvenation of photodamage. Derm. Surg. **28:** 231–236.

24. HUMBERT, P.G., M. HAFTEK, P. CREIDI, *et al.* 2003. Topical ascorbic acid on photoaged skin. Clinical, topographical and ultrastructural evaluation: double-blind study vs. placebo. Exp. Dermatol. **12:** 237–244.

25. GILCHREST, B.A. 1997. Treatment of photodamage with topical tretinoin. J. Am. Acad. Dermatol. **36:** S27–S36.

26. STRATIGOS, A.J. & A.D. KATSAMBAS. 2005. The role of topical retinoids in the treatment of photoaging. Drugs **65:** 1061–1072.
27. KLIGMAN, A.M., D. DOAGADKINA & R.M. LAVKER. 1993. Effects of topical tretinoin on non-sun-exposed protected skin of the elderly. J. Am. Acad. Dermatol. **39:** 25–33.
28. GREEN, L.J., A. MCCORMICK & G.D. WEINSTEIN. 1993. Photoaging and the skin: the effects of tretinoin. Dermatol. Clin. **11:** 97–105.
29. GRIFFITHS, C.E.M., A.N. RUSSMAN, G. MAJMUDAR, *et al.* 1993. Restoration of collagen formation in photodamaged human skin by tretinoin (retinoic acid). N. Engl. J. Med. **329:** 530–535.
30. FISHER, G.J., Z. WANG, S.C. DATTA, *et al.* 1997. Pathophysiology of premature skin aging induced by ultraviolet light. N. Engl. J. Med. **337:** 1419–1427.
31. GILCHREST, B.A. 1997. Treatment of photodamage with topical tretinoin: an overview. J. Am. Acad. Dermatol. **36:** S27–S36.
32. CLUCAS, A., M. BERSCHOORE, V. SORBA, *et al.* 1997. Adapalene 0.1% gel is better tolerated than tretinoin 0.025% gel in acne patients. J. Am. Acad. Dermatol. **36:** S116–S118.
33. LEYDEN, J., G. GROVE & C. ZERWECK. 2004. Facial tolerability of topical retinoid therapy. J. Drugs Dermatol. **3:** 641–651.
34. BRINEY, C. 2005. Industry Growth on the Horizon. Global Cosmetic Industry. June, pp. 41–42.
35. FARRIS, P.K. 2003. A review of the science behind the claims. Cosmetic Dermatol. **16:** 59–70.
36. STILLER, M.J., J. BARTOLONE, R. STERN, *et al.* 1996. Topical 8% glycolic acid and 8% L-lactic acid creams for the treatment of photodamaged skin. Arch. Dermatol. **132:** 631–636.
37. BARCISZEWSKI, J., S.I.S. RATTAN, G. SIBOSKA, *et al.* 1999. Kinetin—45 years on. Plant Sci. **148:** 37–45.
38. RATTAN, S.I. & B.F. CLARK. 1994. Kinetin delays the onset of aging characteristics in human fibroblasts. Biochem. Biophys. Res. Commun. **201:** 665–672.
39. OLSEN, A., G.E. SIBOSKA & B.F.C. CLARK, *et al.* 1999. N6-furfuryladenine, kinetin, protects against Fenton reaction-mediated oxidative damage to DNA. Biochem. Biophys. Res. Commun. **265:** 499–502.
40. VERBEKE, P., G.E. SIBOSKA & B.F.C. CLARK, *et al.* 2000. Kinetin inhibits protein oxidation and glyoxidation in vitro. Biochem. Biophys. Res. Commun. **276:** 1265–1267.
41. MCCULLOUGH, J.L. 1999. Furfuryladenine-A new antiaging topical: research and clinical experience. *In* Skin & Allergy News: Developments in Topical Skin Treatments: An Update 3–5. Skin Disease Education Foundation Symposium.
42. RATTAN, S.I.S. & L. SODAGAM. 2005. Gerontomodulatory and youth-preserving effects of zeatin on human skin fibroblasts undergoing aging *in vitro*. Rejuvenation Res. **8:** 46–57.
43. CARRUTHERS, J.D., N.J. LOWE, M.A. MENTER, *et al.* 2002. A multicenter, double-blind, randomized, placebo-controlled study of the efficacy and safety of botulinum toxin type A in the treatment of glabellar lines. J. Am. Acad. Dermatol. **46:** 840–849.
44. DAVLETOV, B., M. BAJOHRS & T. BINZ. 2005. Beyond BOTOX: advantages and limitations of individual botulinum neurotoxins. Trends Neurosci. **28:** 446–452.
45. WERSCHLER, W.P. & S. WEINKLE. 2005. Longevity of effects of injectable products for soft-tissue augmentation. J. Drugs Dermatol. **4:** 20–27.

46. NELSON, J.S., B. MAJARON & K.M. KELLY. 2002. What is non-ablative photorejuvenation of human skin? Semin. Cutan. Med. Surg. **21:** 238–250.
47. MONHEIT, G.D. 2001. Medium-depth chemical peels. Dermatol. Clin. **19:** 413–425.
48. HOLCK, D.E.E. & J.D. NG. 2003. Facial skin rejuvenation. Curr. Op. Ophthamol. **14:** 246–252.
49. KELLY, K.M., & J.S. NELSON. 1998. Carbon dioxide laser resurfacing of rhytides and photodamaged skin. Lasers Med. Sci. **13:** 232–241.
50. CARRUTHERS, A. 2005. The aging process. Dermatol. Focus **24:** 2.

Kinetin-Induced Differentiation of Normal Human Keratinocytes Undergoing Aging *in Vitro*

ULRICH BERGE, PETER KRISTENSEN, AND SURESH I. S. RATTAN

Laboratory of Cellular Ageing, Danish Centre for Molecular Gerontology, Department of Molecular Biology, University of Aarhus, Denmark

ABSTRACT: Kinetin (N^6-furfuryladenine) is a cytokinin growth factor having several anti-aging effects reported for human cells and fruit flies. We have observed that short-term culturing of human keratinocytes in the presence of 40 to 200 μM kinetin results in a significant inhibition of cell growth. Studies were undertaken to analyze the process of differentiation as a reason for growth inhibition. Keratinocytes at different passage levels were treated with fetal calf serum (FCS) and calcium as differentiation-inducing positive controls, with different concentrations of kinetin, and with a combination of kinetin and calcium. The induction and progression of differentiation was monitored by morphological observations and by using several differentiation markers, including keratins (K10 and K14), involucrin, epidermal transglutaminase, and some new keratinocyte-specific antibodies isolated by the phage display method. In young keratinocytes, two days of calcium treatment reduced the K14 level by 78%, and increased the levels of K10 and involucrin by 40% and 29%, respectively. In comparison, 40 μM kinetin had no effect on the K14 level, but increased the K10 level by 28% and that of involucrin by four-fold. The combination of calcium and 40 μM kinetin led to a decrease by 23% in the K14 level, to an increase in the level of K10 by 55%, and to a two-fold rise in the involucrin level. These results suggest that the rate, extent, and quality of differentiation depend on the inducing agent, and that kinetin may be useful in promoting the differentiation of human keratinocytes, especially in the presence of calcium.

KEYWORDS: cytokinins; skin; aging; anti-aging; epidermal cells; differentiation

Rattan and Clark published the first report of anti-aging effects of N^6-furfuryladenine or kinetin (Kn) on human skin fibroblasts.[1] Later on Sharma *et al.* reported an increased median and maximum life span of the

Address for correspondence: Dr. Suresh I.S. Rattan, Department of Molecular Biology, University of Aarhus, Gustav Wieds Vej 10C, DK8000 Aarhus-C, Denmark. Voice: +45-8942-5034; fax: +45-8612-3178.

e-mail: rattan@mb.au.dk [*or*] ulb@mb.au.dk

Ann. N.Y. Acad. Sci. 1067: 332–336 (2006). © 2006 New York Academy of Sciences.
doi: 10.1196/annals.1354.045

fruit fly *Zaprionuns paravittiger* fed with low levels of Kn.[2] Furthermore, this cytokinin has been found to inhibit oxidative and glycoxidative protein damage *in vitro*,[3] to protect the DNA against oxidative damage,[4] and to be an effective free-radical scavenger *in vitro*.[5] Since there are reports showing that Kn improves the appearance of the skin[6,7] and may induce differentiation in keratinocytes,[8] we investigated the effect of Kn in young human keratinocyte cultures with respect to growth, survival, and differentiation using a battery of biomarkers.

EXPERIMENTAL METHODS

Primary cultures of human epidermal keratinocytes were established from a mammary skin biopsy of a healthy woman (age: 28 years). For serial subculturing, the cells were thawed quickly and grown in proliferative mode-keeping, low-calcium EpiLife medium (Cascade Biologics, Mansfield, UK) with 5% CO_2/95% air and 95% humidity for 3–4 days until the medium had to be changed. When the cells reached 80% confluency, the culture was split using the trypsin/EDTA method (BioWhittacker™ Cambex Bio Science, Vervierts, Belgium). Kn (Olechemim Ltd., Czech Republic) was prepared by dissolving in 1 M HCl (30 mg/mL) followed by dilution in PBS. The effects of Kn on one-step growth, cell survival, and extent of apoptosis were studied by the standard methods described before.[1,9,10]

Differentiation Markers and ELISA

Since *in vitro* differentiation does not lead to fully differentiated corneocytes, four early, suprabasal markers were chosen: cytokeratins, K10 (ab9025, mouse monoclonal; Abcam, Cambridge, UK) and K14 (as single-chain variable fragments [scFv][11]), and involucrin (ab14504, mouse monoclonal; Abcam Cambridge, UK). In addition, the scFvs clone 10, which is specific for keratinocytes, but whose antigen is not known, was also tested.[12] The protocol for the expression and purification of scFv and the scFv-conjugagted phages was as described (*E. coli*: TG1 [supE hsd D5 (lac-pro AB)thi F'{tra D36 pro AB+ lacIq lacZ}]).[12–14] For the enzyme-linked immunosorbent assay (ELISA), 750,000 cells were seeded per T_{25} flask. After 6 h, the medium was changed according to the different treatments: control, 1% FCS, 1.2 mM $CaCl_2$, 40 μM Kn, 80 μM Kn, 200 μM Kn, and 1.2 mM $CaCl_2$ + 40 μM Kn. Cells were harvested after days 1, 2, and 3 with the trypsin/EDTA treatment and were washed twice subsequently with PBS (0.1 M NaCl, 50 mM $Na_xH_yPO_4$). The cell pellets were lysated (0.5 M TrisHCl, pH 8.0; 150 mM NaCl; 10 mM $MgCl_2$; 10% glycerol; 0.25‰ SDS) and stored at $-20°C$ for later use.

Specific protein amounts (0.25 μg to 1 μg, depending on the antibody) in 50 μL lysis buffer were used to coat 96-well plates overnight at 4°C in triplicate. After one or two washing steps with PBS, the wells were blocked with 2% milk in PBS (MPBS) and incubated for 1 h at room temperature (RT). After the incubation time, the blocking MPBS was changed for 100 μL of MPBS containing the antibody and incubated for 1 h at RT. The plates were washed six times with PBS, incubated with 100 μL of the MPBS containing the secondary antibody, and washed again six times. The protein levels were quantified applying OPD, 2 HCl (1,2-phenylenediamine dihydrochloride [OPD, 2 mg for ELISA]: DakoCytomation Denmark A/S, Glostrup, Denmark) as the detection system.

RESULTS AND DISCUSSION

The one-step growth analysis showed that Kn (40–200 μM) inhibited the growth of early-passage keratinocytes (30% life span completed; data not shown). However, there was no induction of apoptosis due to Kn treatment (control: 5–7%; Kn-treated: 3–7%). Studies on cell viability (MTT assay) and DNA-synthesis (5-Bromo-2′-deoxy-uridine [BrdU]) showed that Kn had no negative effects up to concentrations of 80 μM. Thus, Kn-inhibited cell growth in keratinocytes *in vitro* is not due to impaired DNA synthesis or cell viability or increased apoptosis.

In order to study the effects of Kn on differentiation, early-passage young (30% life span completed) keratinocytes were treated either with known inducers of differentiation (10% FCS, 1.2 mM CaCl$_2$), with Kn (40 μM, 80 μM, and 200 μM), or with a combination of Kn and calcium (1.2 mM CaCl$_2$ + 40 μM Kn) for 2 days. TABLE 1 shows that calcium and FCS treatment induced differentiation markers K10 by 41% and 30%, and involucrin by 29% and 89%, respectively. At the same time the levels of the basal cell marker K14 were reduced by 78% and 82%, respectively. The keratinocyte-specific protein recognized by scFv 10 was significantly induced by FCS, whereas its levels were reduced in the presence of calcium.

TABLE 1. Changes in the levels of keratinocyte differentiation markers after different treatments

Differentiation marker	Treatment					
	10% FCS	1.2 mM CaCl$_2$	40 μM Kn	80 μM Kn	200 μM Kn	1.2 mM CaCl$_2$ + 40 μM Kn
Keratin 10	1.30	1.41	1.28	1.12	1.06	1.56
Keratin 14	0.18	0.22	1.04	0.76	0.90	0.77
Involucrin	1.89	1.29	4.25	1.65	1.47	2.09
scFv 10 antibody	2.79	0.70	1.37	1.40	1.75	0.90

NOTE: Data are presented as the ratios of normalized ELISA values for days 2 and 1.

Kn treatment of keratinocytes also increased K10 levels, but to a lower extent than that with calcium and FCS (TABLE 1). The K14 level was unaltered when keratinocytes were treated with 40 μM Kn, but 80 μM Kn caused a decrease by 24% and 200 μM by 10%. Involucrin levels were induced most by 40 μM Kn (four-fold). For 80 μM and 200 μM Kn, the increase in involucrin level was 65% and 47%, respectively. The signals for the scFv 10 revealed increasing levels of this protein with rising concentrations of Kn, suggesting that Kn has some effect on the expression of this protein (TABLE 1).

A combination of Kn and calcium caused expression patterns similar to those of calcium, although in all ELISAs of young cells higher ratios could be observed. Therefore, the highest ratios for K10 were detected (+56%). K14 levels were similarly reduced as in 80 μM Kn (−23%). The involucrin level was elevated two-fold compared with both positive controls (TABLE 1).

Our studies indicate that Kn has a differentiation-modulating property. Although on its own, Kn does not appear to be a strong inducer of keratinocyte differentiation, in combination with calcium, a significant enhancement of differentiation could be observed. This could have implications for the use of Kn in the maintenance and promotion of keratinocyte differentiation during aging when both the calcium levels and the extent of differentiation are generally reduced. This may also explain the skin thickness–promoting effects of Kn in human clinical studies.[7,8]

ACKNOWLEDGMENTS

Thanks are extended to Anne Gylling, Helle Jakobsen, Gunhild Siboska, Regina Gonzalez-Dosal, Rehab El-Sayed Ali, and Lakshman Sodagam for their help and critical discussions. The Laboratory of Cellular Ageing is supported by research grants from the Danish Research Councils, Carlsberg Fund, Senetek PLC, and EU's Biomed Health Programmes.

REFERENCES

1. RATTAN, S.I.S. & B.F.C. CLARK. 1994. Kinetin delays the onset of aging characteristics in human fibroblasts. Biochem. Biophys. Res. Commun. **20:** 665–672.
2. SHARMA, S.P., P. KAUR & S.I.S. RATTAN. 1995. Plant growth hormone kinetin delays ageing, prolongs the lifespan and slows down development of the fruitfly *Zaprionus paravittiger*. Biochem. Biophys. Res. Commun. **216:** 1067–1071.
3. VERBEKE, P., G.E. SIBOSKA, B.F. CLARK, *et al*. 2000. Kinetin inhibits protein oxidation and glycoxidation in vitro. Biochem. Biophys. Res. Commun. **276:** 1265–1270.
4. OLSEN, A., G.E. SIBOSKA, B.F. CLARK, *et al*. 1999. N(6)-furfuryladenine, kinetin, protects against Fenton reaction-mediated oxidative damage to DNA. Biochem. Biophys. Res. Commun. **265:** 499–502.

5. HSIAO, G., M.Y. SHEN, K.H. LIN, *et al.* 2003. Inhibitory activity of kinetin on free radical formation of activated platelets in vitro and on thrombus formation in vivo. Eur. J. Pharmacol. **465:** 281–287.
6. MCCULLOUGH, J.L. & G.D. WEINSTEIN. 2002. Clinical study of safety and efficacy of using topical kinetin 0.1% (Kinerase) to treat photodamaged skin. Cosmet. Dermatol. **15:** 29–32.
7. KIMURA, T. & K. DOI. 2004. Depigmentation and rejuvenation effects of kinetin on the aged skin of hairless descendants of Mexican hairless dogs. Rejuvenation Res. **7:** 32–39.
8. BOLUND, L., P.K.A. JENSEN & P. BJERRING. 1991. Method and composition for treating hyperproliferative skin diseases using 6-aminopurine cytokinins. United Stated Patent Patent Number 5,021,422.
9. VERBEKE, P., G.E. SIBOSKA, B.F. CLARK, *et al.* 2000. Kinetin inhibits protein oxidation and glycoxidation in vitro. Biochem. Biophys. Res. Commun. **276:** 1265–1270.
10. FONAGER, J., R. BEEDHOLM, B.F. CLARK, *et al.* 2002. Mild stress-induced stimulation of heat-shock protein synthesis and improved functional ability of human fibroblasts undergoing aging in vitro. Exp. Gerontol. **37:** 1223–1228.
11. STAUSBOL-GRON, B., K.B. JENSEN, K.H. JENSEN, *et al.* 2001. De novo identification of cell-type specific antibody-antigen pairs by phage display subtraction: isolation of a human single chain antibody fragment against human keratin 14. Eur. J. Biochem. **268:** 3099–3107.
12. JENSEN, K.B., O.N. JENSEN, P. RAVN, *et al.* 2003. Identification of keratinocyte-specific markers using phage display and mass spectrometry. Mol. Cell. Proteomics **2:** 61–69.
13. KRISTENSEN, P. & G. WINTER. 1998. Proteolytic selection for protein folding using filamentous bacteriophages. Fold. Des. **3:** 321–328.
14. JENSEN, K.B. & P. KRISTENSEN. 2005. Isolation of recombinant phage-displayed antibodies recognizing skin keratinocytes. Methods Mol. Biol. **289:** 359–370.

Epidermal and Dermal Characteristics in Skin Equivalent after Systemic and Topical Application of Skin Care Ingredients

JANA VICANOVA,[a] CHARBEL BOUEZ,[b] SOPHIE LACROIX,[b] LARS LINDMARK,[c] AND ODILE DAMOUR[b]

[a] DermData s.r.o, Czech Republic

[b] Banque de Tissus et Cellules, Hôpital Edouard Herriot, Hospices Civils de Lyon, Lyon, France

[c] Imedeen Research, Ferrosan, Denmark

ABSTRACT: Effects of active ingredients from topical and systemic skin-care products on structure and organization of epidermis, dermal–epidermal junction (DEJ), and dermis were examined using an *in vitro* reconstructed skin equivalent (SE). Imedeen Time Perfection (ITP) ingredients (a mixture of BioMarine Complex, grape seed extract, tomato extract, vitamin C) were supplemented systemically into culture medium. Kinetin, an active ingredient from Imedeen Expression Line Control Serum, was applied topically. Both treatments were tested separately or combined. In epidermis, all treatments stimulated keratinocyte proliferation, showing a significant increase of Ki67-positive keratinocytes ($P < 0.05$). Kinetin showed a twofold increase of Ki67-positive cells, ITP resulted in a fivefold, and ITP+kinetin showed a nine-fold increase. Differentiation of keratinocytes was influenced only by kinetin since filaggrin was found only in kinetin and kinetin+ITP samples. At the DEJ, laminin 5 was slightly increased by all treatments. In dermis, only ITP increased the amount of collagen type I. Both kinetin and ITP stimulated formation of fibrillin-1 and elastin deposition. The effect of kinetin was seen in upper dermis. It stimulated not only the amount of deposited fibrillin-1 and elastin fibers but also their organization perpendicularly to the DEJ. ITP stimulated formation of fibrillin-1 in deeper dermis. In summary, the combination of topical treatment with kinetin and systemic treatment with ITP had complementary beneficial effects in the formation and development of epidermis and dermis.

KEYWORDS: Imedeen; Mimeskin; skin equivalent; keratinocyte proliferation; dermal matrix; kinetin

Address for correspondence: Jana Vicanova, Ph.D., Osvobozeni 920, 273 51 Unhost, Czech Republic. Voice: +420 603 468 949; fax: +420 312 699 236.
e-mail: javi@ferrosan.com

Ann. N.Y. Acad. Sci. 1067: 337–342 (2006). © 2006 New York Academy of Sciences.
doi: 10.1196/annals.1354.046

Skin aging is associated with changes of skin structure and skin cell activities. The most prominent modifications were found in dermis, but changes were also observed at the dermal–epidermal junction (DEJ) and in epidermis.[1] In recent years, a search for active ingredients that would prevent, counteract, or reverse degenerative changes in skin aging has been increasing. Among available testing systems, *in vitro* reconstructed three-dimensional skin equivalent model (SE) Mimeskin® proved to be innovative and relevant in testing cosmetic products.[2–4]

This study was aimed to examine the effect of systemic treatment with Imedeen Time Perfection active ingredients (ITP) and of topical treatment with kinetin, an active ingredient present in Imedeen Expression Line control serum, using SE. In epidermis, the investigations focused on potential effect on keratinocyte proliferation (Ki67) and differentiation (filaggrin). In dermis, amount and localization of deposited dermal components such as fibrillin-1, elastin, and collagen type I were examined.

EXPERIMENTAL METHODS

The SE Mimeskin® was prepared as described previously.[5] Dermal equivalents were prepared by adding a suspension of 200,000 fibroblasts/cm^2 originating from healthy 42-year-old female skin on the top of the collagen–glycosaminoglycan–chitosan porous sponge Mimedisk® (Coletica, France). All equivalents were cultured for 21 days in fibroblast medium (Dulbecco's Modified Eagle's Medium (DMEM with Glutamax-1, Invitrogen, Cergy Pontoise, France) with 10% calf serum (HyClone, Logan, UT), 20 μg/mL gentamicin (Panpharma, Fougères, France), 100 IU/mL penicillin (Sarbach, Suresnes, France), 1 μg/mL amphotericin B (Bristol Myers Squibb, Puteaux, France), and 10 μg/mL L-ascorbic acid 2-phosphate (Sigma, St. Quentin Fallavier, France). The medium was changed daily.

Keratinocytes (250,000 cells/cm^2) were seeded on the top of dermal equivalent at day 14. After 7 days of submerged culture in the keratinocyte medium [3:1 mixture of DMEM and Ham's F12 (Invitrogen), with10% calf serum (HyClone), 10 ng/mL epidermal growth factor (EGF) (Austral Biologic, San Ramon, CA), 0.12 IU/mL insulin (Lilly, Saint-Cloud, France), 0.4 μg/mL hydrocortisone (UpJohn, St. Quentin en Yvelines, France), 5 μg/mL triiodo-L-thyronine (Sigma), 24.3 μg/mL adenine (Sigma), and antibiotics as above], the SE were elevated at the air–liquid interface and cultured in a simplified keratinocyte medium containing DMEM supplemented with 10% calf serum, 10 ng/mL EGF, 0.12 IU/mL insulin, 0.4 μg/mL hydrocortisone, antibiotics, and 10 μg/mL L-ascorbic acid, and were changed daily.

ITP ingredients were from Ferrosan A/S (Denmark). The final concentrations in medium were: sodium ascorbate (5 μg/mL), grape seed extract (GE; 2.5 μg/mL), tomato extract (TE; 5 μg/mL), and BioMarine Complex™ (BMC; 35 μg/mL). All ingredients were water-soluble except tomato extract, which was dissolved in tetrahydrofuran (THF). ITP was added from the time of the first culture medium change until harvesting. Kinetin was obtained from Senetek (USA). Solution of 0.1% kinetin in ketrol was applied topically from day 28 (after 1 week of air-exposed epidermis) and reapplied every second day. Final samples were collected at day 49. The culture conditions were: (i) kinetin, (ii) ITP, (iii) ITP+kinetin, (iv) control with systemic THF and topical ketrol, and (v) control without any treatment.

Three samples of material at each condition were fixed in 4% paraformaldehyde for histologic and immunohistochemical study, dehydrated, and embedded in paraffin. Three others were embedded in OCT Tissue-Tek (Miles, Immunotech, Marseille, France). Four histologic vertical 5-μm sections were stained with hematoxylin–phloxin–saffron.

For immunohistochemical study, 6-μm sections were deparaffinized and whitened in glycine–HCl (100 mmol/L). The antibody was directed against Ki67 (monoclonal, raised in mouse, dilution 1:50, DAKO, Glostrup, Denmark). Peroxydase-conjugated goat anti-mouse IgG (1:50 dilution, Santa Cruz Biotechnology, Santa Cruz, CA) was used to detect the immune complexes using diaminobenzidine as substrate (DAKO). Counterstaining was performed using Harris' hematoxylin. For controls, the primary antibody was omitted. Multiple serial sections of each specimen were processed to ensure representative samples. The number of Ki67-positive cells is expressed as percentage of total cell count in a field of 100 cells. Four fields were scored per sample. For statistical analysis, normality test and Mann-Whitney rank sum test were used for multiple comparison versus control group.

For immunofluorescence, 6-μm frozen sections were air dried, blocked in phosphate buffered saline solution containing 1% (wt/vol) bovine serum albumin. Antibodies were directed against human elastin (polyclonal, raised in rabbit, 1:150 dilution, Novotec), human type I collagen (polyclonal, raised in rabbit, 1:40 dilution, Tebu Bio, Le Perray, France), human filaggrin (monoclonal, raised in mouse; 1:100 dilution, Biomedical Technologies, Stoughton, MA), and human fibrillin-1 (monoclonal, raised in mouse, dilution 1:50, Interchim, Neomarkers, France). Secondary antibodies, either anti-rabbit IgG (1:50 dilution, Sanofi Diagnostics Pasteur Chaska, MN) or goat anti-mouse IgG (1:50 dilution, Santa Cruz Biotechnology), labeled with FITC, were mixed with 0.1 % Evans Blue to reduce non-specific staining of the sponge network. For controls, the primary antibody was omitted. The type I collagen antibodies specific for human collagen do not cross-react with the bovine collagen that was used to prepare the dermal substrate.[6]

RESULTS

Effects of ITP, kinetin, and their combination on selected epidermal and dermal markers are summarized in TABLE 1.

TABLE 1. Overall grading of epidermal and dermal markers in skin equivalent after treatment with ITP, kinetin, and ITP+kinetin

	Control	Kinetin	ITP	ITP+Kinetin
Epidermis				
Ki67-positive keratinocytes	+	++	+++	+++++
Filaggrin	0	++	0	++
Basement membrane				
Laminin	+	++	++	++
Dermis				
Fibrillin-1	+	+++	++	++++
Elastin	+	++	++++	++++
Collagen type I	++	++	++++	++++

NOTE: The individual markers were visualized by immunofluorescence and immunohistochemical techniques and evaluated according to semiquantitative scale. 0 = no effect, absent; + = very low; ++ = low; +++ = moderate; ++++ = high; +++++ = very high.

In epidermis, all treatments stimulated keratinocyte proliferation, showing a significant increase of Ki67-positive keratinocytes ($P < 0.05$). Kinetin showed a twofold increase of Ki67-positive cells, ITP resulted in a fivefold increase, and ITP+kinetin showed a ninefold increase (FIG. 1).

Differentiation of keratinocytes was influenced only by kinetin since fillagrin was found only in kinetin and kinetin+ITP samples (TABLE 1). At the dermal–epidermal junction (DEJ), laminin 5 was slightly increased by all treatments. In dermis, only ITP increased the amount of collagen type I. Both kinetin and ITP stimulated formation of fibrillin and elastin deposition. The effect of kinetin was seen in upper dermis. Kinetin stimulates not only the amount but also the organization of fibrillin-1 and elastin fibers perpendicularly to the DEJ. ITP stimulated formation of fibrillin in deeper dermis.

DISCUSSION

The results of this study confirmed a strong effect of ITP actives on formation and deposition of extracellular matrix components such as collagen type I and fibrillin-1 in reconstructed Skin Equivalent (SE) reported previously.[7] *In vivo* human studies confirmed that the effect observed *in vitro* leads to clinically visible improvement of aging skin structure.[8,9]

In this study, we investigated, for the first time, the effect of ITP on epidermal keratinocytes, which showed a stimulation of basal cell proliferation. It is well known that cell proliferation decreases with aging. Such an effect can be mimicked in SE using cells derived from young and aged donors. Stimulation of Ki67 expression in suboptimally proliferating SE generated from aged cells suggests a potential for the tested ingredients to optimize epidermal turnover *in vivo*.

To further enhance positive effects on aging skin tissue, another active, kinetin, was applied topically in combination with systemic supplementation

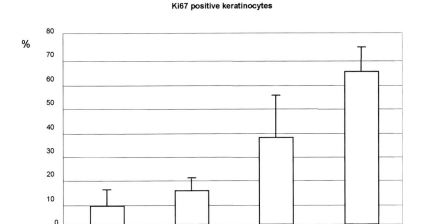

FIGURE 1. Number of Ki67-positive keratinocytes in skin equivalent after treatment with ITP, kinetin, and ITP+kinetin. The number of Ki67-positive cells is expressed as percentage of total cell count in a field of 100 cells. Four fields were scored per sample. For statistical analysis, normality test and Mann-Whitney rank sum test were used for multiple comparison versus control group.

of ITP. Kinetin is a cytokinin that displays a variety of biological effects, including those on cell proliferation and anti-aging effects.[10,11] Human trial on volunteers with moderate signs of skin aging demonstrated objective and statistically significant improvements in several parameters after topical use of kinetin.[12] In our study, kinetin alone influenced keratinocyte proliferation and differentiation as well as formation of basement membrane and elastic network in the upper dermis. Combined treatment of kinetin and ITP seemed to reinforce the effects of each other regarding keratinocyte proliferation and elastic network formation.

In conclusion, treatment with topical kinetin and systemic ITP showed multiple effects on development and organization of epidermis and dermis. ITP and kinetin have complementary beneficial effects on the formation and maintenance of healthy skin tissue.

ACKNOWLEDGMENTS

We thank Sandrine Vidal for her expert technical assistance.

REFERENCES

1. YAAR, M., M. ELLER & B. GILCHREST. 2002. Fifty years of skin aging. J. Invest. Dermatol. Symp. Proc. **7:** 51–58.

2. BLACK, A.F., C. BOUEZ, E. PERRIER, *et al*. 2005. Optimization and characterization of an engineered human skin equivalent. Tissue Eng. **11:** 723–733.

3. DAMOUR, O., C. AUGUSTIN & A.F. BLACK. 1998. Applications of reconstructed skin models in pharmaco-toxicological trials. Med. Biol. Eng. Comput. **6:** 1–8.

4. SCHLOTMANN, K., M. KAETEN, A.F. BLACK, *et al*. 2001. Cosmetic efficacy claims in vitro using a 3D human skin model. Int. J. Cosmet. Sci. **23:** 309–318.

5. DUPLAN-PERRAT, F., O. DAMOUR, C. MONTROCHER, *et al*. 2000. Keratinocytes influence the maturation and organization of the elastin network in a skin equivalent. J. Invest. Dermatol. **114:** 365–370.

6. NOBLESSE, E., V. CENIZO, C. BOUEZ, *et al*. 2004. Lysyl oxidase-like and lysyl oxidase are present in the dermis and epidermis of a skin equivalent and in human skin and are associated to elastic fibers. J. Invest. Dermatol. **122:** 621–630.

7. BOUEZ, C., O. DAMOUR & J. VICANOVA. 2003. Improvement of dermal extracellular matrix structure and composition after treatment with Imedeen Time Perfection in an in vitro skin equivalent. Poster exhibited at meeting of International Society for Bioengineering and International Society for Skin Imaging. May, Hamburg, Germany.

8. KIEFFER, M.E. & J. EFSEN. 1998. Imedeen® in the treatment of photoaged skin: an efficacy and safety trial over 12 months. J. Eur. Acad. Dermatol. Venereol. **11:** 129–136.

9. SIGLER, M.L. & P. RASMUSSEN. 2003. A placebo controlled study of an oral supplement (Imedeen Time Perfection) in improving the appearance of photodamaged skin. Poster exhibited at Meeting of European Academy of Dermato Venereology. October, Barcelona, Spain.

10. RATTAN, S. & B. CLARK. 1994. Kinetin delays the onset of ageing characteristics in human fibroblasts. Biochem. Biophys. Res. Commun. **201:** 665–672.

11. BARCISZEWSKI, J., S. RATTAN, G. SIBOSKA, *et al*. 1999. Kinetin—45 years on. Plant Sci. **148:** 37–45.

12. MCCULLOUGH, J.L. & G.D. WEINSTEIN. 2002. Clinical study of safety and efficacy of using topical kinetin 0.1% (Kinerase) to treat photodamaged skin. Cosmet. Dermatol. **15:** 29–32.

MAP Kinases and Heat Shock–Induced Hormesis in Human Fibroblasts during Serial Passaging *in Vitro*

ELISE R. NIELSEN, YVONNE E.G. ESKILDSEN-HELMOND, AND SURESH I.S. RATTAN

Laboratory of Cellular Ageing, Danish Centre for Molecular Gerontology, Department of Molecular Biology, University of Aarhus, Aarhus, Denmark

ABSTRACT: Adult human skin fibroblasts were exposed repeatedly to 41°C or 42°C heat shock (HS) for 1 h twice a week during serial passaging throughout their replicative life span. On the basis of longevity curves, cell size, and morphology, we observed that repeated mild heat shock (RMHS) at 41,°C had strong anti-aging hormetic effects, including 20% extension of cellular longevity. The basal levels of the MAP kinases JNK1, JNK2, and p38 increased during serial passaging, while that of ERK2 decreased. RMHS further exaggerated these effects, which suggests that age-related changes in MAP kinases may be an adaptive response for better cell survival.

KEYWORDS: stress; hormesis; aging; anti-aging; MAP kinases

INTRODUCTION

Anti-aging hormetic effects of repeated mild heat shock (RMHS) on normal human fibroblasts have been reported earlier from our laboratory.[1-3] Maintenance of youthful morphology, reduced accumulation of oxidized and glycoxidized abnormal proteins, increased ability to decompose H_2O_2, increased activity of the proteosome, reduced accumulation of lipofuscin, and increased resistance to various stresses are some of the main hormetic effects observed.[1-3] Although the beneficial cellular and biochemical effects of RMHS on human cells have been well documented, it is still not clear how cells sense stress and which signaling mechanisms are involved.

The mitogen-activated protein kinases (MAP kinases) are major components of the pathways controlling embryogenesis, cell differentiation, cell proliferation, and cell death. MAP kinases are a family of serine and threonine kinases,

Address for correspondence: Dr. Suresh I.S. Rattan, Department of Molecular Biology, University of Aarhus, Gustav Wieds Vej 10C, DK8000 Aarhus–C, Denmark. Voice: +45 8942 5034; fax: +45 8612 3178.

e-mail: elisernielsen@hotmail.com

Ann. N.Y. Acad. Sci. 1067: 343–348 (2006). © 2006 New York Academy of Sciences.
doi: 10.1196/annals.1354.048

whose function and regulation have been highly conserved throughout evolution in organisms as simple as the unicellular brewer's yeast to complex organisms as humans.[4,5] The MAP kinases can be activated by many different stimuli, such as growth factors, cellular stress, cytokines, hormones, and cell–cell adherence. Most of the substrates for MAP kinases are transcription factors, but MAP kinases are also able to phosphorylate protein kinases, phospholipases, and cytoskeleton-associated proteins, and thereby control gene expression.[4,5] Here we report the effects of RMHS at 41°C and 42°C on the levels of the MAP kinases JNK1, JNK2, p38, and ERK2 in serially passaged human skin fibroblasts.

MATERIALS AND METHODS

Normal adult human mammary skin fibroblast cell line designated ASF2 was established from explant skin biopsy from a healthy young donor (aged 28 years). Cells were cultured in complete medium (Dulbecco's modified Eagle's medium, DMEM, [BioWhittaker; now Cambrex, Copenhagen, Denmark] containing 10% (v/v) fetal calf serum [Hyclone, Bie & Berntsen Copenhagen, Denmark], 1% (v/v) glutamine [BioWhittaker], and 1% (v/v) penicillin/streptomycin [BioWhittaker]) at 37°C at 5% CO_2 and 95% humidity. In this experiment we used a control cell line at 37°C, a RMHS at 41°C cell line, and a RMHS at 42°C cell line. The RMHS cell lines were exposed to 1-h heat shock (HS) at the indicated temperature twice a week throughout the life span of the cells.[1]

Proteins were harvested immediately after the last HS in cold lysis buffer, and soluble protein extracts were prepared by centrifuging the samples for 15 min at 13,000 rpm and collecting the supernatant. Proteins were separated by SDS-PAGE followed by Western blotting (10 μg protein for total MAP kinase assays and 30 μg protein for phosphorylated MAP kinase assays), and analyzed after incubation with following antibodies: ERK2 (sc-154), JNK1 (sc-571), JNK2 (sc-572), p38 (sc-535), p-ERK (sc-7383), p-JNK (sc-6254), all purchased from Santa Cruz Biotechnology.

RESULTS AND DISCUSSION

FIGURE 1 shows the longevity curves of the three cell lines, which grew at a similar rate until cumulative population-doubling level (CPDL) 15, by which time they had received approximately 20 rounds of RMHS, after which a difference in the growth curves of the three lines could be seen. The control line at 37°C slowed down earlier as compared with the other two lines, and the RMHS 41°C cell line grew faster than the RMHS 42°C cell line. 41°C-treated cells reached a CPDL of 30 followed by the other two lines

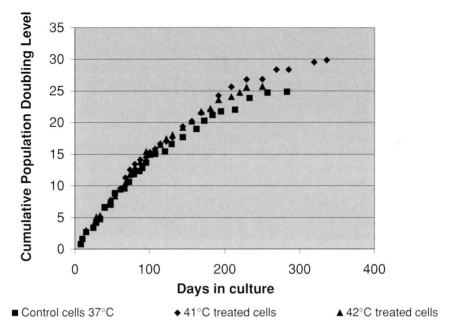

■ Control cells 37°C   ◆ 41°C treated cells   ▲ 42°C treated cells

FIGURE 1. Longevity curves of the three cell lines with or without repeated mild heat shock.

(CPDL = 25). Thus there was 20% increase in proliferative life span of human skin fibroblasts exposed to RMHS at 41°C.

FIGURE 2 shows age-related changes in the morphology of the cells, which became larger, flattened, and irregular with serial passaging and had a typical senescent cell phenotype. RMHS appears to slow down the onset of age-related enlargement and irregularization. Of all the three lines, the RMHS 41°C cell line best maintained a relatively youthful morphology in terms of small size, spindle-shaped cells, fewer multinucleated cells, and a more parallel positioning of the cells. The RMHS 42°C cell line also appeared to prevent age-related changes, but the effect was smaller than at 41°C. On the basis of the longevity curves, morphology, and senescence-associated β-galactosidase activity (data not shown), we conclude that the RMHS 41°C cell line aged more slowly than the other two lines.

FIGURE 3 shows the levels of the MAP kinases JNK1, JNK2, p38, and ERK2. The data are presented for three age groups: early-passage young (less than 30% life span completed), middle-aged (45–70% life span completed), and late-passage senescent (more than 80% life span completed) cells. There are no results for ERK1, because the antibody used in this experiment did not recognize ERK1 sufficiently for reliable quantification.

The amount of the stress-activated protein kinases JNK1, JNK2, and p38 increased with age in the control cells. The most dramatic increase was in

10% lifespan completed   50% lifespan completed   95% lifespan completed

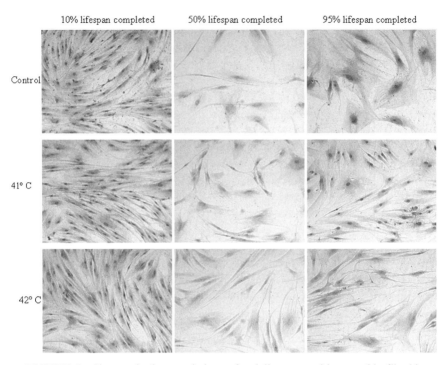

FIGURE 2. Changes in the morphology of serially passaged human skin fibroblasts with or without repeated mild heat shock.

JNK2, where it was more than four times higher in senescent cells than in young cells. In comparison, the levels of JNK1 and p38 increased by 45–70% in senescent cells. In RMHS-treated cells the levels of JNK1, JNK2, and p38 were higher in the middle-aged cells than in the controls. In late-passage senescent cells, the levels of JNK1 and JNK2 were almost similar in all three cell lines, but that of p38 was significantly reduced. In the case of ERK2 the amount was approximately 20% lower in middle-aged and senescent cells as compared to the young cells for all three cell lines (FIG. 3).

Higher levels of MAP kinases in the middle-aged and senescent cells could indicate that the upregulation of the kinases with age may be an adaptive response for cell survival. The increase seen with age can be caused by the constitutive stress coming from the accumulation of damaged proteins. RMHS may therefore act as a signal for enhancing this adaptive response. It will be interesting to find out whether downstream processes affected by MAP kinases are affected in a similar way in normal and RMHS-stressed cells.

We have also determined the basal levels of the phosphorylated (active) form of both ERK1 and ERK2 in serially passaged control cells, which were found to be 4–10 times higher in the middle-aged and senescent cells as compared to the young cells (data not shown). However, the basal activation level of JNK1

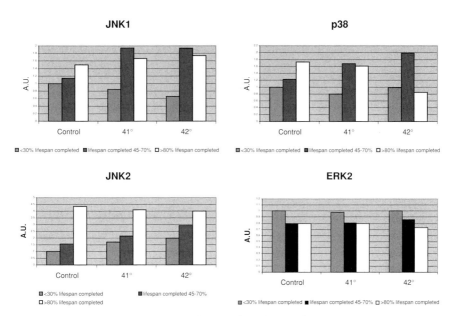

FIGURE 3. Relative amounts (arbitrary units) of MAP kinase proteins in serially passaged human skin fibroblasts with or without repeated mild heat shock.

decreased by 50% in the late-passage cells. This decrease in activated JNK could be due to an increase in Hsp70 levels,[6] which is known to suppress JNK activation. It is believed to be the balance between phosphorylated ERK on one side and phosphorylated JNK and p38 on the other that determines whether the cell will proliferate, differentiate, or undergo apoptosis. The age-related changes observed could indicate that this balance shifts with age, so the senescent cells need a stronger proliferation signal from ERK compared to the apoptotic signals from JNK and p38 than they do at young age.

ACKNOWLEDGMENTS

We thank Anne Gylling, Helle Jakobsen, and Gunhild Siboska for their help and critical discussions. The Laboratory of Cellular Ageing is supported by research grants from the Danish Research Councils, Carlsberg Fund, Senetek PLC, and EU's Biomed Health Programmes.

REFERENCES

1. VERBEKE, P., B.F.C. CLARK & S.I.S. RATTAN. 2001. Reduced levels of oxidized and glycoxidized proteins in human fibroblasts exposed to repeated mild heat shock during serial passaging in vitro. Free Radic. Biol. Med. **31:** 1593–1602.

2. RATTAN, S.I.S. 2004. Aging intervention, prevention, and therapy through hormesis. J. Gerontol. A. Biol. Sci. Med. Sci. **59:** B705–B709.
3. RATTAN, S.I.S. *et al.* 2004. Slowing down aging from within: mechanistic aspects of anti-aging hormetic effects of mild heat stress on human cells. Acta. Biochim. Pol. **51:** 481–492.
4. WIDMANN, C. *et al.* 1999. Mitogen-activated protein kinase: conservation of a three-kinase module from yeast to human. Physiol. Rev. **79:** 143–180.
5. PEARSON, G. *et al.* 2001. Mitogen-activated protein (MAP) kinase pathways: regulation and physiological functions. Endocr. Rev. **22:** 153–183.
6. FONAGER, J. *et al.* 2002. Mild stress-induced stimulation of heat-shock protein synthesis and improved functional ability of human fibroblasts undergoing aging in vitro. Exp. Gerontol. **37:** 1223–1228.

The Roles of Satellite Cells and Hematopoietic Stem Cells in Impaired Regeneration of Skeletal Muscle in Old Rats

SHUICHI MACHIDA,[a,b] AND MITSUO NARUSAWA[b]

[a]*Department of Physical Education, International Budo University, Chiba 299-5295, Japan*

ABSTRACT: Sarcopenia is the involuntary loss of skeletal muscle mass and strength that occurs with aging, resulting in physical frailty. One potential explanation for sarcopenia is the failure of muscle to regenerate after damage, some of which may be due to changes in the function of satellite cells. Recent studies have identified novel populations of adult stem cells in skeletal muscle, such as hematopoietic stem cells. To understand the cellular mechanisms of sarcopenia, we examined the expression of satellite cells and hematopoietic stem cells in old regenerating muscles based on the expression profiles of several markers related to those cells.

KEYWORDS: sarcopenia; satellite cells; hematopoietic stem cells; muscle regeneration

INTRODUCTION

During normal aging in both humans and rodents, a progressive loss of skeletal muscle mass, termed sarcopenia, is observed. The decline in skeletal muscle mass is paralleled by decreased muscle strength and endurance. These changes are functionally important, as they contribute to frailty, functional loss, dependence, disability, high health care costs, and premature death. One concern is that the prevalence of sarcopenia is increasing in the world. There is a great deal of interest in strategies to prevent or reverse sarcopenia in our aging population.

[b]Research Fellow of the Japan Society for the Promotion of Science.

Address for correspondence: Shuichi Machida, Ph.D., Institute for Biomedical Engineering, Consolidated Research Institute for Advanced Science and Medical Care, Waseda University, 2-579-15 Mikajima, Tokorozawa, Saitama, 359-1192, Japan. Voice: +81-4-2949-8113, Ext. 3585; fax: +81-4-2947-6898.

e-mail: machidas@waseda.jp

Ann. N.Y. Acad. Sci. 1067: 349–353 (2006). © 2006 New York Academy of Sciences.
doi: 10.1196/annals.1354.049

SATELLITE CELLS CONTRIBUTE TO MUSCLE
REGENERATION

Sarcopenia is caused by a reduction in the size and number of muscle fibers. Adult skeletal muscle has a remarkable regenerative capacity, largely mediated by satellite cells (SCs). SCs are located in the plasma membrane of myofibers beneath the basement membrane and are mitotically quiescent in adult muscle. During muscle regeneration, SCs are activated, giving rise to myoblasts that proliferate, and fuse together or fuse to preexisting muscle fibers to produce fully mature muscle fibers. Therefore, SCs are integral to the regenerative processes after muscle fiber damage.[1] Skeletal muscle regeneration is markedly impaired with age, some of which may be due to changes in the function of SCs or adult stem cells. Gibson and Schultz (1983) found a decline in the number of SCs in the skeletal muscles of aged rodents compared to that in adult animals.[2] The proliferative potential of SCs *in vitro* decreases with advanced age.[3,4] Therefore, deficits in the regenerative process occur as a function of age, some of which may be due to a decline in function of SCs. However, the cellular mechanisms responsible for the impaired regeneration in old muscle are not well understood. The most reliable way to identify SCs is on the basis of their position using electron microscopy, although this method is not particularly convenient. Therefore, antibodies have been used to identify specific proteins in quiescent (and activated) SCs *in vivo* at the light microscopic level, such as M-cadherin and Pax7.[1] Muscle regeneration from SCs has long been believed to initiate the process of embryonic myogenesis. Supportive evidence includes the findings that proliferating and differentiating SCs reexpress myogenic regulatory factors (MRFs, namely MyoD, Myf5, myogenin, and MRF4) and embryonic myofibrillar genes during muscle regeneration.[5,6] For example, MyoD accumulates in activated SCs and proliferating, undifferentiated myoblasts, whereas myogenin expression increases during differentiation. Embryonic myosin heavy chain (eMyHC) is a specific marker of regenerating myotubes in adult muscle.

To understand the cellular mechanisms of sarcopenia, we examined the expression of SCs in old regenerating muscles based on the expression profiles of several markers related to those cells. In our experiments, muscle mass in young rats had recovered to control values by 14 days after injury, but old muscle mass remained less than that of control values at 21 days after injury. In addition, muscle regeneration in old rats was less successful than that in young rats, based on morphologic properties and expression of eMyHC. Although regenerating muscle in young rats had many MyoD-positive cells, there was an age-related decrease in the number of MyoD-positive cells in regenerating areas from old rats. These results suggest that impaired regeneration in old muscle could be due to a decline in myoblast proliferative capacity, or to loss of factors required for satellite cell activity. In contrast, regenerating muscle in old rats had as many myogenin-positive cells as in young rats. This is in agreement with a report that myogenin mRNA was elevated in regenerating old skeletal muscle.[7] On the basis of the expression of MyoD and myogenin proteins, activation and proliferation of SCs were found to be impaired in old muscle during muscle regeneration; however, differentiation was not affected.

ROLE OF HEMATOPOIETIC STEM CELLS IN OLD REGENERATING MUSCLE

It has long been believed that SCs are the sole population responsible for skeletal muscle regeneration. Recent studies have identified novel populations of adult stem cells that are capable of contributing to muscle regeneration.[8] Adult skeletal muscle contains a novel stem cell population purified as a side population (SP), which actively excludes Hoechst 33342 dye. Muscle SP cells that express the hematopoietic stem cell markers Sca-1 and CD45 can differentiate into hematopoietic cells, skeletal muscle, and SCs following transplantation.[9,10] We previously demonstrated that CD45-positive cells were found in cells isolated from normal rat skeletal muscle, using methods employed to isolate and culture SCs.[11] Interestingly, muscle SP cells *in vitro* readily form hematopoietic colonies, but can also differentiate into muscle cells when cocultured with satellite cell–derived myoblasts.[9] LaBarge and Blau (2002) also found that bone marrow–derived SP cells could give rise to SCs that were capable of contributing to the formation of the regenerated myofibers.[12] A supporting observation for the role of muscle SP (CD45-positive) cells in skeletal muscle repair is the finding that muscle SP cell number increases in response to muscle injury.[13] Furthermore, in a mouse model with impaired muscle regenerative capacity (FoxK1 mutant mice), there was a reduction in its muscle SP cell number, and mobilization of SP cells after injury was suppressed.[14] Muscle SP cells may be mobilized after muscle injury for the purpose of contributing to skeletal muscle regeneration. The question then arises as to whether muscle SP cells in old skeletal muscle might contribute to regenerative processes after muscle damage. Our results indicated that hematopoetic stem (CD45-positive) cells were abundantly present in regenerating areas of both young and old rats. However, there was an age-related decrease in the number of CD45-positive cells in regenerating areas of old rat muscle. This finding is in agreement with the reduction in muscle SP cell number with impaired muscle regeneration.[14] However, it is unclear how much the CD45-positive cells contribute to muscle regeneration. It remains to be confirmed whether muscle SP cells are involved in sarcopenia.

MULTIPOTENCY OF SATELLITE CELLS

An increase in the fat content of muscle occurs with aging and is associated with decreased strength. SCs are thought to be committed myogenic progenitors capable only of contributing to myogenesis. During muscle regeneration, SCs proliferate and then fuse together to form myotubes. More recently, the commitment of SCs to the myogenic lineage has been questioned. Recent experiments have demonstrated that SCs also are capable of differentiation into adipocytes and osteocytes *in vitro*,[15,16] indicating a mesenchymal differentiation potential of SCs. Importantly, clonal analysis of single fiber-derived myogenic cells confirms that single clones are capable of giving rise to both myogenic, osteogenic, and adipogenic cells, verifying that SCs *in vitro* are multifunctional.[16] While the multifunctional nature of SCs has yet to be demonstrated *in vivo*, the accumulation of adipose tissue within aged skeletal muscle suggests that SCs may be capable of nonmyogenic commitment *in vivo*.[8] In our experiments, lipid accumulation was apparent in old muscles, restricted to the regenerating area at 7 days after injury. It is well known that the transcription factor C/EBPα is a key factor involved in differentiation of pre-adipocytes, and promoting lipid storage and stimulating adipocyte-specific gene production during adipogenesis.[17] In old rats, C/EBPα-positive cells were abundant in regenerating areas. Production of lipid in C/EBPα-positive cells in regenerating areas of old rats was observed. In addition, C/EBPα-positive cells were also observed surrounding the eMyHC-positive (nascent) myofibers as well as SCs. Although there was no direct evidence that C/EBPα-positive cells were derived from SCs, our results suggest SCs may convert to adipocytes by expression of C/EBPα. This is consistent with the observation that SCs isolated from old mice exhibited increased adipogenic potential with increased C/EBPα expression.[18] Whether this change in differentiation potential contributes to the increased adiposity that occurs with impaired muscle regeneration with increasing age remains to be determined.

CONCLUSION

Our results indicate that impaired muscle regeneration may be partially attributed firstly to attenuated activation and proliferation of satellite cells, but not differentiation, and secondly to increased adipogenic potential. These results suggest that impaired muscle regeneration might contribute to loss of muscle mass and increased lipid content, both characteristic of aged muscle and the process of sarcopenia.

ACKNOWLEDGMENT

This work was supported by research fellowships of the Japan Society for the Promotion of Science for Young Scientists (to S.M.). We would like to thank Dr. Jonathan Peake for language editing.

REFERENCES

1. HAWKE, T.J. & D.J. GARRY. 2001. Myogenic satellite cells: physiology to molecular biology. J. Appl. Physiol. **91:** 534–551.

2. GIBSON, M.C. & E. SCHULTZ. 1983. Age-related differences in absolute numbers of skeletal muscle satellite cells. Muscle Nerve **6:** 574–580.

3. MACHIDA, S. & F.W. BOOTH. 2004. Increased nuclear proteins in muscle satellite cells in aged animals as compared to young growing animals. Exp. Gerontol. **39:** 1521–1525.

4. SCHULTZ, E. & B.H. LIPTON. 1982. Skeletal muscle satellite cells: changes in proliferation potential as a function of age. Mech. Ageing Dev. **20:** 377–383.

5. LASSAR, A. & A. MUNSTERBERG. 1994. Wiring diagrams: regulatory circuits and the control of skeletal myogenesis. Curr. Opin. Cell Biol. **6:** 432–442.

6. SWYNGHEDAUW, B. 1986. Developmental and functional adaptation of contractile proteins in cardiac and skeletal muscles. Physiol. Rev. **66:** 710–771.

7. MARSH, D.R., D.S. CRISWELL, J.A. CARSON, et al. 1997. Myogenic regulatory factors during regeneration of skeletal muscle in young, adult, and old rats. J. Appl. Physiol. **83:** 1270–1275.

8. CHARGE, S.B. & M.A. RUDNICKI. 2004. Cellular and molecular regulation of muscle regeneration. Physiol. Rev. **84:** 209–238.

9. ASAKURA, A., P. SEALE, A. GIRGIS-GABARDO, et al. 2002. Myogenic specification of side population cells in skeletal muscle. J. Cell Biol. **159:** 123–134.

10. GUSSONI, E., Y. SONEOKA, C.D. STRICKLAND, et al. 1999. Dystrophin expression in the mdx mouse restored by stem cell transplantation. Nature **401:** 390–394.

11. MACHIDA, S., E.E. SPANGENBURG & F.W. BOOTH. 2004. Primary rat muscle progenitor cells have decreased proliferation and myotube formation during passages. Cell Prolif. **37:** 267–277.

12. LABARGE, M.A. & H.M. BLAU. 2002. Biological progression from adult bone marrow to mononucleate muscle stem cell to multinucleate muscle fiber in response to injury. Cell **111:** 589–601.

13. POLESSKAYA, A., P. SEALE & M.A. RUDNICKI. 2003. Wnt signaling induces the myogenic specification of resident CD45+ adult stem cells during muscle regeneration. Cell **113:** 841–852.

14. MEESON, A.P., T.J. HAWKE, S. GRAHAM, et al. 2004. Cellular and molecular regulation of skeletal muscle side population cells. Stem Cells **22:** 1305–1320.

15. ASAKURA, A., M. KOMAKI & M. RUDNICKI. 2001. Muscle satellite cells are multipotential stem cells that exhibit myogenic, osteogenic, and adipogenic differentiation. Differentiation **68:** 245–253.

16. WADA, M.R., M. INAGAWA-OGASHIWA, S. SHIMIZU, et al. 2002. Generation of different fates from multipotent muscle stem cells. Development **129:** 2987–2995.

17. KIRKLAND, J.L., T. TCHKONIA, T. PIRTSKHALAVA, et al. 2002. Adipogenesis and aging: does aging make fat go MAD? Exp. Gerontol. **37:** 757–767.

18. TAYLOR-JONES, J.M., R.E. MCGEHEE, T.A. RANDO, et al. 2002. Activation of an adipogenic program in adult myoblasts with age. Mech. Ageing Dev. **123:** 649–661.

Age-Related Effects of Dexamethasone Administration in Adrenal Zona Reticularis

HENRIQUE ALMEIDA, LILIANA MATOS, JORGE FERREIRA, AND DELMINDA NEVES

Laboratory for Molecular Cell Biology, Faculdade de Medicina do Porto, 4200-319 Porto, Portugal

Instituto de Biologia Molecular e Celular da Universidade do Porto, Rua do Campo Alegre, 4150-180 Porto, Portugal

ABSTRACT: Suppression of adrenocorticotropic hormone results in reduced adrenal steroid output, adrenocortical cell atrophy, and apoptosis in young rats. To verify such effects during aging, dexamethasone was injected into rats for 3 days at five different ages; at day 4, adrenals and blood were collected for morphologic and corticosterone assay. Adrenal structure was similar at all ages, but in dexamethasone-injected animals there were ultrastructural features of apoptosis and a higher percentage of TUNEL and caspase-3-labeled nuclei and cytoplasm; their corticosterone decreased significantly. In both groups, there was age-related decrease in the percentage of apoptotic cells, significant only in dexamethasone-injected rats. The data suggest that aged adrenocortical cells are less susceptible to the lack of adrenocorticotropic hormone (ACTH), possibly as a result of their decreased functional ability.

KEYWORDS: adrenal; age-related; TUNEL; caspase-3; apoptosis; corticosterone

INTRODUCTION

The inner zone (IZ) of the adrenal cortex (AC) comprises the zona fasciculata (ZF) and the zona reticularis (ZR). Under close regulation by the pituitary-originated adrenocorticotropic hormone (ACTH) the IZ cells synthesize and secrete glucocorticoids to the circulation, mostly cortisol in humans and corticosterone in rats.

The administration of ACTH is followed by enhancement of steroidogenic enzyme activity, enlargement of IZ cell volume and mitochondrial and smooth

Address for correspondence: Henrique Almeida, Laboratório de Biologia Molecular e Celular, Faculdade de Medicina do Porto 4200-319 Porto, Portugal. Voice: +351 22 551 3654; fax: +351 22 551 3655.

e-mail: almeidah@med.up.pt

Ann. N.Y. Acad. Sci. 1067: 354–360 (2006). © 2006 New York Academy of Sciences.
doi: 10.1196/annals.1354.050

endoplasmic reticular compartments, and an increase in steroid output.[1,2] However, when ACTH is suppressed, as occurs after hypophysectomy or corticosteroid administration, those effects are reversed[1,2] and notable apoptotic features are observed in ZR and its transition to ZF.[3,4]

So far, to the best of our knowledge, all experimental studies of ACTH suppression were done using rat fetuses or young adult animals. Therefore data are lacking about such effects in the adrenal parenchymal cells of the aged animals or during aging. Yet, a recent study in a setting of ACTH blockade[5] indicated an age-related increase in macrophages, suggesting an increment in the need for the clearance of parenchymal dead cell and debris.

It was thus the purpose of this structural and immunocytochemical study to observe and quantify apoptotic age-related changes in adrenal ZR parenchymal cells.

MATERIAL AND METHODS

Wistar male rats from the colony of the Institute of Molecular and Cell Biology (IBMC, Porto) were maintained with free access to water and laboratory diet. At 2, 6, 12, 18, and 24 months, eight apparently healthy animals were randomly selected and divided into two groups. The first group was injected intramuscularly for three consecutive days with 4 mg/kg of dexamethasone phosphate (Decadron®, Merck, Sharp & Dohme, Portugal), and the second (control) received a similar volume of saline solution. On the fourth day, the animals were sacrificed by decapitation. One adrenal was processed for ultrastructural morphologic study using previously described procedures;[6] the other adrenal was fixed in formalin, embedded in paraffin, and sectioned onto poly-L-lysine–coated slides.

The sections were processed for TUNEL by means of a TdT-FragEL kit from Oncogene Research Products (now Calbiochem) using the manufacturer's instructions; in the immunocytochemical study, a monoclonal antibody, anti-activated caspase-3 (Cell, Signaling Technology), diluted at 1:200, was employed and a streptavidin/biotin/peroxidase system (Dakocytomation) using diaminobenzidine (DAB) was used for the final labeling.

Morphometric study, to assess parenchymal cell volume (CV), nuclear volume (VN), and numerical density (N_v), was done as previously described.[7] The apoptotic index (AI) was quantified in ZR random photographs of TUNEL sections, as the percentage of apoptotic nuclei per total number of nuclei; for each rat a total 2,500–3,000 nuclei were counted.

Trunk blood was collected for corticosterone assay by high-performance liquid chromatography (HPLC).[6]

ANOVA was used to compare the means of measurements at different ages. The statistical significance of differences between individual pairs of means was assessed using the least-significant-difference procedure of Fisher (LSD test). For a comparison between the two groups, the Student *t*-test was used.

RESULTS

Microscopic Study

Light microscopy revealed that the general structure of the AC was conserved throughout aging, allowing the identification of the usual cortical zones and the medulla. In the IZ of dexamethasone (DEX)-treated animals, there was an apparent decrease in cell and nuclear volumes.

The ultrastructural study did not disclose major changes in the cytoplasm and nuclei of DEX animals at any age, but, in contrast to the controls, a substantial number of cells displayed nuclei with a wavy outline and distorted and clumped chromatin, indicating apoptotic changes. In addition, various apoptotic bodies appearing as membrane-bound structures containing packed mitochondria, lipid droplets, and portions of chromatin (some enveloped by nuclear membrane) were observed close to, or within, the capillaries (FIG. 1A). Some of the capillaries had a disrupted structure, allowing direct contact of parenchymal cells with the lumina and access of apoptotic bodies into the lumina.

In the TUNEL sections, several nuclei in the ZR and ZF/ZR transition were shrunken and intensely stained with DAB (FIG. 1B). Clearly, they were more common in DEX animals when compared to controls. Immunocytochemical study of caspase-3 some parenchymal cells of the ZR of DEX rats had a distinctive DAB-stained cytoplasm (FIG. 1C), but in the same zone other cells had faint labeling. In the sections processed either for TUNEL or caspase-3 labeling, the cells from the zona glomerulosa ZG, most of the ZF and medulla presented no labeling.

Quantitative Study

The results for CV (μm^3), VN (μm^3), and N_v ($\times 10^3/mm^3$) are shown in TABLE 1. There was a statistically significant decrease in cell and nuclear volumes of DEX animals when assessed by the Student t-test. However, ANOVA did not reveal any significant age-related trend.

---→

FIGURE 1. (A) Ultrastructure of ZR from a 24-month-old DEX rat displaying an apoptotic body beside a capillary lumen (*black star*). Mitochondria (m), lysosome (*arrow*), and possible fragments of the nucleus (*white star*) are seen; some lipid droplets are extruding from the body (L). N and M: nucleus and mitochondria from a parenchymal cell. Bar: 2 μm. **(B)** ZR from a 24-month-old DEX rat with DAB-stained nuclei (*circles*). M: adrenal medulla. TUNEL. Bar: 50 μm. **(C)** Same material as **(B)**. Several ZR cells have DAB-stained cytoplasm (*arrows*). M: adrenal medulla. Caspase-3 immunocytochemistry. Bar: 50 μm.

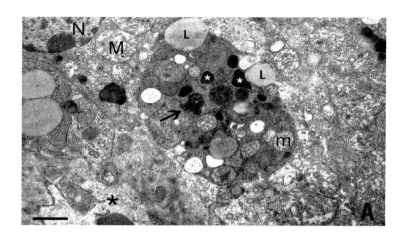

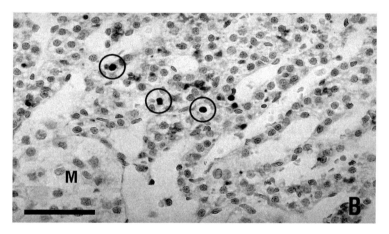

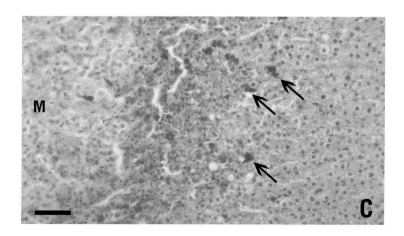

The results for the apoptotic and corticosterone assay are displayed in TABLE 2. There was an age-related decrease of AI in both groups, significant for DEX rats and marginally not significant for controls, and a reduced basal blood corticosterone in older animals compared to young ones. In some DEX animals, the assay failed to detect any corticosterone peak.

DISCUSSION

The pituitary peptide ACTH exerts a trophic action on the IZ of the adrenal cortex. ACTH mobilizes cholesterol obtained from circulating lipoproteins and intracellular lipid stores. Then, the steroidogenic acute regulatory enzyme (StAR) delivers the cholesterol to the mitochondria for glucocorticoid synthesis and ultimate secretion into the blood; in addition, *in vivo* mitogenic effects on the adrenal cortex have been attributed to the peptide. Conversely, this balance is changed when ACTH secretion is blocked by hypophysectomy or corticosteroid administration: steroid output is reduced, adrenals lose weight, the cortex becomes atrophic, and IZ cells decrease in volume[1,8] and display apoptotic features.[3,4]

The present study confirmed a decrement of circulating corticosterone and ZR cell volume, and showed that the effects on ZR cells are maintained during aging. Either ultrastructural observations or the results of the TUNEL study and caspase-3 labeling provided clear evidence that frequent apoptotic phenomena were taking place at any age under these experimental conditions.

The cell migration theory of the adrenal cortex[9] states that cell proliferation occurs in the ZG, or the intermediate zone between ZF and ZG, and, as the cells differentiate, they move centripetally and die at the ZR, where they are removed by the macrophages. Whether for the purpose of clearance or as on additional modulation effect, adrenal macrophages attain their highest numerical density in ZR, where they increase in an age-related fashion.[10] This trend is maintained in DEX-treated animals,[5] supporting their role in removing the dead cells or debris.

This study showed significant quantitative differences between controls and DEX animals in blood corticosterone, ZR nuclear and cellular volumes, and apoptotic indexes at any age. However, in the assessment of differences during aging, the decrease of the apoptotic index in DEX rats was the only significant trend observed. Interestingly, higher levels of AI were observed in the 6-month-old and 12-month-old groups, whereas the lowest level was present in 24-month-old animals. At this age, the lowest levels of corticosterone, either basal or in response to the ACTH challenge, were recorded in a previous study,[6] indicating a lesser functional ability of aged cells eventually due to a decrease in ACTH receptors.[11]

It is conceivable that this lesser ability of aged cells to respond to ACTH enables them to better withstand the lack of ACTH, thus explaining the age-related decrease in the apoptotic index.

TABLE 1. Parenchymal cellular (CV, μm^3) and nuclear (VN, μm^3) volumes and N_v ($\times 10^3/mm^3$) of controls (Ct) and dexamethasone-injected (Dx) rats at different ages

	CV Ct		CV Dx		VN Ct		VN Dx		N_v Ct		N_v Dx	
2 m	1419.01	±48.07	1037.05[b]	±62.77	210.10	±8.07	149.10[b]	±8.25	542.58	±16.85	597.09	±28.25
6 m	1364.15	±68.20	1094.35	±90.83	185.39	±1.95	149.98[a]	±12.24	589.82	±27.12	691.16[a]	±25.73
12 m	1504.86	±113.07	1029.37[b]	±57.44	184.69	±8.61	134.28[b]	±4.37	526.89	±29.17	696.81	±65.03
18 m	1558.79	±156.10	1044.73[a]	±96.30	202.80	±19.31	134.50[a]	±5.07	511.90	±65.72	630.32	±71.70
24 m	1528.21	±181.70	1117.29[a]	±53.68	214.26	±20.97	136.14[a]	±8.91	530.24	±72.93	583.77	±59.85
$P<$	n.s.		n.s.		n.s.		n.s.		n.s.		n.s.	

[a] and [b] refer to comparisons with the controls, respectively, for $P < 0.05$ and $P < 0.01$ in the Student's t-test. Means ± standard error, $n = 4$.

TABLE 2. Apoptotic index (AI, %) in ZR and blood corticosterone (B, ng/mL) of controls (Ct) and dexamethasone-injected (Dx) rats at different ages

	AI Ct		AI Dx		B Ct		B Dx	
2 m	0.39	±0.11	3.07^b	±0.42	285.5*	±25.4	15.1^b	±9.9
6 m	1.25	±0.43	4.80^a	±0.72	236.1	±39.7	0.0^b	±0.0
12 m	0.98	±0.16	4.41^b	±0.67	305.5	±61.8	4.0^b	±4.0
18 m	0.54	±0.12	3.98^b	±0.26	175.0*	±2.0	0.0^b	±0.0
24 m	0.65	±0.10	2.28^a	±0.60	143.4	±41.6	18.4^a	±10.6
$P<$	0.051		0.05		n.s.		n.s.	

[a] and [b] refer to comparisons with the controls, respectively, for $P < 0.05$ and $P < 0.01$ in the Student's t-test. Means ± standard error, $n = 4$ or $n = 2$ (*).

REFERENCES

1. NUSSDORFER, G.G. 1986. Cytophysiology of the adrenal cortex. Int. Rev. Cytol. **98:** 1–405.
2. ESTIVARIZ, F.E., P.J. LOWRY & S. JACKSON. 1992. Control of adrenal growth. In The Adrenal Gland, 2nd edition. V.H.T. James, Ed.:1–42. Raven Press. New York.
3. WYLLIE, A.H., J.F.R. KERR, I.A.M. MACASKILL, et al. 1973. Adrenocortical cell deletion: the role of ACTH. J. Pathol. **111:** 85–94.
4. CARSIA, R.V., G.J. MACDONALD, J.A. GIBNEY, et al. 1996. Apoptotic cell death in the rat adrenal gland: an in vivo and in vitro investigation. Cell Tissue Res. **283:** 247–254.
5. ALMEIDA, H., J. FERREIRA & D. NEVES. 2004. Macrophages of the adrenal cortex— a morphological study of the effects of aging and dexamethasone administration. Ann. N. Y. Acad. Sci. **1019:** 135–140.
6. ALMEIDA, H., M.C. MAGALHÃES & M.M. MAGALHÃES. 1998. Age-related changes in the inner zone of the adrenal cortex of the rat—a morphologic and biochemical study. Mech. Ageing Develop. **105:** 1–18.
7. WEIBEL, E.R. & R.P. BOLENDER. 1973. Stereological techniques for electron microscopic morphometry. In Principles and Techniques of Electron Microscopy, Vol. 3, M.A. Hayat, Ed.: 237–296. Van Nostrand-Reinhold. New York.
8. THOMAS, M., M. KERAMIDAS, E. MONCHAUX, et al. 2004. Dual hormonal regulation of endocrine tissue mass and vasculature by adrenocorticotropin in the adrenal cortex. Endocrinology **145:** 4320–4329.
9. LONG, J.A. 1975. Zonation of the mammalian adrenal cortex. In Handbook of Physiology, Section 7 (Endocrinology), Vol 6. R.O. Greep & E.B. Astwood, Eds.: 13–24. American Physiological Society. Washington, DC.
10. ALMEIDA, H., M.C. MAGALHÃES & M.M. MAGALHÃES. 1995. Adrenal zonation and age-related changes in macrophage number [abstract]. AGE **18:** 194–195.
11. MALAMED, S. & R.V. CARSIA. 1983. Aging of the rat adrenocortical cell: response to ACTH and cyclic AMP in vitro. J. Gerontol. **38:** 130–136.

Does Chronic Glycolysis Accelerate Aging? Could This Explain How Dietary Restriction Works?

ALAN R. HIPKISS

Centre for Experimental Therapeutics, William Harvey Research Institute, Barts' and the London School of Medicine and Dentistry, Charterhouse Square, London EC1M 6BQ, UK

ABSTRACT: The mechanisms by which dietary restriction (DR) suppresses aging are not understood. Suppression of glycolysis by DR could contribute to controlling senescence. Many glycolytic intermediates can glycate proteins and other macromolecules. Methyglyoxal (MG), formed from dihydroxyacetone- and glyceraldehyde-3-phosphates, rapidly glycates proteins, damages mitochondria, and induces a prooxidant state to create a senescent-like condition. *Ad libitum*-fed and DR animals differ in mitochondrial activity and glycolytic flux rates. Persistent glycolysis in the unrestricted condition would increase the intracellular load of glycating agents (e.g., MG) and increase ROS generation by inactive mitochondria. Occasional glycolysis during DR would decrease MG and reactive oxygen species (ROS) production and could be hormetic, inducing synthesis of glyoxalase-1 and anti-glycating agents (carnosine and polyamines).

KEYWORDS: calorie; diet; methylglyoxal; glycation; hormesis

IS GLYCOLYSIS POTENTIALLY DELETERIOUS?

Mitochondria are frequently regarded as major sources of age-associated cellular disorder/dysfunction because of reactive oxygen species (ROS) generated within them. Glycolysis, however, is another source of endogenous molecular toxicity; most glycolytic intermediates possess reactive carbonyl groups (being aldehydes or ketones) that modify protein amino groups and DNA, in the cytosol and mitochondria, via mechanisms similar to those of nonenzymic glycosylation (glycation).[1–4] Glyceraldehyde-3-phosphate and dihydroxyacetone-phosphate rapidly glycate proteins, producing advanced glycosylation end-products (AGEs) that are implicated in age-related pathologies, diabetes[5]

Address for correspondence: Alan R. Hipkiss, Centre for Experimental Therapeutics, William Harvey Research Institute, Barts' and the London School of Medicine and Dentistry, Charterhouse Square, London EC1M 6BQ, UK. Voice: 44-(0)20-7882-6032; fax: 44-(0)20-7882-6037.
e-mail: alanandjill@lineone.net

Ann. N.Y. Acad. Sci. 1067: 361–368 (2006). © 2006 New York Academy of Sciences.
doi: 10.1196/annals.1354.051

and its secondary complications,[5] brain aging,[6] and Alzheimer's disease.[7] Methylglyoxal (MG), generated both spontaneously and enzymically from the glyceraldehyde-3- and dihydroxyacetone-phosphates, as well as from threonine, glycine, and fatty acids,[8] is highly deleterious; it glycates and cross-links proteins, and damages lipids and DNA (see Ref. 8 and references therein). It induces peroxides in cortical neurons,[9] has pro-oxidant effects in smooth muscle cells,[10] inhibits heart mitochondria,[3] and reacts with arginine residues of mitochondrial permeability transition pore proteins[4] to provoke organelle dysfunction and ROS production.[11] MG-induced protein glycation creates active centers for one-electron oxidation/reduction reactions and ROS generation.[12] MG inactivates glutathione peroxidase irreversibly, which increases cellular peroxide concentration and oxidative damage. Prolonged MG administration induces microvascular damage and other diabetes-like complications, even within a normo-glycemic context.[13]

METHYLGLYOXAL AND DIETARY RESTRICTION

Intracellular MG concentration is determined by the rate and duration of glycolytic activity.[14,15] The MG formation rates range between 0.1% and 0.4% of the glycolytic flux; the free intracellular MG concentration ranges from 0.16 μM to 2.4 μM; reversibly bound MG is 2–3 orders of magnitude higher.[8] It is proposed that more MG is produced in *ad libitum*-fed animals during continued (chronic) glycolysis than under food restriction, where glycolysis is both brief and infrequent because of constrained food availability. Low cellular proliferation rates also increase cellular MG concentrations in *ad libitum*-fed animals on account of decreased use of glycolytic intermediates as precursors for DNA and protein synthesis.[8] Deficiency or inactivation of glyceraldehyde-3-phosphate dehydrogenase (GAPDH) raises the concentrations of MG and glycated products. [16]

As MG can provoke many, or most, of the biochemical changes that accompany normal aging (protein carbonyl groups and cross-linking, lipid and DNA damage, mitochondrial dysfunction, ROS production, and apoptosis as described above), it is proposed that chronic glycolysis in *ad libitum*-fed animals is detrimental because of continuous generation of relatively high levels of MG. In DR animals glycolysis is transient; any MG that is generated would persist for only short periods of time. That dietary restriction's effects on aging can be induced by fasting or intermittent (e.g., every other day) feeding, without any decrease in overall caloric intake,[17] is consistent with the current proposal.

NATURALLY OCCURRING PROTECTION AGAINST MG

Most cells possess glyoxalases[18] as well as other aldehyde-scavenging enzymes[19] that detoxify MG. Glyoxalase-1 expression in certain areas of the brain varies during the human life span[20] and a large increase in plasma AGEs is associated with erythrocyte glyoxalase-1 deficiency.[21] Upregulation of glyoxalase-1 activity can lower cell-associated MG and possibly suppress Alzheimer's disease (AD).[22] DR attenuates amyloid-β deposition in an AD animal model,[23] although the mechanisms involved are uncertain.

Glutathione, pyridoxamine, thiamine, the polyamines spermine and spermidine, and carnosine can scavenge MG.[24] Spermine, spermidine, and carnosine are present at high concentrations in many tissues.

Carnosine, present in long-lived tissues (muscles and nerves) particularly, inhibits MG-induced generation of protein carbonyl groups and cross-linking of MG-modified lysine and MG-treated ovalbumin to normal proteins,[25] and forms adducts with MG-induced protein-bound carbonyl groups[26] (see Ref. 25 and references cited therein). Adducts of carnosine with acrolein, MG, and hydroxynonenal (HNE) adducts have been characterized[25] and carnosine–HNE adducts were recently detected in muscle tissue;[25] "carnosinylated" amino-lipid has been detected in human muscle.[25] Carnosine suppresses senescence in cultured human fibroblasts and some antiaging effects were observed in mice and fruit flies;[25] it also delays onset of diabetic complications in mice.[27] Hence, carnosine might protect against reactive carbonyl compounds *in vivo*.

Spermine, spermidine,[28] and pyridoxamine[29] may perform similar antiglycating functions. Millimolar quantities of spermine are present in nuclei that may help protect DNA and histones against glycation.[28] Spermine can inhibit formation of the AGE pyrraline during long-term exposure of albumin to glucose.[30] Pyridoxamine scavenges aldehydes and MG–pyridoxamine adducts have been characterized.[31] Pyridoxamine may act synergistically as it stimulates glyoxalase activity in erythrocytes.[32] Deglycating[33] and trans-glycating[34] roles for fructosamine-3-kinase have been proposed; the enzyme either recycling spermine–carbonyl adducts[33] or the sugar-derived component of Maillard reaction products (Schiff bases) is transferred to taurine, carnosine, anserine, or glutathione. Tissue concentrations of polyamines[33] and carnosine[25] possibly decrease with age, increasing the potential for MG-induced dysfunction in older animals, although more research is needed to substantiate this.

Thiamine, in the form of a lipid-soluble derivative benfotiamine,[35] stimulates transketolase, the rate-limiting enzyme in the pentose pathway, whose substrates are fructose-6-phosphate and glyceraldehyde-3-phosphate, which would decrease MG generation.

DR AND HORMESIS: IS GLYCOLYSIS A STRESSOR?

Transient exposure to stress could induce a hormetic response that increases long-term protection against deleterious age-related changes, such as protein oxidation and glycation.[36] It is suggested that persistent glycolysis is deleterious, but brief glycolysis is hormetic. There is some evidence to support this idea: increased glucose uptake upregulates glyoxalase-1 synthesis in yeast,[37] while a nematode glyoxalase-1 gene promoter region contains an insulin-responsive element and responds to oxidative stress.[38] MG enhances chaperone functions of α-crystallin and Hsp-27 (stress proteins),[39] an action that may be hormetic; the amount of extra protection afforded by MG would be limited by the number of chaperone protein molecules available for modification; excess MG generation during persistant glycolysis in *ad libitum*-fed animals would be deleterious.

Carnosine synthesis is metabolically controlled in astroglia-rich primary cultures, where cAMP downregulates carnosine synthetase by up to 80%.[40] Because the dipeptide suppresses MG reactivity by its glycoxalase-1 mimetic activity,[41] its ability to form adducts with MG (see above), its disaggregation effects on MG-glycated protein,[42] and, when complexed with zinc ions, its ability in rat mucosal tissue to induce synthesis of the stress protein hsp72,[43] short-term glycolysis could increase carnosine synthesis and increase protection against MG. Persistent glycolysis could increase MG production to an extent that overwhelms all the protective activities to increase intracellular glycation potential. Increased carnosine synthesis could help explain the improved cancer resistance observed when DR is imposed[44] because the dipeptide can selectively kill transformed cultured cells.[25]

Spermine synthesis may be stimulated by stress; ornithine decarboxylase (ODC), the first enzyme of polyamine synthesis pathway, is upregulated under oxidative stress and UVB irradiation,[33] conditions that provoke glycoxidation. The increased ODC levels in rat kidney in early diabetes may be a glycation-inhibiting response in this tissue,[33] consistent with the proposal that antiglycating mechanisms are hormetically activated during brief periods of glycolysis.

Macrophages undergo adaptive responses when exposed to glycated serum: exposure to subtoxic amounts of AGE (5%) increases antioxidant activity and protects against subsequent treatment with 10% AGE, while 10% AGE is lethal to nonadapted cells,[45] observations consistent with the suggestion that responses to glycation are hormetic.

In a study of the effects of DR on diurnal rat metabolism, McCarter and Palmer[46] showed that DR and *ad libitum*-fed animals differed in terms of fuel utilization. The restricted animals metabolized more carbohydrate immediately after feeding and then switched to a predominantly lipid/protein-based metabolism. In contrast the *ad libitum*-fed animals' metabolism was substantially glycolytic for the whole 24 hours of each day. These observations are consistent with the assumption in the present report that glycolysis is transient in DR animals but persistent in those fed *ad libitum*.[47]

GLYCOLYSIS AND MECHANISMS OF AGING

It is suggested that under certain circumstances age-related cellular dysfunction may not derive entirely from mitochondrially generated ROS.

Extra-mitochondrial ROS, induced by MG and glycated polypeptides, can damage the mitochondrial membranes, including the permeability transition pore, to produce features characteristic of senescence. Excessive and persistent glycolysis could provide a source of mitochondrial damage and ROS generation in *ad libitum*-fed animals, whereas DR would suppress production of glycating agents such as MG and decrease the occurrence of macromolecular damage, including that to mitochondria.

The present proposals do not exclude the operation of any other mechanism(s) by which DR mediates aging suppression, it being unreasonable to assume that senescence in different tissues and cells is controlled by a single, universal, mechanism. The possible effects of glycolysis, occasional or persistent, outlined here may overlap or supplement other possible mechanisms of DR's effects on aging, such as increased plasma membrane NAD(P)H oxidase activity, decreased electron supply to mitochondria, protein acetylation/deacetylation, protein turnover, stress proteins synthesis, and increased ROS production by underemployed mitochondria.

CONCLUSION

The mechanisms by which DR mediates its protective effects toward aging and related pathologies may be due, at least in part, to infrequent glycolysis, rather than any direct action affecting mitochondrial function. It is suggested that the glycolytic by-product MG, which induces many of the biochemical and subcellular changes associated with ageing and related pathologies, including mitochondrial dysfunction, may play a causal role in the aging of *ad libitum*-fed animals. In DR animals occasional glycolysis could be hormetic, and protective activities (e.g., synthesis of glyoxalase, carnosine, spermine, and other agents as yet unidentified) may be induced. It is interesting that *ad libitum* feeding increases glycolysis and decreases mitochondrial usage, both conditions being deleterious on account of increased MG and ROS generation, while DR suppresses glycolysis and increases mitochondria-mediated transfer of electrons to oxygen to decrease stressor production.

[NOTE ADDED IN PROOF: After submission of this manuscript, Ramasamy *et al.*[48] and Yao *et al.*[49] have provided evidence demonstrating the role of glycolytically derived MG in both protein modification and gene expression, consistant with the ideas outlined here.]

REFERENCES

1. SUJI, G. & S. SIVAKAMI. 2004. Glucose, glycation and aging. Biogerontology **5:** 365–373.
2. BAYNES, J.W. 2000. From life to death—the struggle between chemistry and biology during aging: the Maillard reaction as an amplifier of genomic damage. Biogerontology **1:** 235–246.

3. SINHAROY, S., S. BANERJEE, M. RAY, *et al.* 2005. Possible involvement of glutamic and/or aspartic acid residues and requirement of mitochondrial integrity for the protective effect of creatine against inhibition of cardiac mitochondrial respiration by methyglyoxal. Mol. Cell. Biochem. **271:** 167–176.

4. JOHANS, M., E. MILANESI, M. FRANCK, *et al.* 2005. Modification of permeability transition pore arginine(s) by phenylglyoxal derivatives in isolated mitochondria and mammalian cells. J. Biol. Chem. **280:** 12130–12136.

5. BROWNLEE, M. 2001. Biochemistry and molecular biology of diabetic complications. Nature **414:** 813–820.

6. DUKIC-STEFANOVIC, S., R. SCHINZEL, P. RIEDERER, *et al.* 2001. AGES in brain ageing: AGE-inhibitors as neuroprotective and anti-dementia drugs? Biogerontology **2:** 19–34.

7. REDDY, V.P., M.E. OBRENOVICH, C.S. ATWOOD, *et al.* 2002. Involvement of Maillard reactions in Alzheimer's disease. Neurotox. Res. **4:** 191–209.

8. CHAPLEN, F.W.R. 1998. Incidence and potential implications of the toxic metabolite methylglyoxal in cell culture: a review. Cytotechnology **26:** 173–183.

9. KIKUCHI, S., K. SHINPO, M. TAKEUCHI, *et al.* 2003. Glycation – a sweet tempter for neuronal death. Brain Res. Rev. **41:** 306–323.

10. WU, L. 2005. The pro-oxidant role of methylglyoxal in mesenteric artery smooth muscle cells. Can. J. Physiol. Pharmacol. **83:** 63–68.

11. ROSCA, M.G., T.G. MUSTATA, M.T. KINTER, *et al.* 2005. Glycation of mitochondrial proteins from diabetic rat kidney is associated with excess superoxide formation. Am. J. Physiol. Renal Physiol. **289:** F420–430.

12. YIM, M.B., H.S. YIM, C. LEE, *et al.* 2001. Protein glycation: creation of catalytic sites for free radical generation. Ann. N.Y. Acad. Sci. **929:** 48–53.

13. BERLANGA, J., D. CIBRIAN, I. GUILLEN, *et al.* 2005. Methylglyoxal administration induces diabetes-like microvascular changes and perturbs the healing process of cutaneous wounds. Clin. Sci. (Lond.) **109:** 83–95.

14. BEISSWENGER, P.J., S.K. HOWELL, R.M. O'DELL, *et al.* 2001. α-Dicarbonyls increase in the postprandial period and reflect the degree of hyperglycemia. Diabetes Care **24:** 726–732.

15. NEMET, I., Z. TURK, L. DUVNJAK, *et al.* 2005. Humoral methyglyoxal level reflects glycemic fluctuation. Clin. Biochem. **38:** 379–383.

16. AHMED, N. 2005. Advanced glycation endproducts – role in pathology of diabetic complications. Diabetes Res. Clin. Pract. **67:** 3–21

17. M.P. MATTSON & R. WAN. 2005. Beneficial effects of intermittent feeding and caloric restriction on the cardiovascular and cerebrovascular systems. J. Nutr. Biochem. **16:** 129–137.

18. THORNALLEY, P.J. 1993. The glyoxalase system in health and disease. Mol. Aspects Med. **14:** 287–371.

19. DAVYDOV, V.V., N.M. DOBAEVA & A.I. BOZHKOV. 2004. Possible role of alteration of aldehyde's scavenger enzymes during aging. Exp. Geront. **39:** 11–16.

20. KUHLA, B., K. BOECK, H-J. LUTH, *et al.* 2005. Age-dependent changes of glyoxalase 1 expression in human brain. Neurobiol. Aging. In press.

21. MIYATA, T., C. VAN YPERSELE DE STRIHOU, T. IMASAWA, *et al.* 2001. Glyoxalase 1 deficiency is associated with an unusual level of advanced glycation end products in a hemodialysis patient. Kidney Int. **60:** 2351–2359.

22. CHEN, F., M.A. WOLLMER, F. HOERNDLI, *et al.* 2004. Role of glyoxalase 1 in Alzheimer's disease. Proc. Natl. Acad. Sci. USA **101:** 7687–7692.

23. Patel, N.V., M.N. Gordon, K.E. Conner, *et al*. 2005. Caloric restriction attenuates Aβ-deposition in Alzheimer's transgenic models. Neurobiol. Aging **26:** 995–1000.

24. Monnier, V.M. 2003. Intervention against the Maillard reaction in vivo. Arch. Biochem. Biophys. **419:** 1–15.

25. Hipkiss, A.R. 2005. Glycation, ageing and carnosine: are carnivorous diets beneficial? Mech. Ageing Dev. **126:** 1034–1039.

26. Brownson, C. & A.R. Hipkiss. 2000. Carnosine reacts with a glycated protein. Free Radic. Biol. Med. **28:** 1564–1570.

27. Lee, Y., C. Hsu, M. Lin, *et al*. 2005. Histidine and carnosine delay diabetic deterioration in mice and protect human low density lipoprotein against oxidation and glycation. Eur. J. Pharmacol. **512:** 145–150.

28. Gugliucci, A. & T. Menini. 2003. The polyamines spermine and spermidine protect proteins from structural and functional damage by AGE precursors: a new role for old molecules? Life Sci. **9314:** 1–14.

29. Onorato, J.M., A.J. Jenkins, S.R. Thorpe, *et al*. 2000. Pyridoxamine, an inhibitor of advanced glycation reaction, also inhibits advanced lipoxidation reactions—mechanisms of action of pyridoxamine. J. Biol. Chem. **275:** 21177–21184.

30. Mendez, J.D. & L.I. Leal. 2004. Inhibition of in vitro pyrraline formation by L-arginine and polyamines. Biomed. Pharmacother. **58:** 598–604.

31. Nagaraj, R.H., P. Sarker, A. Mally, *et al*. 2002. Effect of pyridoxamine on chemical modification of proteins by carbonyls in diabetic rats: characterization of a major product from the reaction of pyridoxamine and methylglyoxal. Arch. Biochem. Biophys. **402:** 110–119.

32. Amarnath, V., K. Amarnath, K. Amarnath, *et al*. 2004. Pyridoxamine: an extremely potent scavenger of 1,4-dicarbonyls. Chem. Res. Toxicol. **17:** 410–415.

33. Gugliucci, A. 2005. Alternative antiglycation mechanisms: are spermine and fructosamine-3-kinase part of a carbonyl damage control pathway? Med. Hypoth. **64:** 770–777.

34. Szwergold, B.S. 2005. Intrinsic toxicity of glucose, due to non-enzymatic glycation, is controlled *in vivo* by deglycating systems including: FN3K-mediated deglycation of fructosamines and transglycation of aldoamines. Med. Hypoth. **65:** 337–348.

35. Hammes, H-P., X. Du, D. Edelstein, *et al*. 2003. Benfotiamine blocks three major pathways of hyperglycemic damage and prevents experimental diabetic retinopathy. Nat. Med. **9:** 294–299.

36. Verbeke, P., B.F. Clarke & S.I. Rattan. 2000. Modulating cellular aging in vitro: hormetic effects of repeated mild heat stress on protein oxidation and glycation. Exp. Gerontol. **35:** 787–794.

37. Maeta, K., S. Izawa & Y. Inoue. 2005. Methylglyoxal, a metabolite derived from glycolysis, functions as a signal initiator of the high osmolarity glycerol-mitogen-activated protein kinase cascade and calcineurin/Crz1-mediated pathway in *Sacccharomyces cerevisiae*. J. Biol. Chem. **280:** 253–260.

38. Sommer, A., P. Fischer, K. Krause, *et al*. 2001. A stress-responsive glyoxalase 1 from the parasitic nematode *Onchocerca volvulus*. Biochem. J. **353:** 445–452.

39. Nagaraj, R.H., T. Oya-Ito, P.S. Padayatti, *et al*. 2003. Enhancement of chaperone function of alpha-crystallin by methyglyoxal modification. Biochemistry **42:** 10746–10755.

40. SCHULZ, M., B. HAMPRECHT, H. KLEINKAUF, *et al.* 1989. Regulation by dibutyryl cyclic AMP of carnosine synthesis in astroglial-rich primary cultures kept in serum-free medium. J. Neurochem. **52:** 229–234.
41. BATTAH, S., N. AHMED & P.J. THORNALLY. 2002. Novel anti-glycation therapeutic agents: glyoxylase-1-mimetics. Int. Congress Series **1245:** 107–111.
42. SEIDLER, N.W., G.S. YEARGENS & T.G. MORGAN. 2004. Carnosine disaggregates glycated alpha-crystallin: an *in vitro* study. Arch. Biochem. Biophys. **427:** 110–115.
43. ODASHIMA, M., M. OTAKA, M. JIN, *et al.* 2002. Induction of 72-kDa heat-shock protein in cultured rat gastric mucosal cells and rat gastric mucosa by zinc L-carnosine. Dig. Dis. Sci. **47:** 2799–2804.
44. SPINDLER, S.R. 2005. Rapid and reversible induction of longevity, anticancer and genomic effects of caloric restriction. Mech. Ageing Devel. **126:** 960–966.
45. BASSI, A.M., S. LEDDA, M.C. PASCALE, *et al.* 2005. Antioxidant status in J774A.1 macrophage cell line during chronic exposure to glycated serum. Biochem. Cell Biol. **83:** 176–187.
46. MCCARTER, R.J. & J. PALMER. 1992. Energy metabolism and aging: a lifelong study of Fischer 344 rats. Am J. Physiol. **263:** E448–E452.
47. HIPKISS, A.R. 2006. On the mechanisms of aging suppression by dietary restriction: is persistent glycolysis the problem. Mech. Ageing Dev. **127:** 8–15.
48. RAMASAMY, R., S.F. YAN & A.M. SCHMIDT. 2006. Methylgloxal comes of AGE. Cell **124:** 258–260.
49. YAO, D., T. TAGUCHI, T., MATSUMURA, *et al.* 2006. Methylglyoxal modification of mSin3A links glycolysis to angiopoietin-2 transcription. Cell **124:** 275–286.

Would Carnosine or a Carnivorous Diet Help Suppress Aging and Associated Pathologies?

ALAN R. HIPKISS

Centre for Experimental Therapeutics, William Harvey Research Institute, Barts' and the London School of Medicine and Dentistry, Charterhouse Square, London EC1M 6BQ, UK

ABSTRACT: Carnosine (β-alanyl-L-histidine) is found exclusively in animal tissues. Carnosine has the potential to suppress many of the biochemical changes (e.g., protein oxidation, glycation, AGE formation, and cross-linking) that accompany aging and associated pathologies. Glycation, generation of advanced glycosylation end-products (AGEs), and formation of protein carbonyl groups play important roles in aging, diabetes, its secondary complications, and neurodegenerative conditions. Due to carnosine's antiglycating activity, reactivity toward deleterious carbonyls, zinc- and copper-chelating activity and low toxicity, carnosine and related structures could be effective against age-related protein carbonyl stress. It is suggested that carnivorous diets could be beneficial because of their carnosine content, as the dipeptide has been shown to suppress some diabetic complications in mice. It is also suggested that carnosine's therapeutic potential should be explored with respect to neurodegeneration. Olfactory tissue is normally enriched in carnosine, but olfactory dysfunction is frequently associated with neurodegeneration. Olfactory administration of carnosine could provide a direct route to compromised tissue, avoiding serum carnosinases.

KEYWORDS: glycation; anti glycators; AGEs; carbonyls; chelators

INTRODUCTION

Nonenzymic protein glycosylation or glycation mediated by glucose (and more reactive aldehydes) contributes to aging, neurodegeneration, diabetes, and related complications.[1–3] Aldehydes are major sources of protein modification, while aldehyde-scavenging enzymes[4] and glyoxalase-1 activity, which

Address for correspondence: Alan R. Hipkiss, Centre for Experimental Therapeutics, William Harvey Research Institute, Barts' and the London School of Medicine and Dentistry, Charterhouse Square, London EC1M 6BQ, U.K. Voice: 44-(0)20-7882-6032; fax: 44-(0)20-7882-6037.
e-mail: alanandjill@lineone.net

Ann. N.Y. Acad. Sci. 1067: 369–374 (2006). © 2006 New York Academy of Sciences.
doi: 10.1196/annals.1354.052

detoxify the highly reactive aldehyde methylglyoxal,[5] together with nonenzymic aldehyde scavengers[6] provide protection against these deleterious agents. Diet can influence glycation,[2] and levels of advanced glycosylation end-products (AGEs) in vegetarian diabetic plasma are higher than those detected in omnivores,[7] possibly because of the higher intake of fructose by vegetarians.[7] An alternative explanation, however, is discussed below.

CARNOSINE AND ALDEHYDES

The dipeptide carnosine (β-alanyl-L-histidine), found exclusively in animal tissue, sometimes in millimolar concentrations, inhibits formation of protein carbonyls and cross-links induced by reducing sugars and other reactive aldehydes, such as malondialdehyde and methylglyoxal (see Ref. 6 and references therein). Adducts formed by carnosine and acrolein and hydroxynonenal have been characterized and detected in muscle tissue.[6] The dipeptide reacts with (i.e., carnosinylates) protein carbonyls and suppresses AGE formation, and AGE-induced protein modification.[6] Carnosinylation of carbonyl groups in oxidized muscle tissue phosphatidylcholine has been reported.[6]

DIABETES, CARNOSINE, AND GLYCATION

Secondary complications of diabetes often result from protein glycation and oxidation (glycoxidation)[1,9] caused by agents against which carnosine may, theoretically, protect,[6] as evidenced by the following; plasma carnosine concentration is lower in diabetic rats than in normal animals; erythrocyte carnosine levels are lower in human diabetics than in normal subjects; carnosine protects diabetic rat erythrocytes against acidic hemolysis; and carnosine exerts regulatory effects on rat blood glucose levels.[6] In addition to its glyoxalase-mimetic action,[8] carnosine is a carbonyl scavenger, metal ion chelator, and antioxidant,[6] satisfying the requirements for a putative glycation inhibitor.[1] Its ability to alleviate diabetic deterioration in mice[10] further substantiates this proposal.

PROTECTIVE ROLES OF CARNOSINE

Carnosine can ameliorate aging at cellular and whole-animal levels (see Ref. 6 and citations therein). It suppresses senescence in cultured human fibroblasts and even rejuvenates senescent cells and protects their telomeres against oxidative damage. Beneficial effects of carnosine on survival of senescence-accelerated mice, *Drosophila*, and rodent fibroblasts have been reported, most likely due to carnosine's pluripotency.[6]

COULD CARNOSINE SUPPRESS CARBONYL STRESS-INDUCED PATHOLOGY?

Carnosine can suppress murine diabetes[10] and cataractogenesis, especially when supplied as its acetylated pro-drug, acetyl-carnosine.[6]

Glycoxidation is important in neurodegeneration.[11–14] Glyoxalase activity attenuates neuronal methylglyoxal levels, suppressing aldehyde-mediated tau modification and aggregation in a mouse model of Alzheimer's disease.[3] Theoretically, carnosine could supplement glyoxalase's action, both by dipeptide's aldehyde-scavenging action[6] and its glyoxalase-mimetic activity,[8] and the dipeptide ameliorates aspects of Parkinson's and Alzheimer's diseases.[15–20] The olfactory lobe, an area implicated in the onset of neurodegeneration, is normally carnosine-enriched.[21–23] One therefore speculates whether olfactory administration of carnosine could be beneficial.

CARNOSINE'S EFFECTS ON HUMANS

Carnosine may be beneficial in humans, despite the presence of serum and cellular carnosinases, which destroy the dipeptide as meat and carnosine-supplemented diets increase total antioxidant activity in human sera.[24] Dietary carnosine supplementation improved the behavior of autistic children.[25] The mechanisms involved are unknown, but carnosine's antioxidant and aldehyde-scavenging roles could be involved because the autistic brain shows signs of oxidative injury,[26] possible due to a lowered glyoxalase 1 activity.[27]

DIETS AND CARNOSINE

Macromolecular glycation by sugars and associated glycotoxins, deleterious aldehydes and ketones, together with associated pathologies, might be ameliorated by carnivorous diets containing carnosine and possibly the related peptides, acetyl-carnosine, homocarnosine, and anserine. As an exclusively vegetarian diet would lack carnosine, the observations of Krajcovicova-Kudlackova et al.,[7] who observed more AGEs in vegetarian plasma than in omnivores, might be explained by a deficiency of carnosine in a vegetarian diet, which could permit the increased AGE formation observed in vegetarians.

There is little evidence that either supports or refutes the proposal that either a carnivorous diet or carnosine supplementation suppresses glycation and secondary diabetic complications in humans. This is most likely because the components of human carnivorous diets have yet to be regarded as protective (but see McCarty).[28]

It has very recently been shown, however, that a low activity of the enzyme that destroys carnosine, carnosinase, decreases the susceptibility to diabetic nephropathy,[31] an observation consistent with the proposal that carnosine is protective *in vivo*.

Carnosine-rich diets could be important in old age as tissue levels of the dipeptide apparently decline with age.[6] The related structure, homocarnosine, present in human cerebrospinal fluid, decreases with age by more than 10-fold,[29] which could be important as an association has been reported between Alzheimer's disease and raised levels of protein glycation products in cerebrospinal fluid (CSF).[30] Could homocarnosine suppress protein glycation in young CSF, but does the decline in the concentration of this dipeptide permit increased protein glycation in the CSF?

CONCLUSIONS

Much more research is required to determine whether carnivorous diets or carnosine supplementation suppress protein glycation and the secondary complications of diabetes, and whether carnosine and/or related peptides (e.g., homocarnosine) exert any protection action toward Alzheimer's disease or other human neurodegenerative conditions in which glycoxidative events are involved.

REFERENCES

1. AHMED, N. 2005. Advanced glycation endproducts—role in pathology of diabetic complications. Diabetes Res. Clin. Pract. **67:** 3–21.
2. SUJI, G. & S. SIVAKAMI. 2004. Glucose, glycation and aging. Biogerontology **5:** 365–373.
3. CHEN, F., M.A. WOLLMER, F. HOERNDLI, *et al*. 2004. Role of glyoxalase 1 in Alzheimer's disease. Proc. Natl. Acad. Sci. USA **101:** 7687–7692.
4. DAVYDOV, V.V., N.M. DOBAEVA & A.I. BOZHKOV. 2004. Possible role of alteration of aldehyde's scavenger enzymes during aging. Exp. Gerontol **39:** 11–16.
5. KIKUCHI, S., K. SHINPO, M. TAKEUCHI, *et al*. 2003. Glycation—a sweet tempter for neuronal death. Brain Res. Rev. **41:** 306–323.
6. HIPKISS, A.R. 2005. Glycation, ageing and carnosine: are carnivorous diets beneficial? Mech. Ageing Dev. **126:** 1034–1039.
7. KRAJCOVICOVA-KUDLACKOVA, M., K. SEBEKOVA, R. SCHINZEL, *et al*. 2002. Advanced glycation end products and nutrition. Physiol. Res. **51:** 313–316.
8. BATTAH, S., N. AHMED & P.J. THORNALLY. 2002. Novel anti-glycation therapeutic agents: glyoxylase-1-mimetics. Int. Congress Series **1245:** 107–111.
9. BROWNLEE, M. 2001. Biochemistry and molecular biology of diabetic complications. Nature **414:** 813–820.
10. LEE, Y-T., C-C. HSU, M-H. LIN, *et al*. 2005. Histidine and carnosine delay diabetic deterioration in mice and protect human low density lipoprotein against oxidation and glycation. Eur. J. Pharmacol. **512:** 145–150.
11. SHUVAEV, V.V., I. LAFFONT, M. SEROT, *et al*. 2001. Increased protein glycation in cerebrospinal fluid of Alzheimer's disease. Neurobiol. Aging **22:** 397–402.

12. PICKOLO, M.J., Sr., T.J. MONTINE, V. AMARNATH, *et al*. 2002. Carbonyl toxicology and Alzheimer's disease. Toxicol. Appl. Pharmacol. **184:** 187–197.
13. REDDY, V.P., M.E. OBRENOVICH, C.S. ATWOOD, *et al*. 2002. Involvement of Maillard reactions in Alzheimer's disease. Neurotox. Res. **4:** 191–209.
14. AHMED, N., U. AHMED, P.J. THORNALLEY, *et al*. 2005. Protein glycation, oxidation and nitration adduct residues and free adducts of cerebrospinal fluid in Alzheimer's disease and link to cognitive impairment. J. Neurochem. **92:** 255–263.
15. HIPKISS, A.R. 2005. Could carnosine suppress zinc-mediated proteasome inhibition and neurodegeneration? Therapeutic potential of a non-toxic but non-patentable dipeptide. Biogerontology **6:** 147–149.
16. PRESTON, J.E., A.R. HIPKISS, D.J.T. HIMSWORTH, *et al*. 1998. Toxic effects of β-amyloid (25-35) on immortalised rat brain endothelial cells: protection by carnosine, homocarnosine and β-alanine. Neurosci. Lett. **242:** 105–108.
17. MUNCH, G., S. MAYER, J. MICHAELIS, *et al*. 1997. Influence of advanced glycation end-products and AGE-inhibitors on nucleation-dependent polymerization of β-amyloid peptide. Biochim. Biophys. Acta **1360:** 17–29.
18. KIM, K.S., S.Y. CHOI, H.Y. KWON, *et al*. 2002. The ceruloplasmin and hydrogen peroxide system induces α-synuclein aggregation in vitro. Biochimie **84:** 625–631.
19. MIYATA, T. & C. VAN YPERSELE VAN STRIHOU. 2003. Angiotensin II receptor blockers and angiotensin converting enzyme inhibitors: implications of radical scavenging and transition metal chelation in inhibition of advanced glycosylation end product formation. Arch. Biochem. Biophys. **419:** 50–54.
20. BOLDYREV, A., E. BULYGINA, T. LEINSOO, *et al*. 2003. Protection of neuronal cells against reactive oxygen species by carnosine and related compounds. Comp. Biochem. Physiol. Part B **137:** 81–88.
21. HIPKISS, A.R. 2004. Is carnosine a naturally occurring suppressor of olfactory damage in olfactory neurones? Rejuven. Res. **7:** 253–255.
22. GHANBARI, H.A., K. GHANBARI, P.L.R. HARRIS, *et al*. 2004. Oxidative damage in cultured human olfactory neurons from Alzheimer's disease patients. Aging Cell **3:** 41–44.
23. SASSOE-POGNETTO, M.M., D. CANTINO, P. PANZANELLI, *et al*. 1993. Presynaptic colocalization of carnosine and glutamate in olfactory neurones. Neuroreport **5:** 7–10.
24. ANTONINI, F.M., E. PETRUZZI, P. PINZANI, *et al*. 2002. The meat in the diet of aged subjects and the antioxidant effects of carnosine. Arch. Gerontol. Geriatr. Suppl. **8:** 7–14.
25. CHEZ, M.G., C.P. BUCHANAN & M.C. AIMONOVITCH. 2002. Double-blind, placebo-controlled study of L-carnosine supplementation in children with autistic spectrum disorders. J. Child Neurol. **17:** 833–837.
26. MCGINNIS, W.R. 2004. Oxidative stress in autism. Altern. Ther. Health Med. **10:** 22–36.
27. JUNAID, M.A., D. KOWAL, M. BARUA, *et al*. 2004. Proteomic studies identified a single nucleotide polymorphism in glyoxalase 1 as autism susceptibility factor. Am. J. Med. Genet A. **131:** 11–17.
28. MCCARTY, M.F. 2005. The low-AGE content of low-fat vegan diets could benefit diabetics—though concurrent taurine supplementation may be needed to minimize endogenous AGE production. Med. Hypotheses **64:** 394–398.

29. HUANG, Y., J. DUAN, H. CHEN, *et al.* 2005. Separation and determination of carnosine-related peptides using capillary electrophoresis with laser-induced fluorescence detection. Electrophoresis **26:** 593–599.
30. AHMED, N., U. AHMED, P.J. THORNALLEY, *et al.* 2005. Protein glycation, oxidation and nitration adduct residues and free adducts of cerebrospinal fluid in Alzheimer's disease and link to cognitive impairment. J. Neurochem. **92:** 255–263.
31. JANSSEN, B., D. HOHENADEL, P. BRINKKOETTER, *et al.* 2005. Carnosine as a protective factor in diabetic nephropathy: association with a leucine repeat of the carnosinase gene CNDP1. Diabetes **54:** 2320–2327.

The Necessity of Having a Proper Dose of (−)Deprenyl (D) to Prolong the Life Spans of Rats Explains Discrepancies among Different Studies in the Past

KENICHI KITANI,[a] SETSUKO KANAI,[b] KYOKO MIYASAKA,[b] MARIA CRISTINA CARRILLO,[c] AND GWEN O. IVY[d]

[a]National Institute for Longevity Sciences, 36-3, Gengo, Moriokacho, Obu-shi, Japan

[b]Tokyo Metropolitan Institute of Gerontology, Tokyo 173, Japan

[c]Institute for Experimental Physiology, University Rosario, Rosario, Argentina

[d]University of Toronto at Scarborough, Ontario, Canada

ABSTRACT: (−)Deprenyl (D) has been shown to be effective in prolonging life span in experimental animals, although, there are some discrepancies in its effect on the life span the even within the same species (rats). The present study aims to clarify the reason for these discrepancies. Male F344/DuCrj rats began receiving subcutaneous (s.c.) injections of D at the age of 18 months. Doses used were 0.25, 0.50, and 1.0 mg/kg/injection (inj.), three times a week. Average life spans of animals were significantly longer in male rats given 0.25 and 0.5 mg/kg/inj.; however, rats given a 1.0 mg/kg dose began dying earlier than control rats, leading to an inverse U-shaped dose–efficacy relationship, a hormesis. Old (27-month-old) rats given different doses of D for 1 month showed a typical hormetic response for antioxidant enzyme activities, indicating a significant increase in superoxide dismutase (SOD) and catalase (CAT) activities in brain dopaminergic regions with four lower doses (0.25 to 2 mg/kg/inj., 3 times a week), but a significantly negative response with the highest dose (4 mg/kg/inj.). Our results clearly indicate that a proper dose of D within a certain dose range can significantly increase the life span of rats, but that a greater dose becomes less effective and may actually adversely affect the life span of rats. A similar hormetic response for its effect on antioxidant enzyme activities and the parallel between the two different effects of D suggest a possible causal relationship between these two effects of D. The presence of this effective dose range of D may explain previously reported discrepancies in the effect of D on the life span of animals.

Address for correspondence: Kenichi Kitani, National Institute for Longevity Sciences, 36-3, Gengo, Morioka-cho, Obu-shi, Aichi 474-8522 Japan. Voice: 81-562-44-5651, ext.5274; fax: 81-562-48-6668.
e-mail: kitani@nils.go.jp

Ann. N.Y. Acad. Sci. 1067: 375–382 (2006). © 2006 New York Academy of Sciences.
doi: 10.1196/annals.1354.053

KEYWORDS: antioxidant enzymes; (−)deprenyl; F344/DuCrj male and female rats; optimal dose range; specific pathogen-free rats; survival prolongation

INTRODUCTION

(−)Deprenyl (D) is an MAO-B inhibitor that was initially developed as an antidepressant. Knoll in Hungary first reported that D significantly prolonged the average life expectancy of rats.[1] The life-prolonging effect of the drug has been reported in at least four different animal species.[2,3] At least three studies[4-6] reported a significant effect of the drug on the life span of rats. On the other hand, at least one study reported no significant effect[7] and another[8] reported an adverse effect, that is, a shortening of the life span of rats.

We aimed to clarify the reason for these past discrepancies in the effect of D on the life span of rats.

MATERIALS AND METHODS

Male F344/DuCrj rats were originally obtained from Charles River Japan (Atsugi). They were bred and maintained in the specific pathogen-free (SPF) aging farm of the Tokyo Metropolitan Institute of Gerontology (TMIG). Experimental animals began receiving D at the age of 18 months in the clean conventional facility of the same institute (TMIG), as was described previously.[5] D was dissolved in saline solution and given subcutaneously (s.c.). Doses tested were 0.25, 0.50, and 1.0 mg/kg/inj., three times a week. Control animals received isovolumetric vehicle (saline solution) injection. Antioxidant enzyme activities in different brain regions were determined, as was reported previously.[9] All values were expressed as mean ± SD. When two values were first compared, a one-way analysis of variance (ANOVA) was applied. Next, the result of the ANOVA was subjected to the Student's t-test for a statistical comparison. When values for more than two were compared, Scheffe's F-test was applied. P values lower than 0.05 were considered to be significant.

RESULTS AND DISCUSSION

The life-span studies presented here were performed at varying time intervals and the results were reported previously elsewhere. In rats given 0.25 or 0.5 mg/kg/inj., three times a week, average life spans were significantly increased by 8.1%[6] and 5.6%,[5] respectively. In contrast, rats given a higher dose (1.0 mg/kg/inj.) started to die earlier than control rats. At the end of the 13-month treatment, which had begun at 18 months of age, only 3 out of

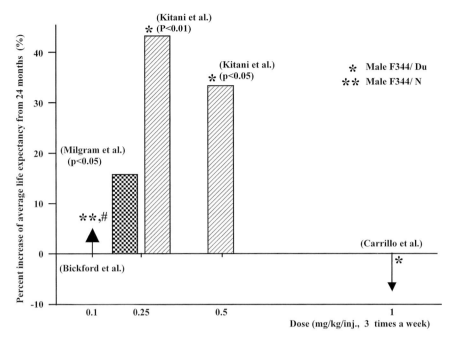

FIGURE 1. Dose–efficacy relationship of (−)deprenyl on survivals of male F344/Du (*) and F344/N (**) rats. The effect is shown as a percentage increase in the average life expectancies after 24 months of age of D-treated rats relative to respective control values, when values were available. D injections (s.c. 3 times a week) in three studies in F344/Du (*) rats were begun at the age of 18 months, while in the study by Milgram *et al.* in F344/N (**) rats injections were begun at the age of 24 months. The dose used in the study by Bickford *et al.*, which was administered daily in drinking water beginning from at 54 weeks of age, was recalculated as a s.c. dose (see the text).

12 D-treated rats survived, while 7 out of 12 control rats still survived at this time.[9] FIGURE 1 shows a dose–response relationship of several life-span studies, using the percentage in the increase of life expectancies after 24 months of age. These calculations were made including rats that died earlier than 24 months using negative days. It is apparent that the effective dose range of D for increasing survival of rats has an upper limit and that above this level, the effect becomes less effective and even shortens the survival of animals. This type of dose–efficacy relationship is called a hormetic response, showing an inverse U shape rather than a sigmoid shape.[10] Two other studies[4,7] reported in the past the effect of D on the life span of male F344/N rats (not F344/Du rats as was used in our studies[5,6]): Milgram *et al.*[4] reported a marginal but significant increase in the average life expectancies of male F344/N rats, that received D injections at 24 months of age at a dose of 0.25 mg/kg/inj., three times a week. Thus the significant effect of this dose (0.25 mg/kg/inj.) is reproduced in two

different studies: Milgram *et al.*[4] and Kitani *et al.*[6] On the other hand, Bickford *et al.*[7] reported no significant effect of D on the life spans of male F344/N rats. They administered D in drinking water every day starting from 54 weeks of age and estimated the amount taken to be approximately 0.5 mg/kg/day. However, since the first-pass effect of D by the liver is very efficient (more than 90%)[11] and since D is inactivated by the liver, the majority of D administered orally does not reach the systemic circulation. Accordingly, the systemic availability of D via the oral route is at least one order of magnitude lower than that via the s.c. route. When calculated as a s.c. dose, it is actually lower than 0.05 mg/inj. Since D was administered daily, it was assumed to be 0.1 mg/kg/inj. as a s.c. dose (FIG. 1). Despite this rather low dose, the figure reported by Bickford *et al.*[6] clearly indicated the shift of the survival curve toward the right in D-treated rats, especially in the second year of the rats age, suggesting a positive effect of D on the survivals of male F344/N rats. In fact, they found a significantly longer mean life span in D-treated rats than in control rats calculated for rats that died before 118 weeks of age, when all rats were sacrificed. However, an analysis that considered the rats that were still living at the time of sacrifice indicated no significant difference in longevity between the two groups ($P = 0.21$), because of the rather quick deaths of D-treated rats after 2 years of age.

F344/Du male rats treated with D for 13 months at a dose of 1.0 mg/kg/inj. (3 times a week) in our study were sacrificed at the age of 31 months and antioxidant enzyme activities were determined.[9] Another group of male rats was treated with five different doses of D for only 1 month at the age of 27 months. FIGURE 2a shows an effective dose range of D on the total superoxide dismutase activities in the striata of 27-month-old rats treated for 1 month.[9] It is quite clear that this effect of D also shows a typical hormetic response. Doses from 0.25 to 2.0 mg/kg/inj., three times a week for 1 month, were similarly effective in increasing the activities of both types of SOD as well as of CAT in striatum, s. nigra, and cerebrum (but not hippocampus); however, the highest dose tested (4.0 mg/kg/inj.) was ineffective or adversely effective (decreased activities).[9] In contrast, a 1.0 mg/kg dose, which is in the middle of the optimal dose range in the study for 1 month, when continued for 13 months (beginning from 18 months), showed no significant increase in enzyme activities relative to respective control values (FIG. 2b).[9] In a previous study we demonstrated that a long-term treatment reduced the optimal dose for increasing antioxidant enzyme activities to one-fourth or less in comparison to the dose for a short-term treatment of 3 to 4 weeks.[2,3,12,13] Apparently, a longer treatment shifts this hormetic response toward the left.[12] Thus, in a longer study, such as a life-span study, the optimal dose range for increasing total antioxidant enzyme activities becomes much lower.

The fact that a 1.0 mg/kg dose was not effective in increasing antioxidant enzyme activities in a long-term treatment study may mean that this dose roughly corresponds to the 4.0 mg/kg dose in the study for 1 month shown in FIGURE 2a. Accordingly, an optimal dose for increasing antioxidant enzyme

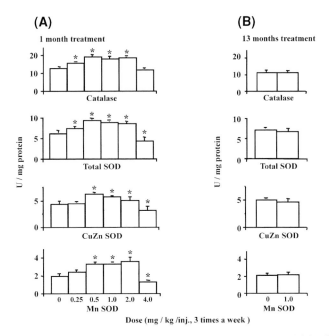

FIGURE 2. The effects of (D) injection on antioxidant enzyme activities in striata at different doses (mg/kg/inj., 3 times a week) for 1 month in 27-month-old F344/Du rats (**a**) and at a dose of 1.0 mg/kg/inj., 3 times a week for 13 months in rats beginning at 18 months of age (**b**). *Significantly different ($P<0.05$) from respective values in control rats given no (−)deprenyl (0 mg/kg). (Reproduced with permission from Carrillo *et al.* 2000.[9])

activities in a life-span study may be at least one-fourth that of the 1.0 mg/kg dose in a 1-month study (0.25 mg/kg/inj.). Although the causal relationship between the two effects of D (on life spans and antioxidant enzyme activities), which we have suggested,[2,3] has no direct proof, we attempted to examine this dose of 0.25 mg/kg, to discern whether it works on the life span of our male F344/Du rats. This dose turned out to be significantly effective in increasing the life span of our rats, suggesting that the effective dose ranges of D are close to each other for these two different effects. In addition, we have also found that a dose of 0.25mg/kg/inj., which was effective in maintaining antioxidant enzyme activities significantly higher than control values for at least 6 months in female rats,[13] also significantly prolonged the life span of female rats.[9]

The hormetic response for the effect of D on life spans of F344/Du rats, as shown in the present study, may explain a negative result of the effect of D in a study by Gallagher *et al.*[8] They used male Wistar rats and began to treat animals with s.c. injections, at the age of 3 months at a dose of 0.5 mg/kg/inj. (3 times a week). They found that treated rats started to die earlier than control rats, as we had observed in our F344/Du rats given 1.0 mg/kg/inj.,[9] but even more drastically than in our study. One major factor to determine an optimal dose of D to increase antioxidant enzyme activities is the hepatic microsomal P-450 function.[2,3,13] D and its metabolites are all known to be inactivated by this system. It is well known that the P-450 function varies widely between male and female rats as well as among different strains and ages of rats.[2,3,14] If we assume that the Wistar rats Gallagher *et al.*[8] used had P-450 functions at least 50% lower than those in our F344/Du rats, this adverse effect of D on life spans of Wistar rats can be explained by the fact that the dose of 0.5 mg/kg they used already exceeded the optimal dose range of D in their Wistar rats. In fact, Gallagher *et al.*[15] reported no effect on SOD activities in their long-term study using a 0.5 mg/kg dose, as we observed in F344/Du rats given a 1.0 mg/kg dose.

Mechanisms for the effect of D on the survival of animals remain unclear. D has a variety of pharmacological effects including an antitumor[16–18] effect and mobilization of various cytokines and other humoral factors involving immunomodulation.[2,3] Until recently the upregulation of antioxidant enzyme activities in transgenic animals has been reported not to be effective in prolonging the life span of rodents. However, a recent study for the first time reported a successful prolongation of the life span of Cu/Zn-SOD-upregulated F344/N rats [Tg(hSod1)$^{+/-}$].[19] Furthermore, mice upregulated for CAT were reported to have a longer life span than their wild-type counterparts.[20] These recent studies may be supportive of our contention that pharmacological upregulation of antioxidant enzyme activities can also prolong the life span of animals.

In conclusion, the discrepancies reported in the past on the effect of D on the life span of rats can be reasonably explained by the fact that this effect of D shows a hormetic response with a lesser effect or even an adverse effect at doses higher than an optimal dose range. Furthermore, a similar dose–efficacy relationship observed for its effect on antioxidant enzyme activities and the fact that effective doses for both effects of D are quite close to each other support our earlier contention that these two effects of D are causally related to each other.

ACKNOWLEDGMENTS

The skillful secretarial work of Ms. T. Ohara is gratefully acknowledged.

REFERENCES

1. KNOLL, J. 1988. The striatal dopamine dependency of life span in male rats: longevity study with (−)deprenyl. Mech. Ageing Dev. **46:** 237–262.

2. KITANI, K., C. MINAMI, K. ISOBE, *et al.* 2002. Why (−)deprenyl prolongs survival of experimental animals: increase of anti-oxidant enzymes in brain and other body tissues as well as mobilization of various humoral factors may lead to systemic anti-aging effects. Mech. Ageing Dev. **123:** 1087–1100.

3. KITANI, K., C. MINAMI, T. YAMAMOTO, *et al.* 2002. Pharmacological interventions in aging and age-associated disorders: potential of propargylamines for human use. Ann. N. Y. Acad. Sci. **959:** 295–307.

4. MILGRAM, N.W., R.J. RACINE, P. NELLIS, *et al.* 1990. Maintenance of L-deprenyl prolongs life in aged male rats. Life Sci. **47:** 415–420.

5. KITANI, K., S. KANAI, Y. SATO, *et al.* 1993. Chronic treatment of (−)deprenyl prolongs the life span of male Fischer 344 rats: further evidence. Life Sci. **52:** 281–288.

6. KITANI, K., S. KANAI, K. MIYASAKA, *et al.* 2005. Dose-dependency of life span prolongation of F344/Du Crj rats injected with (−) deprenyl. Biogerontology **6:** 1–6.

7. BICKFORD, P.C., C.E. ADAMS, S.J. BOYSON, *et al.* 1997. Long-term treatment of male F344 rats with deprenyl: assessment of effects on longevity, behavior, and brain function. Neurobiol. Aging **18:** 309–318.

8. GALLAGHER, I.M., A. CLOW & V. GLOVER. 1998. Long term administration of (−)deprenyl increases mortality in male Wistar rats. J. Neural. Transm. **52**(Suppl.): 315–320.

9. CARRILLO, M.C., S. KANAI, K. KITANI, *et al.* 2000. A high dose of long term treatment with deprenyl loses its effect on antioxidant enzyme activities as well as on survivals of Fischer-344 rats. Life Sci. **67:** 2539–2548.

10. CALABRESE, E.J. & L.A. BALDWIN. 2002. Defining hormesis. Hum. Exp. Toxicol. **21:** 91–97.

11. MAHMOOD, I., D.K. PETERS & W.D. MASON. 1994. The pharmacokinetic and absolute availability of selegiline in the dog. Biopharm. Drug Dispos. **15:** 653–664.

12. CARRILLO, M.C., K. KITANI, S. KANAI, *et al.* 1996. Long term treatment with (−)deprenyl reduces the optimal dose as well as the effective dose range for increasing antioxidant enzyme activities in old mouse brain. Life Sci. **59:** 1047–1057.

13. CARRILLO, M.C., K. KITANI, S. KANAI, *et al.* 1994. The effect of a long term (6 months) treatment with (−)deprenyl on antioxidant enzyme activities in selective brain regions in old female Fischer 344 rats. Biochem. Pharmacol. **47:** 1333–1338.

14. KITANI, K., S. KANAI, G.O. IVY, *et al.* 1998. Assessing the effects of deprenyl on longevity and antioxidant defenses in different animal models. Ann. N. Y. Acad. Sci. **854:** 291–306.

15. GALLAGHER, I.M., A. CLOW, P. JENNER, *et al.* 1999. Effect of long-term administration of pergolide and (−)deprenyl on age related decline in hole board activity and antioxidant enzymes in rats. Biogenic Amines **15:** 379–393.

16. THYAGARAJAN, S., J. MEITES & S.K. AUADRI. 1995. Deprenyl reinitiates estrous cycles, reduces serum prolactin, and decreases the incidence of mammary and pituitary tumors in old acyclic rats. Endocrinology **136:** 1103–1110.

17. THYAGARAJAN, S., S.Y. FELTEN & D.L. FELTEN. 1998. Antitumor effect of L-deprenyl in rats with carcinogen-induced mammary tumors. Cancer Lett. **123:** 177–183.

18. THYAGARAJAN S. & S.K. QUADRI. 1999. L-deprenyl inhibits tumor growth, reduces serum prolactin, and suppresses brain monoamine metabolism in rats with carcinogen-induced mammary tumors. Endocrine **10:** 225–232.
19. IKENO, Y., L. CORTEZ, C. LEW, *et al.* 2005. Abstract, 34th Annual Meeting of the American Aging Association. P. 32.
20. SCHRINER, S.E., N.J. LINFORD, G.M. MARTIN, *et al.* 2005. Extension of murine life span by overexpression of catalase targeted to mitochondria. Science **308:** 1909–1911.

Processing, Lysis, and Elimination of Brain Lipopigments in Rejuvenation Therapies

SORIN RIGA,[a] DAN RIGA,[a] FRANCISC SCHNEIDER,[b] AND FLORIN HALALAU[c]

[a]*Department of Stress Research and Prophylaxis, "Al. Obregia" Clinical Hospital of Psychiatry, RO-041914 Bucharest 8, Romania*

[b]*Center for Applied Physiology and Molecular Biology, RO-310396 Arad, Romania*

[c]*"V. Babes" National Institute of Pathology and Biomedical Sciences, RO-050096 Bucharest 35, Romania*

ABSTRACT: Cerebral lipopigments (LPs)—lipofuscin and ceroid—represent a significant marker in postmitotic normal and pathologic aging, connected with causal and associated neuropathologic damage. Therefore, LP processing, lysis, and elimination may be the main targets in anti-aging and rejuvenation therapies. The regenerative neuroactive factors improve neuron supply with specific nutrients from plasma. They enhance the antioxidative defense, have anti-LP-poietic actions, stimulate brain anabolism, support energetic metabolism, and elevate the reduced lysosomal enzymes. In the second stage, by cytoplasm rehydration, they initiate the breaking up of the neuronal aggregated LP conglomerates, by consecutive disintegration. Then, possibly by the localized exo-endocytosis process between neurons and adjacent glia (especially microglia), intercellular LP transfer can be realized. So, therapeutically activated glia turn into brain garbage collectors and transporters. Therapeutic processing of glial LPs increases in the capillary neighborhood. Highly processed LPs, by glio-endothelial transfer, reach capillary walls before being eliminated. Consequently, neuroactive therapies having these synergistic rejuvenative actions represent new prospects in deceleration of normal and pathological cerebral aging.

KEYWORDS: processing; lipopigments; lipofuscin; glial cells; neuroactive factors; anti-aging

Address for correspondence: Sorin Riga, Department of Stress Research & Prophylaxis, "Al. Obregia" Clinical Hospital of Psychiatry, 10 Berceni Rd., Sector 4, RO-041914 Bucharest 8, Romania. Voice: +40-21-334-3008; fax: +40-21-230-9579.

e-mail: d_s_riga@yahoo.com

Ann. N.Y. Acad. Sci. 1067: 383–387 (2006). © 2006 New York Academy of Sciences.

doi: 10.1196/annals.1354.054

INTRODUCTION

A new direction in anti-aging medicine is the long-term administration of nutraceuticals (functional foods) coupled with regenerative bioactive factors.[1,2] In conformity with their main objectives, these therapies may do one or more of the following: (i) decelerate, antagonize, and remove the "causes of aging," as well as diversify, improve, and efficiently increase the "causes of longevity";[3] (ii) have antistress, anti-impairment, and anti-aging actions;[4] and (iii) synergistically protect, regulate, and recover the three key organs (liver, heart, and brain) of the human being.[5]

In antiaging medicine, the role, characteristics, and functions of the brain determine specific objectives in order to:

- optimize the unbalanced neurono-glial homeostasis,[6] especially by anti-inflammatory and antidegenerative actions;
- restore the balance between oxidative stress damage and antioxidant defense–repair processes;[7]
- ensure mitochondrial protection and remove oxidative mitochondrial decay;[2]
- reconfigurate and intensify the functions of catabolic subcellular systems and accelerate destruction and elimination of subcellular garbage;[8,9]
- increase ribososomal RNA and protein biosynthesis, as well as activate polyribosomes and endoplasmic reticula;[10], and
- protect and offer repair potential for genome damage.[7]

One of the main factors in proteasome–lysosomal aging dysfunction is progressive accumulation and storage of brain lipopigments (LPs).[11] Cerebral LPs—lipofuscin and ceroid—represent a significant marker in postmitotic normal and pathologic aging. Moreover, LPs are connected with important causal and associated neuropathologic damage, generating imbalances in neuronal and glial homeostasis and multiple subcellular impairment, with negative consequences ranging from neuronal function to brain physiology.

Therefore, LP processing, lysis, and elimination[8,9,12] can become the main mechanisms for the reestablishment of metabolic, cellular, and tissue homeostasis, as well as in antistress, anti-aging, and rejuvenation therapies.[13] However, in rejuvenation therapies, these important anti-aging mechanisms are and should be prefigured and followed by other synergistic subcellular revitalizing actions, mechanisms, and effects.[14]

PROCESSING, LYSIS, AND ELIMINATION
OF BRAIN LIPOPIGMENTS

The antistress, anti-impairment, and anti-aging therapy (3A-SIA-T) under consideration corresponds to these objectives and acts at the neuronal subcellular level. 3A-SIA-T is a simultaneous synergistic neurometabolic neurovascular medication with the following complementary composition:[13]

1. *for anabolic rejuvenation:* Hydrooxopyrimidine carboxylates/oxopyrrolidine acetamides (18.8–20.0%), fructose (0.6–0.7%), nicotinic alcohol/acid/amide with prolonged release (4.1–5.3%), lithium (0.025–0.033%), potassium (2.5–2.9%), magnesium (0.3–0.4%), iodide (0.005–0.007%), and monoacide phosphate (2.6–3.5%).

2. *for catabolic homeostasis and garbage scavenging and elimination:* Aminoethanol phenoxyacetates/aminoethyl phenoxyacetamides (31.0–33.1%), methionine (18.0–19.1%), aspartate (9.7–10.6%), fructose (1.1–1.3%), vitamin B_1 (0.9–1.3%), vitamin B_6 (1.2–1.5%), nicotinic alcohol/acid/amide with fast release (1.1–1.3%), magnesium (1.2–1.5%), zinc (0.3–0.7%), and sulfate (0.5–1.0%).

BRAIN METABOLIC PATHWAYS AND LONGEVITY

Two main metabolic pathways of the nervous tissue with the same course, but in the opposite directions, are used in glia–neuron nutrition and metabolism, as well as by rejuvenation therapies. They are: (i) import pathway: arterioles—capillaries → glial cells → neurons, and (ii) elimination pathway: neurons → neuroglial systems → capillary-venule areas.

First, the regenerative neuroactive factors of 3A-SIA-T activate arteriolar precapillary and capillary areas, and improve neuron supply from plasma with anabolites, specific nutrients, and nutraceuticals, and thus better nourish the nerve cells. Then, by acting on neuroglia, they ameliorate glial functions; destroy, dissociate, and dissolve glial LP conglomerates by glioplasm rehydration and glial LP-lytic actions; and optimize glial–neuronal interactions.

In neurons, 3A-SIA-T compounds have the following effects:[15,16]

- enhancing the antioxidative defense and having anti-LP-genesis actions, through their scavenging properties;
- increasing the ribosomal RNA, total RNA, water-soluble proteins, and total proteins, stimulating brain anabolism;
- protecting and augmenting the number of healthy mitochondria and supporting energetic metabolism; and
- regulating proteasome–lysosomal dysfunction and enzymes by neuroplasm rehydration and initiating the break-up of the stored neuronal aggregated LP, followed by LP vacuolation, disintegration, and decrease, and a reduction of water-insoluble proteins.

Second, in neurons, diminished processed LPs are carried by intracellular transport in the neurosomal periphery.[15] Neurono-glial transfer of processed LPs is initiated by activation of circumscribed neurono-glial areas. Then, possibly by localized exo-endocytosis between neurons and adjacent glia (especially parenchymal microglia), the intercellular transfer of the neuronal LPs can be realized.[16]

Thus, therapeutically activated glia (particularly microglia) turn into brain garbage collectors and transporters, moving waste from neuronal proximity, through neuropil, to pericapillary areas.[16] Thus, the microglial paradox appears, that is, cells with a high rate of division have their cytoplasm filled up to 90% with LPs. An explanation for this is the glial mechanism of neuronal LP collecting and transport, besides the phagocytosis with degradation of neuronal apoptotic bodies. Therapeutic processing of glial LPs increases in the capillary neighborhood. Finally, the vacuolated and highly processed LPs (glial end-feet, pericytes, perivascular microglia) are transferred from pericapillary zones into capillaries and venules (postcapillary areas), and eliminated together with catabolites in capillary lumina.[13] The natural impaired and incomplete mechanism of LP transport and elimination is therapeutically reorganized into an activated, complete, and efficient mechanism.

CONCLUSIONS

In the brain, 3A-SIA-T compounds exert their rejuvenative actions and LP processing and lysis by a metabolic route from capillaries through neuroglial cells to neurons. In addition, this simultaneous synergistic antistress and anti-aging therapy also activates the inverse pathway, in which the highly processed LPs are moved, transported, and eliminated from neurons into capillary lumen via glial systems. Morever, long-term administration of neuroactive therapies having these synergistic rejuvenation mechanisms, actions, and effects represents new prospects in the deceleration of normal and pathologic cerebral aging, with increase of neuronal healthy longevity, as well as alternative and complementary treatments in neuro-psycho-geriatrics.

Three different strategies for antistress, anti-aging, and rejuvenation have certain common molecular, cellular actions, mechanisms, and effects: (i) healthy diet, nutraceuticals, regenerative bioactive factors,[13] (ii) regular exercise, daily physical activity,[17] and (iii) hormesis, including low-level stress.[18,19] Their association produces synergistic, amplified, and consolidated effects[5] and represents an efficient direction in anti-aging prophylaxis, therapy, and recovery, as well as in sanogenesis and prolongevity medicine.

REFERENCES

1. RIGA, D. 2003. SENS acquires SENSe: present and future anti-aging strategies. J. Anti-Aging Med. **6:** 231–236.
2. AMES, B.N. 2004. Delaying the mitochondrial decay of aging. Ann. N.Y. Acad. Sci. **1019:** 406–411.

3. CUTLER, R.G. 1991. Human longevity and aging: possible role of reactive oxygen species. Ann. N.Y. Acad. Sci. **621:** 1–28.

4. DIERICK, J-F., C. FRIPPIAT, M. SALMON, *et al.* 2003. Stress, cells and tissue aging. *In* ModulatingAging and Longevity. S. I. S. Rattan, Ed.: 101–125. Kluwer. Dordrecht, NL.

5. ROSENFELDT, F., F. MILLER, P. NAGLEY, *et al.* 2004. Response of the senescent heart to stress: clinical therapeutic strategies and quest for mitochondrial predictors of biological age. Ann. N.Y. Acad. Sci. **1019:** 78–84.

6. GLEES, P. & M. HASAN. 1976. Lipofuscin in Neuronal Aging and Diseases. G. Thieme. Stuttgart, Germany.

7. SITTE, N. & T. VON ZGLINICKI. 2003. Free radical production and antioxidant defence: a primer. *In* Aging at the Molecular Level. T. von Zglinicki, Ed.: 1–10. Kluwer. Dordrecht, NL.

8. NANDY, K. 1979. Experimental studies on centrophenoxine in aging brain. *In* Geriatric Psycho-pharmacology. K. Nandy, Ed.: 247–260. Elsevier/North-Holland. New York, NY.

9. RIGA, S. & D. RIGA. 1974. Effects of centrophenoxine on the lipofuscin pigments in the nervous system of old rats. Brain Res. **72:** 265–275.

10. ZS.-NAGY, I. 1989. Centrophenoxine as OH$^\bullet$ free radical scavenger. *In* CRC Handbook of Free Radicals and Antioxidants in Biomedicine, Vol. 2. J. Miquel, A.T. Quintanilha & H. Weber, Eds.: 87–94. CRC Press. Boca Raton, FL.

11. TERMAN, A. & U.T. BRUNK. 2003. Aging and lysosomal degradation of cellular constituents. *In* Aging at the Molecular Level. T. von Zglinicki, Ed.: 233–242. Kluwer. Dordrecht, NL.

12. ARIVAZHAGAN, P. & C. PANNEERSELVAM. 2004. Alpha-lipoic acid increases Na$^+$K$^+$ ATPase activity and reduces lipofuscin accumulation. Ann. N.Y. Acad. Sci. **1019:** 350–354.

13. RIGA, S. & D. RIGA. 1995. An antistress and antiaging neurometabolic therapy: accelerated lipofuscinolysis and stimulated anabolic regeneration by the Antagonic-Stress synergistic formula. Ann. N.Y. Acad. Sci. **771:** 535–550.

14. ZS.-NAGY, I. 2002. Pharmacological interventions against aging through the cell plasma membrane: a review of the experimental results obtained in animals and humans. Ann. N.Y. Acad. Sci. **959:** 308–320.

15. RIGA, S. & D. RIGA. 1994. Antagonic-Stress: a therapeutic composition for deceleration of aging. I. Brain lipofuscinolytic activity demonstrated by light and fluorescence microscopy. Arch. Gerontol. Geriatr. **19:** 217–226.

16. RIGA, D. & S. RIGA. 1994. Antagonic-Stress: a therapeutic composition for deceleration of aging. II. Brain lipofuscinolytic activity demonstrated by electron microscopy. Arch. Gerontol. Geriatr. **19:** 227–234.

17. GOTO, S., Z. RADAK, C. NYAKAS, *et al.* 2004. Regular exercise. An effective means to reduce oxidative stress in old rats. Ann. N.Y. Acad. Sci. **1019:** 471–474.

18. RATTAN, S.I.S. 2004. Mechanisms of hormesis through mild heat stress on human cells. Ann. N.Y. Acad. Sci. **1019:** 554–558.

19. MINOIS, N. & S.I.S. RATTAN. 2003. Hormesis in aging and longevity. *In* Modulating Aging and Longevity. S. I. S. Rattan, Ed.: 127–137. Kluwer. Dordrecht, NL.

Effect of Dietary Restriction on Learning and Memory Impairment and Histologic Alterations of Brain Stem in Senescence-Accelerated Mouse (SAM) P8 Strain

RYOYA TAKAHASHI, YUKARI KOMIYA, AND SATARO GOTO

Department of Biochemistry, Faculty of Pharmaceutical Sciences, Toho University 2-2-1 Miyama, Funabashi, Chiba, Japan

ABSTRACT: The age-associated spontaneous spongy degeneration in the brain stem of senescence-accelerated mouse (SAM) P8 strain has been suggested to be closely associated with the ability to learn and memorize. In this study, we investigated the effects of dietary restriction (DR) initiated from weaning on learning and memory and histologic changes of the brain stem in P8 and control R1 mice. Although no effect of DR was observed in the retention of the passive-avoidance response in both the P8 and R1 mice, the acquisition of the task was significantly improved by DR in P8 mice. On the other hand, the total area and number of vacuoles in the brain stem was significantly higher in *ad libitum*-fed (AD)-P8 mice than in AD-R1 mice. However, no significant effect was observed on the vacuole formation in the brain stem of P8 mice by DR. These observations suggest that the improvement of the acquisition of the task by DR in P8 mice is possibly due to changes in neuronal function rather than histologic alteration in brain stem.

KEYWORDS: dietary restriction; learning; memory; senescence-accelerated mouse; spongy degeneration; SAMP8

INTRODUCTION

Dietary restriction (DR) has been recognized to inhibit or delay (or both) the appearance and intensity of many late-life age-related cases of functional deterioration and other pathalogic changes, and to prolong mean and maximum life span.[1–4] In addition, DR is known to prevent or delay the occurrence of some

Address for correspondence: Dr. Ryoya Takahashi, Department of Biochemistry, Faculty of Pharmaceutical Sciences, Toho University, 2-2-1 Miyama, Funabashi, Chiba 274-8510, Japan. Voice/Fax: +81-47-472-1562.

e-mail: takahasi@phar.toho-u.ac.jp

Ann. N.Y. Acad. Sci. 1067: 388–393 (2006). © 2006 New York Academy of Sciences.
doi: 10.1196/annals.1354.055

genetic diseases, such as autoimmune diseases of B/W mice[5] and hypertension of SHR rats.[6]

The senescence-accelerated mouse (SAM) was established as an animal model of accelerated aging by Takeda *et al.*[8] SAMP8, a substrain of SAM, has a much shorter life span (approximately 50% that of the control strain the accelerated senescence-resistant strain, R1) and exhibits early deficits in learning and memory in different tasks, such as passive-avoidance response tests,[8,9] active avoidance tasks,[8–10] and spatial learning tasks (including the Morris water maze task).[8,11] For example, the impairment of passive-avoidance behavior in P8 mice began to occur at a much earlier age (about 2 months of age) and increased with age.[12] On the other hand, remarkable histopathologic changes, such as vacuolization, have been found mainly in the brain stem of P8 mice.[13] Yagi *et al.*[12] suggested that such pathologic change in the brain stem of P8 mice is closely associated with memory and the ability to learn.

In this study, therefore, we investigated the effects of DR initiated from weaning on learning and memory and vacuolization in the brain stem in P8 and control R1 mice.

MATERIALS AND METHODS

Animals and Dietary Restriction

SAMP8 and SAMR1 mice obtained from Dr. T. Takeda in 1988 were bred and maintained in our Laboratory Animal Center. The 50% survival of male SAMP8/Toho and SAMR1/Toho was found at about 430 and 780 days of age, respectively.[14]

At the age of 21 days, all mice were housed individually and dietary restriction was started. Restricted mice were fed 60% of the amount of food consumed by the control animals.

Passive Avoidance Task

A two-compartment, step-through passive avoidance test was performed at the age of 6 months according to the method described by Sasaki *et al.*[15] Briefly, a Plexiglas two-compartment, step-through passive avoidance apparatus (Muromachi Kikai, Japan) was used for the test. In a pretraining trial, a mouse was placed in the illuminated chamber, the guillotine door was opened and the mouse was adapted to the apparatus for 4 min and then returned to its home cage. In an acquisition trial 24 h after the pretraining trial, the mouse was placed in the illuminated chamber and the time (acquisition latency) before it entered the dark chamber was recorded. Immediately after the mouse had entered the dark chamber, the door was closed and a scrambled foot shock (0.2 mA at 50 Hz) was applied to the floor grid for 3 s through a shock generator (SGS-003, Muromachi Kagaku, Japan). Training was terminated when the mouse remained in the illuminated chamber for 300 consecutive seconds. The number of trials (entries into the dark chamber) and total training time (acquisition time) were recorded. Retention of avoidance behavior was tested 24 h and more after the foot shock. The mouse was again placed in the illuminated chamber and latency to reenter the dark chamber was recorded up to a maximum of 300 s. If the mouse did not enter the dark chamber within 300 s, the retention test was terminated and a ceiling score of 300 s was assigned.

Spontaneous Activity

Locomotor activity in mice was quantified using an Animex activity meter Type S (LKB, Farad, Sweden) at the same time of day as the passive avoidance test. Spontaneous activity was expressed as signal counts automatically produced by the movement of the animal placed on the top of the Animex activity meter.

Study of Pathologic Changes

After completion of the behavior test, the mice were anesthetized by exposure to ethyl ether, and the brains were removed immediately and immersed in methacarn (methanol: chloroform: acetic acid = 6:3:1). The fixed brains were embedded in paraffin and 3-μm-thick coronal sections were prepared. The sections of brain stem were stained with hematoxylin and eosin and photographed with a light microscope. The number and area of the vacuoles in the brain stem of P8 and R1 mice were measured using an image analyzer.

Statistical Analysis

All experimental results are given as the mean $\pm$ SEM. Analysis of variance, followed by Fisher's protected least significant difference procedure for *post hoc* comparison, were used to verify significance between the two means.

RESULTS

Body Weight

Restriction of the diet was started at the age of 21 days and continued for about 5 months. The body weight of DR mice fed 60% of the amount of food consumed by the control animals (fed *ad libitums*) was consistently lower than that of AD animals in both P8 and R1 mice. However, the general growth pattern was similar for the mice on the two dietary regimens; the body weight increased rapidly during the first 2.5 months of age and increased at a lower rate thereafter.

TABLE 1. Effect of dietary restriction on the acquisition of the passive avoidance test

Strain	Diet	Acquisition time (s)
SAMP8	AD	432 ± 65^a
	DR	234 ± 34^b
SAMR1	AD	95 ± 30
	DR	66 ± 20

Mean $\pm$ SE (n = 25).
[a]Significant difference between P8 and R1 in AD ($P < 0.05$).
[b]Significant difference between AD and DR ($P < 0.05$).

Learning and Memory Abilities

A two-compartment, step-through passive avoidance test was performed at the age of 6 months. AD-P8 mice showed significant impairment in the acquisition of passive avoidance response (TABLE 1) and retention of the acquired response assessed by repeated extinction trials compared with AD-R1 mice.

DR significantly improved the acquisition of the task in P8 mice (TABLE 1). However, no effect of DR was observed on the retention of the acquired response in both P8 and R1 mice.

It is conceivable that the improvement in the acquisition of passive avoidance response might be associated with altered motor activity by DR. Therefore, we next determined the spontaneous activities of AD and DR mice in both strains. The spontaneous activity of individual mice was measured at the same time of day as the passive avoidance test. No significant difference was observed in the spontaneous activity between AD and DR mice in both strains, suggesting that the improvement in the acquisition of the passive avoidance task in P8 mice is not due to changes in the motor activity in response to DR.

Thus, DR improved the impaired acquisition of passive avoidance response but not the extinction of the acquired response in P8 mice.

Spongy Degeneration in Brain Stem

In SAMP8 mice, spongy degeneration (vacuole formation) in the brain stem is closely associated with deterioration of learning and memory.[12] It is interesting how DR alters such pathologic changes of the brain stem in P8 mice.

We determined the total area and number of vacuoles in the brain stem of AD and DR mice in both strains at the age of 6 months. The total area and the number of vacuoles in the brain stem were significantly higher in AD-P8 mice than in AD-R1 mice. However, no significant effect was observed on the vacuole formation in the brain stem of P8 mice by DR.

DISCUSSION

The present study showed that DR from time of weaning significantly improved the acquisition but not the retention of the passive avoidance response in P8 mice. It has been demonstrated that P8 mice exhibit age-related deterioration in learning and memory in passive avoidance response tests,[16] especially in the acquisition stage.[12] However, little is known about the mechanism underlying the acquisition impairment of the task in P8 mice. Yagi *et al.*[12] suggested that vacuolization in brain stem, especially the magnocellular reticular formation, might result in an age-related deterioration of learning and memory in P8 mice because some neurons in the brain stem respond to tasks requiring learning and memory. For example, destruction of pedunculo-pontine nucleus-parabrachial nucleus,[17,18] or median raphe nucleus[19] in the brain stem resulted in the deterioration of maze learning and of active avoidance and visual discrimination learning. In addition, electrophysiological studies have also shown that neurons in the reticular formation of the brain stem have learning and memory functions.[20] Thus, neurons in the reticular formation of the brain stem play important roles in learning and memory. However, in the present study, we could not observe any significant effect of DR on the vacuole formation in the brain stem of P8 mice. These observations suggest that the improvement in the acquisition of the task by DR in P8 mice is possibly due to changes in neuronal function,[21] such as the amount of neurotransmitters and receptors, rather than a histologic alteration in the brain stem. However, possible changes in the cerebellum must also be studied because they may be involved in learning and memory deficit in P8 mice.[21–23] Further study will be required to clarify the effect of DR on the improvement in the acquisition of such tasks in P8 mice.

REFERENCES

1. MASORO, E.J. 2000. Caloric restriction and aging: an update. Exp. Gerontol. **35:** 299–305.
2. WEINDRUCH, R. 1996. Caloric restriction and aging. Sci. Am. **274:** 46–52.
3. WEINDRUCH, R. & R. WALFORD. 1988. The Retardation of Aging and Disease by Dietary Restriction. Charles C Thomas. Springfield, IL.
4. YU, B.P. 1994. Modulation of Aging Processes by Dietary Restriction. CRC Press. Boca Raton, FL.
5. JOLLY, C.A. 2004. Dietary restriction and immune function. J. Nutr. **134:** 1853–1856.
6. LLOYD, T. 1984. Food restriction increases life span of hypertensive animals. Life Sci. **34:** 401–407.
7. TAKEDA, T., M. HOSOKAWA & K. HIGUCHI. 1991. Senescence-accelerated mouse (SAM): a novel murine model of accelerated senescence. J. Am. Geriatr. Soc. **39:** 911–919.

8. MIYAMOTO, M., Y. KIYOTA, N. YAMAZAKI, *et al*. 1986. Age-related changes in learning and memory in the senescence-accelerated mouse (SAM). Physiol. Behav. **38:** 399–406.

9. YAGI, H., S. KATOH, I. AKIGUCH, *et al*. 1988. Age-related deterioration of ability of acquisition in memory and learning in senescence accelerated mouse: SAM-P/8 as an animal model of disturbance in recent memory. Brain Res. **474:** 86–93.

10. FLOOD, J.F. & J.E. MORLEY. 1993. Age-related changes in footshock avoidance acquisition and retention in senescence accelerated mouse (SAM). Neurobiol. Aging **14:** 153–157.

11. MIYAMOTO, M., Y. KIYOTA, M. NISHIYAMA, *et al*. 1992. Senescence-accelerated mouse (SAM): age-related reduced anxiety-like behavior in the SAM-P/8 strain. Physiol. Behav. **51:** 979–985.

12. YAGI, H., I. AKIGUCHI & A. OHTA. 1998. Spontaneous and artificial lesions of magnocellular reticular formation of brainstem deteriorate avoidance learning in senescence-accelerated mouse SAM. Brain Res. **791:** 90–98.

13. YAGI, H., M. IRINO, T. MATSUSHITA, *et al*. 1989. Spontaneous spongy degeneration of the brainstem in SAM-P/8 mice, a newly developed memory-deficient strain. J. Neuropathol. Exp. Neurol. **48:** 577–590.

14. TAKAHASHI, R. & S. GOTO. 2004. Altered gene expression in the brain of senescence accelerated mouse SAMP8. *In* The Senescence-Accelerated Mouse (SAM): an animal model of senescence. International Congress Series **1260:** 85–90.

15. SASAKI, K., I. TOOYAMA, A.J. LI, *et al*. 1999. Effects of an acidic fibroblast growth factor fragment analog on learning and memory and on medial septum cholinergic neurons in senescence-accelerated mice. Neuroscience **92:** 1287–1294.

16. MIYAMOTO, M., Y. KIYOTA & N. YAMAZAKI. 1986. Age-related changes in learning and memory in the senescence-accelerated mouse (SAM). Physiol. Behav. **38:** 399–406.

17. DELLU, F., W. MAYO & J. CHERKAOUI. 1991. Learning disturbances following excitotoxic lesion of cholinergic pedunculo-pontine nucleus in the rat. Brain Res. **544:** 126–132.

18. IVANOVA, S.F. & J. BURES. 1990. Acquisition of conditioned taste aversion in rats is prevented by tetrodotoxin blockade of a small midbrain region centered around the parabrachial nuclei. Physiol. Behav. **48:** 543–549.

19. THOMPSON, R., A. RAMSAY & J. YU. 1984. A generalized learning deficit in albino rats with early median raphe or pontine reticular formation lesions. Physiol. Behav. **32:** 107–114.

20. PRAGAY, E.B., A.F. MIRSKY & C.L. RAY. 1978. Neuronal activity in the brainstem reticular formation during performance of a "go-no go" visual attention task in the monkey. Exp. Neurol. **60:** 83–95.

21. NOMURA, Y. & Y. OKUMA. 1999. Age-related defects in lifespan and learning ability in SAMP8 mice. Neurobiol. Aging **20:** 111–115.

22. OHTA, A., I. AKIGUCHI, N. SERIU, *et al*. 2002. Deterioration in learning and memory of inferential tasks for evaluation of transitivity and symmetry in aged SAMP8 mice. Hippocampus **12:** 803–810.

23. MORLEY, J.E. 2002. The SAMP8 mouse: a model of Alzheimer disease? Biogerontology **3:** 57–60.

Curcumin's Biphasic Hormetic Response on Proteasome Activity and Heat-Shock Protein Synthesis in Human Keratinocytes

REHAB E. ALI AND SURESH I. S. RATTAN

Laboratory of Cellular Ageing, Danish Centre for Molecular Gerontology, Department of Molecular Biology, University of Aarhus, Science Park, DK-8000 Aarhus C, Denmark

ABSTRACT: Curcumin (diferuloylmethane), is a component of the yellow powder prepared from the roots of *Curcuma longa* (Zingiberaceae), also known as tumeric or turmeric. It is widely cultivated and used as a food ingredient in tropical areas of Asia and Central America. Treatment of mid-passage human epidermal keratinocytes with curcumin resulted in a biphasic hormetic dose–response with respect to proteasome activity. Curcumin treatment (up to 1 μM for 24 h) increased chymotrypsin-like activity by 46% compared to that in untreated keratinocytes. However, higher concentrations of curcumin were inhibitory, and at 10 μM the proteasome activity decreased to 46% of its initial value. Furthermore, the preincubation of human keratinocytes at 43°C for 1 h, followed by 24-h treatment with 3 μM curcumin, led to an increase in heat-shock protein (hsp70 and hsp90) levels by 24% and 19%, respectively, and the effect was sustained at concentrations up to 10 μM. On the other hand, the level of the small hsp27 was unaffected by curcumin concentrations of 0.3–1 μM, while it decreased by 34% at 10 μM.

KEYWORDS: aging; hormesis; hormetin; heat shock; stress; protein degradation

The use of medicinal plants in pharmacology has increased significantly in recent times, owing to their affordability and apparent safety, when compared to synthetic drugs. Curcumin (diferuloylmethane), the active constituent of *Curcuma longa*, is one of the best studied natural antioxidant compounds. Curcumin has been used as a spice and coloring agent for centuries, and it is used in India against hepatic disorders, anorexia, diabetic wounds, and rheumatism.[1] Curcumin has been shown to have anti-inflammatory, anti-carcinogenic,

Address for correspondence: Dr. Suresh I. S. Rattan, Department of Molecular Biology, University of Aarhus, Gustav Wieds Vej 10C, DK 8000 Aarhus C, Denmark. Voice: +4589425034; fax: +4586123178.
e-mail: rattan@mb.au.dk

Ann. N.Y. Acad. Sci. 1067: 394–399 (2006). © 2006 New York Academy of Sciences.
doi: 10.1196/annals.1354.056

anti-diabetogenic, antibacterial, antiviral, and antioxidant effects.[2,3] Curcumin has also been shown to induce the heat-shock (HS) response in HeLa cells in a time-dependent and dose-dependent manner,[4] and an enhancement of HS response has been seen in rat liver cells and Swiss 3T3 mouse fibroblasts.[5] In addition, high concentrations of curcumin were reported to inhibit proteasome activity in HeLa cells.[6] Proteasome inhibition was also found to induce HS response of mammalian cells,[7] suggesting that the two mechanisms are related. Therefore, the present investigation was undertaken to test whether curcumin modulates HS response and proteasome activity in cultured human keratinocytes undergoing aging *in vitro*.

EXPERIMENTAL METHODS

Primary cultures of normal diploid human epidermal keratinocytes were established from mammary skin biopsies obtained from a healthy woman donor (age: 28 years). Cells were grown in T_{25} plastic flasks (COSTAR, Cambridge, UK) at 37°C, 5% CO_2 and 95% humidity in Epilife medium (Cascade Biologics, Mansfield, UK) supplemented with 100 ng/mL EGF, 0.18 mg/mL hydrocortisone, 2.4 mg/mL insulin, 2.5 mg/mL transferrin, 0.06 M $CaCl_2$, and 12 mg/mL BPA. The medium was changed twice a week, and when the cells reached 80% confluence, the culture was split using the trypsin/EDTA (Biowhittacker ™ Cambex Bioscience, Verviets, Belgium) method.

Curcumin was purchased from Sigma-Aldrich (St Louis, MO, USA; catalog number: C1386). The naturally occurring ratio for curcuminoids is 5% bisdesmethoxycurcumin, 15% desmethoxycurcumin, and 80% curcumin.[8] A stock solution of curcumin (10 mM; molecular weight 368.39) was dissolved in 100% DMSO. During incubation of cells with curcumin, the final DMSO concentration was 0.08%. Cell survival after exposure to different curcumin concentrations was measured with the 3-(4,5 dimethylthiazol-2-yl)-2,5-diphenyl tetrazolium bromide (MTT) assay.

For proteasome activity assay, cells were washed with cold PBS and harvested using cell scraper and buffer A (50 mM NaCl, 10 mM HEPES, pH 8, 250 mM sucrose, 1 mM EDTA, and 0.2% Triton X-100). Cell suspension was vortexed for 2 min and centrifuged at 15,000 rpm at 4°C. Twenty micrograms of total protein were added to a 96-well plate and mixed with 25 μM Suc-LLVY-AMC (Sigma-Aldrich) in 200 μL 0.1 M HEPES pH 7.4. As a negative control, 800 μM MG132 (Sigma-Aldrich) was incubated with the sample and substrate. The fluorescence intensity was measured at excitation 360 nm and emission 460 nm for 30 min at 37°C, using a fluorimeter (BMG LABTECH, GmbH, Hoffenberg, Germany). The proteolytic activities were expressed as a percentage of control.

For heat-shock response, cells were subjected to 43°C HS for 1 h, treated with curcumin for 24 h, then harvested in 500 μL lysis buffer (5M NaCl, 1M $MgCl_2$,

50% glycerol, 0.5% SDS, 1 M Tris/HCl, pH 8). Cellular proteins were isolated and protein content of the cell extracts was determined by the Lowry method. All samples were heated for 3 min at 95°C. The proteins were transferred to polyvinylidene fluoride (PVDF) membrane (Immobilon-P, Millipore). The membranes were blocked overnight at 4°C in TBS-T containing 5% skim milk, and then incubated with primary antibodies, hsp90, hsp70, and hsp27 (Nordic Biosite, Sweden) for 60 min at room temperature.

RESULTS

Serially passaged middle-aged human epidermal keratinocytes (~50% lifespan completed) were treated with curcumin for 24 h. Curcumin concentrations up to 1 μM did not affect cell viability, whereas at high concentrations (3–10 μM) cell viability decreased to 48% and 53%, respectively (data not shown). FIGURE 1 depicts the effect of curcumin on the chymotrypsin-like

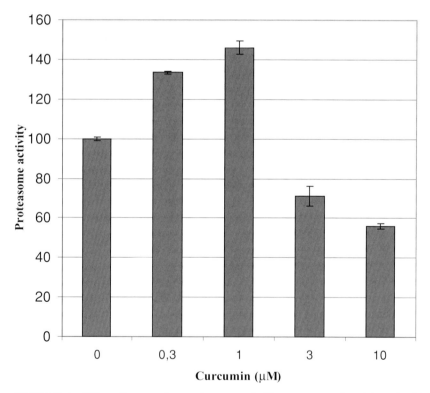

FIGURE 1. Effect of curcumin on chymotrypsin-like proteasomal activity of mid-passage human keratinocytes (50% life span completed). Data are mean ± SD of triplicate measurements and expressed as a percentage of control, measured in the absence of curcumin.

activity of middle-aged cultured keratinocytes, showing that at 0.3 μM and 1 μM curcumin stimulated proteasome activity by 34% and 46%, respectively. On the other hand, significant inhibition of proteasome activity (32% and 46%) was observed at 3 and 10 μM curcumin concentration. To investigate the effect of curcumin on HS response, cells were preincubated at 43°C for 1 hr followed by 24-h curcumin treatment. In HS-exposed cells, treatment with 3 μM curcumin resulted in a marked increase in the levels of hsp90 and hsp70 (19% and 24%, respectively) as compared with HSP levels in untreated cells and this effect of curcumin was additive (data not shown). However, hsp27 levels were not affected by curcumin treatment at concentrations up to 1 μM, and were reduced by 34% at 10 μM.

DISCUSSION

Inhibition of the proteasome by application of high (up to 50 μM) curcumin concentrations was previously reported[6] but the effect of lower concentrations has not been investigated. Our studies have shown that low (up to 1 μM) concentrations of curcumin have a stimulatory effect on proteasome in human keratinocytes, whereas high concentrations of curcumin are inhibitory for the proteasome. We have also observed similar biphasic response of curcumin on the proteasomal activity in other cell types, including human fibroblasts and telomerase-immortalized mesenchymal bone marrow stem cells (data not shown). This biphasic dose response is a typical expression of hormesis, in which low doses of a compound elicit beneficial biological effects, whereas higher doses do have deleterious effects.[9–11] This phenomenon has been shown in other conditions such as irradiation, temperature, hypergravity, pro-oxidants, electric shocks and repeated physical injuries, which have been reported to have several beneficial effects including an extension of life span.[9–11]

With respect to curcumin's effects as a modulator of HS response, previous studies on C6 rat glioma cells had shown that curcumin doses (up to 30 μM) increased the levels of hsp27, hsp70, and αB crystallin.[5] Furthermore, it was shown that proteasome inhibition induced hsp70 and hsp27 expression in mouse embryonic fibroblasts (MEF) cells immortalized by SV-40 transfection.[12] We have also observed in mid-passage human keratinocytes that the synthesis of hsp70 and hsp90, but not of hsp27, was enhanced after preincubation at 43°C for 1 h followed by 24-h curcumin treatment. In this study, the 32% decrease in proteasome activity induced by 3 μM curcumin was accompanied with an increase in the levels of hsp70 and hsp90 by 24% and 19%, respectively. As previously discussed, it seems that the induction of hsp locks 20S proteasome in a latent inactive state and impairs further activation of the 26S proteasome by ATP.[13]

In conclusion, our studies have shown that curcumin modulates the HS response and proteasome activity in cultured human keratinocytes in a biphasic hormetic manner. Thus, curcumin may be a useful "hormetin" as a natural food component by enhancing protective stress response and by stimulating proteasome-mediated removal of abnormal proteins during aging. Further studies are in progress to determine the mechanism of curcumin's hormetic effects on human cells undergoing aging *in vivo*.

ACKNOWLEDGMENTS

David C. Kraft is acknowledged for his help in the proteasome assay. Ulrich Berge and Regina Gonzalez-Dosal are acknowledged for useful discussions. Thanks are extended to Anna Gylling, Helle Jackobsen, and Gunhild Siboska for expert technical assistance. The Laboratory of Cellular Ageing is supported by research grants from The Danish Research Councils, Carlsberg Fund, Senetek PLC, and EU's Biomed Health Programmes.

REFERENCES

1. ARAÚJO, C.A.C. & L.L. LEON. 2001. Biological activities of *Curcuma longa*. Mem. Inst. Oswaldo Cruz. **96:** 723–728.
2. MIQUEL, J., A. BERND, J.M. SEMPERE, *et al.* 2002. The curcuma antioxidants: pharmacological effects and prospects for future clinical use. Arch. Gerontol. Geriatr. **34:** 37–46.
3. JOE, B., M. VIJAYKUMAR & B.R. LOKESH. 2004. Biological properties of curcumin: cellular and molecular mechanisms of action. Crit. Rev. Food Sci. Nutr. **44:** 97–111.
4. DUNSMORE, K.E., P.G. CHEN & H.R. WONG. 2001. Curcumin, a medicinal herbal compound capable of inducing the heat shock response. Crit. Care Med. **29:** 2199–2204.
5. KATO, K., H. ITO, K. KAMEI, *et al.* 1998. Stimulation of the stress-induced expression of stress proteins by curcumin in cultured cells and in rat tissues in vivo. Cell Stress Chaperones **3:** 152–160.
6. JANA, N.R., P. DIKSHIT, A. GOSWAMI, *et al.* 2004. Inhibition of proteasomal function by curcumin induces apoptosis through mitochondrial pathway. J. Biol. Chem. **279:** 11680–11685.
7. BUSH, K.T., A.L. GOLDBERG & S.K. NIGAM. 1997. Proteasome inhibition leads to a heat-shock response, induction of endoplasmic reticulum chaperones, and thermotolerance. J. Biol. Chem. **272:** 9086–9090.
8. IRESON, C., S. ORR & D.J.L. JONES. 2001. Characterization of metabolites of the chemopreventive agent curcumin in human and rat hepatocytes and in the rat *in vivo*, and evaluation of their ability to inhibit phorbol ester-induced prostaglandin E2 production. Cancer Res. **61:** 1058–1064.
9. CALABRESE, E.J. & L.A. BALDWIN. 2001. U-shaped dose-responses in biology, toxicology, and public health. Annu. Rev. Public Health **22:** 15–33.
10. RATTAN, S.I.S. 2004. Aging intervention, prevention, and therapy through hormesis. J. Gerontol. Biol. Sci. **59A:** 705–709.

11. RATTAN, S.I.S. 2005. Anti-ageing strategies: prevention or therapy? EMBO Rep. **6:** S25–S29.

12. KIM, D., S.H. KIM & G.C. LI. 1999. Proteasome inhibitors MG 132 and lactacystin hyperphosphorylate HSF1 and induce hsp70 and hsp27 expression. Biochem. Biophys. Res. Commun. **254:** 264–268.

13. KUCKELKORN, U., C. KNUEHI, B. BOES-FABIAN, *et al*. 2000. The effect of heat shock on 20S/26S proteasomes. Biol. Chem. **381:** 1017–1023.

Nutraceutical Supplementation: Effect of a Fermented Papaya Preparation on Redox Status and DNA Damage in Healthy Elderly Individuals and Relationship with GSTM1 Genotype

A Randomized, Placebo-Controlled, Cross-Over Study

FRANCESO MAROTTA,[a,e] MARK WEKSLER,[b] YASUHIRO NAITO,[c] CHISATO YOSHIDA,[d] MAYUMI YOSHIOKA,[c] AND PAOLO MARANDOLA[e]

[a] HepatoGastroenterology Unit, S. Giuseppe Hospital, Milano, Italy

[b] Geriatrics Department, Cornell University Medical Center, New York, USA

[c] Immunology Research Institute and Clinic, Nagoya, Japan

[d] GAIA, Age-Management Foundation, Pavia, Italy

[e] ORI Bioscience Laboratory, Gifu, Japan

ABSTRACT: Our study group consisted of 54 elderly patients without major invalidating diseases who were randomly divided into two fully matched groups. Group A was given a certified fermented papaya preparation 9 g/day by mouth, while group B received placebo. Treatment was carried out in a cross-over manner with a 3-month supplementation followed by a 6-week washout period. Blood samples were drawn at entry and on a monthly basis to check routine parameters, redox status, and 8-OHdG in circulating leukocyte DNA. Polymorphism analysis of GSTM1 was carried out as well. The glutathune-S transferase M1 (GSTM1) genotype was null (−) in 40% and 46% of groups A and B, respectively. GSTM1 (−) smokers had a significantly higher level of plasma DNA adducts and leukocytes level of 8-OHdG than their GSTM1 (+) counterparts ($P < 0.01$). There was a weak correlation between cigarettes smoked/day and DNA adduct (r: 0.61, $P < 0.05$), which also correlated with antioxidant concentrations, but only in GSTM1 (−) smokers ($P < 0.01$). The fermented papaya preparation (FPP)–supplemented group showed a significant enhancement of the antioxidant protection ($P <$

Address for correspondence: F. Marotta, via Pisanello, 4-20146, Milano, Italy.
e-mail: fmarchimede@libero.it

Ann. N.Y. Acad. Sci. 1067: 400–407 (2006). © 2006 New York Academy of Sciences.
doi: 10.1196/annals.1354.057

0.01 vs. A) within the subgroups with GSTM1 ($-$) and of plasma DNA adduct, irrespective of the GSTM1 genotype. Only the GSTM1 ($-$) subgroup was the one that, under FPP treatment, increased lymphocyte 8-OHdG ($P < 0.01$). Such preliminary data show that FPP is a promising nutraceutical for improving antioxidant-defense in elderly patients even without any overt antioxidant-deficiency state while helping explain some inconsistent results of prior interventional studies.

KEYWORDS: GSTM1; redox status; elderly; fermented papaya; 8-OHdG

INTRODUCTION

Reactive oxygen species have been implicated in the pathogenesis of many chronic diseases since they may cause a different degree of damage to DNA other biological molecules. Such DNA damage can account for the genetic changes that take place along with the progression from dysplastic lesions to precancerous lesions and, eventually, to anaplastic cancerous growth and metastatic dissemination. On the other hand, it is known that, even without any overt disease, oxidative damage to DNA, proteins, and lipids accumulates with age and contributes to degenerative diseases and aging phenomena by disrupting cellular homeostasis.[1] Moreover, this population is more prone to depleted antioxidant defenses on account of poor/improper intake, while a number of elderly may concomitantly suffer from a subclinically impaired gut absorption ability. In this respect, a study conducted among 490 geriatric patients has showed that more than 40% had indeed an occult malabsorption.[2] To make the field of interventional nutrition even more complex, although intriguing, the post-genomic era has opened new avenues in the study of specific genotype-modulated understanding of the interrelationships between food, food components, and xenobiotic exposure with each single individual response. As an example, quite interestingly, Palli *et al.*[3] have recently suggested that the effect of dietary antioxidants in reducing DNA adducts is dependent on the detoxifying activity of the GSTM1 isoenzyme. This finding is of great practical relevance and may help explain some contradictory or inconclusive results of studies tackling the issue of antioxidants and genomic abnormalities when considering that GSTM1 gene deficiency has been shown to occur in approximately half of the population of various ethnic origins, mostly Caucasian, Japanese, and white Americans. GSTM1 deficiency has been shown to increase DNA adduct formation[4] and cytogenetic damage.[5] Indeed, the glutathione S-transferases (GST) represent a crucial enzymatic system of the cellular mechanism of detoxification by protecting cells against reactive oxygen metabolites by means of the conjugation of glutathione with electrophilic compounds. GST enzymes are involved in the metabolism of xenobiotics that include environmental carcinogens, reactive oxygen species, and chemotherapeutic agents.[6] Associations of GSTM1 and/or GSTT1 null genotypes with bladder, lung, and colorectal cancer, as well as head and neck squamous cell carcinoma, have been reported and represent an area of growing intensive research.[7–10]

The aim of the present study was to test in a healthy elderly population the effects of a novel nutraceutical on redox status abnormalities that are likely to take place with advancing age. A number of bench-validated studies of this compound have proved its potent antioxidant and NO-stimulating properties. Moreover, we aimed to get further insights into the role played by GSTM1 genotype status.

PATIENTS AND METHODS

Our study group consisted of 60 generally elderly persons (mean age: 72 years, range 72–84 years; male/female: 36/24). Major invalidating disease that were regarded as exclusion criteria were: prior or ongoing cancer, autoimmune disease, chronic illness requiring steroids or immunosuppressive agents, allopurinol treatment, chronic renal failure, and overt cardio-respiratory abnormality. Thirteen patients (male/female: 9:2) were mild smokers (<10 cigarette/day), 9 were treated for mild hypertension, 10 for osteoporosis, 11 for insomnia, and 4 for mild depression. The patients were randomly divided into two groups matched for age/gender, life style, alcohol/tobacco use, physical activity, and medication. One group was given a GMP-, ISO9001/14000-certified fermented papaya preparation (FPP, Osato Research Institute, Gifu, Japan; 9 g/day) by mouth in the morning, 1 h after breakfast, and fasting for at least a further 30 min, while the control group received the same amount of placebo (flavored powdered sugar). The treatment was carried out in a cross-over manner with a 3-month supplementation period followed by a 6-week washout period between treatments.

As an age-control group for redox status, a group of 10 young/early middle-age healthy nonsmoking patients were also considered.

Diet and Life Style Questionnaire

A detailed life style questionnaire was administered to all patients with particular attention paid to stress factors and physical activity. Moreover, a dietary questionnaire was used, and specific care taken in assessing the daily dietary content of macronutrients and micronutrients. This was re-assessed at the end of the study using the model of 7-day diet history.

Blood Collection and Storage

Blood samples were drawn at entry and on a monthly basis. Studies related to genetic susceptibility were carried out only at entry and at the end of the study.

Assessment of Redox Status

GSH, GSH-Px, and GSSG were measured by means of hemoglobin-catalyzed oxidation of 10-*N*-methylcarmoyl-3,7-dimethylamino-10-H-phenothiazione after treatment with phospholipase. Values were read by a fluorescence detector.

Determination of Plasma Malondialdehyde

Malondialdehyde was measured from frozen, EDTA-containing plasma after thiobarbituric acid (TBA) reaction by high-performance liquid chromatography (HPLC) modified by adding 0.01% butylated-hydroxytoluene to the coloring solution to avoid the generation of TBA-reactive molecules during the procedure. The system was heated at 100°C for 45 min. After cooling, the chromophore was extracted with 2 mL of *N*-butanol by vigorous shaking and dried under constant nitrogen flux. The final powder was resuspended in 100 μL of chromatographic solvent A and added to the HPLC system (solvent A: 10 mmol hexate sulfonic acid and H_3PO_4 adjusted to pH 3; solvent B; methanol). Tetra-ethoxy-propane served as a standard source of malonyldialdehyde (MDA), which is a thiobarbituric acid–reactant substance. All samples were processed in duplicate.

Analysis of 8-OHdG in Circulating Leukocyte DNA

DNA was isolated and purified from leukocytes as described by Fraga *et al.*[11] with minor modifications. The resulting deoxynucleoside mixture was analyzed by means of a HPLC-electrochemical detection (ECD) system and the amounts of 8-OHdG were referred to the quantities of deoxyguanosine detected, in the same sample, by ultraviolet absorbance. The results are expressed as the ratio of the absorbance peak of 8-oxodGuo adducts to that of dGuo adducts $\times 10^5$.

Polymorphism Analysis

This was conducted by the multiple polymerase chain reaction (PCR) method to check the presence of GSTM1 gene in genomic DNA samples. PCR analysis was performed in 25 μL reaction buffer containing 0.5 mmol/L of dNTPs, 2.0 mmol/L of $MgCl_2$, 12.5 pmol of each primer, about 150 ng DNA, and 1.25 U of thermostable Taq DNA polymerase, using a programmable thermocycler. The primers used for GSTM1 were 5′-GAACTCCCTGAAAAGCTAAGC and 5′-GTTGGGGCTCAAATATACGGTGG. The PCR protocol included an initial melting temperature set at 94°C for a 5-min period followed by 35 cycles of amplification (with the apparatus set as follows: 2 min at 94°C, 1 min at 59°C, and extension for 1 min at 72°C). A final 10-min extension step processed at 72°C terminated the process. The final PCR product from co-amplification of GSTM1 (215 bp) was visualized on an ethidium bromide–stained 2.0% agarose gel. The subjects were accordingly classified as either positive (when at least one copy of the gene was present) or null genotypes. The genotype of DNA samples was identified blindly and controls were prepared and set up in association with every single PCR operation as blank control (without DNA template), positive control, and negative control.

Statistics

Data were evaluated by repeated-measures analysis of variance and independent t-tests with a Bonferroni correction for multiple comparisons.

RESULTS

Six participants were excluded during the study for a number of reasons that could theoretically interfere with the understanding of the final data (two participants had flu [complicated in one by transient asthma] and both required drug treatment, one was enrolled in an intensive gym regimen, one moved away, one was hospitalized for an uneventful diverticulitis, and another dropped out spontaneously). As expected, no side effect was reported by participants completing the study beyond a subjective feeling of wellness and mood stabilization. However, such clinical signs were outside the aim of our designed protocol. Elderly patients showed a normal level of the all antioxidants tested, the only abnormalities being a significantly higher level of plasma MDA as well as lower GSH/GSSG ratio ($P < 0.05$ vs. young/middle-age group). At the entry, before the cross-over shift, the two elderly groups proved to be comparable in terms of GSTM1 genotype, which ranged between 40% and 46%. A further finding was that, at baseline assessment, as compared to GSTM1-positive smoker participants, the GSTM1-negative counterpart showed a significantly higher level of DNA adducts (1.8 vs 2.7×10^8 nucleotides, $P < 0.01$) and of 8-OhdG concentration (72 vs 88×10^5 dG, $P < 0.01$) in leukocyte DNA. Moreover, a weak but significant correlation appeared between cigarettes smoked per day and DNA adducts (r: 0.61, $P < 0.05$), but the intrinsic limitation of these data is that a larger number of participants are required. Within the GSTM1-negative smoker subgroup, DNA adducts correlated with MDA and GSH/GSSG ratio (r: 0.78, $P < 0.01$). FPP brought about a trend in improvement of oxidative/antioxidative balance, but this reached statistical significance only in the GSTM1-negative subgroup, irrespective of smoking ($P < 0.01$). Such results were also confirmed when smokers were excluded from the analysis. Similar protective effects on leukocyte DNA adducts ($P < 0.05$) were obtained when

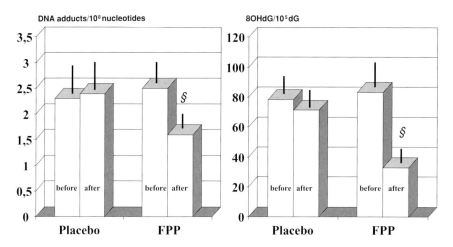

FIGURE 1. *Left:* concentration of DNA adducts in all subjects and of 8-OHdG in circulating leukocytes (only in GSTM1–subjects). *Right:* effect of nutraceutical intervention. $^{\S}P < 0.05$ vs. baseline and vs. placebo.

considered subject as a whole (FIG. 1). These data were paralleled by a significant decrease in leukocyte 8-OhdG concentration, but only when considering GSTM1-negative participants (FIG. 1).

DISCUSSION

Although redox status imbalance is well recognized as an adverse factor in a large number of chronic degenerative diseases and aging, the question still remains as to whether antioxidant supplementations are beneficial if they are to be regarded as potential therapeutic tools (nutraceuticals/nutrigenomics). Indeed, one of the major drawbacks in any supplementation study is the limited population and/or observation time. Moreover, a further limitation in evaluating the clinical impact of epidemiologic and/or interventional studies dealing with antioxidants is represented by the questionable appropriateness of suitable markers of oxidative injury *in vivo*.[12] Among the most convincing evidence of the role of oxidative stress and protection by antioxidants in the disease process is provided by studies conducted in patients with heart diseases.[13] On the other hand, it is becoming all the more important to distinguish the role of oxidants as mediators of disease as well as crucial elements of signal transduct ion pathways.[14] The post-genomic revolution with the study of polymorphisms thus offers unprecedented opportunities to ideally unfold, tailor, and monitor the impact of diet and dietary components with cell signaling/function in physiological and pathologic situations. As a consequence, the design of nutritional studies becomes even more demanding, but with far-reaching expectations. In the present study, among the multifaceted scenarios of polymorphisms, we chose GSTM1 because of its high frequency, which may allow a smaller study sample. Having started from an experimentally and clinically supported nutraceutical,[15–19] we showed that it could significantly improve the oxidative/antioxidative balance that was found to be impaired in elderly people, even in the absence of any overt inflammatory disease. The genetic susceptibility to oxidative stress, as assessed by GSTM1 analysis, further enhanced this result, whereas smokers might prove to get the highest benefit from FPP supplementation. Interestingly, FPP appeared to exert protective effects on leukocyte DNA adducts' formation, irrespective of genotype profile, while also enhancing DNA repair mechanisms against the highly mutagenic base modification, but only in GSTM1-null genotype participants. Although the fundamental epigenetic mechanisms of action of FPP are still a matter of ongoing investigation, and no conclusions can be drawn in the relevance of its beneficial effects on the natural history of the studied population in the long run, the present promising data suggest that there is indeed a role for nutraceutical intervention when supported by proper protocol design and mandatorily bench-validated natural compounds.

REFERENCES

1. SOHAL, R.S. & W.C. ORR. 1995. Is oxidative stress a causal factor in aging? *In* Molecular Aspects of Aging. K. Esser G.M. Martin, Eds.: 109–127. Wiley and Sons. Chichester.

2. HABOUBI, N.Y. & R.D. MONTGOMERY. 1992. Small-bowel bacterial overgrowth in elderly people: clinical significance and response to treatment. Age Ageing **21:** 13–19.

3. PALLI, D., G. MASALA, M. PELUSO, *et al.* 2004. The effect of diet on DNA bulky adducts levels are strongly are strongly modified by GSTM1 genotype: a study on 634 subjects. Carcinogenesis **25:** 1–8.

4. KATO, S., E.D. BOWMAN, A.M. HARRINGTON, *et al.* 1995. Human lung carcinogen-DNA adduct levels mediated by genetic polymorphisms in vivo. J. Natl. Cancer Inst. **87:** 902–907.

5. VAN POPPEL, G., N. DE VOGEL, P. VAN BALDEREN, *et al.* 1992. Increased cytogenetic damage in smokers deficient in glutathione S-transferase isozyme mu. Carcinogenesis (Lond.) **13:** 303–305.

6. AWASTHI, Y.C., R. SHARMA & S.S. SINGHAL. 1994. Human glutathione S-transferases: minireview. Int. J. Biochem. **26:** 295–308.

7. LANDI, S. 2000. Mammalian class theta GST and differential susceptibility to carcinogens: a review. Mut. Res. **463:** 247–283.

8. RESZKA, E. & W. WASOWICZ. 2001. Significance of genetic polymorphisms in glutathione S-transferase multigene family and lung cancer risk. Int. J. Occup. Med. Environ. Health **14:** 99–113.

9. ENGEL, L.S., E. TAIOLI, R. PFEIFFER, *et al.* 2002. Pooled analysis and meta-analysis of glutathione S-transferase M1 and bladder cancer: a HuGE review. Am. J. Epidemiol. **156:** 95–109.

10. COTTON, S.C., L. SHARP, J. LITTLE, *et al.* 2000. Glutathione S-transferase polymorphisms and colorectal cancer: a HuGE review. Am. J. Epidemiol. **151:** 7–32.
11. FRAGA, C.G., J. ONUKI, F. LUCESOLI, *et al.* 1994. 5-Aminolevulinic acid mediates the *in vivo* and *in vitro* formation of 8-hydroxy-2′-deoxyguanosine in DNA. Carcinogenesis **15:** 2241–2244.
12. WÜNSCH FILHO, V. & G.J.F. GATTÁS. 2001. Molecular biomarkers in cancer: implications for epidemiological research and public health. Cadernos de Saúde Pública **17:** 467–480.
13. MCCALL, M.R. & B. FREI. 1999. Can antioxidant vitamins materially reduce oxidative damage in humans? Free Radic. Biol. Med. **6:** 1034–1053.
14. ABE, J. & B.C. BERK. 1988. Reactive oxygen species as mediators of signal transduction in cardiovascular disease. Trends Cardiovasc. Med. **8:** 59–64.
15. RIMBACH, G., Y.C. PARK, Q. GUO, *et al.* 2000. Nitric oxide synthesis and TNF-alpha secretion in RAW 264.7 macrophages: mode of action of a fermented papaya preparation. Life Sci. **67:** 679–694.
16. RIMBACH, G., Q. GUO, T. AKIYAMA, *et al.* 2000. Ferric nitrilotriacetate induced DNA and protein damage: inhibitory effect of a fermented papaya preparation. Anticancer Res. **20:** 2907–2014.
17. COLOGNATO, R., I. FONTANA, F. COPPEDÉ, *et al.* Modulation of the hydrogen peroxide induced DNA damage and cell death in PC12 cells by papaya extract and ergothioneine. Mut. Res. Accepted for publication.
18. MAROTTA, F., R. BARRETO, H. TAJIRI, *et al.* 2004. The aging/precancerous gastric mucosa: a pilot nutraceutical trial. Ann. N. Y. Acad. Sci. **1019:** 195–199.
19. MORI, A., I. YOKOI, Y. NODA & L. J. WILLMORE. 2004. Natural antioxidants may prevent posttraumatic epilepsy; a proposal based on experimental animal studies. Acta Med. Okayama **3:** 111–118.

Redox Status Impairment in Liver and Kidney of Prematurely Senescent Mice

Effectiveness of DTS Phytotherapeutic Compound

F. MAROTTA,[a,d] F. LORENZETTI,[d] M. HARADA,[b] S. K. ONO-NITA,[c] E. MINELLI,[a] AND P. MARANDOLA[d]

[a] WHO-Center for Biotechnology and Traditional Medicine, University of Milano, Milan, Italy

[b] MCH Hospital, Tokyo, Japan

[c] Hepato-Gastroenterology Department, Sao Paulo University, Sao Paulo, Brazil

[d] A. Scarpa-G.A.I.A. Age-Management Foundation, Pavia, Italy

ABSTRACT: T-maze test–selected prematurely senescent mice (PSM) were allocated into two groups: (A) those given DTS (150 mg/kg) orally for 30 days and (B) untreated PSM with age-matched fast T-maze performers as control. After sacrifice, the liver and kidney were analyzed for catalase (CAT) activity, glutathione peroxidase (GPx), superoxide dismutase (SOD), malondyaldehyde (MDA), and plasma thiols. Untreated PSM showed decreased plasma thiols and tissue level of CAT, SOD, GPx, with higher MDA ($P < 0.01$ vs. fast performers), while DTS (Denshichi–Tochiu–Sen) significantly improved glutathione and cysteine ($P < 0.05$) and tissue concentration of the above parameters ($P < 0.05$). Such preliminary data suggest that DTS mitigated oxidative damage in PSM, with likely action on the cytoplasm and mitochondrial matrix.

KEYWORDS: prematurely senescent mice; oxidative stress; DTS

INTRODUCTION

The aging process is associated with a decrease in protein-bound thiol levels and their related antioxidant capacity, with oxidative modification of DNA, proteins, lipids, and small cellular molecules by reactive oxygen species (ROS). In particular, thiol compounds (cysteine 80%, glutathione 17%, and homocysteine 2–3%) have a relevant role as key factors in regulating the intracellular

Address for correspondence: Prof. F. Marotta, M.D., Ph.D., via Pisanello, 4, 20146 Milano, Italy. Voice and fax: +39-0240 77243.
e-mail: fmarchimede@libero.it

Ann. N.Y. Acad. Sci. 1067: 408–413 (2006). © 2006 New York Academy of Sciences.
doi: 10.1196/annals.1354.058

and extracellular redox buffer capacity. Decreased tissue GSH levels are also associated with depressed immunity and the progression of aging, and it may also increase the risk of cancer development. Recently, De la Fuente *et al.*[1] using the T-maze test as a clear-cut parameter, have shown that some mice express overt features of premature aging with immunologic impairment and a shorter life span when compared to their age-matched fast-performing counterparts. The aim of this study was to apply the same methodology in Balb-c mice to test a novel nutraceutical that was shown in preliminary in-house experiments to be endowed with significant antioxidative/anti-inflammatory effects in agreement with the literature.[2–6]

MATERIALS AND METHODS

Balb-c mice (25–30 g) were bred under conventional conditions, housed in a pathogen-free environment at $23 \pm 1°C$ with an alternating 12-h light/dark cycle and supplied food and water *ad libitum*. At 70 weeks of age, the T-maze test was performed once a week for 4 weeks and prematurely senescent mice (PSM) were regarded as those animals that failed at all times to complete the test within the maximum allotted time (60 s). Animals with intermediate performances were excluded so as to obtain a "fast" and a "slow" group, containing 100% and 0%, respectively. Altogether, 28 PSM and 26 non-prematurely senescent mice (NPSM) were chosen. PSM were allocated into two groups: Group A: fed standard food for 4 weeks; Group B: fed standard food added with DTS (*Panax pseudoginseng*, *Eucommia ulmoides*, ginseng radix, kindly donated by the Institute of Health Care Oriental Herbs and Medicine, Tokyo, Japan) 150 mg/kg of body weight daily. After a 4-week supplementation study, the liver and kidney were quickly removed and tissues were kept at $-80°C$ until analysis. A part of the tissues was used to separate the cytosolic and mitochondrial fraction by means of a standard methodology used to measure SOD.

Preparation of Phytotherapeutic Compound

DTS, which is produced under quality-controlled procedures and ISO 9001 and 140001 regulation, was kindly donated by the Institute of Health Care with Oriental Herbs and Medicine, Tokyo, Japan. This compound presents in the form of tiny grains of medium consistency and is palatable and can be easily mixed with food.

Plasma Analysis

The total thiol levels as well as their free and protein-bound fractions were measured by high-performance liquid chromatography (HPLC) after pre-column derivatization with 2-chloro-1-methylquinolinium tetrafluorobo-rate and the samples were reduced with sodium borohydride.

Liver and Kidney Tissue Analysis

Catalase activity was determined at 240 nm by measuring the rate of H_2O_2 utilization with the molar extinction coefficient for H_2O_2 being 43.6 M/cm. The amount of the enzyme utilizing 1 μmol H_2O_2/min was taken as one activity unit.

Glutathione peroxidase (GPx) activity was determined at 340 nm by spec-trophotometry and the amount of the enzyme converting 1 μmol GSH/min was taken as one activity unit.

Glutathione reductase activity was measured at 340 nm by spectrophotom-etry and the amount of the enzyme reducing 1 μmol GSSG/min was taken as one activity unit.

Superoxide dismutase activity (SOD) was measured at 560 nm as the rate of reduction of nitrotetrazolium blue and for one unit of activity, the amount of protein was taken, which provided a 50% inhibition of nitrotetrazolium blue reduction under standard conditions.

Malondyaldehyde Determination

Malondyaldehyde (MDA) in liver and kidney tissues was assayed by spec-trophotometric measurement and the concentration of thiobarbituric acid was calculated by the absorbance coefficient of MDA–TBA complex and expressed as nmol/mL.

Statistical Evaluation

For statistical analyses, normality was investigated first, and it was shown that some values of the parameters did not fit the normal distribution. There-fore, the nonparametric Kruskal-Wallis test and Mann-Whitney U test were used to compare groups.

RESULTS

Plasma Thiol Analysis

As compared to age-matched mice, NPSM mice showed a statistically sig-nificant decreased level of total plasma level of thiols (a decrease of 30–33%, $P < 0.01$), which affected all the separate components of thiol (data not shown). DTS administration yielded a partial (17–23% increase) but signifi-cant improvement of this parameter ($P < 0.05$ vs NPSM) and further analysis identified glutathione and cysteine as the thiol components, which significantly improved (data not shown). The free/bound thiol ratio showed that PSM mice had a statistically higher ratio ($P < 0.05$ vs. NPSM), and this parameter was not influenced by DTS treatment.

Liver and Kidney Tissue Analysis

The activity of antioxidant enzymes did not show any difference when testing the cytosolic fraction of both tissues. As compared to NPSM, PSM showed a number of significant modifications ($P < 0.01$), that is, a decrease of GSH (μmol/g tissue: 4.7 ± 0.02 vs. 5.4 ± 0.02 in liver; 2.9 ± 0.09 vs. 4.1 ± 0.04 in kidney), of GSH-Px (U/mg protein: 148 ± 7.3 vs. 163 ± 8.3 in liver; 135 ± 3.6 vs. 168 ± 5.7 in kidney) and of GSH/GSSG ratio (25–40% in both tissues). DTS administration yielded a partial but significant ($P < 0.05$) improvement of these parameters and a normalization of GSH redox, expressed as GSH redox $GSSG/(GSH + GSSG) \times 100$ ($P < 0.05$). As shown in TABLE 1, besides kidney SOD, the tested oxidative/antioxidative parameters were improved by DTS administration ($P < 0.05$). Subcellular analysis revealed that while cytosol SOD was unaltered in PSM, the mitochondrial compartment was significantly ($P < 0.01$) depleted in both tested tissues (units/mg protein: 7.4 ± 2.7 vs. 12.6 ± 1.4 in liver; 6.5 ± 1.0 vs. 10.6 ± 0.9 in kidney). Both parameters were partially improved by DTS (units/mg protein: 11.2 ± 1.1 and 9.8 ± 0.7, respectively, $P < 0.05$).

CONCLUSION

Aging is associated with a decrease in the level of the most relevant antioxidant, glutathione, and of cysteine, which can be a result of both an elevated

TABLE 1. Effect of DTS on catalase, SOD, and MDA in control and PSM mice

Group	Catalase U/mg protein	SOD U/mg protein	MDA nmol/mg protein
	Liver		
NPSM/Balb-c	276 ± 6.4	25.6 ± 3.32	55 ± 55
PSM			
Untreated	$255 \pm 5.8^*$	24.7 ± 2.82	$0.83 \pm 0.06^*$
+ DTS	$271 \pm 5.8^{**}$	24.9 ± 2.01	$0.62 \pm 0.02^{**}$
	Kidney		
NPSM/Balb-c	187 ± 6.9	18.9 ± 2.66	0.21 ± 0.01
PSM			
Untreated	$164 \pm 4.1^*$	$16.4 \pm 3.21^*$	$0.32 \pm 0.03^*$
+ DTS	$171 \pm 5.1^*$	$18.0 \pm 3.42^{**}$	$0.26 \pm 0.02^{**}$

$^*P < 0.01$ vs. NPSM; $^{**}P < 0.05$ vs. untreated PSM.

demand and inhibited GSH biosynthesis. In particular, glutathione is an important defense mechanism in living cells and, as a substrate for the antioxidant enzyme glutahione peroxidase, GSH protects cellular constituents from the damaging effects of peroxides formed by metabolism and through other ROS reactions. Thus, a change in the thiol:disulfide ratio (i.e., an alteration of the thiols redox status), significantly affects the morphology and function of cellular and extracellular proteins. By applying previously described selection criteria to detect mice with prematurely aging features,[1] we found that such animals have a defective redox status due to an unbalanced enzymatic antioxidant apparatus. Although specific immunologic deficits have been shown in these animals,[1] the damaging effects on cellular macromolecules and functions by such sustained oxidative stress are likely to argue for a further mechanism for explaining their defective behavioral responses and life span. On the other hand, the same group[7] has shown that an antioxidant intervention with thioproline or N-acetylcysteine would significantly improve the immunologic function in such animals. Nonetheless, the observed increased level of endogenous GSH together with the decrease of GSH redox ratio, which represents the degree of H_2O_2 generation, when PSM were given DTS suggest that this nutraceutical might act directly on the regulation of GSH/GSSG redox status while also increasing glutathione reductase activity. In particular, the mitochondrial SOD fraction was significantly improved. Interestingly, although outside the aim of this study, it has been shown that some saponins contained in DTS might exert beneficial immunologic effects and potent anti-inflammatory properties.[8,9] While senescence-accelerated mice represent a valuable source of investigations in aging research, the present model in normal strain animals may provide useful insights into the "physiological" aging process that is potentially amenable to clinically oriented therapeutic interventions. While more detailed studies on the mechanisms of action of DTS are in progress, given its inner components' variety as well,[10] DTS seems a promising nutraceutical in old age.

REFERENCES

1. DE LA FUENTE, M., M. MIÑANO, V.M. VICTOR, et al. 1998. Relation between exploratory activity and immune function in aged mice: a preliminary study. Mech. Ageing Dev. **102:** 263–277.
2. HSIEH, C.L. & G.C. YEN. 2000. Antioxidant actions of Du-Zhong (*Eucommia ulmoides* oliv.) towards oxidative damage in biomolecules. Life Sci. **66:** 1387–1400.
3. KEUM, Y.S., K.K. PARK, J.M. LEE, et al. 2000. Antioxidant and anti-tumor promoting activities of the methanol extract of heat-processed ginseng. Cancer Lett. **150:** 41–48.
4. KONOVALOVA, G.G., A.K. TIKHASE & V.Z. LANKIN. 2000. Antioxidant activity of parapharmaceutics containing natural inhibitors of free radicals. Bull. Exp. Biol. Med. **130:** 658–660.

5. CHAN, P., C.S. NIU, B. TOMLINSON, *et al*. 1997. Effect of trilinolein on superoxide dismutase activity and left ventricular pressure in isolated rat hearts subjected to hypoxia and normoxic perfusion. Pharmacology **55:** 252–258.
6. NG, T.B., F. LIU & H.X. WANG. 2004. The antioxidant effects of aqueous and organic extracts of *Panax quinquefolium*, *Panax notoginseng*, *Codonopsis pilosula*, *Pseudostellaria heterophylla* and *Glehnia littoralis*. J. Ethnopharmacol. **93:** 285–288.
7. GUAYERBAS, N., M. PUERTO, M.D. FERRANDEZ, *et al*. 2002. A diet supplemented with thiolic anti-oxidants improves leucocyte function in two strains of prematurely ageing mice. Clin. Exp. Pharmacol. Physiol. **29:** 1009–1014.
8. YOSHIKAWA, M., T. MORIKAWA, K. YASHIRO, *et al*. 2001. Bioactive saponins and glycosides. XIX. Notoginseng (3): immunological adjuvant activity of notoginsenosides and related saponins: structures of notoginsenosides-L, -M, and -N from the roots of *Panax notoginseng* (Burk.) F. H. Chen. Chem. Pharm. Bull. (Tokyo) **49:** 1452–1456.
9. ZHANG, Y., Q.F. YE, L. LU, *et al*. 2005. *Panax notoginseng* saponins preconditioning protects rat liver grafts from ischemia/reperfusion injury via an antiapoptotic pathway. Hepatobiliary Pancreat. Dis. Int. **4:** 207–212.
10. LI, L., J.L. ZHANG, Y.X. SHENG, *et al*. 2005. Simultaneous quantification of six major active saponins of *Panax notoginseng* by high-performance liquid chromatography-UV method. J. Pharm. Biomed. Anal. **38:** 45–51.

A Dietary Supplement Improves Outcome in an Experimental Influenza Model in Old Mice

J. CERVI,[a] F. MAROTTA,[b] C. BATER,[a] K. MASULAIR,[a] E. MINELLI,[b] M. HARADA,[c] AND P. MARANDOLA[d]

[a]SFJO Labs, Paris, France

[b]WHO-Center for Traditional Medicine, Milan University, Milan, Italy

[c]MCH Hospital, Tokyo, Japan

[d]GAIA, Age-Management Foundation, Pavia, Italy

ABSTRACT: Twenty-month-old Swiss mice were allocated into three groups: (A) control; (B) infected group; and (C) infected but treated with 5 mg of the phytocompound MMT. Mice were infected intranasally with 30 μL of 75 HA viral units. MMT markedly blunted the nasal signs of virus infection and the febrile response. Formazan-positive cells, lung and plasma lipoperoxides, and TNF-α in lung tissue increased during viral infection, but improvement was seen in the MMT-treated group ($P < 0.05$). MMT also normalized SOD, catalase activities, and ascorbic acid and determined a significant decrease of lung but not nasal viral titer, although nasal inflammatory infiltrate dropped significantly. MMT has potential clinical applications with and has an excellent safety profile even in old animals.

KEYWORDS: influenza model; old mice; TNF-alpha; RANTES; phytocompound

INTRODUCTION

The available options for the prevention and treatment of influenza and flu syndromes still have several limitations, especially in the elderly. Although inflammatory and oxidative phenomena seem to cause and perpetuate tissue injury in this condition, there are only scanty reports in the literature on the efficacy of antioxidants as therapeutic agents during an influenza virus infection. Thus, in the present study we tested a natural compound, MMT (Kyotsu Jigyo Inc., Tokyo, Japan), containing a number of herbal ingredients with known antioxidant and anti-inflammatory properties.[1–5]

Address for correspondence: Prof. F. Marotta, WHO-Center for Traditional Medicine, Milan University, Milan, Italy. Voice and fax: +39-0240 77243.
e-mail: fmarchimede@libero.it

Ann. N.Y. Acad. Sci. 1067: 414–419 (2006). © 2006 New York Academy of Sciences.
doi: 10.1196/annals.1354.059

MATERIALS AND METHODS

Experimental Design

Twenty-month-old Swiss mice (25–30 g) were housed and fed in a pathogen-free environment and were allocated into three groups: (A) healthy control; (B) infected group; and (C) MMT-treated infected group. Under ether anesthesia, mice were infected intranasally with 30 µL of 75 HA units of virus (A/Hong Kong/8/68 propagated in the allantoic fluid). The control group was given the same quantity of sterile allantoic fluid. The MMT group received 15 mg of a dietary supplement orally divided into three doses daily (MMT: ginger, *Strobilanthes cusia*, *Panax pseudoginseng*, *Eucommia ulmoides*, *Momordicae grosvenori*, licorice root, *Allium fistulosum*) from the day of inoculation till the day they were killed. Clinical signs of infection were observed throughout the study period, while total inflammatory cell counts in nasal washings, as well as virus titers in lung homogenates, were determined for 8 days.

Bronchoalveolar Lavage Fluid (BALF) Collection and Lung Tissue Storage

On the fourth day, BALF was collected and centrifuged to obtain a cell pellet. Quantitative analysis using real-time polymerase chain reaction (PCR) was also performed to determine regulated activation of normal T cell expressed and secreted (RANTES) and PCR products were quantified by densitometric analysis. Soon afterward, the rats were killed by cervical dislocation and the lungs were obtained after perfusion with cold PBS.

Assessment of Superoxide Radical Production

Cell suspensions were mixed with 50 µL of 0.2% nitroblue-tetrazolium (NBT) and after incubation were counterstained with Leishman's stain. Formazan-positive cells (F+) were blindly scored and all results in triplicate were expressed as the number of F+ cells per 200 cells.

Cellular and Biochemical Determination

1. Whole lungs were homogenized and supernatants were analyzed for ascorbate by high-performance liquid chromatography/electrochemical detection. TNF-α activity from tissue culture supernatants was assessed by quantitating cytolytic activity against the L929 target cell line. Plasma antioxidant status was studied by plasma malonyldialdehyde determination.

Toxicological Studies

A separate group of mice received once-daily doses of MMT (5–30 g/kg of body weight per day) or sterile water via oral gavage for 14 consecutive days, and signs of toxicity in 10 predefined tissues (brain, lungs, heart, liver, spleen, pancreas, stomach, small and large intestine, kidneys, bone marrow) were evaluated.

Statistical Analysis

Statistical comparisons between groups were made by "paired t test" and P values lower than 0.05 were accepted as statistically significant.

RESULTS

Infected mice developed a febrile response beginning about 12 h after infection and lasted approximately 48 h. Oral administration of MMT markedly blunted the nasal signs of viral infection as well as the decrease in motor activity and caused a 46% reduction in the area-under-the-curve measurement for the increase in body temperature over baseline values ($P < 0.05$ vs. untreated infected animals). Formazan-positive cells were increased by 80% during viral infection but decreased to 44% after supplementation ($P < 0.01$). Plasma SOD, catalase activities, and ascorbic acid were significantly decreased in the infected groups (9.8 ± 1.2, 23.7 ± 2.3, and 52.2 ± 8.2 vs. 14.2 ± 1.1, 29.7 ± 1.9, and 79.7 ± 7.9, respectively, $P < 0.05$); however, supplemented groups showed activities similar to those of the control group ($P < 0.05$). The levels of MDA in the lung extract and at the plasma level as well as of TNF-α in lung tissue significantly increased during viral infection when compared with the control group (>twofold and >sevenfold, respectively; $P < 0.01$ vs. healthy control). However, the supplementation with MMT enabled a significant reduction of all these parameters (nearly 50%, $P < 0.05$). Virus titer in the nasal wash rapidly increased 36 h after the virus inoculation and reached a maximum of 50% of tissue culture infective doses ($TCID_{50}$) on the third day of observation after infection (3.88 ± 0.33 $\log_{10}$ $TCID_{50}^s$/ml). MMT-treated animals did not show any significant difference. On the contrary, the total count of inflammatory cells in the nasal washing showed an early significant decrease that was maintained throughout the study period ($P < 0.05$). MMT was also found to yield a significant 37% reduction in either the expression or the production of RANTES in mice BAL-collected epithelial cells ($P < 0.05$ vs. untreated mice). Although viral activity in the lung homogenate was not as high as in the nasal washing, it significantly decreased in MMT-supplemented animals ($P < 0.05$ vs. untreated group, FIG. 1).

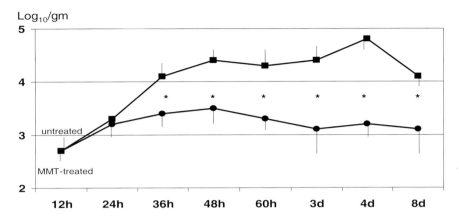

Log$_{10}$/gm

FIGURE 1. Lung virus titer in influenza model: effect of MMT (mean ± SD). *$P < 0.05$ vs. untreated mice

MMT Toxicology Tests

MMT, at dosages up to 30 g/kg/day (i.e., over 50-fold higher than needed to protect mice against the effects of influenza virus infection) was not associated with any drug-related toxicity.

DISCUSSION

Elderly patients who often have an immunocompromised status while taking multidrug prescriptions are known to be at a higher risk of complicated viral infections. Accumulation in the lung of neutrophils and macrophages could play a role in the development of the disease. Indeed, early studies have reported that influenza infection impairs the levels of endogenous concentration of vitamin E and glutathione[6] and an increase in the levels of xanthine oxidase.[7] Accordingly, in our study a significant increase of superoxide radical production together with a decrease of SOD and catalase occurred in the BAL pellets. This process was paralleled by an increase of MDA in the bloodstream and, in particular, in the lung. Lung homogenates also showed a decrease in ascorbic acid and an increase in TNF-α, which is known to trigger the recruitment of leukocytes by the expression of IL-8 and intracellular adhesion molecules. All the above phenomena were significantly prevented, either partially or totally, when the phytocompound MMT was added to the diet. Although the precise mechanism of each single component cannot be clarified at the moment, many of its ingredients have either anti-inflammatory or antioxidant properties.[1–5] Such properties, together with the anti-asthmatic effect exerted by the alk(en)ylsulfinothioic acid alk(en)yl-ester component of *Allium fistolosum*[8] might also help in explaining the symptomatic improvement of infected mice when administered MMT. As a matter of fact, dietary antioxidant deficiency can further impair the function of the lung immune system and vitamin E supplementation has been proven to improve Th1 cytokine production in influenza-infected mice.[9] Interestingly, MMT significantly decreased RANTES levels that are associated with a Th1-related immune response and this might have been the result of the inhibition of phosphorylation of the nuclear transcription NF-κB regulatory molecule IκB-α and the p38 MAP kinase, as recently suggested for one of MMT's ingredients.[10] Finally, while MMT did not alter the high virus titer in the nasal washing, it significantly decreased the viral load in the lung. One can speculate that, due to the lack of any specific antiviral activity, MMT could not interfere with the rapid viral growth into the nasal cavity soon after inoculation, although it decreased the local inflammatory cell recruitment. However, the improved endogenous and anti-inflammatory properties exerted at a systemic and lung level might have played a role in limiting viremia in the lungs. On the basis of the above experiment, it is suggested that a safe natural compound, that is, MMT, has the potential to be applied in clinical practice, while further studies are ongoing to elucidate its mechanism of action in more detail.

REFERENCES

1. HSIEH, C.L. & G.C. YEN. 2000. Antioxidant actions of Du-Zhong (*Eucommia ulmoides* oliv.) towards oxidative damage in biomolecules. Life Sci. **66:** 1387–1400.
2. KEUM, Y.S., K.K. PARK, J.M. LEE, *et al.* 2000. Antioxidant and anti-tumor promoting activities of the methanol extract of heat-processed ginseng. Cancer Lett. **150:** 41–48.
3. TERAO, J., M. HIWADA, K. TAGUCHI, *et al.* 2005. Glutathione peroxidase mimics as novel antioxidants from vegetables. Biofactors **23:** 1–6.
4. SHI, H., M. HIRAMATSU, M. KOMATSU, *et al.* 1996. Antioxidant property of *Fructus Momordicae* extract. Biochem. Mol. Biol. Int. **40:** 1111–1121.
5. CHAN, P. & B. TOMLINSON. 2000. Antioxidant effects of Chinese traditional medicine: focus on trilinolein isolated from the Chinese herb sanchi (*Panax pseudoginseng*). J. Clin. Pharmacol. **40:** 457–461.
6. HENNET, T., E. PETERHANS & R. STOCKER. 1992. Alterations in antioxidant defenses in the lung and liver of mice infected with influenza A virus. J. Gen. Virol. **73:** 39–46.
7. AKAIKE, T., M. ANDO, T. ODA, *et al.* 1990. Dependence of O_2 generation by xanthine oxidase of pathogenesis of influenza virus infection in mice. J. Clin. Invest. **85:** 739–745.
8. WAGNER, H., W. DORSCH, T. BAYER, *et al.* 1990. Antiasthmatic effects of onions: inhibition of 5-lipoxygenase and cyclooxygenase in vitro by thiosulfinates and "Cepaenes." Prostaglandins Leukot. Essent. Fatty Acids **39:** 59–62.

9. HAN, S.N., D. WU, W.K. HA, *et al.* 2000. Vitamin E supplementation increases T helper 1 cytokine production in old mice infected with influenza virus. Immunology **100:** 487–493.
10. MAK, N.K., C.Y. LEUNG, X.Y. WEI, *et al.* 2004. Inhibition of RANTES expression by indirubin in influenza virus-infected human bronchial epithelial cells. Biochem. Pharmacol. **67:** 167–174.

Preincubation with the Proteasome Inhibitor MG-132 Enhances Proteasome Activity via the Nrf2 Transcription Factor in Aging Human Skin Fibroblasts

DAVID CHRISTIAN KRAFT,[a] CUSTER C. DEOCARIS,[b,c]
RENU WADHWA,[b] AND SURESH I. S. RATTAN[a]

[a]Laboratory of Cellular Ageing, Danish Centre for Molecular Gerontology, Department of Molecular Biology, University of Aarhus, Aarhus, Denmark

[b]Gene Function Research Center, National Institute of Advanced Industrial Science and Technology (AIST), 1-1-1 Higashi, Tsukuba, Japan

[c]Cancer Research and Radiation Biology Laboratory, Philippine Nuclear Research Institute, Quezon City, Philippines

ABSTRACT: Strategies that lead to the upregulation of the proteasome are known to elicit beneficial consequences to the organism by countering oxidative stress–associated disorders, such as protein conformational diseases, cancer, and aging. Mild treatment with proteasome inhibitors has been previously demonstrated to stimulate proteasome activity and cellular resistance against oxidative injury. However, the mechanism for this action has not been clearly defined. We examined the role of the nuclear factor-E2-related factor 2 (Nrf2) in fibroblasts, a key transactivator of the antioxidant response pathway, in the regulation of the proteasome by its inhibitor MG-132. Here, we demonstrate that the stimulation of the proteasome by low levels of MG-132 can be abrogated by small interfering RNAs (siRNAs) targeted against Nrf2. Consistently, cells that constitutively express Nrf2 exhibit elevated levels of proteasome activities. We further investigate how its beneficial effects, that is, proteasome stimulation, are manifested in young and replicative-senescent cells. Our data underscore that manipulation of Nrf2 by the administration of pharmacologically low levels of proteasome inhibitors may prove to be an alternatively potent strategy for inducing long-term protective effects against oxidative stress.

KEYWORDS: Nrf2; proteasome; MG-132; fibroblast; hormesis; aging

Address for correspondence: Dr. Suresh I.S. Rattan, Department of Molecular Biology, University of Aarhus, Gustav Wieds Vej 10C, DK8000 Aarhus–C, Denmark. Voice: +45 8942 5034; fax: +45 8612 3178.
  e-mail: rattan@mb.au.dk

Ann. N.Y. Acad. Sci. 1067: 420–424 (2006). © 2006 New York Academy of Sciences.
doi: 10.1196/annals.1354.060

INTRODUCTION

Long-term exposure to proteasome inhibitors leads to severe oxidative stress, cell cycle arrest, downregulation of the proteasome, accumulation of protein aggregates, and appearance of senescence-like phenotypes.[1–5] It is widely accepted that the induction of cell cycle arrest is mainly attributed to the inhibition of the ubiquitin 26S proteasome pathway, which controls cell cycle regulators.[5,8] Analysis of gene expression in neural cells subjected to 12-week proteasome inhibition showed a wide range of cellular changes, such as reduced proteasome expression, and a weakened oxidative defense mechanism accompanied by the downregulation of glutathione S-transferase among others.[6] Such reduction in oxidative defense in response to proteasome inhibition is also evident from the increased levels of DNA and RNA oxidation.[7]

Short-term proteasome inhibition, on the other hand, results in an opposing effect that leads to improved cellular fitness accompanied by the induction of glutathione S-transferase (GST), heat-shock proteins (HSPs), and several proteasome genes.[9] The activation of oxidative-defense genes is known to occur through transcription factors like heat-shock factor 1 (HSF1), activator protein 1 (AP-1), and Nrf2.[9,10] Recently, it has been found that the proteasome is also transcriptionally regulated by Nrf2, suggesting a role for a proteasomal degradation pathway in the cellular adaptive response to oxidative stress.[11] In fact, the promoter regions of 20S and 19S, but not the immunoproteasome, harbor two antioxidant response elements (AREs).[12]

The Nrf2 is a cap-n-collar family of transcription factors that regulates cellular defenses against ROS. Under normal physiologic conditions, it exists in its inactive form because of sequestration by the cytoplasmic nuclear translocation-inhibitor KEAP1, which delivers it to proteasomal degradation.[13–15] Upon oxidative stress, Nrf2 is released from KEAP1 and translocates to the nucleus and initiates transcription of some 200 genes with the *cis*-acting antioxidant response element (ARE). Most of these genes have known roles in protecting the cell against oxidative and electrophilic stressors.[11] As activity of the proteasome is shown to be stimulated by short-term or low-dose exposure to proteasome inhibitors, we wanted to test whether Nrf2 is the transcription factor that controls this negative feedback loop of proteasome activity and gene expression. Furthermore, we tested whether the response to proteasome inhibition differs between young and replicative-senescent human cells.

RESULTS AND DISCUSSION

Normal adult human fibroblasts were co-transfected with the pNQR-ARE, a firefly luciferase reporter construct controlled by an ARE in the promoter region, and pRL-RSV, a constitutive *Renilla* luciferase expression plasmid. After incubation for 12 h with increasing amounts of MG-132 (2.5–30 nM),

(A)

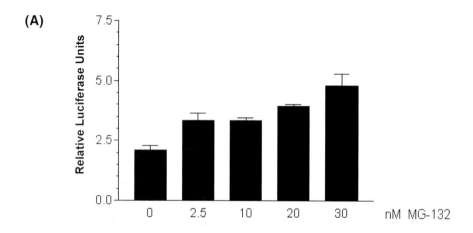

(B)

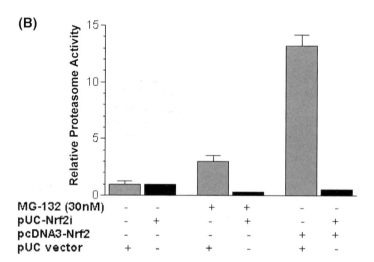

FIGURE 1. Pretreatment with the proteasome-inhibitor MG-132 leads to an increased Nrf2, an upregulated proteasome activity in young cells, which was abolished by Nrf2 siRNA. (**A**) Dual-luciferase reporter (pNQR-ARE, pRL-RSV) on TIG-1 cells treated with different concentrations of the MG-132 for 12–16 h resulted in the upregulation of the Nrf2. (**B**) Assay for the chymotrypsin-like proteasome activity of young cells after treating with 30 nM MG-132 for 16 h and Nrf2 shRNA.

a dual-luciferase assay was performed using a commercial kit from Promega (Madison, WI). The increasing levels of MG-132 resulted in a dose-dependent elevation of Nrf2 activity with the highest induction at 30 nM (FIG. 1A). After 12 h of incubation with 30 nM MG-132, proteasome activity was increased but not to the extent of the cells transfected with the pcDNA3-Nrf2, a

CMV-driven Nrf2 expression cassette (FIG. 1B). The increase in proteasome activity in Nrf2-overexpressing transfectants and in cells treated with 30 nM MG-132 was abolished after (co-)transfection with pUC-Nrf2i, a U6 promoter–driven short hairpin RNA against Nrf2 (FIG. 1B). These results demonstrated that proteasome activity could be stimulated by MG-132 and this proteasome-stimulatory effect may be controlled by the Nrf2 transcription factor.

Finally, we tested the reactivity of young and replicative-senescent cells to mild and severe treatment with MG-132. Proteasome activity was induced by 30 nM (mild) MG-132 treatment both in replicative-senescent (old) and young cells. However, in the old cells induction was only about one-third of the increase in proteasome activity exhibited by young cells. Treatment with MG-132 (30 μM for 1 h) induced severe cell death in the rapidly growing young cells ($\sim$84% death), whereas the replicative-senescent cells were less affected ($\sim$33% death) (data not shown). These data suggest that MG-132-induced protective effects against oxidative stressors via Nrf2 activation may be differentially regulated in young and senescent cells.[16–19]

In summary, our data underscore that the manipulation of the Nrf2 pathway by pharmacologically low levels of proteasome inhibitors could prove to be an alternative potent strategy for inducing long-term protective effects against oxidative stress and aging. We are further investigating how such beneficial effects, that is, proteasome stimulation and increased fitness, are manifested during replicative senescence.

ACKNOWLEDGMENTS

We acknowledge the support of the Gene Function Research Laboratory, National Institute for Advanced Industrial Science and Technology (AIST), for travel and research fellowship to David Christian Kraft, and Professor Masayuki Yamamoto, Tara Institute, University of Tsukuba, Japan for providing the Nrf2 expression and reporter plasmids, and for helpful technical discussion. The Laboratory of Cellular Ageing (University of Aarhus) is supported by research grants from the Danish Research Councils, Carlsberg Fund, Senetek PLC, and EU's Biomed Health Programmes.

REFERENCES

1. YANO, M. *et al.* 2005. Chaperone activities of the 26S and 20S proteasome. Curr. Protein Pept. Sci. **6:** 197–203.
2. BAJOREK, M., D. FINLEY & M.H. GLICKMAN. 2003. Proteasome disassembly and downregulation is correlated with viability during stationary phase. Curr. Biol. **13:** 1140–1144.
3. DING, Q. *et al.* 2003. Characterization of chronic low-level proteasome inhibition on neural homeostasis. J. Neurochem. **86:** 489–497.

4. CHONDROGIANNI, N. *et al.* 2003. Central role of the proteasome in senescence and survival of human fibroblasts: induction of a senescence-like phenotype upon its inhibition and resistance to stress upon its activation. J. Biol. Chem. **278:** 28026–28037.

5. YIN, D. *et al.* 2004. Proteasome inhibitor PS-341 causes cell growth arrest and apoptosis in human glioblastoma multiforme (GBM). Oncogene **24:** 344–354.

6. DING, Q. *et al.* 2004. Analysis of gene expression in neural cells subject to chronic proteasome inhibition. Free Radic. Biol. Med. **36:** 445–455.

7. DING, Q. *et al.* 2004. Proteasome inhibition increases DNA and RNA oxidation in astrocyte and neuron cultures. J. Neurochem. **91:** 1211–1218.

8. IMAI, J. *et al.* 2003. The molecular chaperone Hsp90 plays a role in the assembly and maintenance of the 26S proteasome. EMBO J. **22:** 3557–3567.

9. KIM, D., S.H. KIM & G.C. LI. 1999. Proteasome inhibitors MG132 and lactacystin hyperphosphorylate HSF1 and induce hsp70 and hsp27 expression. Biochem. Biophys. Res. Commun. **254:** 264–268.

10. TACCHINI, L. *et al.* 2001. Influence of proteasome and redox state on heat shock-induced activation of stress kinases, AP-1 and HSF. Biochim. Biophys. Acta **1538:** 76–89.

11. KWAK, M.K. *et al.* 2003. Modulation of gene expression by cancer chemopreventive dithiolethiones through the Keap1-Nrf2 pathway: identification of novel gene clusters for cell survival. J. Biol. Chem. **278:** 8135–8145.

12. KWAK, M.K. *et al.* 2003. Antioxidants enhance mammalian proteasome expression through the Keap1-Nrf2 signaling pathway. Mol. Cell Biol. **23:** 8786–8794.

13. MOI, P. *et al.* 1994. Isolation of NF-E2-related factor 2 (Nrf2), a NF-E2-like basic leucine zipper transcriptional activator that binds to the tandem NF-E2/AP1 repeat of the beta-globin locus control region. Proc. Natl. Acad. Sci. USA **91:** 9926–9930.

14. ITOH, K. *et al.* 1999. Keap1 represses nuclear activation of antioxidant responsive elements by Nrf2 through binding to the amino-terminal Neh2 domain. Genes Dev. **13:** 76–86.

15. DINKOVA-KOSTOVA, A.T. *et al.* 2002. Direct evidence that sulfhydryl groups of Keap1 are the sensors regulating induction of phase 2 enzymes that protect against carcinogens and oxidants. Proc. Natl. Acad. Sci. USA **99:** 11908–11913.

16. LEE, C.S. *et al.* 2004. A proteasomal stress response: pre-treatment with proteasome inhibitors increases proteasome activity and reduces neuronal vulnerability to oxidative injury. J. Neurochem. **91:** 996–1006.

17. LI, J. *et al.* 2005. Stabilization of Nrf2 by tBHQ confers protection against oxidative stress-induced cell death in human neural stem cells. Toxicol. Sci. **83:** 313–328.

18. WAKABAYASHI, N. *et al.* 2004. Protection against electrophile and oxidant stress by induction of the phase 2 response: fate of cysteines of the Keap1 sensor modified by inducers. Proc. Natl. Acad. Sci. USA **101:** 2040–2045.

19. MOTOHASHI, H. & M. YAMAMOTO. 2004. Nrf2-Keap1 defines a physiologically important stress response mechanism. Trends Mol. Med. **10:** 549–557.

Exercise and Hormesis

Activation of Cellular Antioxidant Signaling Pathway

LI LI JI,[a] MARIA-CARMEN GOMEZ-CABRERA,[b] AND JOSE VINA[c]

[a]University of Wisconsin-Madison, Madison, Wisconsin, USA

[b]Catholic University of Valencia, Valencia, Spain

[c]University of Valencia, Valencia, Spain

ABSTRACT: Contraction-induced production of reactive oxygen species (ROS) has been shown to cause oxidative stress to skeletal muscle. As an adaptive response, muscle antioxidant defense systems are upregulated after heavy exercise. Nuclear factor (NF) κB and mitogen-activated protein kinases (MAPKs) are the major oxidative stress–sensitive signal transduction pathways in mammalian tissues. Activation of NF-κB signaling cascade has been shown to enhance the gene expression of important enzymes, such as mitochondrial superoxide dismutase (MnSOD) and inducible nitric oxide synthase (iNOS). MAPK activations are involved in a variety of cellular functions including growth, proliferation, and adaptation. We investigated the effect of an acute bout of exercise on NF-κB and MAPK signaling, as well as on the time course of activation, in rat skeletal muscle. In addition, we studied the role of ROS in the exercise-induced upregulation of MnSOD and iNOS, and the potential interactions of NF-κB and MAPK in the signaling of these enzymes. Our data suggest that ROS may serve as messenger molecules to activate adaptive responses through these redox-sensitive signaling pathways to maintain cellular oxidant-antioxidant homeostasis during exercise.

KEYWORDS: antioxidant; exercise; MAPK; nuclear factor (NF) kappa B; reactive oxygen species

There is now an abundance of literature indicating that generation of reactive oxygen and nitrogen species (RONS) is increased in skeletal muscle and myocardium during strenuous physical exercise.[1–3] The increased RONS have important implications in tissue and cell oxidative damage and aging, as well as in the functional performance of the organs. However, it is also becoming clear that animals and humans engaged in long-term heavy exercise are more resistant to oxidative stress, mainly due to the adaptation of their antioxidant

Address for correspondence: Li Li Ji, Ph.D., The Biodynamics Laboratory, 2000 Observatory Drive, Madison, WI 53706. Voice: 608-262-7250; fax: 608-262-1656.

e-mail: ji@education.wisc.edu

Ann. N.Y. Acad. Sci. 1067: 425–435 (2006). © 2006 New York Academy of Sciences.

doi: 10.1196/annals.1354.061

defense systems.[4–7] It is in this context that we postulate that the concept of hormesis can be applied to exercise-induced gene expression of antioxidant enzymes. We hereby provide research data to demonstrate that several redox-sensitive signal transduction pathways play an important role in conferring the signaling of adaptation in the skeletal muscle in rats.

The key to understanding exercise-induced hormetic response lies in the fact that mammalian cells are endowed with signaling pathways that are sensitive to intracellular redox environment and can be activated by oxidative stress. Those include NF-κB, heat-shock transcriptional factor 1 (HSF-1), and P53 pathways, as well as mitogen-activated protein kinase (MAPK) and PI(3)K/Akt that regulate the first three pathways through phosphorylation.[8] The mechanism of NF-κB-induced signaling in response to oxidative stress is well defined.[9–11] In brief: activating signals, such as proinflammatory cytokines (TNF$_\alpha$ or IL-1,6), irradiation, endotoxins, and ROS may converge on IκB kinase (IKK), which phosphorylates serine residue 19 and 23 on the inhibitory subunit (IκB) of NF-κB, causing its ubiquitination and release from the NF-κB complex. The p50 and p65 dimer subsequently translocate into the nucleus and bind to the κB domain of the target gene promoter, leading to transcriptional activation. Upstream of the IKK, several enzymes of the MAP3K family of kinases have been identified that are thought to convey signals from receptor complexes, including MAPK/ERK kinase (MEKK1) and the NF-κB-inducing kinase (NIK).

Several antioxidant enzymes contain NF-κB binding sites in the gene promoter region, such as MnSOD, inducible nitric oxide synthetase (iNOS), and γ-glumatylcysteine synthetase (GCS).[8] Therefore, they can be potential targets for exercise-activated upregulation via the NF-κB signaling pathway. Hollander et al.[12] first reported that an acute bout of treadmill running activated MnSOD gene expression in rat skeletal muscle, along with enhanced NF-κB binding in muscle nuclear extracts ~2 h after exercise. Messenger RNA abundance for MnSOD was increased in the exercised rats, whereas a significant increase in MnSOD protein level was observed only after 48 h. Vider et al[13] showed that physical exercise (80% maximal O_2 consumption for 1 h) resulted in NF-κB activation in peripheral blood lymphocytes of physically fit young men. Plasma levels of TNF-α and IL-2 receptor in these subjects were also elevated. Adam et al.[14] detected NF-κB activation in the skeletal muscle of patients with chronic heart failure. Interestingly, the activation of NF-κB correlated with the expression of muscle iNOS mRNA levels.

Recently, we have investigated the effect of rigorous muscular contraction on NF-κB signaling pathway in rat skeletal muscle in two separate studies. In the first study,[15] a group of rats was run on the treadmill at 25 m/min, 5% grade, for 1 h or until exhaustion, and compared with a second group subjected to the same exercise regimen and injected with two doses of pyrrolidine dithiocarbamate (PDTC), a well-known NF-κB inhibitor. Three additional groups of rested rats were treated with either lipopolysaccharide (LPS), t-butylhydroperoxide (tBHP), or saline solution, as positive or negative

(A)

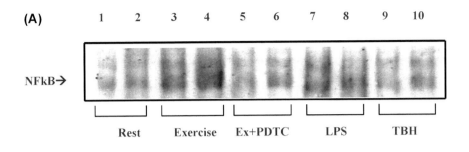

NF-kB

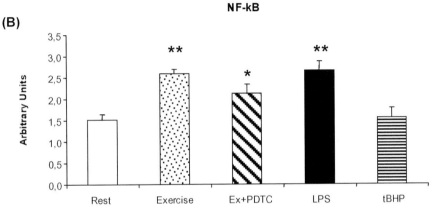

FIGURE 1. (**A**) EMSA sample using NF-κB probe end-labeled with digoxigenin-11-ddUTP, shown with two muscle samples randomly selected from each treatment group ($N =$ 6). *Lanes* 1 and 2: Rest. *Lanes* 3 and 4, run on treadmill at 25 m/min, 5% grade for 1 h, or until exhaustion. *Lanes* 5 and 6, exercised and injected with pyrrolidine dithiocarbamate (PDTC, 100 mg/kg, i.p.) 24 and 1 h prior to killing. *Lanes* 7 and 8, injected with lipopolysaccharride (LPS, 8 mg/kg, i.p.) 1 h prior to killing. *Lanes* 9 and 10, injected with *t*-butylhydroperoxide (tBHP, 1 mmol/kg, i. p.) 1 h prior to killing. (**B**) Mean $\pm$ SEM ($N = 6$) of NF-κB binding intensity derived from densitometry. *$P < 0.05$; **$P < 0.01$ versus rest.

controls, respectively. Electrophoretic mobility shift assay (EMSA) shows that exercised rats showed significantly higher levels of NF-κB binding in the muscle nuclear extracts compared to control rats (FIG. 1). The exercise-induced activation of the NF-κB signaling was partially abolished by PDTC treatment, whereas LPS, but not *t*BHP treatment, mimicked the effects observed in the exercised rats. Consistent with the above observations, Western blot analysis indicates that P50 content in the nuclear extracts of the exercised and LPS-treated rats was dramatically increased compared to resting controls, whereas the exercise effect was abolished by PDTC treatment.[15] We investigated the various components of the NF-κB signaling cascades in response to those treatments. Cytosolic IκBα content was decreased, whereas phospho-IκBα content was increased, comparing exercised with control rats (FIG. 2). Further, exercised and LPS-treated rats showed a marked reduction of IKKα and an

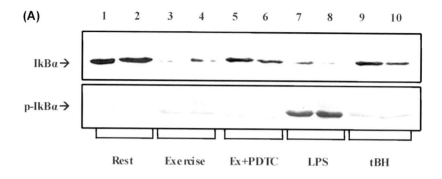

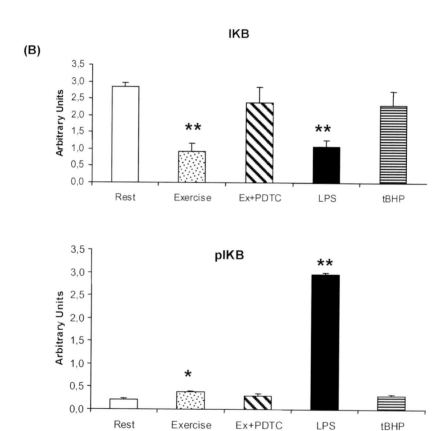

FIGURE 2. (**A**) Western blot analysis of IκBα and phospho-IκBα in the cytosolic fraction of DVL muscle. Two muscle samples were randomly selected from each treatment group ($N = 6$). Lane descriptions are identical to those in FIG. 1. The assay was performed per product instructions from Cell Signaling Technology Inc. (Beverly, MA, USA). (**B**) Mean ± SEM ($N = 6$) of IκBα and phospho-IκBα contents derived from densitometry. $^*P < 0.05$; $^{**}P < 0.01$ versus rest.

increase in phospho-IKKα (not shown), indicating that the exercise and LPS activation of the NF-κB pathway was mediated by IKK phosphorylation and activation. In order to examine the time course of the exercise-induced NF-κB activation, we conducted another experiment wherein six groups of rats were randomly assigned to an exercise protocol—running on treadmill at 25 m/min, 5% grade for 1 h, or until exhaustion—and killed either immediately (0 h), or at 1, 2, 4, 24, or 48 h after the cessation of exercise.[15] Six additional groups of rats were killed at the matching time points at rest as controls. The highest levels of NF-κB binding were observed at 2 h post exercise (FIG. 3), whereas decreased cytosolic IκBα and increased phospho-IκBα content were found at 0–1 h post exercise (not shown. Ref. 15). Further, P65 content in the nuclear extraction reached the peak at 4 h post exercise (not shown). These data suggest that the NF-κB signaling pathway can be activated in a redox-sensitive manner in response to muscular contraction. Previously, we demonstrated that an acute bout of treadmill running at similar intensity significantly increased ROS production in rat hindlimb muscles.[16] Presumably, increased ROS lead to IKK activation, causing phosphorylation and dissociation of IkB, unleashing p50/p65 into the nucleus and binding with the NF-κB motif of the target genes, such as MnSOD. Signals upstream of IKK were not reviewed in this

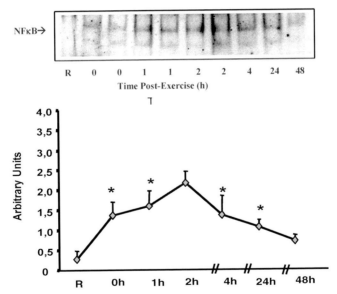

FIGURE 3. (**A**) Representative EMSA samples using NF-κB probe end-labeled with digoxigenin-11-ddUTP. Muscle nuclear extracts were from pooled muscle of rats at rest (R), or at 0, 1, 2, 4, 24, and 48 h after an acute bout of treadmill run at 25 m/min, 5% grade for 1 h, or until exhaustion. (**B**) Time course of NF-κB-binding intensity derived from densitometry. Each point represents mean ± SEM ($N = 4$). *$P < 0.05$; **$P < 0.01$ versus rest.

study; however, it is likely that activation of NIK and other kinases capable of responding to ROS are involved. At present we cannot tell whether activation of the NF-κB pathway was the cause of, rather than a coincidence with, the exercise activation of MnSOD gene expression, as we reported earlier.[15] However, our work provided *in vivo* data that were consistent with a study by Zhou *et al.*,[17] who examined the role of NF-κB in H_2O_2-induced antioxidant gene expression in C2C12 muscle cells. In that study, H_2O_2 stimulated GPX mRNA expression in the wild-type cells but not in an IkB mutant cell line. The time course for peak NF-κB binding was 2 h at the concentration of 1–2 mM H_2O_2. Given the critical role of MnSOD in removing superoxide anion to prevent hydroxyl radical formation, it is likely that the cell uses H_2O_2 as a signaling molecule to upregulate intracellular antioxidant defense through the NF-κB pathway, so as to reduce potential oxidative stress and damage to the mitochondria.

It is becoming increasingly clear that an optimal ROS level is essential for the cell's survival. Too much ROS may cause impaired physiological function due to either random cellular damage or programmed cell death (apoptosis), whereas too few ROS may lead to decreased proliferative response and defective host defense capacity.[18] If hormetic response is indeed beneficial to the oxidative-antioxidant homeostasis in the cell, then the suppression of the ROS source is expected to attenuate not only oxidative damage, but also the cell's ability to adapt under oxidative stress. To test this hypothesis, we employed an experimental model wherein mitochondrial ROS generation was marginalized, whereas cytosolic ROS was derived from xanthine oxidase (OX), an enzyme involved in hypoxia-reperfusion-induced ROS production.[19] A group of rats was subjected to an acute bout of sprinting exercise at progressive speed and grade on treadmill until exhaustion (SP, total exercise time 58 ± 7 min).[20] A second group of rats was subjected to the same exercise protocol except that allopurinol (ALP, 32mg/kg body weight), a competitive inhibitor of XO, was administered (i.p.) to reduce ROS production. A third group of rats was treated with ALP but rested as controls (C). It was found that the sprinting exercise significantly increased NF-κB binding in the nuclear extracts of rat gastrocnemius muscle (FIG. 4), accompanied by increased XO activity and ROS concentration (data not shown). ALP treatment reduced XO activity and completely abolished exercise-induced NF-κB binding. Thus, it is clear that cytosolic ROS are involved in NF-κB signaling in response to muscle contraction, which could be reversed by inhibiting the key ROS source XO. To assess the physiological significance of NF-κB activation and suppression, we examined the gene expression of two well-known target enzymes, MnSOD and iNOS, in the rat skeletal muscle. MnSOD mRNA level was significantly increased by ~2.5-fold in SP versus C rats (FIG. 5A), whereas this effect was not seen in the ALP-treated rats. Similarly, exercise resulted in 2.5-fold increase in muscle mRNA of iNOS in SP, but not in ALP rats (FIG. 5B). These data strongly supported the notion that ROS are the required agents in the

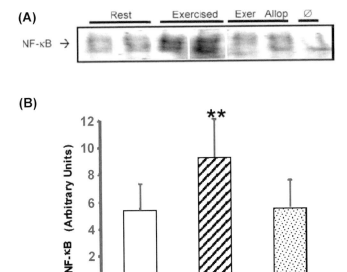

FIGURE 4. Exercise activates NF-κB: prevention by allopurinol. (**A**) EMSA analysis of NF-κB in the nuclear extracts of rat gastrocnemius. (Ø, competition assay: unlabeled competitor probe was added in 100-fold molar excess). (**B**) densitometry analysis of NF-κB ($N = 4$). Values are means ± S.D. **$P < 0.01$ versus rest.

exercise-induced gene expression of antioxidant enzymes and that suppression of ROS generation may attenuate or abolish such hormetic responses. MnSOD plays an important role in controlling mitochondrial H_2O_2, as well as •OH formation. Cells increase MnSOD expression in response to hypoxic reoxygenation in a relatively short period of time. It has been shown that myocardial preconditioning composed of short episodes of ischemic shocks could increase MnSOD activity and protein content.[21,22] It is possible that anaerobic exercise (sprinting) may create a cellular milieu similar to that of an ischemic heart and activate antioxidant gene expression, which facilitates protection in subsequent oxidative insult in the mitochondria. Increased NO synthesis is known to be a double-edged sword. It improves blood perfusion due to its vasodilative effect, but NO can also react with $O_2^{•-}$ to form peroxynitrite, a lethal ROS that can cause damage.[23]

It is well documented that a single episode of muscular contraction can activate the MAPK pathway in human skeletal muscle.[24-26] Also, extracellular signal-regulated kinase (ERK) and p38 MAPK activity was increased in rat slow- and fast-twitch skeletal muscle after electrically stimulated contraction.[27] Nader and Esser[28] showed that immediately after an acute bout of treadmill running, ERK and p38 were activated in rat soleus and tibialis muscles. Activation

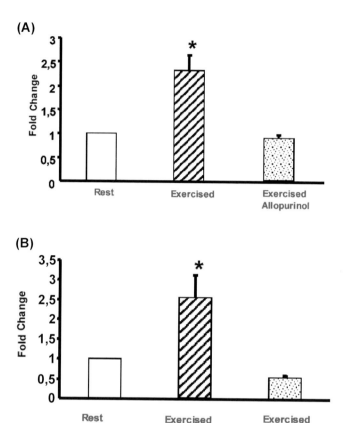

FIGURE 5. Exercise-induced upregulation of MnSOD and iNOS is prevented by allopurinol. Expression of MnSOD (**A**) and iNOS (**B**) measured by real-time RT-PCR from gastrocnemius muscle of rats at rest, after exercise, and after exercise but pretreated with allopurinol ($N = 9$).

of various kinases involved in the MAPK pathway can lead to the sequential phosphorylation of a series of proteins, resulting in increased expression of c-Jun, a subunit of the transcription factor activator protein-1 (AP-1).[29] In order to gain some insight into the role of the MAPK pathway in exercise activation of NF-κB and antioxidant signaling, we measured two important enzymes in this family, ERK1/ERK2 and p38 MAPK. Western blot revealed significant increases in protein levels for both ERK1/ERK2 and p38 in the SP rats, compared to C rats.[20] ALP-treated exercised rats showed severe reductions of both enzyme protein levels, compared to SP rats treated with saline solution. Our data provided evidence that ROS produced by XO may be involved in MAPK signaling, because inhibition of ROS with ALP attenuated phosphorylation of these enzymes. Whether weakened MAPK signaling was related to the lowered MnSOD and iNOS expression remains to be investigated. However, it is

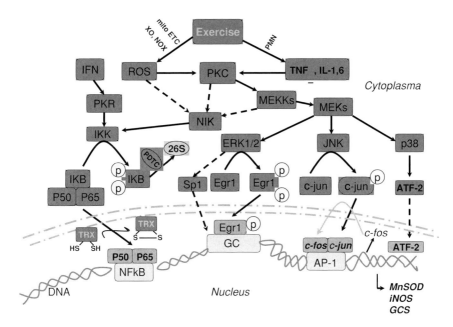

FIGURE 6. Schematic representation of proposed antioxidant enzyme gene expression controlled by NF-κB and MAPK signal transduction pathways. Dotted links denote potential actions. Abbreviations: ATF, activating transcription factor; Egr-1, early growth response-1 transcription factor; IFN, interferon; MEK, MAPK kinase; MEKK, MAPK kinase kinase; NOX, NADPH oxidase; PKC, protein kinase C; PKR, double-stranded RNA-activated protein kinase; PMN, polymorphoneutrophil; TRX, thioredoxin. Other abbreviations: see text.

plausible that integrated inputs from both NF-κB and MAPK signaling pathways are required to mediate gene expression of MnSOD and/or iNOS in the muscle cells in response to exercise stress. FIGURE 6 is a postulated pathway of exercise-induced antioxidant signaling pathway based on available knowledge gained primarily from, but not limited to, skeletal muscle. Attenuation of ROS production, either by direct inhibition with chemical agents (such as ALP), or by large-dose supplementation of antioxidants, will not only reduce oxidative damage, but also block cellular adaptations deemed beneficial to oxidant-antioxidant homeostasis. The pros and cons of such manipulations will likely be a debatable topic in this field.

REFERENCES

1. DAVIES, K.J., A.T. QUINTANILHA, G.A. BROOKS, *et al.* 1982. Free radicals and tissue damage produced by exercise. Biochem. Biophys. Res. Commun. **107:** 1198–1205.
2. SEN, C.K. 1995. Oxidants and antioxidants in exercise. J. Appl. Physiol. **79:** 675–686.

3. JI, L.L. 1999. Antioxidants and oxidative stress in exercise. Proc. Soc. Exp. Biol. Med. **222:** 283–292.

4. HIGUCHI, M., L.J. CARTIER, M. CHEN, *et al.* 1985. Superoxide dismutase and catalase in skeletal muscle: adaptive response to exercise. J. Gerontol. **40:** 281–286.

5. LAUGHLIN, M.H., T. SIMPSON, W.L. SEXTON, *et al.* 1990. Skeletal muscle oxidative capacity, antioxidant enzymes, and exercise training. J. Appl. Physiol. 682337–682343.

6. POWERS, S.K., D. CRISWELL, J. LAWLER, *et al.* 1994. Influence of exercise and fiber type on antioxidant enzyme activity in rat skeletal muscle. Am. J. Physiol. **266:** R375–R380.

7. HOLLANDER, J., R. FIEBIG, M. GORE, *et al.* 1999. Superoxide dismutase gene expression in skeletal muscle: fiber-specific adaptation to endurance training. Am. J. Physiol. **277:** R856–R862.

8. ALLEN, R.G. & M. TRESINI. 2000. Oxidative stress and gene regulation. Free Radic. Biol. Med. **28:** 463–499.

9. BAEUERLE, P.A. & D. BALTIMORE. 1988. Activation of DNA-binding activity in an apparently cytoplasmic precursor of the NF-κB transcriptional factor. Cell **53:** 211–217.

10. SCHRECK, R., K. ALBERMANN & P.A. BAEUERLE. 1992. Nuclear factor kB: an oxidative stress responsive transcriptional factor of eukaryotic cells. Free Rad. Res. Commun. **17:** 221–237.

11. BAEUERLE, P.A. & T. HENKEL. 1994. Function and activation of NF-κB in the immune system. Ann. Rev. Immunol. **12:** 141–179.

12. HOLLANDER, J., R. FIEBIG, T. OOKAWARA, *et al.* 2001. Superoxide dismutase gene expression is activated by a single bout of exercise. Pflug. Arch. (Eur. J. Physiol.) **442:** 426–434.

13. VIDER, J., D.E. LAAKSONEN, A. KILK, *et al.* 2001. Physical exercise induces activation of NF-κB in human peripheral blood lymphocytes. Antiox. Redox Signaling **3:** 1131–1137.

14. ADAMS, V., U. SPATE, N. KRANKEL, *et al.* 2003. Nuclear factor-kappa B activation in skeletal muscle of patients with chronic heart failure: correlation with the expression of inducible nitric oxide synthase. Eur. J. Cardiovas. Prev. Rehab. **10:** 273–277.

15. HOLLANDER, J., R. FIEBIG, T. OOKAWARA, *et al.* 2001. Superoxide dismutase gene expression is activated by a single bout of exercise. Pflug. Arch. (Eur. J. Physiol.) **442:** 426–434.

16. BEJMA, J., P. RAMIRES & L.L. JI. 2000. Free radical generation and oxidative stress with aging and exercise: differential effects in the myocardium and liver. Acta Physiol. Scand. **169:** 343–351.

17. ZHOU, L.Z., A.P. JOHNSON & T.A. RANDO. 2001. NF kappa B and AP-1 mediate transcriptional responses to oxidative stress in skeletal muscle cells. Free Radic. Biol. Med. **31:** 1405–1416.

18. FINKEL, T. & N. HOLBROOK. 2000. Oxidants, oxidative stress and the biology of ageing. Nature **408:** 239–247.

19. BINDOLI, A., A. CAVALLINI, M.P. RIGOBELLO, *et al.* 1988. Modification of the xanthine-converting enzyme of perfused rat heart during ischemia and oxidative stress. Free Radic. Biol. Med. **4:** 163–167.

20. GOMEZ-CABRERA, M-C., C. BORRAS, G. SANTANGELO, *et al.* 2005. Decreasing xanthine oxidase mediated oxidative stress prevents useful cellular adaptations to exercise in rats. J. Physiol. (London) **567:** 113–120.

21. YAMASHITA, N., S. HOSHIDA, N. TANIGUCHI, *et al.* 1998. Whole-body hyperthermia provides biphasic cardioprotection against ischemia/reperfusion injury in the rat. Circulation **98:** 1414–1421.

22. YAMASHITA, N., S. HOSHIDA, N. TANIGUCHI, *et al.* 1998. A "second window of protection" occurs 24 h after ischemic preconditioning in the rat heart. J. Mol. Cell. Cardiol. **30:** 1181–1189.

23. REID, M.B. 1998. Role of nitric oxide in skeletal muscle: synthesis, distribution and functional importance. Acta Physiol. Scand. **162:** 401–409.

24. ARONSON, D., M.A. VIOLAN, S.D. DUFRESNE, *et al.* 1997. Exercise stimulates the mitogen-activated protein kinase pathway in human skeletal muscle. J. Clin. Invest. **99:** 1251–1257.

25. BOPPART, M.D., D. ARONSON, L. GIBSON, *et al.* 1999. Eccentric exercise markedly increases c-Jun NH_2-terminal kinase activity in human skeletal muscle. J. Appl. Physiol. **87:** 1668–1673.

26. WIDEGREN, U., X.J. JIANG, A. KROOK, *et al.* 1998. Divergent effects of exercise on metabolic and mitogenic signaling pathways in human skeletal muscle. FASEB J. **12:** 1379–1389.

27. WRETMAN, C., U. WIDEGREN, A. LIONIKAS, *et al.* 2000. Differential activation of mitogen-activated protein kinase signalling pathways by isometric contractions in isolated slow- and fast-twitch rat skeletal muscle. Acta Physiol. Scand. **170:** 45–99.

28. NADER, G. & K. ESSER. 2001. Intracellular signaling specificity in skeletal muscle in response to different modes of exercise. J. Appl. Physiol. **90:** 1936–1942.

29. PULVERER, B.J., J.M. KYRIAKIS, J. AVRUCH, *et al.* 1991. Phosphorylation of c-Jun mediated MAP kinases. Nature **353:** 670–674.

Stem Cells

Potential Therapy for Age-Related Diseases

MOUSTAPHA KASSEM

Department of Endocrinology and Metabolism, University Hospital of Odense, DK-5000 Odense C, Denmark

ABSTRACT: Aging is associated with a progressive failing of tissues and organs of the human body leading to a large number of age-related diseases. Regenerative medicine is an emerging clinical discipline that aims to employ cellular medicines (normal cells, *ex vivo* expanded cells, or tissue-engineered organs) to restore the functions of damaged or defective tissues and organs and thus to "rejuvenate" the failing aging body. One of the most important sources for cellular medicine is embryonic and adult (somatic) stem cells (SSCs). One example of SCCs with enormous clinical potential is the mesenchymal stem cells (MSCs) that are present in the bone marrow and are able to differentiate into cell types such as osteoblasts, chondrocytes, endothelial cells, and probably also neuron-like cells. Because of the ease of their isolation and their extensive differentiation potential, MSCs are among the first stem cell types to be introduced in the clinic. Some recent studies have demonstrated the possible use of MSCs in systemic transplantation for systemic diseases, local implantation for local tissue defects, as a vehicle for genes in gene therapy protocols, or to generate transplantable tissues and organs in tissue-engineering protocols. However, several challenges confront the use of these cells in the clinic, ranging from biological challenges (e.g., how to isolate a homogenous populations of the cells with specific criteria from the bone marrow and how to expand them *ex vivo* without affecting their differentiation potential) to biotechnological challenges (e.g., how to develop easy methods for quality control of the cellular-based products). While it is expected that cellular medicines will decrease the burden of several age-related diseases, it is not clear whether they can change the course of the aging process itself and thus prolong human life.

KEYWORDS: stem cells; regenerative medicine; mesenchymal stem cells; differentiation; therapy

INTRODUCTION

The hallmark of aging is the gradual and progressive failing of tissues and organs of human body due to a multitude of causes. During steady-state

Address for correspondence: Prof. Moustapha Kassem, M.D., Ph.D., D.Sc., Department of Endocrinology and Metabolism, University Hospital of Odense, DK-5000 Odense C, Denmark. Voice: +45-6541 1606; fax: +45-6591 9653.
e-mail: mkassem@health.sdu.dk

Ann. N.Y. Acad. Sci. 1067: 436–442 (2006). © 2006 New York Academy of Sciences.
doi: 10.1196/annals.1354.062

conditions, damaged tissues are replaced by continuous recruitment and differentiation from stem cells in the body. However, with aging, the body's ability for regeneration becomes impaired. Regenerative medicine is an emerging discipline in clinical medicine that aims at restoring tissue and organs' failing functions due to aging or degenerative diseases by transplantation of cellular medicines. These are cell-based products of either autologous or allogeneic normal cells, *ex vivo* expanded cells, or tissue-engineered organs. One of the main sources for cellular medicine is stem cells.

What are Stem Cells?

Stem cells are undifferentiated cells that are defined by their ability to both self-renew and to differentiate to produce mature progeny cells, including both non-renewing progenitors and terminally differentiated effector cells.[1,2] Classically, stem cells can be classified into either pluripotent human embryonic stem cells (hESCs), derived from inner cell mass of blastocysts of early embryos[3] or primitive germ cells of around 2-month-old fetal tissues,[4] or human adult (somatic) stem cells (hSSCs), derived through specific isolation procedures from nearly every organ in the body (e.g., bone marrow, liver, pancreas, adipose tissue). Among hSSCs, human mesenchymal stem cells (hMSCs) are the first hSSCs to be introduced in the clinic.

Human Mesenchymal Stem Cells (hMSCs)

hMSCs are clonogenic, nonhematopoietic stem cells that exist in bone marrow and have been recognized for many years. However, Friedenstein *et al.* were the first to develop *in vitro* culture methods for isolation and testing of their differentiation potential.[5] In recent years, a large number of investigators have studied the biological characteristics of hMSCs and the cells have been given different names by different investigators, including marrow stromal cells, bone marrow fibroblasts, and skeletal stem cells.

Isolation and Biological Characteristics of hMSCs

No prospective markers exclusively defining MSCs are currently available. Thus, cell populations obtained by the current methods are essentially heterogenous. Traditionally, MSCs have been isolated from the bone marrow mononuclear cell fraction based on their selective adherence, compared to hematopoietic cells, to plastic surfaces.[6–8] Other investigators tried different methods to isolate a more homogenous cell population. Gronthos *et al.* developed a monoclonal antibody, Stro-1, which has been used to isolate a population of cells with MSC characteristics.[9] Reyes *et al.* isolated a mesodermal progenitor cell (MPC) and the same group later characterized a similar population of cells termed Multipotent Adult Progenitor Cells (MAPCs) from $CD45^-$/glycoprotein A^-

depleted bone marrow–derived mononuclear cell fraction that selectively adhered to laminin-coated plates under low serum conditions. Finally, MIAMI (marrow-isolated adult multilineage inducible) cells were isolated from the whole bone marrow cells by selective adhesion to fibronectin-coated plates in the presence of reduced serum conditions and under low oxygen tension.[12] The biological differences among these different cell populations are not clear.[13] Newer studies have also demonstrated the possibility of isolating MSC-like cells from the "stroma" of a number of organs including synovial membranes[14] and deciduous teeth.[15] MSCs were detected circulating in peripheral blood[16] and in umbilical cord blood.[17]

Morphologically, MSCs are mostly fusiform and cuboidal fibroblast-like cells. Their initial growth *in vitro* is characterized by the formation of colonies (termed *colony-forming unit-fibroblasts* [CFU-f]). The cells are negative for hematpoietic surface markers: CD34, CD45, CD14, CD31, CD133 and positive for CD63, CD105, CD166, CD54, CD55, CD13, and CD44.[10,12,18] Differences exist among the reported studies in the surface marker characteristics that may be explained by variations in culture methods and/or differentiation stage of the cells. The most important characteristic of MSCs is their ability to differentiate into several cell types *in vitro* depending on culture conditions (e.g., osteoblasts,[19] adipocytes,[20] chondrocytes,[21] and non-mesoderm-type cells, such as neuron-like and endoderm-like cells).[11,12,22,23] The classical assay for detecting the "stemness" nature of MSCs is based on transplanting the cells subcutaneously in immunodeficient mice and demonstrating their ability to form bone, adipocytes, and hematopoietic bone marrow–supporting stroma.[24,25]

FROM BIOLOGY TO CLINICAL APPLICATIONS

hMSCs can potentially be used in therapy in a variety of conditions on the basis of their demonstrated efficiency in animal models of human diseases and also in some clinical human studies. Among these, the use of hMSCs in repair of nonhealed bone or cartilage defect,[26–28] treatment of systemic bone diseases such as osteogenesis imperfecta,[29] or use of the cells for gene transfer (e.g., factor VIII or IL-3)[30] or tissue engineering.[31] However, several biological and biotechnological challenges need to be overcome before cells can be routinely used in therapy. For this review two issues will be discussed: the limited growth potential of the *in vitro*-cultured hMSCs and the control of differentiation of hMSCs.

In Vitro *Expansion of hMSCs*

A large number of normal cells are needed for any clinical use of hMSCs. Unfortunately, under current *in vitro* culture conditions that include fetal bovine serum, hMSCs obtained from young donors can undergo 24–40 population doublings (PDs) *in vitro* and the proliferative potential of MSCs obtained from older donors is more compromised.[32] Similar to other diploid cells, hMSCs exhibit senescence-associated growth arrest, a phenomenon termed as *replicative senescence*.[32,33] Replicative senescence of cultured diploid cells, including MSC cells, is caused by several factors including progressive telomere shortening during continuous subculture *in vitro* due to absence of telomerase activity.[34,35] We have demonstrated that it is possible to overcome the senescence phenotype of cultured hMSCs by forced expression of human telomerase reverse transcriptase gene (hTERT) in MSCs thus restoring telomerase activity.[35] The telomerized MSC cells exhibited extended life span and maintained a robust bone-forming ability when transplanted *in vivo* in immunodeficient mice. Similar results were obtained recently from telomerized smooth muscle cells used in forming tissue-engineered arteries. Thus, telomerase activation of hMSCs is a potential strategy for obtaining a large number of biologically competent cells for clinical use. However, the extensive cell proliferation of hMSCs-TERT *in vitro* led to genetic instability and resulted in MSC transformation.[36] Thus, conditional or intermittent activation of the hTERT gene is a more appropriate approach.

Control of Differentiation of hMSCs

Currently, the clinical use of hMSCs is envisaged to entail an *ex vivo* stage, where the cells are expanded to form a large number of undifferentiated cells, followed by induction of differentiation into specific cell types needed for therapy. To accomplish this task, understanding the molecular mechanisms that maintain self-renewal of the undifferentiated stem cells or progenitor cells versus differentiation need to be understood. We have studied the role of Dlk1/Pref-1(delta-like 1/preadipocyte factor-1) in the control of hMSCs differentiation. Dlk1/Pref-1 is a member of epidermal growth factor (EGF)-like protein family that includes Notch-Delta-Serrata proteins characterized by the presence of EGF-like motifs in their extracellular domain and are known to control cell fate decision and cell differentiation processes in a variety of tissues. Dlk1/Pref-1 was found to be expressed in fetal and adult bone, hMSC and some osteoblastic cell lines. Overexpression of Dlk1/Pref-1 did not affect the proliferation rate of hMSC but the ability of the cells to differentiate into osteoblasts and adipocytes were impaired suggesting that Dlk1/Pref-1 maintains the size of the undifferentiated progenitor cell pool.[37] Thus, our current hypothesis is that for hMSC differentiation to proceed, downregulation of Dlk1/Pref-1 is necessary. We are testing this hypothesis in animal models *in vivo* currently.

Induction of differentiation of hMSCs into a specific cell type is based on modulating the microenvironment of the cells through the addition of a variety of hormones, growth factors, and extracellular matrix components. We have recently demonstrated that closely related growth factors (epidermal growth factor [EGF] and platelet-derived growth factor [PDGF], both of which use receptor-tyrosine kinase-based intracellular signaling) exert differential effects on hMSCs differentiation. EGF enhances osteoblastic differentiation of hMSCs but PDGF does not.[38] To understand the molecular mechanisms causing this differential effect on osteoblast differentiation, the entire EGF and PDGF tyrosine phospho-proteomes were determined using quantitative proteomics. Interestingly, 90% of the signaling proteins were used by both ligands. The PI3K pathway was exclusively activated by PDGF, implicating it as a control point for osteoblast differentiation. Using chemical inhibitors of PI3K in PDGF-stimulated cells led to the disappearance of the differential effect of the two growth factors. It seems thus that cell fate decisions can be made by preferentially activating a small subset of the signaling network. It will be important to discover these control points that influence cell fate in order to more precisely direct stem cell differentiation to cells needed for therapy.

In addition to these biological challenges, several biotechnological challenges must be overcome before hMSC therapy is introduced into the clinic. These problems, which face the whole field of cellular medicine, include issues related to long-term safety, absence of assays for quick quality control of the cells to be administered to patients, and problems related to immunologic responses if allogeneic cell transplantation is to be employed. Finally, the efficiency of cellular therapies (including hMSC-based therapies) in controlled clinical trials of sufficient power needs to be demonstrated before these therapies are accepted in the clinic. It is hoped that these issues will be solved during the coming years.

CAN STEM CELL–BASED THERAPY PROLONG HUMAN LIFE SPAN?

Stem cell therapy has the potential of providing a causal treatment for several age-related degenerative diseases and will, if realized, improve the quality of life of a large segment of the aging population. It is also claimed that "rejuvenation" by stem cell transplantation and cellular therapies may emerge as a causal treatment for the aging process itself. However, since aging is associated with failure of several homeostatic mechanisms, it is not plausible that cellular therapies will change the course of the aging process itself or prolong the life span of the general population. Testing these ideas and realization of their full therapeutic potential will be an intensive topic of biomedical research in the coming years.

REFERENCES

1. WAGERS, A.J. & I.L. WEISSMAN. 2004. Plasticity of adult stem cells. Cell **116:** 639–648.
2. WATT, F.M. & B.L. HOGAN. 2000. Out of Eden: stem cells and their niches. Science **287:** 1427–1430.

3. ODORICO, J.S., D.S. KAUFMAN & J.A. THOMSON. 2001. Multilineage differentiation from human embryonic stem cell lines. Stem Cells **19:** 193–204.

4. SHAMBLOTT, M.J., J. AXELMAN, S.P. WANG, et al. 1998. Derivation of pluripotent stem cells horn cultured human primordial germ cells. Proc. Natl. Acad. Sci. USA **95:** 13726–13731.

5. FRIEDENSTEIN, A.J. 1991. Osteogenic stem cells in the bone marrow. Bone Miner. **7:** 243–272.

6. LURIA, E.A., A.F. PANASYUK & A.Y. FRIEDENSTEIN. 1971. Fibroblast colony formation from monolayer cultures of blood cells. Transfusion **11:** 345–349.

7. KASSEM, M., L. MOSEKILDE & E.F. ERIKSEN. 1993. 1,25-dihydroxyvitamin D3 potentiates fluoride-stimulated collagen type I production in cultures of human bone marrow stromal osteoblast-like cells. J. Bone Miner. Res. **8:** 1453–1458.

8. RICKARD, D.J., M. KASSEM, T.E. HEFFERAN, et al.1996. Isolation and characterization of osteoblast precursor cells from human bone marrow. J. Bone Miner. Res. **11:** 312–324.

9. GRONTHOS, S., S.E. GRAVES, S. OHTA & P.J. SIMMONS. 1994. The STRO-1+ fraction of adult human bone marrow contains the osteogenic precursors. Blood **84:** 4164–4173.

10. REYES, M., T. LUND, T. LENVIK, et al. 2001. Purification and ex vivo expansion of postnatal human marrow mesodermal progenitor cells. Blood **98:** 2615–2625.

11. JIANG, Y., B.N. JAHAGIRDAR, R.L. REINHARDT, et al. 2002. Pluripotency of mesenchymal stem cells derived from adult marrow. Nature **418:** 41–49.

12. D'IPPOLITO, G., S. DIABIRA, G.A. HOWARD, et al. 2004. Marrow-isolated adult multilineage inducible (MIAMI) cells, a unique population of postnatal young and old human cells with extensive expansion and differentiation potential. J. Cell Sci. **117:** 2971–2981.

13. LODIE, T.A., C.E. BLICKARZ, T.J. DEVARAKONDA, et al. 2002. Systematic analysis of reportedly distinct populations of multipotent bone marrow-derived stem cells reveals a lack of distinction. Tissue Eng. **8:** 739–751.

14. DE BARI, C., F. DELL'ACCIO, P. TYLZANOWSKI, et al. 2001. Multipotent mesenchymal stem cells from adult human synovial membrane. Arthritis Rheum. **44:** 1928–1942.

15. MIURA, M., S. GRONTHOS, M. ZHAO, et al. 2003. SHED: stem cells from human exfoliated deciduous teeth. Proc. Natl. Acad. Sci. USA **100:** 5807–5812.

16. KUZNETSOV, S.A., M.H. MANKANI, S. GRONTHOS, et al. 2001. Circulating skeletal stem cells. J. Cell Biol. **153:** 1133–1140.

17. ROSADA, C., J. JUSTESEN, D. MELSVIK, et al. 2003. The human umbilical cord blood: a potential source for osteoblast progenitor cells. Calcif. Tissue Int. **72:** 135–142.

18. PITTENGER, M.F., A.M. MACKAY, S.C. BECK, et al.1999. Multilineage potential of adult human mesenchymal stem cells. Science **284:** 143–147.

19. KASSEM, M., W. BLUM, J. RISTELLI, et al. 1993. Growth hormone stimulates proliferation and differentiation of normal human osteoblast-like cells in vitro. Calcif. Tissue Int. **52:** 222–226.

20. JUSTESEN, J., K. STENDERUP, E.F. ERIKSEN, et al. 2002. Maintenance of osteoblastic and adipocytic differentiation potential with age and osteoporosis in human marrow stromal cell cultures. Calcif. Tissue Int. **71:** 36–44.

21. JOHNSTONE, B., T.M. HERING, A.I. CAPLAN, et al. 1998. In vitro chondrogenesis of bone marrow-derived mesenchymal progenitor cells. Exp.Cell Res. **238:** 265–272.

22. ZHAO, L.R., W.M. DUAN, M. REYES, *et al*. 2002. Human bone marrow stem cells exhibit neural phenotypes and ameliorate neurological deficits after grafting into the ischemic brain of rats. Exp. Neurol. **174:** 11–20.

23. SANCHEZ-RAMOS, J., S. SONG, F. CARDOZO-PELAEZ, *et al*. 2000. Adult bone marrow stromal cells differentiate into neural cells in vitro. Exp. Neurol. **164:** 247–256.

24. STENDERUP, K., C. ROSADA, J. JUSTESEN, *et al*. 2004. Aged human bone marrow stromal cells maintaining bone forming capacity in vivo evaluated using an improved method of visualization. Biogerontology **5:** 107–118.

25. FRIEDENSTEIN, A.J. 1980. Stromal mechanisms of bone marrow: cloning in vitro and retransplantation in vivo. Hamatol. Bluttransfus. **25:** 19–29.

26. QUARTO, R., M. MASTROGIACOMO, R. CANCEDDA, *et al*. 2001. Repair of large bone defects with the use of autologous bone marrow stromal cells. N. Engl. J. Med. **344:** 385–386.

27. OHGUSHI, H., V.M. GOLDBERG & A.I. CAPLAN. 1989. Repair of bone defects with marrow cells and porous ceramic: experiments in rats. Acta Orthop. Scand. **60:** 334–339.

28. BRUDER, S.P., D.J. FINK & A.I. CAPLAN. 1994. Mesenchymal stem cells in bone development, bone repair, and skeletal regeneration therapy. J. Cell Biochem. **56:** 283–294.

29. HORWITZ, E.M., D.J. PROCKOP, L.A. FITZPATRICK, *et al*. 1999. Transplantability and therapeutic effects of bone marrow-derived mesenchymal cells in children with osteogenesis imperfecta. Nat. Med. **5:** 309–313.

30. ALLAY, J.A., J.E. DENNIS, S.E. HAYNESWORTH, *et al*. 1997. LacZ and interleukin-3 expression in vivo after retroviral transduction of marrow-derived human osteogenic mesenchymal progenitors. Hum. Gene Ther. **8:** 1417–1427.

31. BIANCO, P. & P.G. ROBEY. 2001. Stem cells in tissue engineering. Nature **414:** 118–121.

32. STENDERUP, K., J. JUSTESEN, C. CLAUSEN, *et al*. 2003. Aging is associated with decreased maximal life span and accelerated senescence of bone marrow stromal cells. Bone **33:** 919–926.

33. RATTAN, S.I.S. 2003. Aging outside the body: usefulness of the Hayflick system. **1:** 1–8.

34. ZIMMERMANN, S., M. VOSS, S. KAISER, *et al*. 2003. Lack of telomerase activity in human mesenchymal stem cells. Leukemia **17:** 1146–1149.

35. SIMONSEN, J.L., C. ROSADA, N. SERAKINCI, *et al*. 2002. Telomerase expression extends the proliferative life-span and maintains the osteogenic potential of human bone marrow stromal cells. Nat. Biotechnol. **20:** 592–596.

36. SERAKINCI, N., P. GULDBERG, J. BURNS, *et al*. 2004. Adult human mesenchymal stem cell as a target for neoplastic transformation. Oncogene **23:** 5095–5098.

37. ABDALLAH, B.M., C.H. JENSEN, G. GUTIERREZ, *et al*. 2004. Regulation of human skeletal stem cells differentiation by Dlk1/Pref-1. J. Bone Miner. Res. **19:** 841–852.

38. KRATCHMAROVA, I., B. BLAGOEV, M. HAACK-SORENSEN, *et al*. 2005. Mechanism of divergent growth factor effects in mesenchymal stem cell differentiation. Science **308:** 1472–1477.

Heat Shock–Induced Enhancement of Osteoblastic Differentiation of hTERT-Immortalized Mesenchymal Stem Cells

RUNE NØRGAARD,[a] MOUSTAPHA KASSEM,[b]
AND SURESH I. S. RATTAN[a]

[a]*Laboratory of Cellular Ageing, Danish Centre for Molecular Gerontology, Department of Molecular Biology, University of Aarhus, Aarhus, Denmark*

[b]*Department of Endocrinology, University of Southern Denmark, Odense, Denmark*

ABSTRACT: Heat shock (HS)–induced stress response in human cells results in a variety of biological effects and is known to induce the transcription of heat-shock proteins, which help the cells to cope with different kinds of stress. We have studied the effects of HS on the differentiation of human mesenchymal stem cells (hMSCs) into osteoblastic cells. As a model for hMSCs we used a telomerase-immortalized hMSC line designated hMSC-TERT. Cells were exposed to 1 h HS at 41°C, 42.5°C, or 44°C prior to incubation in a medium containing either 10^{-8} M 1α,25-dihydroxy-vitamin-D_3 (calcitriol) or 10^{-8} M calcitriol, 50 μg/mL L-ascorbic acid, and 10 mM β-glycerophosphate followed by an analysis of induction of osteoblast differentiation and the formation of mineralized matrix, respectively. Our results indicate that the exposure of cells to mild heat stress enhances the extent of differentiation of hMSCs by 12% to 42%. These effects are an expression of the phenomenon of mild stress-induced hormesis.

KEYWORDS: osteoblast; differentiation; stress; hormesis; human mesenchymal stem cells

INTRODUCTION

Human mesenchymal stem cells (hMSCs) can differentiate into a variety of cell types including osteoblasts, adipocytes, chondrocytes, and endothelial-like cells.[1] In order to improve therapeutic use of stem cells it is important to find

Address for correspondence: Dr. Suresh I.S. Rattan, Department of Molecular Biology, University of Aarhus, Gustav Wieds Vej 10C, DK-8000 Aarhus C, Denmark. Voice: +45 8942 5034; fax: +45 8612 3178.
e-mail: rattan@mb.au.dk

Ann. N.Y. Acad. Sci. 1067: 443–447 (2006). © 2006 New York Academy of Sciences.
doi: 10.1196/annals.1354.063

ways to enhance the qualitative and quantitative extent of differentiation, and thereby increase the chances of the cells to grow into the right kind of tissue or structure. Therefore, we have examined the effects of heat shock (HS) on the differentiation of hMSCs as measured by the synthesis of an osteoblastic marker, alkaline phosphatase (ALP), and cell matrix mineralization. As a model for hMSCs we used a telomerase-immortalized hMSC line designated hMSC-TERT. The results indicate that hyperthermia could be used as a differentiation promoter and an efficient way of making stem cells differentiate to a greater extent.

EXPERIMENTAL METHODS

The hMSC cultures were established from bone marrow aspirates taken from the iliac crest of young donors (men and women between 25 and 30 years old).[2] The establishment and characterization of the hMSC-TERT cell line have been described previously.[3] For cell differentiation assays, cells were seeded in 6- or 96-well plates at a density of 10^4 cells/cm^2 and incubated at 37°C until 50–60% cell confluence. For osteoblast differentiation studies, cells were grown in medium containing 10^{-8} M calcitriol (1α,25-dihydroxy-vitamin-D$_3$–Leo, Ballerup, Denmark). For *in vitro* mineralized matrix formation studies, cells were grown in medium containing 10^{-8}M calcitriol, 50 μg/mL L-ascorbic acid, and 10 mM β-glycerophosphate. The medium was replaced every second or third day. The number of cells in each well was estimated by either MTT assay, crystal violet assay, or by using a standard growth curve. Control cells were counted in triplicate every day from day 0 to day 8 using a Coulter Counter.

For HS studies the cultures were exposed to 41°C, 42.5°C, or 44°C HS for 1 h using a thermostatic water bath controlled to ±0.1°C. To avoid any possible loss of water caused by hyperthermia, the medium was removed and substituted after HS. Alkaline phosphatase (ALP) was quantified using a colorimetric assay using *p*-nitrophenol phosphate (PNP) as a substrate.[4] When exposed to ALP enzyme a yellow reaction product is formed by the dephosphorylation of PNP into *p*-nitrophenol. Cells were washed twice with PBS and incubated with 100 μL of an alkaline buffer solution and 200 μL of ALP substrate solution (alkaline buffer solution containing 5 mM PNP) for 30 min at 37°C. The cells were washed with distilled water and specific ALP activity (expressed as nanomoles of PNP/min/10^4 cells) was measured at 410 nm and quantified against a standard curve of *p*-nitrophenol.

The mineralized matrix was stained with Alizarin red S and the amount of the mineralized matrix was quantified by modification of previously described methods.[5,6] Alizarin red S is a dye that binds selectively to calcium salts and is widely used for calcium mineral histochemistry.[7] Alizarin red S (1 mole) binds 2 mole of calcium in an Alizarin red S-calcium complex. The cells were washed with PBS and fixed in ice-cold 70% ethanol for 30 min followed by staining with Alizarin red S for another 30 min and washed again. Finally, the stained cells were incubated in 10% (wt/vol) cetylpyridinium chloride to elute bound stain. The dye was collected and absorbance was measured at 570 nm. Alizarin red S in samples was quantified according to a standard curve and expressed as micromoles of bound cetylpyridinium chloride per 10^4 cells.

RESULTS AND DISCUSSION

Previous studies with hTERT-MSC in our laboratory have shown that the maximum level of HS protein 70 (Hsp70) is reached 3 h post HS (data not shown). Therefore, the cells were treated with HS 3 h prior to adding the medium promoting osteoblast differentiation and mineralized matrix formation, respectively. Three sets of similar experiments were carried out using HS temperatures of 41°C, 42.5°C, or 44°C.

Level of ALP after HS

FIGURE 1 shows that untreated control cell cultures produced a basic amount of ALP after 8 days in culture. Adding calcitriol to the medium showed more than a doubling of the amount of ALP in control cells after incubation for 8 days. However, cells preexposed to hyperthermia had higher levels of

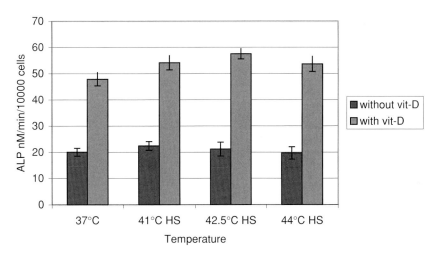

FIGURE 1. Effect of heat shock on calcitriol-induced differentiation of hTERT-MSCs as measured by the levels of alkaline phosphatase (ALP).

calcitriol-induced ALP, which were 12% to 20% higher depending on the temperature. These results suggest that a 1-h HS of 42.5°C is the most beneficial pretreatment to give to hMSC-TERT cells while inducing them to differentiate into osteoblasts.

Amount of Mineralized Matrix Formation After HS

FIGURE 2 shows that untreated control cell cultures had a low level of mineralized matrix formation after 8 days in culture. Adding calcitriol, L-ascorbic acid, and β-glycerophosphate to the medium showed a large increase in the amount of mineralized matrix after incubation for 8 days. As in the case of ALP, the formation of a mineralized matrix was 28% to 42% higher in cells preexposed to hyperthermia. These results suggest that a 1-h HS of 42.5°C is the most beneficial pretreatment to give to hMSC-TERT cells while inducing them to form a mineralized matrix.

Finally, it seems that mild heat stress-induced increase in the levels of Hsps enhances the responsiveness of stem cells to differentiate. These results have practical applications in the therapeutic use of stem cells where a preexposure of cells to mild stress may improve their biological activity and function. Such beneficial effects of mild heat stress on stem cell differentiation are novel examples of the phenomenon of hormesis.[8] Our studies are in progress to elucidate the exact mechanism of the hormetic effects of mild stress on stem cells and during aging.

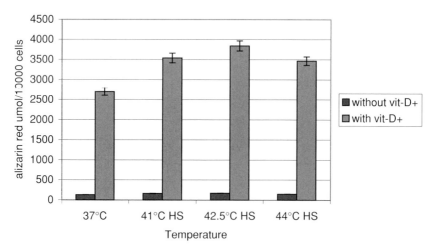

FIGURE 2. Effect of heat shock on the mineralized matrix formation by hTERT-MSCs treated with calcitriol, L-ascorbic acid, and β-glycerophosphate (vit-D+).

ACKNOWLEDGMENTS

We thank Helle Jakobsen, Regina Gonzalez-Dosal, Elise Røge Nielsen, and Gunhild Siboska for their help and critical discussions. The Laboratory of Cellular Ageing is supported by research grants from the Danish Research Councils, Carlsberg Fund, Senetek PLC, and EU's Biomed Health Programmes.

REFERENCES

1. ABDALLAH, B.M., M. HAACK-SORENSEN, J.S. BURNS, *et al.* 2005. Maintenance of differentiation potential of human bone marrow mesenchymal stem cells immortalized by human telomerase reverse transcriptase gene despite extensive proliferation. Biochem. Biophys. Res. Commun. **326:** 527–538.
2. KASSEM, M., L. MOSEKILDE & E.F. ERIKSEN. 1993. 1,25-dihydroxyvitamin D3 potentiates fluoride-stimulated fluoride-stimulated collagen type I production in cultures of human bone marrow stromal osteoblast-like cells. J. Bone Miner. Res. **8:** 1453–1458.
3. SIMONSEN, J.L., C. ROSADA, N. SERAKINCI, *et al.* 2002. Telomerase expression extends the proliferative life-span and maintains the osteogenic potential of human bone marrow stromal cells. Nat. Biotechnol. **20:** 592–596.
4. ABDALLAH, B.M., C.H. JENSEN, G. GUTIERREZ, *et al.* 2004. Regulation of human skeletal stem cells differentiation by Dlk1/Pref-1. J. Bone Miner. Res. **19:** 841–852.
5. STANTON, L.-A., S. SABARI, A.V. SAMPAIO, *et al.* 2004. p38 MAP kinase signalling is required for hypertrophic chondrocyte differentiation. Biochem. J. **378:** 53–62.
6. WANG, W. & T. KIRSCH. 2002. Retinoic acid stimulates annexin-mediated growth plate chondrocyte mineralization. J. Cell. Biol. **157:** 1061–1069.
7. MCGEE-RUSSEL, S.M. 1958. Histochemical method for calcium. J. Histochem. Cytochem. **6:** 22–42.
8. RATTAN, S.I.S. 2004. Aging intervention, prevention, and therapy through hormesis. J. Gerontology. Biol. Sci. **59A:** 705–709.

Selective PPAR Agonists for the Treatment of Type 2 Diabetes

JAN O. NEHLIN, JOHN P. MOGENSEN, INGRID PETTERSON, LONE JEPPESEN, JAN FLECKNER, ERIK M. WULFF, AND PER SAUERBERG

Novo Nordisk A/S, Novo Nordisk Park, 2760 Måløv, Denmark

ABSTRACT: Type 2 diabetes is a metabolic disease characterized by increased plasma glucose and insulin as well as dyslipidemia. If left untreated, chronic diseases will develop that are associated with neuropathic damage and higher mortality risk. Using a rational drug design, novel compounds have been developed that selectively activate the human PPAR receptors, leading to lessening of hyperglycemia and hyperinsulinemia as well as reduction of lipid levels in conjunction with an increase of the beneficial HDL-cholesterol. These PPAR agonists showed increased potency and efficacy compared to previously marketed insulin sensitizers. Lead compounds with desirable pharmacokinetic properties were chosen for further testing in several animal models. The *in vivo* activity of some synthetic ligands, capable of activating two or all three members of peroxisome proliferator-activated receptors (PPAR) family of receptors, suggested that they may have improved efficacy in type 2 diabetes therapy. Here, we briefly summarize the development of some novel PPAR agonists identified by our group in recent years.

KEYWORDS: diabetes type 2; PPAR; insulin sensitizers; triple agonists; hyperglycemia; dyslipidemia

BACKGROUND

Type 2 diabetes (also known as noninsulin-dependent diabetes mellitus, T2DM) is a life-long disease developing in adulthood as a consequence of an unhealthy lifestyle (e.g., physical inactivity, consumption of energy-rich foods, etc.) and genetic predisposition.[1] Obesity is considered to be a major risk factor, evidenced by a strong correlation between body mass index (BMI) and T2DM incidence. It afflicts close to 4% of the human population, with the number of cases expected to nearly double over the next 25 years.[1-3] The accompanying insulin resistance, a state whereby the action of insulin in promotion of cellular uptake of glucose is low, leads to high glucose levels and

Present address and address for correspondence: Dr. Jan O. Nehlin, Department of Clinical Immunology, Centre for Stem Cell Treatment, Odense University Hospital & University of Southern Denmark, SdR. Boulevard 29, 5000 Odense, Denmark. Voice: +45-65-413673; fax: +45-66-127975.
e-mail: jan.nehlin@ouh.fyns-amt.dk

Ann. N.Y. Acad. Sci. 1067: 448–453 (2006). © 2006 New York Academy of Sciences.
doi: 10.1196/annals.1354.064

compensatory hyperinsulinemia. Eventually, the insulin-producing pancreatic beta cells fail to overcome the defect, resulting in cellular failure and a drop in insulin levels, leading to impaired glucose tolerance. If left untreated, the chronic hyperglycemia is associated with long-term damage to various organs, particularly the retina, nerves, and kidney. Elevated plasma triglycerides lead to atherosclerosis and an increase in the mortality rate.[3]

The marketed insulin sensitizers (rosiglitazone and pioglitazone), which are glucose-lowering compounds and the fibrates, (bezafibrate, fenofibrate, and clofibrate) which are triglyceride-lowering compounds, are agonists of the nuclear PPARγ and PPARα receptors, respectively.[4,5] The peroxisome proliferator-activated receptors (PPARs) are ligand-dependent transcription factors belonging to the nuclear receptor superfamily. The PPAR receptors heterodimerize with retinoid X receptor (RXR) upon ligand binding and recruit co-activator(s) to modulate expression of target genes after binding to specific peroxisome proliferator response elements (PPREs).[6–8]

Three different PPAR members have been identified—PPARα, PPARγ, and PPARδ[9–12]—having different tissue-specific expression profiles. There is no marketed drug available that targets PPARδ selectively. However, recent findings link PPARδ function with lipid transport and metabolism.[12] Indeed, treatment of obese rhesus monkeys with the PPARδ-selective agonist GW501516 resulted in a dramatic decrease in plasma triglycerides and LDL-cholesterol, and increase in plasma HDL-cholesterol.[13]

The fibrates lower serum triglycerides and raise HDL-cholesterol.[4] The insulin sensitizers decrease hepatic gluconeogenesis and hepatic glucose output, increase glucose uptake in muscle, and reduce the release of fatty acids from adipocytes. These events result in a decrease in the insulin resistance, with reduced blood glucose and triglyceride levels.[5]

Several approaches have been undertaken over the last decade to improve the agonist activity of PPAR binding ligands. Here, we provide a brief summary of our findings on the development of novel PPAR-agonists with different selectivity and efficacy at either one or more of the three PPAR receptors.

SYNTHETIC PPAR-LIGANDS: DESIGN, AND *IN VITRO* AND *IN VIVO* CHARACTERIZATION

In comparison to natural PPAR ligands,[14–17] synthetic ligands may have improved pharmacokinetic properties, such as enhanced metabolic stability and better oral bioavailability. They will therefore often constitute better drug candidates than natural ligands.

Whereas benefits of the fibrates in the treatment of hyper-triglyceridemia are evident, they exhibit relatively low receptor potency, which in fact may limit their clinical efficacy.[18] Similarly, insulin sensitizers modulate glucose levels, while lipid levels are only mildly affected. Thus, it was anticipated that dual PPARα,γ receptor agonists would have an improved efficacy when compared to PPAR subtype-selective agonists. Synthesis of molecules derived from the structure of the alkoxy-propionic acid class of insulin sensitizers was performed using a rational drug design.[19]

The molecules were screened on HEK293 cells, transiently expressing chimeric constructs composed of the ligand-binding domains of either human PPARα, PPARγ, or PPARδ isoforms fused with the yeast GAL4 DNA-binding domain. Using a luminescent-based PPAR *in vitro* transactivation assay (see FIG. 1), it was possible to characterize these compounds in terms of potency and efficacy.[19,20] Vector control or vectors expressing hybrid proteins were transfected into HEK293 cells together with a transfection-control vector encoding beta-galactosidase and a luciferase-reporter vector (see Refs. 19,20 for details).

Novel tricyclic-α-alkyloxyphenylpropionic acids were generated that exhibited potent dual PPARα,γ activities. Next, the compounds were tested in various animal models. Male db/db obese mice (lacking the leptin receptor) were used as the primary *in vivo* model for blood glucose measurements and assessing improvement of insulin sensitivity. Male Sprague-Dawley (SD) rats were used to study the pharmacokinetics of the various compounds and as a high cholesterol-fed animal model. Several dual PPAR-activating compounds showed good pharmacokinetics.[19] One of the novel dual PPARα,γ agonists

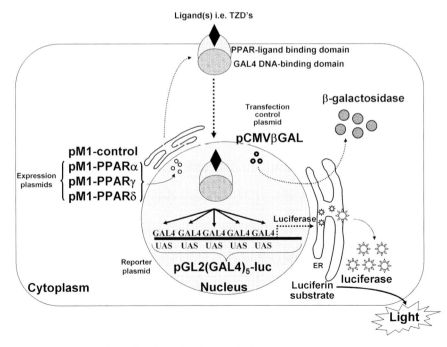

FIGURE 1. Schematic view of an *in vitro* PPAR-transactivation assay.

was 100 times more potent in the *in vitro* PPARα transactivation assay than was bezafibrate. Furthermore, a long half-life in rats is assumed to contribute to the efficacy of the compound *in vivo*, suggesting that the best improvement of hypertriglyceridemia is obtained using drugs with long exposure. Treatment of db/db mice with this compound greatly improved their insulin sensitivity, as measured by an oral glucose tolerance test. In fact, the efficacy was even better than what can be obtained with rosiglitazone or pioglitazone. In summary, it was possible to obtain potent and efficacious dual PPARα,γ agonists in both *in vitro* and *in vivo* assays. The dual PPARα,γ activators combined the agonist activity of both the PPARα activity resulting in hypolipidemic effects and the PPARγ activity resulting in hypoglycemic effects and increased insulin sensitivity.[19,20]

In spite of the high sequence homology of the three PPAR receptor subtypes, it was shown that PPAR subtype selectivity could be achieved by only modifying the lipophilic part of the ligands. Systematic structural changes in the lipophilic part of NNC 61–0029/DRF2725 (ragaglitazar)[21] in combination with docking experiments into the ligand-binding domain (LBD) of the PPARα, PPARγ, and PPARδ receptors led to the design of selective PPARα, PPARγ, dual PPARα,γ and triple PPARα,γ,δ agonists with various degrees of potency and efficacy.[19,20]

The design of dimeric ligands has proven to be advantageous on account of improved receptor subtype selectivity and/or improved potency when compared to their monomeric counterparts. Dimeric ligands contain two recognition units linked covalently through a spacer or a common group.[22] Using a triple PPAR activator as a start template, bivalent molecules were obtained that still retained triple agonist activity. In spite of their large molecular weight (above 500 g/mol) and bulky structures, these molecules exhibited favorable pharmacokinetic properties in SD rats. These included very high maximal plasma concentrations, very high oral bioavailability, very low plasma clearances, very low volume of distributions, and the desired long plasma half-lives. These properties resulted in a potent and efficacious lowering of plasma triglycerides, blood glucose, and plasma insulin levels in db/db mice, confirming that dimeric PPAR activators might be suitable drug candidates.[22] A full structure–activity analysis on dimeric ligands revealed an altered PPAR subtype profile compared to the monomeric ligands, and their enhanced potency could in part be explained by means of molecular receptor modeling.[23]

CONCLUSIONS

Selective PPARα, PPARγ, dual PPARα,γ and triple PPAR α,γ,δ agonists were designed and tested.[19,20,22] The dual PPARα,γ activators showed higher potency and efficacy than the selective PPARγ agonist rosiglitazone and the PPARα agonist fenofibrate.[19] Dimeric ligands were developed that resulted in effective PPARγ agonist activity with retained or increased potency as compared to rosiglitazone.[22,23] The preclinical effects of the triple PPARαγδ agonist warrants further animal testing and eventually clinical studies.

ACKNOWLEDGMENTS

We thank all past and present members of the PPAR team whose dedicated contributions to the development and characterization of novel PPAR agonists have been instrumental to the project.

REFERENCES

1. WORLD HEALTH ORGANISATION. 2005. http://www.who.int/en/.
2. WILD, S. *et al*. 2004. Global prevalence of diabetes: estimates for the year 2000 and projections for 2030. Diabetes Care **27:** 1047–1053.
3. STUMVOLL, M., B.J. GOLDSTEIN & T.W. VAN HAEFTEN. 2005. Type 2 diabetes: principles of pathogenesis and therapy. Lancet **365:** 1333–1346.
4. ETGEN, G.H. & N. MANTLO. 2003. PPAR ligands for metabolic disorders. Curr. Top. Med. Chem. **3:** 1649–1661.
5. WILLSON, T.M. *et al*. 1996. The structure-activity relationship between peroxisome proliferator-activated receptor gamma agonism and the antihyperglycemic activity of thiazolidinediones. J. Med. Chem. **39:** 665–668.
6. EVANS, R.M., G.D. BARISH & Y.X. WANG. 2004. PPARs and the complex journey to obesity. Nat. Med. **10:** 355–361.
7. FERRE, P. 2004. The biology of peroxisome proliferator-activated receptors: relationship with lipid metabolism and insulin sensitivity. Diabetes **53**(Suppl 1): S43–S50.
8. BERGER, J.P., T.E. AKIYAMA & P.T. MEINKE. 2005. PPARs: therapeutic targets for metabolic disease. Trends Pharmacol. Sci. **26:** 244–251.
9. VAN RAALTE, D.H. *et al*. 2004. Peroxisome proliferator-activated receptor (PPAR)-alpha: a (PPAR)-alpha: a pharmacological target with a promising future. Pharm. Res. **21:** 1531–1538.
10. RANGWALA, S.M. & M.A. LAZAR. 2004. Peroxisome proliferator-activated receptor gamma in diabetes and metabolism. Trends Pharmacol. Sci. **25:** 331–336.
11. ROSEN, E.D. & B.M. SPIEGELMAN. 2001. PPARgamma: a nuclear regulator of metabolism, differentiation, and cell growth. J. Biol. Chem. **276:** 37731–37734.
12. FREDENRICH, A. & P.A. GRIMALDI. 2005. PPARdelta: an incompletely known PPAR nuclear receptor. Diabetes Metab. **31:** 23–27.
13. OLIVER, W.R. *et al*. 2001. A selective peroxisome proliferator-activated receptor delta agonist promotes reverse cholesterol transport. Proc. Natl. Acad. Sci.USA **98:** 5306–5311.
14. FORMAN, B.M. *et al*. 1995. 15-Deoxy-delta 12, 14-prostaglandin J2 is a ligand for the adipocyte determination factor PPAR gamma. Cell **83:** 803–812.
15. KLIEWER, S.A. *et al*. 1995. A prostaglandin J2 metabolite binds peroxisome proliferator-activated receptor gamma and promotes adipocyte differentiation. Cell **83:** 813–819.

16. Fu, J. *et al.* 2003. Oleylethanolamide regulates feeding and body weight through activation of the nuclear receptor PPAR-alpha. Nature **425:** 90–93.
17. Lo Verme, J. *et al.* 2004. The nuclear receptor peroxisome proliferator-activated receptor-alpha mediates the anti-inflammatory actions of palmitoylethanolamide. Mol. Pharmacol. **67:** 15–19.
18. English, P. & G. Williams. 2001. Type 2 diabetes. Martin Dunitz Ltd. Taylor & Francis, London.
19. Sauerberg, P. *et al.* 2002. Novel tricyclic-α-alkyloxyphenylpropionic acids: dual PPARalpha/gamma agonists with hypolipidemic and antidiabetic activity. J. Med. Chem. **45:** 789–804.
20. Mogensen, J.P. *et al.* 2003. Design and synthesis of novel PPARalpha/gamma/delta triple activators using a known PPARalpha/gamma dual activator as structural template. Bioorg. Med. Chem. Lett. **13:** 257–260.
21. Lohray, B.B. *et al.* 2001. (−)3-[4-[2-(Phenoxazin-10-yl)ethoxy]phenyl]-2-ethoxypropanoic acid [(−)DRF 2725]: a dual PPAR agonist with potent anti-hyperglycemic and lipid modulating activity. J. Med. Chem. **44:** 2675–2678.
22. Sauerberg, P. *et al.* 2003. Large dimeric ligands with favorable pharmacokinetic properties and peroxisome proliferator-activated receptor agonist activity *in vitro* and *in vivo*. J. Med. Chem. **46:** 4883–4894.
23. Sauerberg, P. *et al.* 2005. Structure-activity relationships of dimeric PPAR agonists. Bioorg. Med. Chem. Lett. **15:** 1497–1500.

Alzheimer's Disease Pathogenesis

Role of Aging

DENHAM HARMAN

*Department of Medicine, University of Nebraska College of Medicine,
984635 Nebraska Medical Center, Omaha, Nebraska 68198–4635, USA*

ABSTRACT: Alzheimer's disease (AD) is the chief cause of dementia, and
age is its major risk factor. The majority of cases (90–95%) are sporadic (SAD), and the remainder are familial (FAD). AD is characterized
by two brain lesions, intraneuronal fibrillary tangles and extracellular
plaques. The lesions are identical in SAD and FAD as well as to those in
persons with Down's syndrome (DS). The same lesions are also observed
frequently in elderly non-demented individuals (E-ND). Both AD lesions
may stem from the normal progressive increases in oxidative stress (OxS)
throughout the body with age. Onset of dementia due to the accumulating lesions is around 40 years for DS, 40–60 years for FAD, over about
65 years for SAD, while that for E-ND is unknown. The lesions are made
clinically manifest with time by the normal increase with age of OxS,
"the dementia of old age," or by a process specific for each AD category,
which enhances the normal OxS so as to lower the unknown onset age of
dementia for E-ND individuals to that associated with the AD category. A
plausible process can be advanced for each AD category. The hypothesis
suggests convenient, effective measures to prevent and treat, for example, by decreasing brain OxS levels with oral antioxidants such as lipoic
or dehydroascorbic acids that are capable of passing the blood–brain
barrier.

KEYWORDS: aging; oxidative stress; mutations; Alzheimer's disease;
Down's syndrome

INTRODUCTION

Alzheimer's disease (AD) is the chief cause of dementia.[1] Age is the major
risk factor for the disease.[1,2]

The majority of cases[3] (90–95%) are sporadic (SAD). The remainder are
familial (FAD).[3] Most FAD cases are associated with mutations in the gene
for presenilin 1 (PS1) on chromosome 14,[4] some with mutations in the gene

Address for correspondence: Denham Harman, M.D., Ph.D., Department of Medicine, University
of Nebraska College of Medicine, 984635 Nebraska Medical Center, Omaha, Nebraska 68198-4635,
USA. Fax: 402-559-7330.
e-mail: vcerino@unmc.edu

Ann. N.Y. Acad. Sci. 1067: 454–460 (2006). © 2006 New York Academy of Sciences.
doi: 10.1196/annals.1354.065

for presenilin 2 (PS2) on chromosome 1,[5] while a few have mutations in the gene for the amyloid precursor protein (APP) on chromosome 21.[6]

AD is characterized by two lesions[1,2,7]: intraneuronal fibrillary tangles and extracellular plaques. Major steps in pathogenesis have been summarized.[8,9] Plaques are either diffuse or neuritic; Congo red stains the latter but not the former. Diffuse plaques contain the majority of brain βA peptides, mainly βA42. These plaques can form quickly—within a few days after head injury,[10] and early in life—as early as 12 years in patients with Down's syndrome (DS).[11] Amyloid plaques, that is, neuritic plaques, stained by Congo red, are formed by oxidative-polymerization free radical reactions involving preamyloid plaques.[12] Amyloid formation is generally associated with the clinical manifestations of AD.

The AD brain lesions in SAD and FAD are the same, and have the same distribution pattern. Identical lesions are present in the brains of individuals with DS,[1,11] and are frequently observed in elderly non-demented persons (E-ND).[13] The latter suggests that AD lesions may be a normal accompaniment of aging, and that in these E-ND individuals the number of lesions had not risen to clinically significant levels before death.

Dementia onset, due to the accumulating AD lesions, is at around 40 years for DS,[11] 40–60 years for FAD,[3] over about 65 years for SAD,[3] while that for E-ND is not known. Lower dementia onset ages are associated with shorter life spans.

Extensive studies of AD over the past 10–15 years have not resulted in a generally accepted hypothesis on pathogenesis.[14] Major emphasis has been placed on the role of amyloid,[9] the neurotoxin formed by the action of free radicals on preamyloid.[12]

HYPOTHESIS ON PATHOGENESIS OF ALZHEIMER'S DISEASE

The two lesions associated with AD are a normal part of aging; they stem from the progressive increases in oxidative stress throughout the body with advancing age. The lesions are made clinically manifest by time, "the dementia of old age," or by a process specific for each AD category, which enhances OxS.

Formation of AD Lesions

Intraneuronal Fibrillary Tangles

The progressive increase throughout the body of more-or-less random free radical reactions with advancing age (oxidative stress)—owing to the presence of O_2 in the tissues, formation of superoxide radicals (SO) by mitochondria in the course of normal metabolism and their spontaneous/enzymatic dismutation to H_2O_2,[15,16] decreasing availability of ATP for reductive synthesis, and the likely progressive increases in tissue peroxidizability—should,[8] like that caused by menadione,[17] eventually cause sustained elevation of calcium concentrations in the intracellular compartments. This leads[18] to disruption of the cytoskeleton and activation of calcium-dependent catabolic enzymes including phospholipases, kinases, proteases, and endonucleases. In the case of neurons, the foregoing may be exacerbated by overstimulation of receptors for excitatory amino acids.[19] Some neurons may be expected to undergo apoptosis and die.

Activation of kinases such as CaMK may be expected to progressively phosphorylate tau and thereby decrease the strength of its binding with microtubules. The latter permits phosphorylated tau to self-assemble and form paired helical filaments and, in turn, neurofibrillary tangles, while concomitantly the destabilized microtubules break down. Accordingly, elevation of the intracellular Ca^{2+} levels in cultured human cortical neurons[20] causes ultrastructural and antigenic changes in the cytoskeleton similar to those seen in neurons with neurofibrillary tangles.

Neuritic Plaques

Conversion of the fibril form of the βA peptides present in diffuse plaques to that in amyloid probably normally increases slowly and progressively with advancing age owing in part to increasing oxidative stress.[8] At some age in brain locations associated with elevated metabolic rates, that is, AD areas,[8] the oxidative stress may exceed the threshold for the activation of microglial cells; this occurs in the late 20s or early 30s for those with DS,[11] in a manner akin to the upregulation of the synthesis of cytokines IL-8 and TNF-α by the action of H_2O_2 on dendritic cells.[21] Then, free radicals formed by activated microglia could serve to catalyze the oxidative conversion of preamyloid in the microglial area to amyloid, and simultaneously initiate the inflammation[22] involved in neuritic plaque formation and neuronal cell loss.

How apolipoprotein E4 lowers AD onset age is apparently not known. The O_2-mediated interaction between apoE4[23] and preamyloid (probably facilitated by the presence of the two arginines in apoE4[24]) suggests a possible explanation: reaction of tissue O_2 with apoE4 may serve as a catalyst to further increase the normally slow formation of oxidative changes in preamyloid, a process, which results eventually in formation of amyloid. Thus, when H_2O_2-induced microglial activation occurs, less time is required to complete the transformation. Hence, the age of onset of clinical symptoms of AD is decreased, more so the longer the period of apoE4-associated changes prior to microglial activation.

Augmentation of the Innate Rate of AD Lesion Formation

Sporadic AD

Some of the accumulating mutation(s) in one or more of the approximately 1,000 mtDNA and nucDNA genes involved in mitochondrial biogenesis and function[25]—ignoring those involved in "the mitochondrial diseases"—would be expected to have adverse effects on mitochondrial function, thereby increasing oxidative stress and the rate of formation of AD lesions. The latter lowers the onset age of the dementia of the E-ND group into that associated with SAD.

Familial AD

APP, PS1, and PS2, as well as their mutated forms, undergo proteolytic processing in the endoplasmic reticulum (ER) membrane.[9] The calcium-buffering activity of the ER is modulated by the ATPase calcium pumps,[26] located in the ER membrane, and by the associated Ca^{2+} release channels.[27] Many compounds influence ER calcium content,[28] including (1) phospholamban, (2) the ganglioside GM1 and GM3, (3) 6-gingerol and ellagic acid, (4) procaine, caffeine, thapsigargin, and dantrolene, and (5) the erythrocyte isoenzyme of acylphosphatase (this enzyme inhibits the Ca^{2+} pump by hydrolyzing the phosphointermediate formed during the catalytic cycle of the calcium ATPase).

It seems very likely that mutations in APP or the presenilins decrease ER calcium buffering, in a manner akin to that of one or more of the substances known to influence it, resulting in compensatory increases in other calcium pools, particularly in mitochondria. The foregoing is strongly supported by studies with cultured neurons.[29]

Increases in mitochondrial calcium content enhance SO formation, and hence that of H_2O_2.[30] This, in turn, lowers the age of onset of dementia of the E-ND group and the life span.

Down's Syndrome

Individuals with Down's Syndrome disorder have three copies of chromosome 21 rather than the normal two.[31]

The early onset of AD in individuals with DS is attributed to an enhanced rate of H_2O_2 formation[31] as a result of a defect in complex 1 of the respiratory chain. Thus, the early appearance of AD in individuals with DS, as with SAD and FAD, may be largely caused by a higher than normal rate of increase of H_2O_2 with age.

COMMENT

Oxidative stress increases with age; a major contributor to this is the H_2O_2 derived from superoxide radicals formed by mitochondria in the course of

TABLE 1. Processes specific for each AD category.[a]

AD category	Processes
SAD	Accumulation of mutation(s) in one or more of the approximately 1,000 mtDNA and nucDNA genes involved in mitochondrial biogenesis and function.
FAD	Mutations in APP or the presenilins that downregulate ER calcium-buffering capacity. This increases mitochondrial calcium levels, resulting in enhanced H_2O_2 formation.
DS	Defective complex 1 of the mitochondrial respiratory chain.

[a]These augment to different degrees the innate cellular formation of hydrogen peroxide, thus lowering the potential dementia onset age of the innate AD process into that associated with the AD category.

normal metabolism. Augmentation of the innate rate of H_2O_2 formation by a process (TABLE 1) specific for each AD category increases the rate of AD lesion formation and accumulation, so as to lower the age of onset of dementia of the EN-D group into that associated with the AD category.

The above suggests effective measures for prevention and treatment, for example, by decreasing brain H_2O_2 levels by oral antioxidants capable of passing the blood–brain barrier such as lipoic acid[32] or dehydroascorbic acid.[33]

REFERENCES

1. KATZMAN, R. 1986. Alzheimer's disease. N. Engl. J. Med. **314:** 964–973.
2. KATZMAN, R. & T. SAITOH. 1991. Advances in Alzheimer's disease. FASEB J. **5:** 278–286.
3. GOEDERT, M., J. STRITTMATTER & A.D. ROSES. 1994. Risky apolipoprotein in brain. Nature **372:** 45–46.
4. SCHELLENBERG, G.D., T.D. BIRDD, E.M. WIJSMAN, et al. 1992. Genetic linkage evidence for a familial Alzheimer's disease locus on chromosome 14. Science **258:** 668–671.
5. LEVY-LAHAD, E.W., E.M. WIJSMAN, E. NEMENS, et al. 1995. A familial Alzheimer's disease locus on chromosome 1. Science **269:** 970–973.
6. GOATE, A., M.-C. CHARTIER-HARLIN, M. MULLAN, et al. 1991. Segregation of a missense mutation in the amyloid precursor protein gene with familial Alzheimer's disease. Nature **349:** 704–706.
7. KATZMAN, R. & J.E. JACKSON. 1991. Alzheimer's disease: basic and clinical advances. J. Am. Geriatr. Soc. **39:** 516–525.
8. HARMAN, D. 1995. Free radical theory of aging: Alzheimer's disease pathogenesis. AGE **18:** 97–119.
9. SELKOE, D.J. 1999. Translating cell biology into therapeutic advances in Alzheimer's disease. Nature **399** (Suppl, June 24): A23–A31.
10. ROBERTS, G.W., S.M. GENTLEMEN, A. LYNCH, et al. 1991. βA4 amyloid protein deposition in brain after head trauma. Lancet **338:** 1422–1423.
11. MANN, D.M.A. & M.M. ESIRI. 1989. The pattern of acquisition of plaques and tangles in the brains of patients under 50 years of age with Down's syndrome. J. Neurol. Sci. **89:** 169–179.

12. DYRKS, T., E. DYRKS, T. HARTMANN, *et al*. 1992. Amyloidogenicity of βA4-bearing amyloid protein precursor fragments by metal-catalyzed oxidation. J. Biol. Chem. **267:** 18210–18217.

13. ARRIAGADA, P.V., K. MARZLOFF & B.T. HYMAN. 1992. Distribution of Alzheimer-type pathologic changes in nondemented elderly individuals matches the pattern in Alzheimer's disease. Neurologia **42:** 1681–1688.

14. EDITORIAL. 1998. Amyloid and Alzheimer's disease. Nature Med. **4:** 745.

15. SOHAL, R.S. & B.H. SOHAL. 1991. Hydrogen peroxide release by mitochondria increases during aging. Mech. Aging Dev. **57:** 187–202.

16. BARJA, G. 1999. Mitochondrial oxygen radical generation and leak: sites of production in states 4 and 3, organ specificity, and relation to aging and longevity. J. Bioenerg. Biomembr. **31:** 347–366.

17. MIRABAELLI, F., A. SALIS, M. VAIRETTI, *et al*. 1989. Cytoskeletal alterations in human platelets exposed to oxidative stress are mediated by oxidative and Ca^{2+}-dependent mechanisms. Arch. Biochem. Biophy. **270:** 478–489.

18. ORRENIUS, S., D.J. MCCONKEY & P. NICOTERA. 1991. Role of calcium in toxic and programmed cell death. Adv. Exper. Med. Biol. **283:** 419–425.

19. LIPTON, S.A. & P.A. ROSENBERG. 1994. Excitatory amino acids as a final common pathway for neurologic disorders. N. Engl. J. Med. **330:** 613–622.

20. MATTSON, M.D., D. RYCHLIK & M.G. ENGLE. 1990. Possible involvement of calcium and inositolphospholipid signaling pathways in neurofibrillary degeneration. *In* Alzheimer's Disease: Basic Mechanisms, Diagnosis and Therapeutic Strategies. K. Iqbal, D.R.C. McLachlan, B. Winblad & H.W. Wisniewski, Eds.: 191–198. John Wiley & Sons. New York.

21. VERHASSELT, V., M. GOLDMAN, F. WILLEMS, *et al*. 1998. Oxidative stress up-regulates IL-8 and TNF-α synthesis by human dendritic cells. Eur. J. Immunol. **28:** 3886–3890.

22. LUE, L.-F., L. BRACHOVA, W.H. CIVIN, *et al* 1996. Inflammation, Aβ deposition, and neurofibrillary tangle formation as correlates of Alzheimer's disease neurodegeneration. J. Neuropathol. Exper. Neurol. **55:** 1083–1088.

23. STRITTMATTER, W. J., K.H. WEISGRABER, D.Y. HUANG, *et al*. 1993. Binding of human apolipoprotein E to synthetic amyloid β-peptide: isoform-specific effects and implications for late-onset Alzheimer's disease. Proc. Natl. Acad. Sci. USA **90:** 8098–8102.

24. SANAN, D.A., K.H. WEISGRABER, S.J. RUSSELL, *et al*. 1994. Apolipoprotein E associates with β-amyloid peptide of Alzheimer's disease to form novel monofibrils: apoE4 associates more efficiently than apoE3. J. Clin. Invest. **94:** 860–869.

25. LARSSON, N.-G. & R. LUFT. 1999. Revolution in mitochondrial medicine. FEBS LETT. **455:** 199–202.

26. MACLENNAN, D.H., W.J. RICE & N.M. GREEN. 1997. The mechanism of Ca^{2+} transport by sarco(Endo)plasmic reticulum Ca^{2+}-ATPases. J. Biol. Chem. **272:** 28815–28818.

27. XU, L., J.P. EU, G. MEISSNER, *et al*. 1998. Activation of the cardiac calcium release channel (ryanodine receptor) by poly-S-nitrosylation. Science **279:** 234–237.

28. MILLER, R.J. 1991. The control of neuronal Ca^{2+} homeostasis. Prog. Neurobiol. **37:** 255–285.

29. MATTSON, M.P., H. ZHU, J. YU, *et al*. 2000. Presenilin-1 mutation increases neuronal vulnerability to focal ischemia *in vivo* and to hypoxia and glucose deprivation in cell culture: involvement of perturbed calcium homeostasis. J. Neurosci. **20:** 1358–1364.

30. RICHTER, C., V.L. GOGVADZE, R. SCHLABACH, *et al*. 1995. Oxidants in mitochondria: from physiology to disease. Biochem. Biophys. Acta **1271:** 67–74.
31. SCHUCHMANN, S. & U. HEINEMANN. 2000. Increased mitochondrial superoxide generation in neurons from trisomy 16 mice: a model of Down's syndrome. Free Radic. Biol. Med. **28:** 235–250.
32. ZHANG, L., G.Q. XING, J.L. BARKER, *et al*. 2001. α-lipoic acid protects rat cortical neurons against cell death induced by amyloid and hydrogen peroxide through the Akt signalling pathway. Neurosci. Lett. **312:** 125–128.
33. HUANG, J., D.B. AGUS, C.J. WINFREE, *et al*. 2001. Dehydroascorbic acid, a blood-brain barrier transportable form of vitamin C, mediates potent cerebroprotection in experimental stroke. Proc. Natl. Acad. Sci. USA **98:** 11720–11724.

RNA Regulation in Mammals

MACIEJ SZYMANSKI AND JAN BARCISZEWSKI

*Institute of Bioorganic Chemistry of the Polish Academy of Sciences,
Noskowskiego 12, 61-704 Poznan, Poland*

ABSTRACT: Noncoding RNAs (ncRNA) are ubiquitous regulatory factors
affecting gene expression in all organisms. In eukaryotes ncRNAs have
been shown to operate on virtually every level of transmission of genetic
information. They are implicated in processes that are crucial for the
correct growth and development of multicellular organisms. Changes in
their expression are often related to stress conditions or associated with
diseases or developmental disorders.

KEYWORDS: RNA; noncoding transcripts; antisense; epigenetics

NONCODING RNAs

In recent years, we have witnessed an increasing interest in regulation of
gene expression by RNA molecules. It is now widely accepted that non-protein-
coding RNAs (noncoding RNAs, ncRNAs) constitute very important elements
of cellular mechanisms, which together with protein transcription factors are
responsible for precise control of the repertoire of expressed genes in virtually
all living organisms. The support for this view comes from two lines of evidence. On one hand, the analyses of sequenced genomes revealed significantly
lower than expected numbers of protein-coding genes.[1] This is especially the
case for higher eukaryotes, in which the open reading frames (ORFs), or the
sequences, which are actually translated into proteins, account only for a very
small fraction of total genomic DNA. In mammals, the ORFs constitute less
than 2% of nuclear genomes. This number is higher in less complex organisms like insects (18%), nematodes (25%), or fungi (60–80%). Within the
whole transcriptomes of human and mouse, the ratio of coding to noncoding
sequences is 1:47 and 1:43, respectively, which means that 98% of the whole
transcriptional output is not protein coding. This contrasts with the ratios found
in *Drosophila* and *Caenorhabditis* genomes, which are 1:2.4 and 1:1.3, respectively.[2] One can, therefore, easily notice that the amount of DNA, which does
not code for proteins, increases with the complexity of organisms. There is also

Address for correspondence: Prof. Jan Barciszewski, Institute of Bioorganic Chemistry of the Polish
Academy of Sciences, Noskowskiego 12, 61-704 Poznan, Poland. Voice: 0048-61-8528503; fax: 0048-
61-8520532.

  e-mail: jbarcisz@ibch.poznan.pl

Ann. N.Y. Acad. Sci. 1067: 461–468 (2006). © 2006 New York Academy of Sciences.
doi: 10.1196/annals.1354.066

a growing amount of experimental evidence that indicates that non-protein-coding genes are very abundant in mammalian cells. An expression analysis of human chromosomes 21 and 22 using microarrays as well as an analysis of transcription factor-binding sites revealed that transcripts that do not code for proteins constitute a significant fraction of RNA originating from these chromosomes.[3] In a more direct approach, a large number of noncoding transcripts have been identified in large-scale sequencing projects of human and mouse cDNAs.[4,5] Also, the detailed analysis of the male-specific region of Y chromosome revealed that a half of transcription units do not yield proteins.[6] Most of these studies were, however, restricted to the analysis of polyadenylated transcripts. Recently, it has been found that most of the transcripts from the human genome do not possess poly(A) tails. Moreover, approximately 50% of all transcripts is not exported to the cytoplasm and remains sequestered in the nucleus. The majority of these RNAs lacks annotation and their functions remain a mystery.[7] It is also interesting that, contrary to initial views on the organization of genetic information, there is a significant amount of genomic DNA that undergoes transcription from both strands and gives rise to pairs of sense–antisense transcripts.[7,8] The obvious conclusion from these data is that the number of non-protein-coding genes may actually be at least equal to that of protein-coding ones.

FUNCTIONS OF NONCODING RNAs

The term *noncoding RNA* can be interpreted as any transcript, or part thereof, which is not used as a template in protein synthesis. Such definition encompasses all housekeeping RNAs that are necessary for the transmission of genetic information (rRNAs, tRNA), RNA processing and modifications (RnaseP RNA, snoRNAs, snRNAs), or constitutively expressed RNA components of various ribonucleoprotein particles (e.g., vault RNAs or signal-recognition particle RNA). It is now evident that the vast majority of noncoding transcripts in eukaryotes are not expressed in all cells and in all stages of development and differentiation. These regulatory RNAs, which are sometimes called riboregulators or RNA regulators, seem to play a crucial role in numerous mechanisms controlling expression of genes.

Most of eukaryotic ncRNAs identified so far are products of transcription by RNA polymerase II. Apparently, their expression is regulated in much the same manner as the expression of the majority of protein-coding genes. This became evident from the analysis of Pol II transcription factor-binding sites on human chromosomes 21 and 22.[3] The expression of genes for a few examples of regulatory RNAs transcribed by Pol III is also tightly regulated. Unlike other genes transcribed by Pol III (tRNA, 5S rRNA), these genes are usually controlled by external promoter elements recognized by transcription factors, which also cooperate with Pol II.[9]

As discussed in the preceding section, the number of potential ncRNAs encoded by mammalian genomes is very large, and still probably underestimated. This contrasts with a relatively small number of RNAs for which there are at least hints as to what their functions are.

One of the well-established functions of ncRNAs is their participation in the regulation of epigenetic features of the chromatin and thereby global influence on the expression of genes on the levels of the structure of chromosomal domains or even entire chromosomes. In the simplest form of epigenetic regulation, ncRNAs may influence the DNA methylation within promoter regions of target genes and thereby control their transcription. The expression of different, tissue-specific isoforms of sphingosine kinase-1 encoded by the *Sphk1* locus depends on the use of alternative transcription start sites and splicing of the alternative first exons. This process is controlled by a 3.7-kb CpG island, which contains a tissue-dependent, differentially methylated region (T-DMR). The methylation status of T-DMR is regulated by an antisense transcript, Khps1, which overlaps the T-DMR. Expression of Khps1 induces demethylation of CG sites and methylation of non-CG sites within T-DMR.[10] It suggests that tissue-specific expression of *Sphk1* subtypes may depend on transcription of specific variants of the antisense RNA directing different methylation patterns of the T-DMR. This mechanism may be more widespread in mammalian genomes since there are numerous CpG islands, which include T-DMRs.[11] Their methylation and tissue-specific expression of adjacent genes may be also regulated by antisense RNAs.

The best studied, and by far the most spectacular, epigenetic phenomenon described in mammals, is the X-chromosome inactivation. This process leads to the equalization of dosage of X-linked genes in XY males and XX females. In mammals, this is accomplished by almost complete transcriptional silencing of all but one X chromosome in female cells.[12] A key element in X-chromosome inactivation is the XIC locus (X-inactivation center), from which a long spliced and polyadenylated Xist RNA is expressed. Xist RNA marks the X chromosome from which it is expressed for silencing by association with its chromatin.[13] Xist RNA is absolutely required for the initiation of silencing as demonstrated by the analysis of Xist deletion from X chromosomes[14] and silencing of autosomes carrying transcriptionally active *Xist* transgene during embryonic stem cells differentiation.[15] The Xist RNA associated with X chromosome serves as a beacon recruiting proteins responsible for chromatin modification and remodeling.[12,13,16,17]

Although X inactivation in the embryo is a random process, extra embryonic tissues of rodents show imprinted expression whereby the paternal allele of Xist is expressed, which leads to preferential silencing of paternal X chromosome.[12] Expression of Xist RNA from the maternal allele depends on the expression of another ncRNA, Tsix, which partially overlaps Xist in antisense orientation. It has been proposed that the repression of *Xist* function may depend on sense–antisense interactions between Xist and Tsix RNAs. However, current data indicate that Tsix represses Xist transcription by induction of chromatin structure modifications, but the details of this process remain unknown.[18,19]

A similar mechanism is probably involved in the imprinted expression of genes. In mouse, maternal expression of insulin-like growth factor type-2 receptor (*Igf2r*) gene and three genes (*Igf2r*, *Slc22a2,* and *Slc22a3*) on chromosome 17 depends on the presence of a 3.7-kb Region 2, which plays a role of imprinting control element (ICE). Region 2, harboring a maternally methylated CpG island, is located within the second intron of *Igf2r*. This CpG island serves as a promoter for expression of the antisense RNA Air (antisense *Igf2r* RNA). Air is unspliced, 108-kb long RNA, and it is expressed exclusively from the paternal allele.[20] It overlaps ∼30 kb of *Igf2r* gene, its promoter, and extends over 70 kb further upstream. Air RNA expression is required not only for repression of *Igf2r*, but also for the silencing of two genes, *Slc22a2* and *Slc22a3* located 110 and 155 kb downstream from the *Igf2r*. Because the promoter regions of silenced genes are located on either sides of the Air transcription start site, it was proposed to act as a bidirectional silencer affecting an approximately 400-kb long region. It has been suggested that the mechanism of silencing may be similar to the one observed in X chromosome inactivation. It depends on the association of RNA with chromatin in *cis* followed by recruitment of factors responsible for chromatin modification and establishment of its silent state.[21] Such a mechanism may be common for mammalian imprinted clusters. Antisense, ncRNA LIT-1 is expressed from the CpG island within the intron of a paternal allele of *KCNQ1* gene. Its deletion affects imprinting status of several genes at chromosomal region 11p15.5, which is implicated in the origin of Beckwith–Wiedemann syndrome.[22]

NcRNAs have been also shown to affect expression of genes directly on the level of transcription. A steroid receptor activator RNA (SRA RNA) is a spliced, polyadenylated transcript, which plays a role of a coactivator of nuclear receptors of steroid hormones (progestins, estrogens, androgens, and glucocorticoids).[23] Alternatively spliced SRA RNA isoforms share a common core region flanked by variable sequences. Mutations disrupting the RNA secondary structure of the core region reduce the activity of SRA RNA.[24] SRA RNA binds a subfamily of DEAD-box RNA-binding proteins, p72/p68, which probably mediate its association with SRC-1.[25] Another protein partner of SRA RNA is SHARP (SMRT/HDAC1-associated repressor protein), a hormone-induced transcriptional repressor, involved in the recruitment of histone deacetylases. Competition between transcriptional activators and repressors may therefore provide means for fine-tuning expression of hormone-responsive genes.[26] It is noteworthy that SRA is the first example of a gene that can produce two distinct end products. Recently, it has been shown that there are protein-coding isoforms of SRA RNA. The extension at the 5′-end provides an initiation codon and renders the RNA translatable.[27]

Two ncRNAs expressed from Pol III-dependent genes have been shown to directly interact with transcriptional machinery and to influence its activity.

Mouse B2 RNA originates from short interspersed elements (SINEs) and was shown to be involved in cells' responses to heat shock. The increase of B2 RNA transcription upon heat shock is followed by inhibition of transcription of Pol II-dependent genes.[28] This is a result of a tight association of B2 RNA with the core Pol II before pre-initiation complexes assembly.[29] Although there are no B2 element counterparts of the human genome, it has been proposed that similar functions may be performed by Alu RNA, which shows features similar to B2 including Pol III transcription and induction by heat shock and other stress conditions.[28] Another Pol III transcript involved in transcription is 7SK RNA, which is an inhibitor of positive transcription elongation factor b (P-TEFb).[30,31] 7SK RNA forms a complex with P-TEFb and HEXIM1/MAQ1 protein inhibiting the kinase activity of Cdk9. Upon stress, P-TEFb is released from the complex and becomes available for the transcription of stress-induced genes.[32]

One of the most intensively studied aspects of RNA-dependent regulation of gene expression is the role of microRNAs. MicroRNAs, initially discovered in nematodes as factors regulating development, have since been identified in all animals and plants, and are also encoded by certain viral genomes. The mature microRNAs (20–25 nt long) are processed from longer stem-loop precursors and are involved in the posttranscriptional regulation of gene expression. The complementary interaction between microRNA and mRNA affects either mRNAs' stability or its translation.[33] A majority of animal microRNAs act as specific translational repressors. This depends on binding of microRNA to specific sites within 3′-UTRs of target mRNA, but the details on how such an interaction influences translation inhibition are not known. The binding sites within the 3′-UTRs and microRNAs are not fully complementary, which result in imperfect duplexes featuring bulges and interior loops and allow single microRNA to recognize multiple sequences. The unpaired nucleotides within microRNA-mRNA duplex were shown to be crucial for microRNA's regulatory activity.[34] In addition to the reduction of translation, it has been observed that microRNAs also reduce the levels of target transcripts.[35]

It is estimated that approximately 10% of human genes, which possess at least two potential microRNA binding sites within 3′-UTRs, may be subject to translational regulation.[36] Most of microRNAs target a limited number of genes, but there are microRNAs that can potentially regulate expression of hundreds of mRNAs. Some mRNAs may be regulated by more than one microRNA. It has been proposed that the repertoire of microRNAs expressed in specific cells is analogous to the repertoire of transcription factors. Each of these sets acts on different levels, yet together they provide a highly specific mechanism, which ensures correct gene expression patterns and their combinations can be regarded as determinants of cellular complexity.[37]

The key role of microRNAs for development and differentiation is evident from the observations that virtually every cell type shows distinct microRNA expression profile.[38] It has been also shown that a significant number of microRNA encoding genes are located at chromosomal regions linked to various types of human cancer.[39] In fact, abnormalities in expression of micro-RNAs may be responsible for the induction of tumorigenesis.[40]

Posttranscriptional regulation affecting the stability of mRNA has been demonstrated for mouse *Makorin1* gene. In the mouse genome there is *Makorin1-p1,* an expressed pseudogene derived from *Makorin1.* Low expression or deletion of *Makorin1-p1* is lethal. It has been shown that lack of expression of pseudogene results in increased turnover rate of the *Makorin1* mRNA. The degradation of *Makorin1* mRNA depends on the RNA decay element within its 5'-UTR, which is conserved in the pseudogene. Expression of the processed pseudogene results in competition for the protein factors binding to the decay element between *Makorin1* and *Makorin1-p1* mRNAs.[41] Processed pseudogenes are abundant in both human and mouse genomes,[42] and some of them may be expressed,[43] which suggests that such regulatory mechanism may be more general and apply to other gene-processed pseudogene pairs.

PERSPECTIVES

The recent progress in studies on noncoding RNAs clearly demonstrates a growing interest in RNA biology. It is now evident that without resolving the intricacies of RNA-based regulation we will not be able to fully understand the mechanisms of growth, development, and differentiation. The chemical nature of RNA and its intrinsic instability makes it an ideal candidate for a regulatory molecule, but also makes it difficult to analyze experimentally. Thus the researchers working in the field face new challenges of characterizing in detail the expression profiles and functions of individual ncRNAs.

REFERENCES

1. LANDER, E.S. *et al.* 2001. Initial sequencing and analysis of the human genome. Nature **409:** 860–921.
2. FRITH, M.C., M. PHEASANT & J.S. MATTICK. 2005. Genomics: the amazing complexity of the human transcriptome. Eur. J. Hum. Genet. **13:** 894–897.
3. CAWLEY, S. *et al.* 2004. Unbiased mapping of transcription factor binding sites along human chromosomes 21 and 22 points to widespread regulation of noncoding RNAs. Cell **116:** 499–509.
4. NUMATA, K. *et al.* 2003. Identification of putative noncoding RNAs among the RIKEN mouse full-length cDNA collection. Genome Res. **13:** 1301–1306.
5. OTA, T. *et al.* 2004. Complete sequencing and characterization of 21.243 full-length human cDNAs. Nat. Genet. **36:** 40–45.
6. SKALETSKY, H. *et al.* 2003. The male-specific region of the human Y chromosome is a mosaic of discrete sequence classes. Nature **423:** 825–837.
7. CHEN, J. *et al.* 2005. Genome-wide analysis of coordinate expression and evolution of human cis-encoded sense-antisense transcripts. Trends Genet. **21:** 326–329.

8. CHENG, J. *et al*. 2005. Transcriptional maps of 10 human chromosomes at 5-nucleotide resolution. Science **308:** 1149–1154.

9. TEICHMANN, M., Z. WANG & R.G. ROEDER. 2000. A stable complex of a novel transcription factor IIB- related factor, human TFIIIB50, and associated proteins mediate selective transcription by RNA polymerase III of genes with upstream promoter elements. Proc. Natl. Acad. Sci. USA **97:** 14200–14205.

10. IMAMURA, T. *et al*. 2004. Non-coding RNA directed DNA demethylation of Sphk1 CpG island. Biochem. Biophys. Res. Commun. **322:** 593–600.

11. IMAMURA, T. *et al*. 2001. CpG island of rat sphingosine kinase-1 gene: tissue-dependent DNA methylation status and multiple alternative first exons. Genomics **76:** 113–125.

12. HEARD, E. 2004. Recent advances in X-chromosome inactivation. Curr. Opin. Cell Biol. **16:** 247–255.

13. PLATH, K. *et al*. 2003. Role of histone H3 lysine 27 methylation in X inactivation. Science **300:** 131–135.

14. NEWALL, A.E. *et al*. 2001. Primary non-random X inactivation associated with disruption of Xist promoter regulation. Hum. Mol. Genet. **10:** 581–589.

15. LEE, J.T. & R. JAENISCH. 1997. Long-range cis effects of ectopic X-inactivation centres on a mouse autosome. Nature **386:** 275–279.

16. MAK, W. *et al*. 2002. Mitotically stable association of polycomb group proteins Eed and Enx1 with the inactive X chromosome in trophoblast stem cells. Curr. Biol. **12:** 1016–1020.

17. HELBIG, R. & F.O. FACKELMAYER. 2003. Scaffold attachment factor A (SAF-A) is concentrated in inactive X chromosome territories through its RGG domain. Chromosoma **112:** 173–182.

18. SADO, T., Y. HOKI & H. SASAKI. 2005. Tsix silences Xist through modification of chromatin structure. Dev. Cell **9:** 159–165.

19. SHIBATA, S. & J.T. LEE. 2004. Tsix transcription- versus RNA-based mechanisms in Xist repression and epigenetic choice. Curr. Biol. **14:** 1747–1754.

20. SLEUTELS, F., R. ZWART & D.P. BARLOW. 2002. The non-coding Air RNA is required for silencing autosomal imprinted genes. Nature **415:** 810–813.

21. SLEUTELS, F. *et al*. 2003. Imprinted silencing of Slc22a2 and Slc22a3 does not need transcriptional overlap between Igf2r and Air. EMBO J. **22:** 3696–3704.

22. HORIKE, S. *et al*. 2000. Targeted disruption of the human LIT1 locus defines a putative imprinting control element playing an essential role in Beckwith-Wiedemann syndrome. Hum. Mol. Genet. **9:** 2075–2083.

23. LANZ, R. *et al*. 1999. A steroid receptor coactivator, SRA, functions as an RNA and is present in an SRC-1 complex. Cell **97:** 7–27.

24. LANZ, R. *et al*. 2002. Distinct RNA motifs are important for coactivation of steroid hormone receptors by steroid receptor RNA activator (SRA). Proc. Natl. Acad. Sci. USA **99:** 16081–16086.

25. WATANABE, M. *et al*. 2001. A subfamily of RNA-binding DEAD-box proteins acts as an estrogen receptor alpha coactivator through the N-terminal activation domain (AF-1) with an RNA coactivator, SRA. EMBO J. **20:** 1341–1352.

26. SHI, Y. *et al*. 2001. SHARP, an inducible cofactor that integrates nuclear receptor repression and activation. Genes Dev. **15:** 1140–1151.

27. EMBERLEY, E. *et al*. 2003. Identification of new human coding steroid receptor RNA activator isoforms. Biochem. Biophys. Res. Commun. **301:** 509–515.

28. ALLEN, T.A. *et al*. 2004. The SINE-encoded mouse B2 RNA represses mRNA transcription in response to heat shock. Nat. Struct. Mol. Biol. **11:** 816–821.

29. Espinoza, C.A. *et al*. 2004. B2 RNA binds directly to RNA polymerase to repress transcript synthesis. Nat. Struct. Mol. Biol. **11:** 822–829.

30. Nguyen, V.T. 2001. 7SK small nuclear RNA binds to and inhibits the activity of CDK9/cyclin T complexes. Nature **414:** 322–325.

31. Yik, J.H. *et al*. 2004. A human immunodeficiency virus type 1 Tat-like arginine-rich RNA-binding domain is essential for HEXIM1 to inhibit RNA polymerase II transcription through 7SK snRNA-mediated inactivation of P-TEFb. Mol. Cell. Biol. **24:** 5094–5105.

32. Yik, J.H. *et al*. 2003. Inhibition of P-TEFb (CDK9/Cyclin T) kinase and RNA polymerase II transcription by the coordinated actions of HEXIM1 and 7SK snRNA. Mol. Cell **12:** 971–982.

33. Bartel, D.P. 2004. MicroRNAs: genomics, biogenesis, mechanism, and function. Cell **116:** 281–297.

34. Vella, M.C., K. Reinert & F.J. Slack. 2004. Architecture of a validated microRNA: target interaction. Chem. Biol. **11:** 1619–1623.

35. Lim, L.P. *et al*. 2005. Microarray analysis shows that some microRNAs downregulate large numbers of target mRNAs. Nature **433:** 769–773.

36. John, B. *et al*. 2004. Human microRNA targets. PLoS Biol. **2:** e363.

37. Hobert, O. 2004. Common logic of transcription factor and microRNA action. Trends Biochem. Sci. **9:** 462–468.

38. Lu, J. *et al*. 2005. MicroRNA expression profiles classify human cancers. Nature **435:** 834–838.

39. Calin, G.A. *et al*. 2004. Human microRNA genes are frequently located at fragile sites and genomic regions involved in cancers. Proc. Natl. Acad. Sci. USA **101:** 2999–3004.

40. He, L. *et al*. 2005. A microRNA polycistron as a potential human oncogene. Nature **435:** 828–833.

41. Hirotsune, S. *et al*. 2003. An expressed pseudogene regulates the messenger-RNA stability of its homologous coding gene. Nature **423:** 91–96.

42. Adel, K., D. Laurent & M. Dominique. 2005. HOPPSIGEN: a database of human and mouse processed pseudogenes. Nucleic Acids. Res. **33** [Database Issue]: D59–D66.

43. Yano, Y. *et al*. 2004. A new role for expressed pseudogenes as ncRNA: regulation of mRNA stability of its homologous coding gene. J. Mol. Med. **82:** 414–422.

Quantum Dot-Based Protein Imaging and Functional Significance of Two Mitochondrial Chaperones in Cellular Senescence and Carcinogenesis

ZEENIA KAUL,[a,b] TOMOKO YAGUCHI,[a] SUNIL C. KAUL,[a] AND RENU WADHWA[a]

[a]National Institute of Advanced Industrial Science & Technology (AIST), 1-1-1 Higashi, Tsukuba, Ibaraki – 305 8562, Japan

[b]International Christian University (ICU), 10-2, Osawa 3-chome, Mitaka-shi, Tokyo – 181 8585, Japan

ABSTRACT: Mortalin/mtHSP70 and HSP60 are heat-shock proteins that reside in multiple subcellular compartments, mitochondria being the dominant compartment. We present here biochemical evidence for their *in vivo* and *in vitro* interactions. By the use of quantum dots (powerful tools used for simultaneous imaging of multiple proteins), we visualized minute differences in the subcellular niche of these two proteins in normal and cancer cells. Knockdown of either of these two by shRNA expression plasmids caused growth arrest of osteosarcoma cells. However, interestingly, whereas an overexpression of mortalin extended *in vitro* life span of normal fibroblasts (TIG-1), overexpression of HSP60 was neutral. We demonstrate the minute differences in subcellular distribution of mortalin and HSP60, their involvement in tumorigenesis, and functional distinction in pathways involved in senescence.

KEYWORDS: mortalin; HSP60; quantum dot; imaging; localization

INTRODUCTION

Mortalin/mtHSP70 and HSP60 are the heat-shock proteins that reside in multiple subcellular sites, mitochondria being the most prominent site.[1–6] The staining pattern of mortalin differs in normal and transformed human cells: uniform pancytoplasmic in a normal cell and perinuclear pattern in transformed cells.[2] It is likely that the differential niche of mortalin controls its interactions

Address for correspondence: Renu Wadhwa, National Institute of Advanced Industrial Science & Technology (AIST), Central 4, 1-1-1 Higashi, Tsukuba, Ibaraki, 305-8562, Japan. Voice: +81 29 861 9464; fax: +81 29 861 2900.

e-mail: renu-wadhwa@aist.go.jp

Ann. N.Y. Acad. Sci. 1067: 469–473 (2006). © 2006 New York Academy of Sciences.
doi: 10.1196/annals.1354.067

with other proteins and thus its functional attributes in normal and cancer cells.[7] The molecular basis of the differential staining patterns in normal and cancer cells and their functional significance in response to stress conditions has not been well studied. These studies require visualization tools such as specific antibodies. We have previously showed that Qdot immunoconjugates provide more stable images than are obtained with the conventional organic fluorescent dyes.[8,9] In the present study, we used Qdot-conjugated anti-HSP60 and anti-mortalin antibodies to examine their subcellular distribution in transformed human cells.

EXPERIMENTAL METHODS

Osteosarcoma (U2OS) cells were cultured in Dulbecco's modified Eagle's minimal essential medium (DMEM) supplemented with 10% fetal bovine serum (FBS), penicillin, streptomycin, and fungizone (GIBCO, USA) at 37°C in an atmosphere of 5% CO_2 and 95% air in a humidified incubator. For immunofluorescence studies, cells were plated on glass coverslips placed in a 12-well culture dish. After 24 h, cells were washed with cold phosphate-buffered saline (PBS), and fixed with prechilled methanol/acetone (1/1, v/v) mixture for 5 min on ice. Fixed cells were washed with PBS, permeabilized with 0.5% Triton-X 100 in PBS for 15 min, and blocked with blocking reagent (Sigma, USA) for 1 h. They were incubated with anti-HSP60 antibody (N-20, Santa Cruz, USA) and anti-mortalin antibodies (monoclonal anti-mthsp70; Affinity Bioreagents, USA) for 1 h at room temperature, washed thrice with 0.2% Triton X-100 in PBS, and then incubated with Alexa-conjugated secondary antibodies (Molecular Probes, USA) followed by washings with 0.2% Triton X-100 in PBS. For quantum dot staining, cells were incubated with QD (Qdot^{TM} 525 Streptavidin Conjugate, Qdot^{TM} 655 rabbit IgG, and Qdot^{TM} 655 mouse IgG; Qantum Dot Corporation, USA) in Qdot incubation buffer (1:2000). After three washings of 10 min each with 0.2% Tx-100 in PBS and a final wash with PBS, the coverslips were mounted on glass slides with Fluoromount (Difco, USA). The cells were examined on a Carl Zeiss microscope attached with either photomerics synsys monochrome charge-coupled device (CCD) or an AxioCam HRC color camera (Zeiss, Germany). Confocal images were taken with a LSM510 microscope (Zeiss, Germany) attached with photomultiplier (PMT) detection system. The extent to which the two proteins overlapped was assessed by combining the two images using either Metamorph or AxioVision software.[10]

Overexpression and Gene Silencing by shRNA

Overexpression of mortalin and HSP60 in normal cells was obtained by CMV promoter-driven expression plasmids.[10] U2OS cells were transfected with mortalin and HSP60-specific shRNA vectors followed by selection in puromycin. Selected cells were examined for their proliferation in comparison with the control cells as described.[10]

RESULTS AND DISCUSSION

In vivo binding assays for mortalin and HSP60 proteins have revealed that the two proteins occur in complexes that involve N-terminal region (amino acid residues 150-252) of mortalin.[10] We next examined the subcellular localization of mortalin and HSP60 by fluorescent and Qdot-conjugated antibodies. Quantum dots were used in cellular imaging because of their higher photostability, broad absorption, and narrow and symmetrical emission spectrum.[8,9] Simultaneous excitation of different sizes of quantum dots with a single excitation light source yields different colors, making it possible to have simultaneous imaging of multiple proteins. As shown in FIGURES 1 and 2, Qdot images of transformed (U2OS) cells revealed that in addition to their co-localization (seen as yellow color), each protein has a specific locale. The data implied that the two proteins exist together at some, but not all, subcellular localizations.

To investigate the functional significance of mortalin or HSP60 for growth of tumor cells, these were knocked down in human osteocarinoma (U2OS) cells with specific shRNA plasmids.[10] Cells compromised for HSP60 or mortalin expression showed strong growth arrest. The data revealed that these are essential for the growth of tumor cells and silencing of either of these

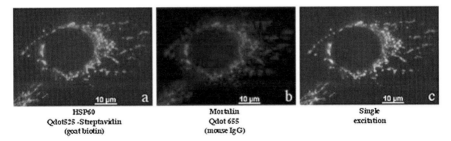

HSP60
Qdot525 -Streptavidin
(goat biotin)

Mortalin
Qdot 655
(mouse IgG)

Single
excitation

FIGURE 1. Double labeling of mortalin and HSP60 with Qdot 655 and Qdot 525, respectively. HSP60 and mortalin in fixed human osteosarcoma (U2OS) cells were labeled with Qdot^{TM} 525 Streptavidin conjugate (**a**) and Qdot^{TM} 655 goat F (ab')2 anti-mouse IgG conjugate (H+L) (**b**). The cells were examined on a Carl Zeiss microscope attached with either photomerics synsys monochrome charge-coupled device (CCD) or an AxioCam HRC color camera (Zeiss). Visualization of HSP60 (Qdot 525, green) and mortalin (Qdot 655, red) with a single excitation and a single long-pass emission filter (**c**). The two colors green (*left panel*) and red (*center panel*) were distinguished and the co-localization of two proteins can be seen as yellow (Color in online version only). The two proteins overlap by about 70% (seen as yellow; *right panel*). Distinct red and green staining was visible.

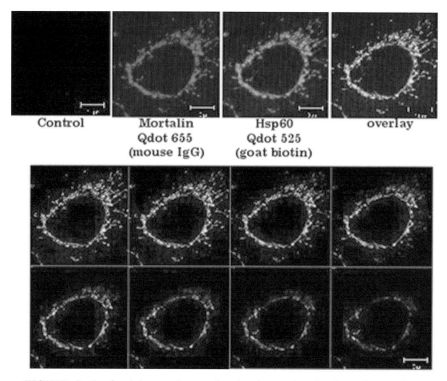

FIGURE 2. Confocal laser micrographs showing co-localization of mortalin and HSP60 proteins labeled with Qdot 655 and Qdot 525 in optical sections of cells.

two is sufficient for their growth arrest. Their data were consistent with their increased expression observed in human transformed cells.[11–13]

The functional significance of mortalin and HSP60 in normal human skin fibroblasts (TIG-1) was also investigated by their overexpression. TIG-1 cells (PD24) were transfected with expression plasmids encoding for either human mortalin (hmot-2) or HSP60 proteins. Selected cells were passaged *in vitro* until they reached senescence and stopped dividing. Whereas mortalin over-expressing cultures underwent about 71 population doublings, the HSP60 and vector-transfected control cells senesced at 58 population doublings.[10] Cells were maintained in a senescent stage for more than 4 weeks. Overexpression of mortalin, but not HSP60, caused temporary escape from senescence, resulting in *in vitro* life-span extension of normal cells. The data revealed functional divergence of mortalin and HSP60 and may involve a function of mortalin as a mitochondrial import motor in addition to its chaperone function similar to HSP60.[14,15]

In the present study, we have shown that Qdots provide a high resolution and stable imaging tool that has revealed that mortalin and HSP60 have common and exclusive localizations. Functional analysis showed that although the two proteins are required for continued proliferation of cancer cells, overexpression of mortalin only endowed normal cells with extended longevity.

REFERENCES

1. WADHWA, R., S.C. KAUL, Y. IKAWA, *et al.* 1993. Identification of a novel member of mouse hsp70 family: its association with cellular mortal phenotype. J. Biol. Chem. **268:** 6615–6621.
2. WADHWA, R., S.C. KAUL, Y. MITSUI, *et al.* 1993. Differential subcellular distribution of mortalin in mortal and immortal mouse and human fibroblasts. Exp. Cell Res. **207:** 442–448.
3. RAN, Q., R. WADHWA, R. KAWAI, *et al.* 2000. Extramitochondrial localization of mortalin/mtHSP70/PBP74/GRP75. Biochem. Biophys. Res. Commun. **275:** 174–179.
4. WADHWA, R., K. TAIRA & S.C. KAUL. 2002. An hsp70 family chaperone, mortalin/mtHSP70/PBP74/Grp75: what, when and where? Cell Stress Chaperones **7:** 309–316.
5. SOLTYS, B.J. & R.S. GUPTA. 2000. Mitochondrial proteins at unexpected cellular locations: export of proteins from mitochondria from an evolutionary perspective. Int. Rev. Cytol. **194:** 133–196.
6. SOLTYS, B.J. & R.S. GUPTA. 1999. Mitochondrial-matrix proteins at unexpected locations: are they exported? Trends Biochem. Sci. **24:** 174–177.
7. WADHWA, R., K. TAIRA & S.C. KAUL. 2002. An HSP70 family chaperone, mortalin/mtHSP70/PBP74/Grp75: what, when and where? Cell Stress Chaperones **7:** 309–316.
8. KAUL, Z., T. YAGUCHI, S.C. KAUL, *et al.* 2003. Mortalin imaging in normal and cancer cells with quantum dot immuno-conjugates. Cell Res. **13:** 503–507.
9. ARYA, H., Z. KAUL, R. WADHWA, *et al.* 2005. Quantum dots in bio-imaging: revolution by the small. Biochem. Biophys. Res. Commun. **329:** 1173–1177.
10. WADHWA, R., S. TAKANO, K. KAUR, *et al.* 2005. Identification and characterization of molecular interactions between mortalin/mtHSP70 and hsp60. Biochem. J. **391:** 185–190.
11. DUNDAS, S.R., L.C. LAWRIE, P.H. ROONEY, *et al.* 2004. Mortalin is over-expressed by colorectal adenocarcinomas and correlates with poor survival. J. Pathol. **205:** 74–81.
12. FARIED, A., M. SOHDA, M. NAKAJIMA, *et al.* 2004. Expression of heat-shock protein HSP60 correlated with the apoptotic index and patient prognosis in human oesophageal squamous cell carcinoma. Eur. J. Cancer **40:** 2804–2811.
13. CAPPELLO, F., M. BELLAFIORE, A. PALMA, *et al.* 2003. 60KDa chaperonin (HSP60) is over-expressed during colorectal carcinogenesis. Eur. J. Histochem. **47:** 105–110.
14. VOOS, W. & K. ROTTGERS. 2002. Molecular chaperones as essential mediators of mitochondrial biogenesis. Biochim. Biophys. Acta. **1592:** 51–62.
15. LIU, Q., J. KRZEWSKA, K. LIBEREK, *et al.* 2001. Mitochondrial HSP70 Ssc1: role in protein folding. J. Biol. Chem. **276:** 6112–6118.

Phage-Displayed Antibodies for the Detection of Glycated Proteasome in Aging Cells

REGINA GONZALEZ-DOSAL, MORTEN DRÆBY SØRENSEN,
BRIAN F.C. CLARK, SURESH I. S. RATTAN, AND PETER KRISTENSEN

*Danish Centre of Molecular Gerontology, Department of Molecular Biology,
University of Aarhus, Aarhus, Denmark*

ABSTRACT: Accumulation of posttranslationally damaged proteins during aging could explain the decline of cell performance with age. N^{ε}-carboxymethyllysine (CML) is the major glycation product on damaged proteins, causing dysfunction and cross-linking. The proteasome, a multicatalytic degradation complex, is one of the pathways for eliminating damaged proteins, and thus regulating their accumulation within the cell. However, the proteinase activities of the proteasome decline during aging. This may be due to posttranslational modifications of the subunits forming the proteasome complex. Using phage display technology, we have selected 16 single-chain variable fragments (scFv) recognizing the CML-modified $\alpha 7$ subunit of the proteasome. Using one of them, Ab3, we have observed a five-fold increase of CML-$\alpha 7$ in old human skin fibroblasts in comparison with young fibroblasts and telomerase-immortalized bone marrow cells (hTERT-BMCs).

KEYWORDS: proteasome; fibroblasts; bone marrow; protein modification; phage display

Advanced glycated end-products (AGEs) are irreversible posttranslational protein modifications that result from an intricate network of complex and spontaneous nonenzymatic reactions. These modifications can result in loss of functionality, misfolding, and cross-linking of proteins.[1] AGE accumulation has been reported to be associated with several pathological conditions, such as diabetes, uremia, atherosclerosis, and Alzheimer's disease, as well as with the normal aging process. AGE levels are considered to be good biochemical markers of the progression of these pathologies, and are thought to be the cause of some complications. Among AGEs are the glycoxidative products, $N\alpha$-(carboxymethyl)lysine (CML) and pentosidine, which require oxidation

Address for correspondence: Dr. Peter Kristensen, Department of Molecular Biology, University of Aarhus, Gustav Wieds Vej 10C, DK8000 Aarhus-C, Denmark. Voice: +45 8942 5032; fax: +45 8612 3178.
   e-mail: pk@mb.au.dk

Ann. N.Y. Acad. Sci. 1067: 474–478 (2006). © 2006 New York Academy of Sciences.
doi: 10.1196/annals.1354.068

for their formation.[2,3] CML is the major AGE product on account of the numerous pathways leading to the formation of this glycoxidative product.[4,5] However, the reaction of glyoxal with the ε-NH2 group of a lysine is the main pathway leading to the generation of CML adducts.

One of the main defenses against accumulation of AGEs and other damaged proteins is the protein degradation machinery, the proteasome, which is a nonlysosomal multicatalytic proteinase ubiquitous in living forms.[6,7]

The activity of the proteasome has been observed to decrease with aging,[8] leading to the accumulation of damaged proteins. Several explanations have been proposed in order to explain this reduction of activity: downregulation of the expression of the proteasome subunits,[9] inhibition of the proteasome by damaged proteins,[10] and loss of activity by posttranslational modifications.[11] Posttranslational modification leading to the formation of AGEs occurs randomly, so it is difficult to determine which modifications cause the loss of function of certain macromolecule, such as the proteasome. The generation of antibodies by use of the phage display technology allows the production of a diverse range of different monoclonal antibodies specific for a given antigen. When antibodies are generated using damaged protein as antigen, molecular tools become available, making it possible to study the influence of single modifications on proteins.

The basic principle in phage display relies on the introduction of a foreign DNA into the bateriophage genome, creating fusion proteins between coat proteins of the filamentous bacteriophage and the foreign protein, which subsequently will be expressed on the surface of the phage particle.[12] When the foreign DNA is introduced in the phage genome code for fragments of human antibodies, large libraries of human antibody fragments will be displayed on the surface of the phage, thus allowing us to perform selections in which specific antibodies are isolated on the basis of their affinity for the antigen. In this study we used the phage display technology to select specific antibodies against the CML-modified α7 subunit of the proteasome.

SELECTION OF SPECIFIC scFv ANTIBODIES

Four micrograms of CML-modified α7 subunit were used to coat an immunotube and were subsequently incubated with the Tomlinson J scFv repertoire.[13] After washing off the nonbinding phages, specific binders were eluted and were able to infect a TG-1 bacterial culture. More than 2,000 colonies were obtained and 768 were monoclonally reproduced. Phages from one plate were tested for specificity in enzyme-linked immunosorbent assay (ELISA) against α7 and CML-α7, using GST and CML-GST as negative control. Fifty positive signals were obtained in the ELISA recognizing either α7 or CML-α7, of which 16 were specific against the CML-α7. One of the 16 specific clones against CML-α7, Ab3, was recloned in the pKBJ3 expression vector,[14]

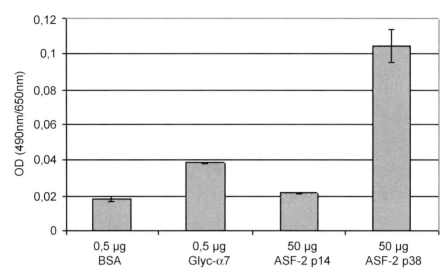

FIGURE 1. Analysis of the presence of CMLα7 in different cellular extracts in ELISA using Ab3. ELISA of old (p36) and young (p14) fibroblasts extract, with BSA as negative control, and glyc-α7 as positive control.

allowing an efficient expression of soluble antibody in bacteria, which were then purified using a his-tag. The activity of the purified Ab3 was tested and used in the analysis of the importance of CML modifications on a specific site of the proteasome.

CML-α7 ACCUMULATES IN FIBROBLAST DURING AGING

Cell extracts of serially passaged old ($>90\%$ of the life span completed) and young ($<25\%$ life span completed) human skin fibroblast ASF-2 were coated in an ELISA plate and the ELISA was performed using Ab3. In young human skin fibroblast and in fast-dividing hTERT-MSC cells (human telomerase immortalized mesenchymal stem cells) minute amounts of CML-α7 could be detected. Following serial passing of fibroblast we observed an increase in the accumulation of CML-α7, resulting in a five-fold accumulation of CML-α7 in fibroblasts, which have reached more than 90% of their life span (FIG. 1).

In conclusion, we have observed an age-related increase in glycated α7 subunit of the proteasome, or in other words damaged proteasome, in human cells undergoing aging *in vitro*. The absence of accumulation of damaged proteasome in the hTERT-MSCs and young fibroblasts in comparison with the old fibroblasts could be due to a faster dispersion of the possible damaged proteins into the daughter cells. On the contrary, old cells with a lower replication rate accumulate damaged proteins. Finally, we have developed a tool for analyzing a marker of proteasomal malfunction, cellular viability, and a potential marker of aging. Additionally, the proteasome condition can be determined by using this antibody after a detrimental or beneficial treatment of cells, such as the addition of glyoxal, cytokinins, and heat shock. Moreover, Ab3 will allow us to determine whether decreasing cellular proliferation will result in the accumulation of damaged proteasome and inhibition of *de novo* synthesis of proteasome.

ACKNOWLEDGMENTS

We thank Geraldine Carrard and Bertrand Friguet (Laboratoire de Biologie et Biochimie Cellulaire du Vieillissement, University of Paris, 7-Denis Diderot, France) for providing the glycated α7 subunit of the proteasome, and to Moustapha Kassem (Department of Endocrinology and Metabolism, University Hospital of Odense, Denmark) for providing the hTERT-MSC cell line. The Laboratory of Cellular Ageing is supported by research grants from the Danish Research Councils, Carlsberg Fund, Senetek PLC, and EU's Biomed Health Programmes.

REFERENCES

1. EBLE, A.S., S.R. THORPE & J.W. BAYNES. 1983. Nonenzymatic glucosylation and glucose-dependent cross-linking of protein. J. Biol. Chem. **258:** 9406–9412.
2. AHMED, M.U., S.R. THORPE & J.W. BAYNES. 1986. Identification of N epsilon-carboxymethyllysine as a degradation product of fructoselysine in glycated protein. J. Biol. Chem. **261:** 4889–4894.
3. DUNN, J.A. *et al.* 1990. Reaction of ascorbate with lysine and protein under autoxidizing conditions: formation of N epsilon-(carboxymethyl)lysine by reaction between lysine and products of autoxidation of ascorbate. Biochemistry **29:** 10964–10970.
4. DUNN, J.A. *et al.* 1991. Age-dependent accumulation of N epsilon-(carboxymethyl)lysine and N epsilon-(carboxymethyl)hydroxylysine in human skin collagen. Biochemistry **30:** 1205–1210.
5. REDDY, S. *et al.* 1995. N epsilon-(carboxymethyl)lysine is a dominant advanced glycation end product (AGE) antigen in tissue proteins. Biochemistry **34:** 10872–10878.
6. LUPAS, A., P. ZWICKL & W. BAUMEISTER. 1994. Proteasome sequences in eubacteria. Trends Biochem. Sci. **19:** 533–534.
7. GROLL, M. *et al.* 1997. Structure of 20S proteasome from yeast at 2.4 A resolution. Nature **386:** 463–471.
8. CARRARD, G. *et al.* 2003. Impact of ageing on proteasome structure and function in human lymphocytes. Int. J. Biochem. Cell. Biol. **35:** 728–739.
9. CHONDROGIANNI, N. *et al.* 2003. Central role of the proteasome in senescence and survival of human fibroblasts: induction of a senescence-like phenotype upon

its inhibition and resistance to stress upon its activation. J. Biol. Chem. **278:** 28026–28037.

10. FRIGUET, B., L.I. SZWEDA & E.R. STADTMAN. 1994. Susceptibility of glucose-6-phosphate dehydrogenase modified by 4-hydroxy-2-nonenal and metal-catalyzed oxidation to proteolysis by the multicatalytic protease. Arch. Biochem. Biophys. **311:** 168–173.

11. ANSELMI, B. *et al.* 1998. Dietary self-selection can compensate an age-related decrease of rat liver 20 S proteasome activity observed with standard diet. J. Gerontol. A. Biol. Sci. Med. Sci. **53:** B173–B179.

12. SMITH, G.P. 1985. Filamentous fusion phage: novel expression vectors that display cloned antigens on the virion surface. Science **228:** 1315–1317.

13. DE WILDT, R.M. *et al.* 2000. Antibody arrays for high-throughput screening of antibody-antigen interactions. Nat. Biotechnol. **18:** 989–994.

14. JENSEN, K.B. *et al.* 2002. Functional improvement of antibody fragments using a novel phage coat protein III fusion system. Biochem. Biophys. Res. Commun. **298:** 566–573.

Techniques Used in Studies of Age-Related DNA Methylation Changes

TOMASZ K. WOJDACZ AND LISE LOTTE HANSEN

The Danish Centre for Molecular Gerontology, Institute of Human Genetics, The Bartholin Building 240, University of Aarhus, DK-8000 Aarhus C, Denmark

ABSTRACT: Epigenetic modification of CpG islands (CGIs) in promoter regions is an important regulatory mechanism of gene expression in eukaryotic cells. Hypermethylation of CGIs may silence a gene, whereas hypomethylation of previously methylated CGIs allows gene expression. The pattern of methylation is cell-type-specific and established during development of the organisms. Changes in the methylation pattern have been found in all cancer forms and in aging cells. The epigenetic-related alternations of gene expression status may significantly contribute to the initiation and maintenance of malignant growth. Cancer incidence increases dramatically with age and correlates strongly with age-related methylation changes. Many techniques have been developed to analyze the genome-wide methylation content and the methylation status of specific loci. The majority of methylation screening protocols utilizes methylation-sensitive endonuclease digestion or bisulfite treatment of the template followed by subsequent PCR amplification of a specific sequence. All methods either examine only one specific DNA sequence at a time, or provide limited genomic information on the screened sequences. The principle of our new approach is to combine methylation-sensitive enzyme digestion with the comparative genomic hybridization (CGH) technique to develop an array-based method to screen the entire genome for changes of methylation pattern. The new technique will serve as an efficient tool in understanding the nature of epigenetic changes and their significance to the aging process and cancer development.

KEYWORDS: epigenetic; hyper-hypomethylation; CpG-island

INTRODUCTION

Epigenetics (which means outside genetic) describes the inheritance of information based on gene expression level without changes of the primary DNA

Address for correspondence: Tomasz K. Wojdacz, The Danish Centre for Molecular Gerontology, Institute of Human Genetics, The Bartholin Building 240, University of Aarhus, DK-8000 Aarhus C, Denmark. Voice: +45 89421992; fax: +45 86123173.
e-mail: wojdacz@humgen.au.dk

Ann. N.Y. Acad. Sci. 1067: 479–487 (2006). © 2006 New York Academy of Sciences.
doi: 10.1196/annals.1354.069

sequence. The epigenetic modifications of genetic information occur during development of the organism, are reproduced during DNA replication, and stably transmitted to the daughter cells.

The three epigenetic processes: DNA methylation, histone modifications, and ATP-dependent modifications of chromatin, can influence gene expression.[1] In recent years epigenetic changes in the human genome have been increasingly recognized as a very important part of normal and pathologic aging. A small percentage of the human genes (2.8%) have been shown to be differently expressed in young and old individuals,[2] but the question as to what extent the epigenetic events contribute to the aging process still remains unanswered.

METHYLATION MECHANISMS

In the human genome methylation is restricted to palindromic CpG dinucleotides. DNA regions with a relatively high density of CpG dinucleotides are called CpG-islands (CGIs), and the human genome contains roughly 28,000 CGIs spread throughout the genome in a nonrandom pattern. Most of the CGIs are located in the promoter region and the first exon of approximately half of all human protein-coding genes and remain free of methylation. In the normal cell only imprinted genes, genes whose expression is restricted to male or female germ line and tissue-specific genes, are silenced by methylation mechanisms.[3] Methylation has also been implicated in the silencing of transposable genomic sequences and inactivation of the X chromosome.[3]

Hypermethylation of regulatory elements abolishes gene expression, whereas genome-wide hypomethylation causes ectopic expression of the genes, release of parasitic genomic sequences, and increase in recombination events leading to extended genomic instability.[4,5]

Enzymatic addition of methyl groups to cytosines within palindromic CpG dinucleotide sequences suppresses transcription by at least three mechanisms. First, methylation of promoter CGIs reduces the binding affinity of sequence-specific transcription factors.[6,7] Second, some of the sequence-specific methyl-CpG-binding proteins (MBPs) may act as transcriptional repressors[8] and third, sequence-independent MBPs can recruit protein complexes containing transcriptional co-repressors and histone deacethylases to the corresponding methylation sites and initiate chromatin remodeling.[9,10] Histone deacethylases (HDACs) remove acetyl groups from core histones, triggering nucleosomal packing and conversion of the chromatin from open into closed structure, no longer accessible to the transcriptional machinery (FIG. 1).[8,11] As opposed to gene silencing by methylation, demethylation of previously methylated sequences allows ectopic gene expression.

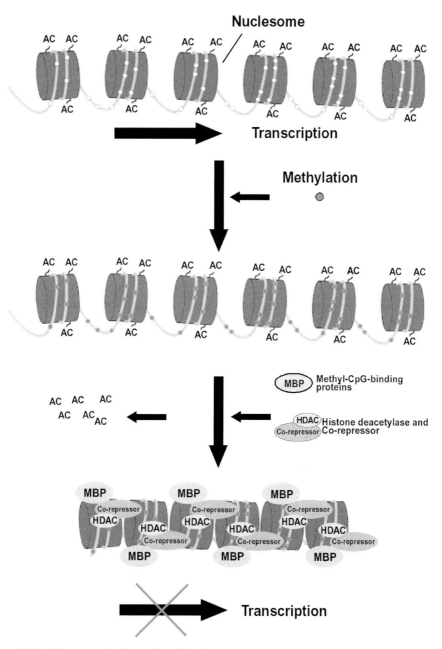

FIGURE 1. Mechanism of methylation-dependent gene silencing. The changes of chromatin structure from transcriptional active (*top*) to inactive (*bottom*). See text for explanation of the mechanism. Modified from Worm and Guldberg.[38]

AGE-RELATED METHYLATION CHANGES

The methylation pattern of postdevelopment cells is very stable; it is reproduced during DNA replication and stably transmitted to the daughter cells.
De novo methylation and demethylation of CGIs are normally rare events. In
recent years an increasing number of autosomal genes has been reported to be
affected by methylation changes during aging. The estrogen receptor (ER) gene
undergoes age-related methylation in the normal human colonic mucosa.[12] Furthermore, up to 70% of CGIs found to be hypermethylated in primary colon
tumors, was due to an age-related increase in hypermethylation of the normal
colon.[13] Simultaneously with hypermethylation of specific CGIs, the genome-
wide and locus-specific loss of methylation occurs as a direct function of age.
The *in vitro* global methylation content in normal human fibroblasts decreases
with increasing population doublings.[14] *In vivo* age-related global hypomethylation was observed in the thymus of cows[15] and T lymphocytes of aging
humans.[16] The direct contribution of epigenetic alternations to the life-span
process has already been confirmed in yeast nematodes and *Drosophila*.[17,18]

GENOME-WIDE METHYLATION CONTENT AND LOCUS-SPECIFIC METHYLATION ANALYSES

The significance of DNA methylation in the aging process and its implication
in many disorders have lead to the development of a wide range of techniques
for methylation studies.

Most frequently used procedures of quantification of genomic 5-
methylcytosine content involve enzymatic hydrolysis of genomic DNA followed by a high-resolution separation of DNA base fractions and calculation
of the 5-metylcytosine and cytosine ratio. Other approaches employ DNA

TABLE 1. Genome-wide methylation content techniques

Technique	Description
HPLC and related techniques	Following an enzymatic hydrolysis, the DNA is separated and the base composition is determined.[23]
SssI acceptance assay	The test DNA and radioactive-labeled methyl groups are incubated with *SssI* methyltansferase. The level of incorporated radioactive methyl groups is measured.[24]
Chloroacetaldehyde assay	Sodium bisulfite-treated DNA is depurinated and incubated with chloroacetaldehyde, which yields a fluorescence-detectable derivative of 5-methyl cytosine.[25]
Immunochemical analyses	Genomic DNA is incubated with a 5-methylcytosine antibody and the staining patterns from the chromosomes are scanned.[26]

methylotransferase and 5-methylcytosine-specific antibodies. An overview of these techniques is presented in TABLE 1.

Analyses of locus-specific methylation status utilize two protocols: methylation-sensitive enzyme digestion and PCR amplification (TABLE 2). The methylation information is erased during PCR amplification, so an initial modification of the DNA with sodium bisulfite is required. Sodium bisulfite deaminates unmethylated cytosine residues to uracil, leaving the 5-methylcytosines intact. In the subsequent PCR reaction the methylated cytosines will be amplified as thymines or cytosines according to their methylation status.

TABLE 2. Gene-specific methylation analysis techniques

Technique	Description
Methylation-sensitive enzyme digestion (MSRE and MSRE-PCR)	Digestion of DNA with MSRE followed by Southern blotting or PCR analysis.[27]
Bisulfite sequencing	Direct sequencing of bisulfite-treated DNA.[28]
Methylation-specific PCR (MS-PCR)	PCR based discrimination between unmethylated and methylated alleles in bisulfite-treated DNA.[29]
Methylation-sensitive single-nucleotide primer extension (MS-SnuPE)	Strand-specific PCR amplification of bisulfite-treated DNA.[30]
MethyLight	PCR amplification of bisulfite-treated DNA in the presence of a fluorescent probe flanked by primers that do not discriminate between unmethylated and methylated alleles.[31]
Methylation-specific single-strand conformation analysis (MS-SSCA)	PCR amplification of a bisulfite-treated target sequence with nondiscriminating primers and electrophoresis in a nondenaturing polyacrylamide gel.[32]
Combined bisulfite restriction analyses (COBRA)	Digestion with MSRE of PCR products obtained from amplification of a bisulfite-treated target sequence using nondiscriminating primers.[33]
Methylation-specific denaturing gradient gel electrophoresis (MS-DGGE)	Nondiscriminatory amplification of bisulfite-treated DNA followed by electrophoresis in a polyacrylamide gel containing a gradient of urea and formamide.[34]
Methylation-specific melting curve analysis (MS-PCR)	Nondiscriminatory amplification of bisulfite-treated DNA and determination of melting temperature of PCR product, which is different for unmethylated and methylated alleles.[35]
Methylation-specific denaturing high-performance liquid chromatography (MS-DHPLC)	DHPLC analysis of a nondiscriminatory amplified bisulfite-treated target sequence in which the G:C content differs between the unmethylated and methylated alleles.[36]
Methylation-specific microarray (MSO)	PCR amplification of bisulfite-treated DNA and the hybridization to glass slides with printed allele-specific oligonucleotides.[37]

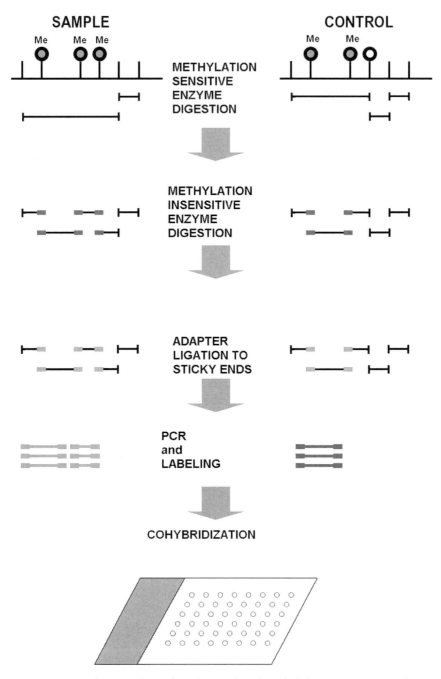

FIGURE 2. The procedure of BAC-array-based methylation-screening experiment. See text for details.

GENOME-WIDE CGI METHYLATION ANALYSES

Up till now there have been three techniques allowing global CGI methylation analyses: restriction landmark genomic scanning (RLGS),[19] methylated CpG island amplification-representational difference analysis (MCA-RDA),[20] and methylation-sensitive arbitrarily primed PCR (MS-AP-PCR).[21] All the above-mentioned techniques reveal genome-wide changes in the methylation pattern. The information obtained is, however, limited and not precise; moreover, the protocols are time and labor consuming.

A NEW APPROACH TO THE ANALYSIS OF GENOME-WIDE METHYLATION CHANGES

The need for new efficient methods of screening for precise genome-wide methylation changes intensifies as the significance of methylation alternations in the development of many disorders and the aging process is clarified. The aim of our project is to combine methylation-sensitive enzyme digestion with comparative genomic hybridization (CGH) to develop an array-based method of screening the entire genome for changes in the methylation pattern. The methodology involves enzymatic digestion of genomic DNA, linker-adapter amplification (LA-PCR) of the digested fragments, and hybridization of the test and control material to tiling BAC arrays covering the entire genome (FIG. 2).[22] The advantages of our method include genome-wide screening for methylation changes in genomes and precise genomic localization of the methylation sites of each spotted clone, leading to a fast identification of the affected sequences. Furthermore, the LA-PCR protocol is not limited to a low amount of test material.

REFERENCES

1. BANDYOPADHYAY, D. & E.E. MEDRANO. 2003. The emerging role of epigenetics in cellular and organismal aging. Exp. Gerontol. **38:** 1299–1307.
2. GEIGL, J.B., S. LANGER, S. BARWISCH, et al. 2004. Analysis of gene expression patterns and chromosomal changes associated with aging. Cancer Res. **64:** 8550–8557.
3. PAULSEN, M. & A.C. FERGUSON-SMITH. 2001. DNA methylation in genomic imprinting, development, and disease. J. Pathol. **195:** 97–110.
4. CHEN, R.Z., U. PETTERSSON, C. BEARD, et al. 1998. DNA hypomethylation leads to elevated mutation rates. Nature **395:** 89–93.
5. WALSH, C.P., J.R. CHAILLET & T.H. BESTOR. 1998. Transcription of IAP endogenous retroviruses is constrained by cytosine methylation. Nat. Genet. **20:** 116–117.
6. CLARK, S.J., J. HARRISON & P.L. MOLLOY. 1997. Sp1 binding is inhibited by (m)Cp(m)CpG methylation. Gene **195:** 67–71.

7. PRENDERGAST, G.C. & E.B. ZIFF. 1991. Methylation-sensitive sequence-specific DNA binding by the c-Myc basic region. Science **251:** 186–189.
8. ASIEDU, C.K., L. SCOTTO, R.K. ASSOIAN, *et al.* 1994. Binding of AP-1/CREB proteins and of MDBP to contiguous sites downstream of the human TGF-beta 1 gene. Biochim. Biophys. Acta **1219:** 55–63.
9. NAN, X., H.H. NG, C.A. JOHNSON, *et al.* 1998. Transcriptional repression by the methyl-CpG-binding protein MeCP2 involves a histone deacetylase complex. Nature **393:** 386–389.
10. JONES, P.L., G.J. VEENSTRA, P.A. WADE, *et al.*1998. Methylated DNA and MeCP2 recruit histone deacetylase to repress transcription. Nat. Genet. **19:** 187–191.
11. BESTOR, T.H. 1998. Gene silencing: methylation meets acetylation. Nature **393:** 311–312.
12. ISSA, J.P., Y.L. OTTAVIANO, P. CELANO, *et al.* 1994. Methylation of the oestrogen receptor CpG island links ageing and neoplasia in human colon. Nat. Genet. **7:** 536–540.
13. TOYOTA, M. & J.P. ISSA. 1999. CpG island methylator phenotypes in aging and cancer. Semin. Cancer Biol. **9:** 349–357.
14. VERTINO, P.M., J.P. ISSA, O.M. PEREIRA-SMITH, *et al.* 1994. Stabilization of DNA methyltransferase levels and CpG island hypermethylation precede SV40-induced immortalization of human fibroblasts. Cell Growth Differ. **5:** 1395–1402.
15. ZIN'KOVSKAIA, G.G., G.D. BERDYSHEV & B.F. VANIUSHIN. 1978. [Tissue-specific decrease and change in the character of DNA methylation in cattle with aging]. Biokhimiia **43:** 1883–1892.
16. GOLBUS, J., T.D. PALELLA & B.C. RICHARDSON. 1990. Quantitative changes in T cell DNA methylation occur during differentiation and ageing. Eur. J. Immunol. **20:** 1869–1872.
17. TISSENBAUM, H.A. & L. GUARENTE. 2002. Model organisms as a guide to mammalian aging. Dev. Cell **2:** 9–19.
18. CHANG, K.T. & K.T. MIN. 2002. Regulation of lifespan by histone deacetylase. Ageing Res. Rev. **1:** 313–326.
19. COSTELLO, J.F., M.C. FRUHWALD, D.J. SMIRAGLIA, *et al.* 2000. Aberrant CpG-island methylation has non-random and tumour-type-specific patterns. Nat. Genet. **24:** 132–138.
20. TOYOTA, M., C. HO, N. AHUJA, *et al.* 1999. Identification of differentially methylated sequences in colorectal cancer by methylated CpG island amplification. Cancer Res. **59:** 2307–2312.
21. GONZALGO, M.L., G. LIANG, C.H. SPRUCK III, *et al.* 1997. Identification and characterization of differentially methylated regions of genomic DNA by methylation-sensitive arbitrarily primed PCR. Cancer Res. **57:** 594–599.
22. INAZAWA, J., J. INOUE & I. IMOTO. 2004. Comparative genomic hybridization (CGH)-arrays pave the way for identification of novel cancer-related genes. Cancer Sci. **95:** 559–563.
23. KUO, K.C., R.A. MCCUNE, C.W. GEHRKE, *et al.* 1980. Quantitative reversed-phase high performance liquid chromatographic determination of major and modified deoxyribonucleosides in DNA. Nucleic Acids Res. **8:** 4763–4776.
24. WU, J., J.P. ISSA, J. HERMAN, *et al.* 1993. Expression of an exogenous eukaryotic DNA methyltransferase gene induces transformation of NIH 3T3 cells. Proc. Natl. Acad. Sci. USA **90:** 8891–8895.

25. OAKELEY, E.J., F. SCHMITT & J.P. JOST. 1999. Quantification of 5-methylcytosine in DNA by the chloroacetaldehyde reaction. Biotechniques **27**: 744–750, 752.

26. OAKELEY, E.J., A. PODESTA & J.P. JOST. 1997. Developmental changes in DNA methylation of the two tobacco pollen nuclei during maturation. Proc. Natl. Acad. Sci. USA **94**: 11721–11725.

27. SINGER-SAM, J., J.M. LEBON, R.L. TANGUAY, *et al.* 1990. A quantitative HpaII-PCR assay to measure methylation of DNA from a small number of cells. Nucleic Acids Res. **18**: 687.

28. FROMMER, M., L.E. McDONALD, D.S. MILLAR, *et al.* 1992. A genomic sequencing protocol that yields a positive display of 5-methylcytosine residues in individual DNA strands. Proc. Natl. Acad. Sci. USA **89**: 1827–1831.

29. HERMAN, J.G., J.R. GRAFF, S. MYOHANEN, *et al.* 1996. Methylation-specific PCR: a novel PCR assay for methylation status of CpG islands. Proc. Natl. Acad. Sci. USA **93**: 9821–9826.

30. GONZALGO, M.L. & P.A. JONES. 1997. Rapid quantitation of methylation differences at specific sites using methylation-sensitive single nucleotide primer extension (Ms-SNuPE). Nucleic Acids Res. **25**: 2529–2531.

31. EADS, C.A., K.D. DANENBERG, K. KAWAKAMI, *et al.* 2000. MethyLight: a high-throughput assay to measure DNA methylation. Nucleic Acids Res. **28**: e32.

32. MAEKAWA, M., K. SUGANO, H. KASHIWABARA, *et al.* 1999. DNA methylation analysis using bisulfite treatment and PCR-single-strand conformation polymorphism in colorectal cancer showing microsatellite instability. Biochem. Biophys. Res. Commun. **262**: 671–676.

33. XIONG, Z. & P.W. LAIRD. 1997. COBRA: a sensitive and quantitative DNA methylation assay. Nucleic Acids Res. **25**: 2532–2534.

34. AGGERHOLM, A., P. GULDBERG, M. HOKLAND, *et al.* 1999. Extensive intra- and interindividual heterogeneity of p15INK4B methylation in acute myeloid leukemia. Cancer Res. **59**: 436–441.

35. WORM, J., A. AGGERHOLM & P. GULDBERG. 2001. In-tube DNA methylation profiling by fluorescence melting curve analysis. Clin. Chem. **47**: 1183–1189.

36. BAUMER, A., U. WIEDEMANN, M. HERGERSBERG, *et al.* 2001. A novel MSP/DHPLC method for the investigation of the methylation status of imprinted genes enables the molecular detection of low cell mosaicisms. Hum. Mutat. **17**: 423–430.

37. ADORJAN, P., J. DISTLER, E. LIPSCHER, *et al.* 2002. Tumour class prediction and discovery by microarray-based DNA methylation analysis. Nucleic Acids Res. **30**: e21.

38. WORM, J. & P. GULDBERG. 2002. DNA methylation: an epigenetic pathway to cancer and a promising target for anticancer therapy. J. Oral Pathol. Med. **31**: 443–449.

Geroprotection by Glycerol

Insights to Its Mechanisms and Clinical Potentials

CUSTER C. DEOCARIS,[a,b] BHUPAL G. SHRESTHA,[a] DAVID C. KRAFT,[c] KAZUHIKO YAMASAKI,[a] SUNIL C. KAUL,[a] SURESH I. S. RATTAN,[c] AND RENU WADHWA[a,b]

[a]*National Institute of Advanced Industrial Science & Technology (AIST), 1–1-1 Higashi, Tsukuba, Japan*

[b]*Department of Chemistry & Biotechnology, School of Engineering, The University of Tokyo, Hongo, Tokyo, Japan*

[c]*Laboratory of Cellular Ageing, Danish Centre for Molecular Gerontology, Department of Molecular Biology, University of Aarhus Laboratory of Biochemistry & Molecular Cell Biology, Aarhus, Denmark*

ABSTRACT: Chaperones, particularly the heat-shock proteins, are considered as key players in the maintenance of protein homeostasis and are associated with longevity and cellular immortalization. In this study, we investigated the geroprotective activity of the chemical chaperone glycerol. Glycerol showed significant chaperoning activity in refolding heat-denatured luciferase *in vivo* and in protecting cells from heat stress-induced cytotoxicity. This was accompanied by decrease in p53, an up-regulation of a stress chaperone mortalin/mtHsp70, and an increase in proteasome activity in the presence of oxidative stress.

KEYWORDS: glycerol; chemical chaperone; protection; antiaging; life-span extension

INTRODUCTION

Accumulation of protein aggregates and misfolded moieties is a nearly universal phenomenon during aging. Such aggregates have been specifically referred to as amyloids, lysosomal lipofuscin, ceroid bodies, advanced glycation end-products (AGEs), and cytoplasmic inclusions observed in senescent cells, as well as in affected tissues of age-associated diseases such as diabetes and Alzheimer's disease.[1] Although it is not exactly clear how these protein aggregates are formed, the dysregulation of innate chaperoning forces, involving

Address for correspondence: Renu Wadhwa, Gene Function Research Center, National Institute of Advanced Industrial Science & Technology (AIST), Central 4, 1-1-1 Higashi, Tsukuba, Japan. Voice: +81 29 861 9464; fax: +81 29 861 2900.
e-mail: renu-wadhwa@aist.go.jp

Ann. N.Y. Acad. Sci. 1067: 488–492 (2006). © 2006 New York Academy of Sciences.
doi: 10.1196/annals.1354.070

mainly the heat-shock proteins (HSPs), have emerged to be the major critical factors. These HSPs are evolutionarily conserved life-essential housekeeping molecules that play a protective role against proteotoxic stress. Several studies further suggest that an increase in the levels of the molecular chaperones is a common denominator for the extension of cellular life span, immortalization and species' longevity.[2]

Recently, chemical chaperones that are of commercial and medical relevance have been introduced to aid protein refolding of various aggregation-prone proteins. A group of these small molecules comprise the osmolytes, such as glycerol, which are known to stabilize native proteins by altering solvent properties of water, protein polarity, and diffusion, and favor formation of native protein oligomers.[3] The chaperone activity of glycerol, specifically, has been used to repair various mutant or misfolded proteins of p53,[4] prions from familial Creutzfeldt-Jakob disease,[5] and the cystic fibrosis transmembrane conductance regulator protein (CFTR),[6] among others. In this study, we provide evidence in support of the action of glycerol as a potential stress modulator.

CHAPERONE ACTIVITY OF GLYCEROL

To establish the minimal levels of glycerol to be used for this study, we first performed an *in vivo* chaperone assay using human osteosarcoma (U2OS) cells transfected with the firefly luciferase construct pGL3.[7] Our observations indicated that 0.4 M glycerol ($P < 0.05$) is sufficient to refold luciferase after heat denaturation at $45°C$ (FIG. 1A). Meng *et al.* have indicated higher concentration requirements (>1.25 M) to effectively inhibit heat-induced aggregation of creatine kinase. Such levels, albeit, are suitable for maintaining integrity of proteins during purification and long-term storage and are otherwise toxic for cells.[8] Glycerol concentrations higher than 0.5 M were progressively toxic to cells (FIG. 1B). Alternatively, we found that the lower doses of glycerol are effective refolding aids *in vivo* as opposed to *in vitro*. Biologically, this was also evident from the survival curves of heat-stressed ($45°C$) cells treated with 0.4 M glycerol (FIG. 1C). The increased tolerance of cells to thermal as well as oxidative killing (data not shown) in the presence of 0.4 M glycerol could likely be due to cellular mechanisms other than direct chaperoning effects of glycerol with a target protein.

DOES GLYCEROL MODULATE PROTEASOME AND MORTALIN?

Diamant *et al.* demonstrated that the protection by osmolytes also occurs in the same low physiologic concentrations that also activate the molecular

(A)

(B)

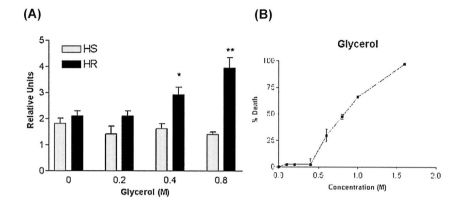

(C)

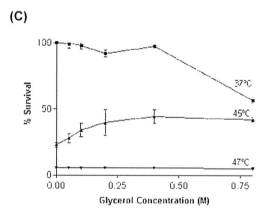

FIGURE 1. Chaperone activity of glycerol protects cells from heat stress. (**A**) *In vivo* chaperone assay in U2OS cells in the presence of different concentrations of glycerol in the medium. After heating cells at 45°C for 30 min (HS), plates were placed back in the CO_2-incubator for 3 h to allow recovery/refolding of heat-denatured luciferase at 37°C (HR). Refolding values were obtained by dividing luciferase activity of heat-shocked and heat-recovered cells by activity of nonheated (control) cells. (**B**) Effect of increasing concentrations of glycerol on survival of U2OS cells. (**C**) Effect of glycerol on survival of heat-shocked cells.

chaperones GroEL, DnaK, and ClpB in *E. coli.*[3] We observed that glycerol causes a modest upregulation of the molecular chaperone mortalin (also known as mthsp70 or grp75) and proteasome activity in the presence of doxorubicin (data not shown). Interestingly, mortalin overexpression has also been associated with longevity and immortalization in human fibroblasts.[9] Both chaperone upregulation and enhancement of proteasome indicate that glycerol, independent of its chemical chaperone activity, may stimulate innate homeostatic maintenance systems that may be useful for healthy aging.

GLYCEROL THERAPY FOR HUMAN LONGEVITY?

The osmotic effect of glycerol has been exploited therapeutically for the acute treatment of brain cortical infarct and edema. Improvement in survival time of patients under glycerol therapy was achieved without serious adverse effects, except for mild, subclinical hemolysis. Stroke patients treated with intravenous 10% glycerol solution experienced only a brief period of plasma hyperosmolarity that returned to baseline levels after a few hours. Its beneficial effects, however, have been facilitated by the rapid glycerol accumulation in the brain.[10,11]

As clinical findings support that glycerol therapy is effective in managing brain pathologies and is well tolerated in humans, a study by Bai *et al.* showed, however, that the concentration of supplemental oral dosing of 10% glycerol in mice would unlikely result in the targeted serum concentration of 0.4 M.[12] The obstacle of increasing systemic availability is mainly due to the rapid metabolism of glycerol resulting to an estimated circulating half-life ($T_{1/2}$) of only 3.8 h both in mice and humans.[12] Because several tissues in the brain, trachea, kidney, eye, nasopharnx, digestive tract, skeletal (but not smooth or cardiac) muscles, and the skin express high levels of the aquaporins, a family of transmembrane transporters that rapidly transports exogenous glycerol into a cell,[13] a rapid intracellular accumulation of glycerol may likely offset the difficulty in maintaining high glycerol serum levels. In light of our preliminary data, glycerol can be tested as a potential antiaging drug.

REFERENCES

1. SHRINGARPURE, R. & K.J. DAVIES. 2002. Protein turnover by the proteasome in aging and disease. Free Radic. Biol. Med. **32:** 1084–1089.
2. SOTI, C. & P. CSERMELY. 2003. Aging and molecular chaperones. Exp. Gerontol. **38:** 1037–1040.
3. DIAMANT, S., N. ELIAHU, D. ROSENTHAL, *et al.* 2001. Chemical chaperones regulate molecular chaperones in vitro and in cells under combined salt and heat stresses. J. Biol. Chem. **276:** 39586–39591.
4. OHNISHI, K., I. OTA, K. YANE, *et al.* 2002. Glycerol as a chemical chaperone enhances radiation-induced apoptosis in anaplastic thyroid carcinoma cells. Mol. Cancer **1:** 4.
5. GU, Y. & N. SINGH. 2004. Doxycycline and protein folding agents rescue the abnormal phenotype of familial CJD H187R in a cell model. Brain Res. Mol. Brain Res. **123:** 37–44.
6. BROWN, C.R., L.Q. HONG-BROWN, J. BIWERSI, *et al.* 1996. Chemical chaperones correct the mutant phenotype of the delta F508 cystic fibrosis transmembrane conductance regulator protein. Cell Stress Chaperones **1:** 117–125.
7. NOLLEN, E.A., F.A. SALOMONS, J.F. BRUNSTING, *et al.* 2001. Dynamic changes in the localization of thermally unfolded nuclear proteins associated with chaperone-dependent protection. Proc. Natl. Acad. Sci. USA **98:** 12038–12043.

8. MENG, F., Y. PARK & H. ZHOU. 2001. Role of proline, glycerol, and heparin as protein folding aids during refolding of rabbit muscle creatine kinase. Int. J. Biochem. Cell Biol. **33:** 701–709.

9. KAUL, S.C., T. YAGUCHI, K. TAIRA, *et al.* 2003. Overexpressed mortalin (mot-2)/mtHSP70/GRP75 and hTERT cooperate to extend the in vitro lifespan of human fibroblasts. Exp. Cell Res. **286:** 96–101.

10. BERGER, C., O.W. SAKOWITZ, K.L. KIENING, *et al.* 2005. Neurochemical monitoring of glycerol therapy in patients with ischemic brain edema. Stroke **36:** e4–e6.

11. SAKAMAKI, M., H. IGARASHI, Y. NISHIYAMA, *et al.* 2003. Effect of glycerol on ischemic cerebral edema assessed by magnetic resonance imaging. J. Neurol. Sci. **209:** 69–74.

12. BAI, C., J. BIWERSI, A.S. VERKMAN, *et al.* 1998. A mouse model to test the in vivo efficacy of chemical chaperones. J. Pharmacol. Toxicol. Methods **40:** 39–45.

13. FRIGERI, A., M.A. GROPPER, F. UMENISHI, *et al.* 1995. Localization of MIWC and GLIP water channel homologs in neuromuscular, epithelial and glandular tissues. J. Cell Sci. **108:** 2993–3002.

Age-Dependent Effects of *in Vitro* Radiofrequency Exposure (Mobile Phone) on CD95+ T Helper Human Lymphocytes

MIRIAM CAPRI,[a,b] STEFANO SALVIOLI,[a,b] SERENA ALTILIA,[a,b] FEDERICA SEVINI,[a,b] DANIEL REMONDINI,[a,c] PIETRO MESIRCA,[a,d] FERDINANDO BERSANI,[a,d] DANIELA MONTI,[e] AND CLAUDIO FRANCESCHI[a,b,f]

[a]*CIG, Interdepartmental Center "L.Galvani," University of Bologna, Bologna, Italy*

[b]*Department of Experimental Pathology, University of Bologna, Bologna, Italy*

[c]*DIMORFIPA, University of Bologna, Bologna, Italy*

[d]*Department of Physics, University of Bologna, Bologna, Italy*

[e]*Department of Experimental Oncology and Pathology, University of Firenze, Firenze, Italy*

[f]*INRCA, National Institute for Research on Aging, Ancona, Italy*

ABSTRACT: Recent studies on "nonthermal" effects of mobile phone radiofrequency (RF) suggest that RF can interact with cellular functions and molecular pathways. To study the possible RF effects on human lymphocyte activation, we analyzed CD25, CD95, CD28 molecules in unstimulated and stimulated CD4+ e CD8+ T cells *in vitro*. Peripheral blood mononuclear cells (PBMCs) from young and elderly donors were exposed or sham-exposed to RF (1,800 MHz, Specific Absorption Rate 2 W/kg) with or without mitogenic stimulation. No significant changes in the percentage of these cell subsets were found between exposed and sham-exposed lymphocytes in both young and elderly donors. Nevertheless, after RF exposure we observed a slight, but significant, downregulation of CD95 expression in stimulated CD4+ T lymphocytes from elderly, but not from young donors. This age-related result is noteworthy given the importance of a such molecule in regulation of the immune response.

KEYWORDS: mobile phone; radiofrequency; aging; human lymphocyte; CD95

Address for correspondence: Dr. Miriam Capri, Ph.D., CIG-Centro Interdipartimentale Galvani, University of Bologna, Via S. Giacomo, 12, 40126 Bologna, Italy. Voice: +39 051 2094740; fax: +39 051 2094747.
  e-mail: miriam.capri2@unibo.it

Ann. N.Y. Acad. Sci. 1067: 493–499 (2006). © 2006 New York Academy of Sciences.
doi: 10.1196/annals.1354.071

INTRODUCTION

During the last 30 years, the attention focused on the biological effects of radiofrequency (RF) electromagnetic fields (EMF) has dramatically increased because of the concomitant increase of EMF sources, in particular mobile phones and base stations.

The recent literature suggests that RF, even at nonthermal levels, could interact with cellular functions and molecular pathways.[1,2] Our previous work showed that RF radiation interfered with lymphocyte proliferation and phosphatidylserine membrane exposure,[3] but did not affect apoptosis.[4] The aim of the present work was to better clarify whether RF, at a Specific Absorption Rate (SAR) comparable to that related to mobile phone radiation exposure, is able to affect *in vitro* activation in human lymphocytes from young and elderly donors. Specifically, we studied CD25, CD95, and CD28 molecules on CD4+ helper and CD8+ cytotoxic T lymphocytes with and without mitogenic stimulation. Concomitantly, data resulting from the comparison between young and old subjects, in the absence of RF exposure, will be discussed for age-dependent effects.

MATERIALS AND METHODS

Peripheral blood (PB) was obtained by venipuncture from 10 young (26 ± 5 years) and 8 elderly donors (88 ± 2 years). These subjects were randomly selected from a district of Bologna (Italy) and enrolled after informed consent. PBMCs were separated by Ficoll gradient according to the standard protocol. Cells were seeded at the concentration of 1×10^6/mL of complete medium with or without mitogenic stimulation (10 ng/mL anti-CD3 monoclonal antibody) and harvested after 44 h of culture. During this time the cell cultures were intermittently (10 min ON and 20 min OFF) exposed or sham-exposed to RF (1,800 MHz, SAR 2W/kg, talk-modulated GSM signal).

Exposure set-up, dosimetry, and quality control were provided by the IT'IS Foundation (Zurich, Switzerland). The exposure system is described in detail in our previous work.[4] Basically, it consisted of two single-mode resonant cavities placed within a CO_2 incubator, one of which was used for the true exposure, while the other was used for sham exposure. All the experiments were performed in blind: exposure and sham conditions were blindly assigned to the two waveguides by the computer-controlled signal unit. The temperature was strictly controlled during the experiments.

Phenotypical analysis of CD4, CD8, CD25, CD95, CD28 markers was done on freshly collected PB or PBMCs after 44 h of culture. In particular, CD25 is the alpha chain of interleukin-2 receptor; CD95 (or APO-1-FAS) is an important membrane receptor for apoptosis induction and a marker of activation; CD28 is a fundamental costimulatory molecule for lymphocyte activation. Analysis was performed by standard flow cytometry techniques by means of FACScalibur cytometer (Becton Dickinson, San Jose, CA, USA) and fluorochrome-conjugated monoclonal antibodies (Serotec, Oxford, UK). Acquired samples were analyzed by Cell Quest® and Paint-A-Gate® software for the simultaneous analysis of two and three fluorescences, respectively. Data were analyzed by two-way ANOVA (followed by HSD post hoc test) and paired *t* Student's test for age and RF effects, respectively.

RESULTS

Results were analyzed on the basis of the following criteria: (1) age-dependent effects (TABLE 1), (2) RF effects (TABLE 2), and (3) RF and age-dependent effects (FIG. 1). First, in PBMCs of old donors the percentage of $CD4^+$ cell (31 ± 1) was significantly lower with respect to the young donors (41.7 ± 0.2), while $CD8^+$ cell percentage appeared to be well preserved (33 ± 2 in old subjects; 29.3 ± 0.6 in young subjects). Thus the ratio CD4/CD8 in young and elderly subjects was 1.4 and 0.9, respectively.

$CD25$ molecules on $CD4^+$ and $CD8^+$ lymphocytes were upregulated by mitogenic stimulation, as expected; moreover, age-dependent differences in the percentage of both $CD4^+CD25^+$ and $CD8^+CD25^+$ cell subsets were observed, as shown in TABLE 1. In addition, a downregulation of CD25 molecules in $CD4^+$ lymphocytes from elderly subjects was found after 44 h of culture without mitogenic stimulation. $CD8^+CD25^+$ cell percentage depended on age, time of culture, and stimulus. The age-related differences were mostly relative to CD95 molecules, as shown in TABLE 1. The frequencies of $CD4^+CD95^{+/-}$ and $CD8^+CD95^{+/-}$ cells are found to be different in PB of the two groups. The mitogenic stimulation induced a complete expression of CD95 in almost all the cells from old donors, but not in young donors. Regarding the CD28 molecule, major differences were found in PB, since elderly subjects have a greater amount of $CD4^+CD28^-$ and $CD8^+CD28^-$ lymphocytes in comparison with young people, as shown in TABLE 1. Age-dependent effects were also found in $CD4^+CD28^+$ cells and, interestingly, this cell subset decreased after 44 h of stimulation only in cells from young subjects.

No difference in the percentage of $CD25^{+/-}$, $CD95^{+/-}$, and $CD28^{+/-}$ on $CD4^+$ and $CD8^+$ lymphocytes was found between sham- and RF-exposed lymphocytes from both young and elderly donors, as shown in TABLE 2 (data of unstimulated cells were not shown). When the fluorescence brightness in stimulated $CD4^+CD95^+$ lymphocytes was considered, two cell populations with different levels of $CD95^+$ (bright or high level and dim or low level) were observed (FIG. 1) both in young and old donors. Their percentages were different in the two groups of donors studied ($P < 0.05$). A difference in $CD95^{Bright}$ and $CD95^{Dim}$ cells between old and young subjects was found.

TABLE 1. CD25$^{+/-}$, CD95$^{+/-}$, CD28$^{+/-}$ on CD4+, and CD8+ T lymphocytes in peripheral blood (PB) and after 44 h of culture with or without anti-CD3 stimulation

Lymphocytes	PB		44 h unstimulated		44 h stimulated		Statistical analysis		
	Y % ± SE	O % ± SE	Y % ±SE	O % ± SE	Y % ± SE	O % ±SE	Age	Culture	Stimulus
CD4+CD25−	25.8 ± 0.7	18 ± 1	27 ± 1	26 ± 1	15.1 ± 0.9	11 ± 1	n.s.	n.s.	<0.01
CD4+CD25+	16.2 ± 0.5	14.1 ± 0.6	14.4 ± 0.7	8.9 ± 0.3	23.0 ± 0.6	20.6 ± 0.9	0.04	n.s.	<0.01
CD8+CD25−	24.0 ± 0.9	23 ± 2	27 ± 1	24 ± 2	14.7 ± 0.6	15.4 ± 0.6	n.s.	n.s.	0.01
CD8+CD25+	4.7 ± 0.5	9.0 ± 0.8	0.8 ± 0.1	3.0 ± 0.3	11.6 ± 0.5	13 ± 1	0.05	<0.01	<0.01
CD4+CD95−	25 ± 0.6	5.3 ± 0.6	25.9 ± 0.9	13 ± 1	22 ± 1	1.3 ± 0.2	<0.001	n.s.	0.04
CD4+CD95+	16.5 ± 0.4	26 ± 1	15.3 ± 0.6	22 ± 1	15 ± 1	30 ± 1	<0.001	n.s.	n.s.
CD8+CD95−	25.7 ± 0.8	14 ± 1	21 ± 1	11 ± 1	17.6 ± 0.7	0.9 ± 0.1	<0.001	n.s.	n.s.
CD8+CD95+	3.7 ± 0.2	21 ± 2	4.2 ± 0.3	19 ± 2	7.6 ± 0.5	28 ± 1	<0.001	n.s.	n.s.
CD4+CD28−	0.9 ± 0.1	5.5 ± 0.8	0.8 ± 0.1	3.2 ± 0.6	3.4 ± 0.5	7 ± 1	0.015	n.s.	n.s.
CD4+CD28+	40.9 ± 0.8	24 ± 1	40 ± 1	33 ± 1	33 ± 1	24.8 ± 0.8	<0.001	n.s.	n.s.
CD8+CD28−	15.5 ± 0.5	23 ± 1	14.8 ± 0.8	18 ± 1	14.8 ± 0.6	21.1 ± 0.7	0.02	n.s.	n.s.
CD8+CD28+	14.3 ± 0.4	10.7 ± 0.9	11.4 ± 0.7	11 ± 2	10.0 ± 0.5	7.1 ± 0.4	n.s.	n.s.	n.s.

NOTE: Data are expressed as % mean ± SE of 10 young (Y) and 8 old (O) donors.

TABLE 2. $CD25^{+/-}$, $CD28^{+/-}$ and $CD95^{+/-}$ molecules on $CD4^+$ and $CD8^+$ T lymphocytes, from 10 young and 8 old donors

Lymphocytes	Young			Old		
	Sham % ± SE	RF % ± SE	P	Sham % ± SE	RF % ± SE	P
CD4+CD25−	15.1 ± 0.9	15.2 ± 0.9	n.s.	11 ± 1	10.3 ± 0.9	n.s.
CD4+CD25+	23.0 ± 0.6	22.8 ± 0.5	n.s.	20.6 ± 0.9	21 ± 1	n.s.
CD8+CD25−	14.7 ± 0.6	15.5 ± 0.6	n.s.	15.4 ± 0.6	14.8 ± 0.6	n.s.
CD8+CD25+	11.6 ± 0.5	11.1 ± 0.5	n.s.	13 ± 1	15 ± 1	n.s.
CD4+CD95−	22 ± 1	22 ± 1	n.s	1.3 ± 0.2	1.0 ± 0.1	n.s.
CD4+CD95+	15 ± 1	15.6 ± 0.9	n.s.	30 ± 1	31 ± 1	n.s.
CD8+CD95−	17.6 ± 0.7	18.1 ± 0.8	n.s.	0.9 ± 0.1	0.7 ± 0.1	n.s.
CD8+CD95+	7.6 ± 0.5	7.2 ± 0.6	n.s.	28 ± 1	28 ± 1	n.s.
CD4+CD28−	3.4 ± 0.5	2.4 ± 0.4	n.s.	7 ± 1	6.1 ± 0.8	n.s.
CD4+CD28+	33 ± 1	32 ± 1	n.s	24.8 ± 0.8	25 ± 1	n.s.
CD8+CD28−	14.8 ± 0.6	14.9 ± 0.7	n.s.	21.1 ± 0.7	22.5 ± 0.8	n.s.
CD8+CD28−	10.0 ± 0.5	9.3 ± 0.5	n.s.	21.1 ± 0.7	22.5 ± 0.8	n.s.

NOTE: Cells were anti-CD3 stimulated and RF-exposed or sham exposed. Data are expressed as % mean ± SE of all the experiments.

Moreover, after RF exposure a slight downregulation of CD95 was found only in old donors ($P = 0.05$).

Effects due to interactions among age, culture time, and stimulus were never detected in all the cases investigated.

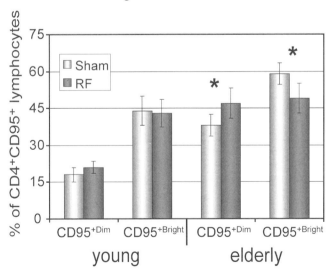

FIGURE 1. Analysis of CD95 fluorescence brightness in stimulated CD4+CD95+ cells from 10 young and 8 elderly donors, after sham exposure and RF exposure (SAR 2 W/kg). *$P = 0.05$. Data are expressed as mean ± SE. Bright and dim CD95 distribution on CD4+ lymphocytes is significantly different between young and old donors, $P < 0.05$. The analysis of CD95 +Bright–Dim cells is reported considering all $CD4^+CD95^+$ lymphocytes as 100%.

DISCUSSION

Human T lymphocytes are affected by age. A wide literature in this field is available and recently the possibility of identifying an immune-risk phenotype (IRP) predictor of mortality has been envisaged.[5] During aging, the two major subsets of T lymphocytes, that is, CD4+ and CD8+ cells, change their ratio, their activity, and their phenotype.

In this paper, we analyzed the phenotype of T lymphocytes from a small sample of unselected elderly donors and we found that the CD4/CD8 ratio is <1, and this is considered as one of the risk factors that, in combination with others, can be a predictor of mortality in the proposed IRP.[5] Moreover, we observed an increase of CD28⁻ T cells and CD95⁺ activated T lymphocytes, which is a characteristic marker of human T lymphocyte immunosenescence; furthermore, the increase of CD28⁻ lymphocytes is another parameter of the IRP.[5] Thus, we confirmed that CD28 and CD95 molecules are important markers for immunosenescence, as previously reported.[6,7] Here, we also show that almost all CD4⁺ and CD8⁺ cells were CD95⁺ activated after 44 h of stimulation, in comparison with cells from young donors. This was likely due to the presence, before the stimulation, of a much higher percentage of activated cells in the elderly than in the young group. Recent data regarding the CD4⁺CD25⁺ lymphocytes, which have a very important immunoregulatory role, suggest that they increase with age.[8] On the contrary, in this work CD4⁺CD25⁺ cells were found to be slightly decreased in the elderly with respect to young group, both before and after stimulation. Surprisingly, CD25 molecules were found to be downregulated in unstimulated, cultured CD4⁺ and CD8⁺ T lymphocytes with respect to PB, and this effect was evident only on cells from elderly donors but not in cells from young subjects. These data suggest that the age of the donor can affect the duration of the activation state, likely through modifications of phosphorylation protein activity or gene expression.

As far as RF effects are concerned, only a slight age-related downregulation of CD95 was found in stimulated CD4⁺ T cells from elderly individuals. This is noteworthy given the importance of such molecule in the immune-response regulation, as an activator of apoptosis. On the basis of such results one can hypothesize that RF exposure could decrease the susceptibility to Fas-induced apoptosis in elderly subjects. If this result will be further confirmed in functional studies and on a larger experimental sample, it should be taken into account for possible implications on human health risk, or benefit for old people.

On the whole, the literature on this topic is still scanty and much more data are needed to draw definitive conclusions, especially if one wants to rule out a possible oncogenic potential of RF, which is still controversial.[9]

ACKNOWLEDGMENTS

We acknowledge support through the REFLEX project (EU 5th Framework Programme) "Risk Evaluation of Potential Environmental Hazards From Low Energy Electromagnetic Field (EMFs) eXposure Using Sensitive *in vitro* Methods." We are also grateful for ISPESL grants C20/DIPIA/03 and for a grant to C.F. from the "Fondazione del Monte di Bologna e Ravenna."

We also thank Professor Niels Kuster and his team (IT'IS, Zurich, Switzerland) for the exposure system set up and quality control.

REFERENCES

1. LESZCZYNSKI, D., S. JOENVAARA, J. REIVINEN, *et al.* 2002. Non-thermal activation of the HSP27/p38MAPK stress pathway by mobile phone radiation in human endothelial cells: molecular mechanism for cancer- and blood-brain barrier-related effects. Differentiation **70:** 120–129.

2. CZYZ, J., K. GUAN, Q. ZENG, *et al.* 2004. High frequency electromagnetic fields (GSM signals) affect gene expression levels in tumor suppressor p53-deficient embryonic stem cells. Bioelectromagnetics **25:** 296–307.

3. CAPRI, M., E. SCARCELLA, C. FUMELLI, *et al.* 2004a. In vitro exposure of human lymphocytes to 900 MHz CW and GSM modulated radiofrequency: studies of proliferation, apoptosis and mitochondrial membrane potential. Radiat. Res. **162:** 211–218.

4. CAPRI, M., E. SCARCELLA, E. BIANCHI, *et al.* 2004b. 1800 MHz radiofrequency (mobile phones, different global system for mobile communication modulations) does not affect apoptosis and heat shock protein 70 level in peripheral blood mononuclear cells from young and old donors. Int. J. Radiat. Biol. **80:** 389–397.

5. PAWELEC, G., A. AKBAR, C. CARUSO, *et al.* 2004. Is immunosenescence infectious? Trends Immunol. **25:** 406–410.

6. ZANNI, F., R. VESCOVINI, C. BIASINI, *et al.* 2003. Marked increase with age of type 1 cytokines within memory and effector/cytotoxic CD8+ T cells in humans: a contribution to understand the relationship between inflammation and immunosenescence. Exp. Gerontol. **38:** 981–987.

7. FAGNONI, F.F., R. VESCOVINI, G. PASSERI, *et al.* 2000. Shortage of circulating naive CD8(+) T cells provides new insights on immunodeficiency in aging. Blood **95:** 2860–2868.

8. GREGG, R., C. M. SMITH, F. J. CLARK, *et al.* 2005. The number of human peripheral blood CD4+ CD25 high regulatory T cells increases with age. Clin. Exp. Immunol. **140:** 540–546.

9. MOULDER, J.E., K. R. FOSTER, L. S. ERDREICH, *et al.* 2005. Mobile phones, mobile phone base stations and cancer: a review. Int. J. Radiat. Biol. **81:** 189–203.

Severe Acute Respiratory Syndrome (SARS)

Development of Diagnostics and Antivirals

MORTEN DRÆBY SØRENSEN,[a] BRIAN SØRENSEN,[a]
REGINA GONZALEZ-DOSAL,[a] CONNIE JENNING MELCHJORSEN,[a]
JENS WEIBEL,[a] JING WANG,[b] CHEN WIE JUN,[b] YANG HUANMING,[b]
AND PETER KRISTENSEN[a]

[a]Department of Molecular Biology, University of Aarhus, Aarhus, Denmark

[b]Beijing Genomics Institute, Beijing, China

ABSTRACT: The previously unknown coronavirus that caused severe acute respiratory syndrome (SARS-CoV) affected more than 8,000 persons worldwide and was responsible for more than 700 deaths during the first outbreak in 2002–2003. For reasons unknown, the SARS virus is less severe and the clinical progression a great deal milder in children younger than 12 years of age. In contrast, the mortality rate can exceed 50% for persons at or above the age of 60. As part of the Sino-European Project on SARS Diagnostics and Antivirals (SEPSDA), an immune phage-display library is being created from convalescent patients in a phagemid system for the selection of single-chain fragment variables (scFv) antibodies recognizing the SARS-CoV.

KEYWORDS: SARS; phage display; antibodies; antiviral agents

INTRODUCTION

In February 2003, the new and previously unknown deadly coronavirus causing severe acute respiratory syndrome (SARS-CoV) was brought to the attention of the World Health Organization (WHO) by Dr. Carlo Urbani and his colleagues.[1]

The SARS virus originated in the province of Guangdong in southern China in November 2002 where it initially was thought to cause atypical pneumonia.[2] However, within a short time the virus spread to Hong Kong, Singapore, Vietnam, Canada, the United States, Taiwan, and several European countries.

Address for correspondence: Dr. Peter Kristensen, Department of Molecular Biology, University of Aarhus, Gustav Wieds Vej 10C, DK8000 Aarhus−C, Denmark. Voice: +45 8942 5032; fax: +45 8612 3178.

e-mail: pk@mb.au.dk

Ann. N.Y. Acad. Sci. 1067: 500–505 (2006). © 2006 New York Academy of Sciences.
doi: 10.1196/annals.1354.072

Concerted efforts of the scientific community led to a very rapid identification of a novel coronavirus as the etiological agent of SARS and the full genome sequencing of the virus.[3–9] The SARS-CoV genome is ~30 kb in length and contains 14 potential open reading frames (ORFs).[7,10]

According to the WHO, the SARS-CoV affected more than 8,000 individuals worldwide and was responsible for over 700 deaths during the first outbreak in 2002–2003. For reasons unknown the SARS virus is less severe and the clinical progression a great deal milder in children younger than 12 years of age.[11] In contrast, the mortality rate was highest among patients >65 years[12] and can exceed 50% for persons at or above the age of 60 years.[13] In Hong Kong, where 298 people died from SARS, the mortality rate for children (age 0–14 years) was 0%. On the other hand, 63.9% of the cases were in persons older than 65 years, most of whom showed a history of chronic disease (http://www.hku.hk/ctc/sars_hk_23). At present no experimental evidence can explain the observed age distribution. However, it should be noted that a recently discovered coronavirus strain, NL63, exhibits a markedly different age distribution with regard to clinical symptoms.

The coronaviruses are a group of viruses that have a crown-like (coronal) appearance. The SARS-CoV are positive-strand RNA viruses and the virion consists of a nucleocapsid core encapsulated by the three envelope glycoproteins: spike (S), membrane (M), and envelope (E) proteins that are common to all members of the genus. The RNA is packaged by the nucleocapsid (N) protein into a helical nucleocapsid.[14] The SARS virus N protein has only a 32% identity with the other known coronaviruses and has been suggested to be a major immunogen.[15] The S protein is known to be a major target of the cellular immune response and plays an important role in the initial roles of infection.

SARS DIAGNOSIS AND THERAPY

Continuous work is being performed to find an early diagnosis and therapy of SARS. Several different approaches have been taken. Diagnosis has been performed by serologic testing using indirect fluorescent antibody or enzyme-linked immunosorbent assays (ELISA) specific for SARS-CoV antibody.[16,17] Detection of the SARS-CoV itself has been done using clinical specimens of serum, nasal secretions, and stool. This was done through viral isolation and electron microscopy, viral culture, or reverse transcription polymerase chain reaction (RT-PCR) to test for viral RNA.[3,8]

Neutralizing antibodies (NAbs) have been found against the SARS virus. One of the targets of these NAbs is the S glycoprotein, especially toward the metallopeptidase angiotensin-converting enzyme 2 (ACE2) binding domain [S(318-510)].[18] NAbs have been selected against the ACE2 domain.[19,20]

SINO-EUROPEAN PROJECT ON SARS DIAGNOSTICS AND ANTIVIRALS (SEPSDA)

Within the SEPSDA consortium significant progress has been made, with regard to both a structural understanding of the SARS-CoV[21-23] and the development of putative therapies.[24]

To further increase the understanding of viral biology and to help devise novel therapies, an effort to harvest the protective immunity generated by convalescent patients has been initiated. Antibodies against the SARS proteins can be obtained in different ways. The most commonly used are hybridomas to make monoclonal antibodies[25] and immunization followed by collection of antiserum.[26] Selections using phage display have been performed, selecting scFv antibodies from semi-synthetic (nonimmune) libraries[27-29] and with immune library.[30]

The first time a fusion protein was displayed on the surface of filamentous bacteriophages was in 1985 by G.P. Smith,[31] who showed that foreign DNA fragments could be inserted in the middle of gene III to create a fusion protein. The phage particle displays a protein or peptide on the surface and carries the gene for the displayed protein or peptide inside the particle, giving a linkage between phenotype and genotype.[31] This allows for the selection of phage displaying a protein or peptide with affinity for a given target, and at the same time the gene encoding the protein or peptide is co-selected. In this way, it is possible to screen millions of different displayed proteins or peptides.

In 1990 a single-chain antibody fragment (scFv) was displayed on the surface of filamentous bacteriophage for the first time by McCafferty et al.[32] In 1991 came the first publications displaying libraries of fragment antigen-binding (Fab) fragments on gIIIp[33,34] and on gVIIIp.[35] Subsequently, better and larger libraries have been constructed and used for selection of antibodies against numerous different antigens.

The creation of large phage-display libraries gives the potential of isolating human antibodies against most antigens,[36] making it possible to bypass both hybridoma technology and immunization.[37] In addition, because no immune system is involved in the selection of antibodies by phage display, it is possible to select antibodies against toxic compounds, lethal pathogens, and highly conserved antigens.[38]

In general two kinds of antibody libraries can be created from donors: immune and naïve (nonimmune) libraries. The immune libraries are made from immunoglobulin (Ig) variable region (V) genes derived from immunized donors.[37] An immune library is biased toward a specific antigen, which leads to the selection of higher-affinity antibodies (compared to naïve libraries of the same size). The naïve libraries are made from Ig V genes derived from non-immunized donors or from synthetic V-genes.[36] The naïve library is unbiased and can therefore select antibodies against virtually any antigen.

Creation of immune phage-display libraries for immunized donors has shown a particular efficiency in selecting neutralizing antibodies (NABs) against different viruses, for example, rabies,[39] varicella-zoster,[40] hepatitis A[41] and E,[42] measles,[43] and respiratory syncytial virus.[44]

The use of phage display seems ideal for the selection of antibodies against the SARS-CoV. Creating an immune library, based on peripheral blood lymphocytes from convalescent patients in a phagemid system, would provide the possibility of developing an early diagnosis and therapy of SARS. NAb has been selected, but an early and fast diagnosis is still important, should another outbreak occur.

ACKNOWLEDGMENT

This work was supported by the Sino-European Project on SARS Diagnostics and Antivirals (EU Contract Number 003831).

REFERENCES

1. WORLD HEALTH ORGANIZATION. 2003. Severe acute respiratory syndrome (SARS): multi-country outbreak. http://www.who.int/csr/don/2003_03-16/en/.
2. ROSLING, L. & M. ROSLING. 2003. Pneumonia causes panic in Guangdong province. Br. Med. J. **326:** 416.
3. DROSTEN, C. *et al.* 2003. Identification of a novel coronavirus in patients with severe acute respiratory syndrome. N. Engl. J. Med. **348:** 1967–1976.
4. RUAN, Y.J. *et al.* 2003. Comparative full-length genome sequence analysis of 14 SARS coronavirus isolates and common mutations associated with putative origins of infection. Lancet **361:** 1779–1785.
5. PEIRIS, J.S. *et al.* 2003. Coronavirus as a possible cause of severe acute respiratory syndrome. Lancet **361:** 1319–1325.
6. ROTA, P.A. *et al.* 2003. Characterization of a novel coronavirus associated with severe acute respiratory syndrome. Science **300:** 1394–1399.
7. MARRA, M.A. *et al.* 2003. The genome sequence of the SARS-associated coronavirus. Science **300:** 1399–1404.
8. KSIAZEK, T.G. *et al.* 2003. A novel coronavirus associated with severe acute respiratory syndrome. N. Engl. J. Med. **348:** 1953–1966.
9. FOUCHIER, R.A. *et al.* 2003. Aetiology: Koch's postulates fulfilled for SARS virus. Nature **423:** 240.
10. THIEL, V. *et al.* 2003. Mechanisms and enzymes involved in SARS coronavirus genome expression. J. Gen. Virol. **84:** 2305–2315.
11. LEUNG, C.W. *et al.* 2004. Severe acute respiratory syndrome among children. Pediatrics **113:** e535–e543.
12. LIANG, W. *et al.* 2004. Severe acute respiratory syndrome, Beijing, 2003. Emerg. Infect. Dis. **10:** 25–31.
13. DONNELLY, C.A. *et al.* 2003. Epidemiological determinants of spread of causal agent of severe acute respiratory syndrome in Hong Kong. Lancet **361:** 1761–1766.

14. TAN, Y.J., S.G. LIM & W. HONG. 2005. Characterization of viral proteins encoded by the SARS-coronavirus genome. Antiviral Res. **65:** 69–78.

15. KROKHIN, O. *et al.* 2003. Mass spectrometric characterization of proteins from the SARS virus: a preliminary report. Mol. Cell Proteomics **2:** 346–356.

16. LI, G., X. CHEN & A. XU. 2003. Profile of specific antibodies to the SARS-associated coronavirus. N. Engl. J. Med. **349:** 508–509.

17. CHEN, W. *et al.* 2004. Antibody response and viraemia during the course of severe acute respiratory syndrome (SARS)-associated coronavirus infection. J. Med. Microbiol. **53:** 435–438.

18. WONG, S.K. *et al.* 2004. A 193-amino acid fragment of the SARS coronavirus S protein efficiently binds angiotensin-converting enzyme 2. J. Biol. Chem. **279:** 3197–3201.

19. SUI, J. *et al.* 2004. Potent neutralization of severe acute respiratory syndrome (SARS) coronavirus by a human mAb to S1 protein that blocks receptor association. Proc. Natl. Acad. Sci. USA **101:** 2536–2541.

20. YI, C.E. *et al.* 2005. Single amino acid substitutions in the severe acute respiratory syndrome coronavirus spike glycoprotein determine viral entry and immunogenicity of a major neutralizing domain. J. Virol. **79:** 11638–11646.

21. ANAND, K. *et al.* 2003. Coronavirus main proteinase (3CLpro) structure: basis for design of anti-SARS drugs. Science **300:** 1763–1767.

22. ZHAI, Y. *et al.* 2005. Insights into SARS-CoV transcription and replication from the structure of the nsp7-nsp8 hexadecamer. Nat. Struct. Mol. Biol. **12:** 980–986.

23. YANG, H. *et al.* 2003. The crystal structures of severe acute respiratory syndrome virus main protease and its complex with an inhibitor. Proc. Natl. Acad. Sci. USA **100:** 13190–13195.

24. CHEN, L. *et al.* 2005. Cinanserin is an inhibitor of the 3C-like proteinase of severe acute respiratory syndrome coronavirus and strongly reduces virus replication in vitro. J. Virol. **79:** 7095–7103.

25. WEN, K. *et al.* 2004. Preparation and characterization of monoclonal antibodies against S1 domain at N-terminal residues 249 to 667 of SARS-associated coronavirus S1 protein. Di Yi Jun Yi Da Xue Xue Bao. **24:** 1–6.

26. LIN, Y. *et al.* 2003. Identification of an epitope of SARS-coronavirus nucleocapsid protein. Cell Res. **13:** 141–145.

27. LIU, H. *et al.* 2004. Recombinant scFv antibodies against E protein and N protein of severe acute respiratory syndrome virus. Acta. Biochim. Biophys. Sin. (Shanghai). **36:** 541–547.

28. ZHONG, X. *et al.* 2005. B-cell responses in patients who have recovered from severe acute respiratory syndrome target a dominant site in the S2 domain of the surface spike glycoprotein. J. Virol. **79:** 3401–3408.

29. VAN DEN BRINK, E.N. *et al.* 2005. Molecular and biological characterization of human monoclonal antibodies binding to the spike and nucleocapsid proteins of severe acute respiratory syndrome coronavirus. J. Virol. **79:** 1635–1644.

30. DUAN, J. *et al.* 2005. A human SARS-CoV neutralizing antibody against epitope on S2 protein. Biochem. Biophys. Res. Commun. **333:** 186–193.

31. SMITH, G.P. 1985. Filamentous fusion phage: novel expression vectors that display cloned antigens on the virion surface. Science **228:** 1315–1317.

32. MCCAFFERTY, J. *et al.* 1990. Phage antibodies: filamentous phage displaying antibody variable domains. Nature **348:** 552–554.

33. BARBAS, C.F. III *et al.* 1991. Assembly of combinatorial antibody libraries on phage surfaces: the gene III site. Proc. Natl. Acad. Sci. USA **88:** 7978–7982.

34. HOOGENBOOM, H.R. *et al.* 1991. Multi-subunit proteins on the surface of filamentous phage: methodologies for displaying antibody (Fab) heavy and light chains. Nucleic Acids Res. **19:** 4133–4137.
35. KANG, A.S. *et al.* 1991. Linkage of recognition and replication functions by assembling combinatorial antibody Fab libraries along phage surfaces. Proc. Natl. Acad. Sci. USA **88:** 4363–4366.
36. MARKS, J.D. *et al.* 1991. By-passing immunization: human antibodies from V-gene libraries displayed on phage. J. Mol. Biol. **222:** 581–597.
37. CLACKSON, T. *et al.* 1991. Making antibody fragments using phage display libraries. Nature **352:** 624–628.
38. HUST, M. & S. DUBEL. 2004. Mating antibody phage display with proteomics. Trends Biotechnol. **22:** 8–14.
39. KRAMER, R.A. *et al.* 2005. The human antibody repertoire specific for rabies virus glycoprotein as selected from immune libraries. Eur. J. Immunol. **35:** 2131–2145.
40. KAUSMALLY, L. *et al.* 2004. Neutralizing human antibodies to varicella-zoster virus (VZV) derived from a VZV patient recombinant antibody library. J. Gen. Virol. **85:** 3493–3500.
41. KIM, S.J. *et al.* 2004. Neutralizing human monoclonal antibodies to hepatitis A virus recovered by phage display. Virology **318:** 598–607.
42. SCHOFIELD, D.J. *et al.* 2003. Monoclonal antibodies that neutralize HEV recognize an antigenic site at the carboxyterminus of an ORF2 protein vaccine. Vaccine **22:** 257–267.
43. DE CARVALHO NICACIO, C. *et al.* 2002. Neutralizing human Fab fragments against measles virus recovered by phage display. J. Virol. **76:** 251–258.
44. NGUYEN, H. *et al.* 2000. Efficient generation of respiratory syncytial virus (RSV)-neutralizing human MoAbs via human peripheral blood lymphocyte (hu-PBL)-SCID mice and scFv phage display libraries. Clin. Exp. Immunol. **122:** 85–93.

Index of Contributors